LUBKIN'S CHRONIC ILLNESS

IMPACT AND INTERVENTION

NINTH EDITION

EDITED BY

PAMALA D. LARSEN, PhD, RN

Professor Emeritus
Fay W. Whitney School of Nursing
University of Wyoming
Laramie, Wyoming

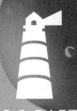

JONES & BARTLETT
LEARNING

World Headquarters
Jones & Bartlett Learning
5 Wall Street
Burlington, MA 01803
978-443-5000
info@jblearning.com
www.jblearning.com

Jones & Bartlett Learning books and products are available through most bookstores and online booksellers. To contact Jones & Bartlett Learning directly, call 800-832-0034, fax 978-443-8000, or visit our website, www.jblearning.com.

Substantial discounts on bulk quantities of Jones & Bartlett Learning publications are available to corporations, professional associations, and other qualified organizations. For details and specific discount information, contact the special sales department at Jones & Bartlett Learning via the above contact information or send an email to specialsales@jblearning.com.

05791-1

Production Credits
VP, Executive Publisher: David Cella
Executive Editor: Amanda Martin
Associate Acquisitions Editor: Rebecca Myrick
Production Editor: Keith Henry
Senior Marketing Manager: Jennifer Stiles
VP, Manufacturing and Inventory Control: Therese Connell
Manager of Photo Research, Rights & Permissions: Lauren Miller
Composition: Cenveo Publisher Services
Cover Design: Kristin E. Parker
Cover Image: © Madredus/Shutterstock, Inc.
Printing and Binding: Edwards Brothers Malloy
Cover Printing: Edwards Brothers Malloy

Library of Congress Cataloging-in-Publication Data
Larsen, Pamala D., 1947- , author.
  Lubkin's chronic illness : impact and intervention / Pamala D. Larsen.—9th edition.
    p. ; cm.
  Chronic illness
  Preceded by Chronic illness / edited by Ilene Morof Lubkin, Pamala D. Larsen. 8th ed. c2013.
  Includes bibliographical references and index.
  ISBN 978-1-284-04900-8 (casebound)
  I. Title. II. Title: Chronic illness.
  [DNLM: 1. Chronic Disease—psychology. 2. Professional-Family Relations. 3. Professional-Patient Relations. 4. Therapeutics.   WT 500]
  RC108

  616'.044—dc23
                                    2014031568
6048
Printed in the United States of America
18 17 16 15   10 9 8 7 6 5 4 3 2

Dedication

For Randy,
We gave cancer a good fight.

And in honor of my 12 grandchildren:
Cody, Kai, Dane, Ben, and Lainey Larsen
Jonah, Temesgen, Landon, Abuzaid, and Kalid Fanning
Abby and Carter Larsen

This text was developed by and originated with Ilene Morof Lubkin in 1986 and was the first work of its kind to address the psychosocial concepts of chronic illness. Pamala Larsen joined the project in its fourth edition in 1998. It remains a landmark work in the healthcare field.

Contents

Preface

As I write the preface for the current edition, my mind wanders back to writing the preface for the eighth edition. Ascribing my feelings to "paper" for that edition and sharing those feelings was cathartic in many ways. And in the 3 years since that time, there have been other life changes: the death of my beloved husband, Randy, on May 10, 2012; the adoption of Temesgen, my 12th grandchild; my retirement from the university; the publication of this text; and the publication of my journal, *Finding a Way Through Cancer, Dying, and Widowhood: A Memoir*, which chronicles my husband's and my life with chronic illness and ultimately tells of the darkness and aloneness of widowhood.

The preface for this edition is a sequel to that of the eighth edition, and because of that I have chosen to reprint the prior one for those not previously familiar with this text.

A View from That Other Place

The first draft of the preface for this edition covered the usual topics—our expensive healthcare system providing limited access to some Americans, falling behind in life expectancy in the world and also in infant mortality, and a plea that we can't keep putting our head in the sand, merely hoping that something will change, along with my usual plea that everyone with chronic illness needs a nurse as a case manager. Yes, it was very preachy, but how I feel.

During this past year, however, my husband of 42 years was diagnosed with esophageal cancer. As Susan Sontag (1988) notes, "Illness is the night-side of life; there is a kingdom of the well and a kingdom of the sick, and that eventually everyone is obligated, at least for a spell, to identify ourselves as citizens of that other place" (p. 3). My husband and I are now in "that other place"— the land of chronic illness. One would think that being a registered nurse for 42 years and caring for those with chronic illness in many settings would have made me an expert in this land. This is my area; I teach about it, know about it, and edit this text. This is "me." However, I didn't realize how little I knew about the kingdom of the sick. In the past, I was confident that I knew what my patients and families were going through. I was supportive. I was empathetic. I was working with them for optimal wellness. But I didn't *know*.

From the day of diagnosis, the day before Thanksgiving 2010 (funny, I don't even remember the date, just the relationship with Thanksgiving), you think your loved one's tests have been mixed up with someone else's, that it must be a mistake. These things happen to other people. You just had Christmas family pictures taken the prior weekend with all 11 grandchildren . . . you are happy, healthy, alive. This diagnosis isn't real. But it soon becomes your reality.

I think of the chapters in this text and how my husband and I can now relate to most of them. I've added a few quotes of my own in some of the chapters, but in reality, I could have added a thousand quotes about our experience. Luckily my husband's hospitalizations, surgeries, chemotherapy, radiation, and care have been in two Magnet hospitals. The nursing and medical care has been fantastic. We've been actively involved in care decisions and have never felt like outsiders. But that care doesn't touch "that other place."

As nurses, we advocate that a person's illness shouldn't take over that individual's life, that illness is just part of who the person is. That is a lofty goal, but the reality is that your life is often your illness. They are one and the same. Your life revolves around how many times you've vomited today; endless doctor appointments; electrolytes are off, need a bag of IV fluids and some potassium as an outpatient; titrating nocturnal jejunostomy feedings with oral intake; IV antibiotics for an infection of some kind; fatigue and weakness; and iatrogenic effects of treatment, to name just a few of the new additions to daily life. Hospitalizations become a blur as to what happened when. Some things, however, are permanently recorded in my brain, such as the night my husband had a cardiac arrest in SICU. Then the thought surfaces that none of this treatment will make any difference, and you talk, again, about advance directives, wills, and so on.

That other place. I didn't know until now.

Pamala D. Larsen
July 2011

References

Sontag, S. (1988). *Illness as metaphor*. Toronto, Canada: Collins Publishers.

The Lived Experience of Chronic Illness

Three years ago this summer, I wrote the preface for the eighth edition of this text. My husband, Randy, was recovering from another surgery, a cardiac arrest, and many days in the SICU—all a result of complications of his esophageal cancer. I wrote about the dark side of chronic illness and how illness—in this case, cancer—exhausts every part of oneself. I also wrote about not "knowing" about the dark side of illness and how as professional caregivers we really have little knowledge or understanding of what the patient and family are experiencing.

Little did I know (although don't we intuitively know, somehow?) that Randy's valiant fight with cancer would last only 18 months. We talk a lot about "survivors" and celebrate their lives, but little about those who don't "win" the battle. However, their experiences and outcomes still contribute to the body of knowledge of chronic illness.

With Randy's cancer diagnosis, our family began a journey to find a "new normal" for our lives. Nothing would be the same again. And then with his death, we sought another "new normal." Randy's illness and death have taught me countless personal lessons: Live each day to its fullest; life is not all about your profession or career; play more, work less; take some risks; get out of your comfort zone; and cherish each moment that you have with your loved ones. I look back and can't believe what I once took for granted.

In addition to the personal revelations, there were other lessons that I learned through my lens as a registered nurse. These lessons and comments are shared throughout the text. In the eighth edition, I began ghost writing Randy's and my experiences as "Jenny" and have continued that activity in this edition. Jenny is me, and those thoughts and comments are mine as Randy and I navigated the roller coaster of chronic illness. Throughout the chronic illness journey, I identified interventions and suggestions in caring for individuals and families with chronic illness. Randy and I experienced some of these interventions during our journey—yet most we did not. Each is listed here, and later are elaborated on in the text:

- Use mindful attentiveness as a nursing intervention.
- Focus on "being" with a patient and family versus "doing."
- You don't know what the patient and family are going through, so don't pretend that you do.
- Listen more; talk less.
- The illness is about the individual and family, not you.

Caring for individuals with chronic illness continues to be a challenge for many professional caregivers. I ask that each of you thoughtfully consider how you care for patients and families with such illnesses and ask yourself, "Is this what the patient and family want or need, or is this what is important to me as a professional caregiver?" Talk with your patients and families and, most importantly, listen.

Pamala D. Larsen
July 2014

Contributors

Jill Berg, PhD, RN
Associate Professor Emeritus
Program in Nursing Science
University of California, Irvine
Irvine, California

Rebecca Carron, PhD, RN, NP-C
Assistant Professor
Fay W. Whitney School of Nursing
University of Wyoming
Laramie, Wyoming

Anne Deutsch, PhD, RN, CRRN
Clinical Research Scientist
Rehabilitation Institute of Chicago *and*
Senior Research Public Health Analyst
RTI International *and*
Research Assistant Professor
Department of Physical Medicine and
Rehabilitation, Feinberg School of Medicine
Northwestern University
Chicago, Illinois

Jacqueline M. Dunbar-Jacob, PhD, RN, FAAN
Dean, School of Nursing
Professor, Nursing, Psychology, Epidemiology,
and Occupational Therapy
Director, Center for Research in Chronic
Disorders
University of Pittsburgh
Pittsburgh, Pennsylvania

Lorraine S. Evangelista, PhD, RN
Professor
Program in Nursing Science
University of California, Irvine
Irvine, California

Cheryl Gies, DNP, MSN, CNP
Associate Professor
College of Nursing
University of Toledo
Toledo, Ohio

Ann Marie Hart, PhD, RN, FNP-BC
Associate Professor
Coordinator, DNP Program
Fay W. Whitney School of Nursing
University of Wyoming
Laramie, Wyoming

Alicia Huckstadt, PhD, APRN, FNP-BC, GNP-BC, FAANP
Professor and Director of Graduate Programs
School of Nursing
Wichita State University
Wichita, Kansas

Faye I. Hummel, PhD, RN, CTN-A
Professor and Interim Director
School of Nursing
University of Northern Colorado
Greeley, Colorado

Cynthia S. Jacelon, PhD, RN-BC, CRRN, FAAN
Associate Professor
Director, PhD Program
College of Nursing
University of Massachusetts
Amherst, Massachusetts

Pamala D. Larsen, PhD, RN
Professor Emeritus
Fay W. Whitney School of Nursing
University of Wyoming
Laramie, Wyoming

Raeann G. LeBlanc, DNP, GNP-BC, ANP-BC
Assistant Clinical Professor
College of Nursing
University of Massachusetts
Amherst, Massachusetts

Barbara J. Lutz, PhD, RN, CRRN, APHN-BC, FAHA, FNAP, FAAN
McNeill Distinguished Professor
School of Nursing
University of North Carolina, Wilmington
Wilmington, North Carolina

Kristin L. Mauk, PhD, DNP, RN, CRRN, GCNS-BC, GNP-BC, FAAN
Professor of Nursing and Kreft Endowed Chair
Valparaiso University
Valparaiso, Indiana *and*
President/CEO, Senior Care Central
Valparaiso, Indiana

Elaine T. Miller, PhD, RN, CRRN, FAHA, FAAN
Professor
College of Nursing
University of Cincinnati
Cincinnati, Ohio

Nicholas R. Nicholson, Jr., PhD, MPH, RN, PHCNS-BC
Assistant Professor
School of Nursing
Quinnipiac University
Hamden, Connecticut

Linda L. Pierce, PhD, RN, CNS, CRRN, FAHA, FAAN
Professor
College of Nursing
University of Toledo
Toledo, Ohio

Barbara M. Raudonis, PhD, RN, FNGNA, FPCN
Associate Professor
College of Nursing
University of Texas, Arlington
Arlington, Texas

Susan K. Rice, PhD, RN, CPNP, CNS
Professor
College of Nursing
University of Toledo
Toledo, Ohio

Robynn Zender, MS
Research Associate
Program in Nursing Science
University of California, Irvine
Irvine, California

PART I

Impact of the Disease to the Individual and Family

Chronicity

Pamala D. Larsen

Addressing the issues of chronic illness is a global challenge. In September 2011, for the first time, the United Nations discussed the topic of chronic disease as a principal theme at a plenary gathering (Institute of Medicine [IOM], 2012). The prevalence of chronic disease on a worldwide basis is similar to, if not greater than, it is in the United States. The World Health Organization (WHO) views chronic disease as a silent pandemic spreading to all parts of the world. Coronary heart disease, stroke, cancer, chronic obstructive pulmonary disease, diabetes mellitus type 2, neurodegenerative disease, and renal failure accounted for more than 62% of all deaths worldwide in 2011 (Harris, 2013). Twenty percent of chronic disease deaths occur in high-income countries, whereas the remaining 80% occur in low- and middle-income countries (WHO, 2013a).

The global pandemic of chronic disease has emerged in tandem with the changing demography of the world population. Throughout the world, the birth rate exceeds the death rate; in addition to having better access to treatment, more people are living to advanced ages, creating a phenomenon of "global aging" (Harris, 2013, p. 1). These epidemiologic transitions are dynamic, wherein some diseases may disappear while others reoccur; for example, infectious diseases are reemerging in high-income countries as bacteria develop resistance to antibiotics. Whereas many healthcare professionals might consider the increase in chronic disease

to be largely attributable to aging of the population, the real situation is much more complex. Epidemiological transitions reflect dynamic patterns of health and disease due to demographic, socioeconomic, technologic, cultural, environmental, and biologic changes (p. 8).

Chronic diseases are common and costly, but preventable. Four health-damaging, but modifiable, behaviors—tobacco use, insufficient physical activity, poor nutrition, and excessive alcohol use—are currently responsible for much of the illness, disability, and premature death related to chronic disease (Centers for Disease Control and Prevention [CDC], 2009).

Introduction

The most current prevalence data for U.S. chronic disease were collected in 2005, when it was estimated that 133 million individuals in the United States were living with at least one chronic disease (CDC, 2009; IOM, 2012; National Health Council, 2013), and that 7 of every 10 Americans who died each year—more than 1.7 million people—died of a chronic disease. Chronic disease accounts for one-third of the years of potential life lost before age 65. Statistics that quantify the costs from chronic disease are sobering:

- The direct and indirect costs of diabetes amounted to $245 billion in 2012 (American

Diabetes Association, 2013). These costs have increased 41% over the last 5 years.

- In 2011, the cost of heart disease totaled $108.9 billion (CDC, 2014).
- In 2010 the total direct and indirect costs of cardiovascular disease and stroke in the United States were estimated to be $314.4 billion (American Heart Association, 2014).
- The direct cost of cancer care amounted to $124.7 billion in 2010 (National Cancer Institute, 2011).
- The medical costs of people with chronic disease account for more than 75% of the United States' $2 trillion medical care costs each year (CDC, 2009).
- By 2030, the global economic burden of noncommunicable diseases is estimated to be $47 trillion (Bloom et al., 2011).

In 2000, minorities represented 16.3% (5.7 million) of older American adults. By 2011, their number had risen to 8.5 million, and projections indicate that the minority older-adult population will increase to 20.2 million by 2030 (28% of the elderly) (Administration on Aging [AOA], 2012). How will the current system or a future system cope with this diverse group of seniors and their accompanying chronic conditions?

Multiple factors have combined to increase the number of individuals with chronic disease. Advances in the fields of public health, genetics, immunology, technology, and pharmacology have led to a significant decrease in mortality from acute disease. This medical success has contributed, in part, to the unprecedented growth of chronic illness by extending life expectancy and by facilitating earlier detection of disease in general. Living longer, however, leads to greater vulnerability to the occurrence of accidents and disease events that can become chronic in nature. The client who may have died from a myocardial infarction in the past now needs continuing health care for heart failure. The cancer survivor has healthcare needs related to the iatrogenic results of the life-saving treatment. The adolescent who is a quadriplegic because of an

accident may live a relatively long life, but needs a lifetime of preventive and maintenance care from the healthcare system. Children with cystic fibrosis have benefited from lung transplantation, but need care for the rest of their lives. As these examples suggest, many previously fatal conditions, injuries, and diseases have become chronic in nature.

Disease Versus Illness

Although the terms *disease* and *illness* are often used interchangeably, there is a distinct difference between them. "Disease" refers to the pathophysiology of a condition. "Illness," in contrast, is the human experience of a disease and refers to how the disease is perceived, lived with, and responded to by individuals, their families, and healthcare professionals. The pathophysiology of the disease is important, but it is just as important to recognize the illness experience in providing holistic care.

Today is the 19th day in a row that Randy has seen a healthcare professional, and actually a couple of those days, he saw two different ones on the same day. It's either radiation therapy, receiving IV fluids and/or replacement potassium, an IV antibiotic for a resistant infection, receiving blood as an outpatient, persistent vomiting, … something every day. Will this ever stop? Will we ever have a normal life again? Right now I don't even remember what normal is.

—Jenny

It is Sunday, 2:08 a.m. I am wheeled into a sterile white examination room, obviously used for "codes," patients like me, deemed to be in serious trouble. I look at the reinforced glass in the windows separating my room from the other side. The curtains are drawn and I cannot see out, but on my side I can read the words on the glass, changing with each window:

O_2 ___L-m___by___
Medication Dose Time
IV Fluid Rate
Defibrillation

Beth puts her arms around me and holds me. She doesn't deserve this, I think. Why must she go through all of this again? (Hsi, 2004, pp. 164–165)

Patient stories chronicle the illness experience; the illness experience is also nursing's domain. Thus, the focus of this book is on the chronic illness experience of individuals and families, and not specific disease processes. While chronic disease cannot be cured, nursing can make a difference in the illness experience with care instead of cure.

Acute Conditions Versus Chronic Conditions

When an individual develops an acute disease, there is typically a sudden onset, with signs and symptoms related to the pathophysiology itself. Acute diseases end in a relatively short time, either with recovery and resumption of prior activities, or with death.

Chronic illness, by comparison, continues indefinitely. Although a welcome alternative to death in most, but not all, cases, the illness may be seen as a mixed blessing to the individual and the family. In addition, the illness often becomes the person's identity. For example, an individual having any kind of cancer, even in remission, may acquire the label of "that person with cancer." Chronic conditions take many forms, and there is no single onset pattern. A chronic disease can appear suddenly or through an insidious process, be associated with episodic flare-ups or exacerbations, or remain in remission with an absence of symptoms for long periods of time. Maintaining wellness or keeping symptoms in remission is a juggling act of balancing treatment regimens, maintaining quality of life, and having a normal life.

Defining Chronicity

Defining chronicity is complex. Initially, the characteristics of chronic diseases were identified by the Commission on Chronic Illness as all impairments or deviations from normal that included one or more of the following: permanency; residual disability; nonpathologic alteration; required rehabilitation; or a long period of supervision, observation, and care (Mayo, 1956). The extent of a chronic disease further complicates attempts in defining this term. Disability may depend not only on the kind of condition and its severity, but also on the implications it holds for the person. The degree of disability and altered lifestyle—part of traditional definitions—may relate more to the client's *perceptions and beliefs* about the disease than to the disease itself.

Long-term and iatrogenic effects of some treatment may constitute chronic conditions in their own right, making them eligible to be defined as a chronic illness. Life-saving procedures create other problems. Of particular note are the chemotherapies and radiation therapy treatments for cancer. Studies have demonstrated that these life-saving treatments that may have occurred many years ago often lead to the development of a new cancer.

Chronic illness, by its very nature, is never completely cured. Biologically, the human body wears out unevenly. Older adults need a progressively wider variety of specialized services for increasingly complicated conditions. In the classic words of Emanuel (1982), "Life is the accumulation of chronic illness beneath the load of which we eventually succumb" (p. 502).

Although definitions of chronic disease are important, from a nursing perspective we are far more interested in how the disease psychosocially affects the client and family. What is the illness experience of the client and family? Perhaps the onus of defining chronic illness—and similarly, quality of life—should be placed on the client, as only the client understands and "knows" the illness experience. However, that aside, the following definition of chronic illness is offered:

Chronic illness is the lived experience of the individual and family diagnosed with chronic disease. The individual's and family's values impact their perceptions and beliefs of the condition and thus their illness and wellness behaviors. Their values are influenced by demographic, socioeconomic, technological, cultural, and environmental variables. The lived experience is "known" only to the individual and family.

Impact of Chronic Illness

The impact and interventions cited in this chapter examine chronic disease from an aggregate perspective, using a public health lens to view chronic disease and potential interventions.

The Older Adult

Although chronic diseases and conditions exist in children, adolescents, and young and middle-aged adults, the bulk of these conditions occur in adults age 65 years and older. Since 1900, the percentage of the U.S. population made up by older Americans has tripled. According to *A Profile of Older Americans: 2012*, the older population (65 years and older) numbered 41.4 million in 2011, an increase of 18% since 2000. By 2030, it is projected there will be 72.1 million adults in the United States who are older than 65 years, and by 2040 the population will reach 79.7 million (AOA, 2012).

Medicare Part A beneficiaries had more chronic conditions, on average, in 2010 than in 2008 (Erdem, 2014). The percentage increase in the average number of chronic conditions was larger for dual-eligible beneficiaries (2.8%) than for non-dual-eligible beneficiaries (1.2%). During the time period of 2008–2010, the prevalence of some chronic conditions decreased, such as congestive heart failure, ischemic heart disease, and stroke. The deterioration of average health, therefore, was due to other chronic conditions: chronic kidney disease, depression, diabetes, osteoporosis, and rheumatoid arthritis/osteoarthritis.

The report *State of Aging and Health in America 2013* (CDC, 2013) provides a snapshot of the impact of chronic illness on older adults. With two out of every three older Americans

having multiple chronic conditions (MCC), the need for action is apparent. The National Report Card on Healthy Aging reports on 15 indicators of older adult health, 8 of which are identified in *Healthy People 2020*. On a positive note, older adults have met six of the *Healthy People 2020* targets—those dealing with leisure-time physical activity, obesity, current smoking, taking medications for high blood pressure, mammograms within the past 2 years, and colorectal cancer screenings. However, three areas need improvement in this population: receiving a flu vaccine, receiving pneumonia vaccine, and up-to-date preventive services. Consequently, *State of Aging and Health in America 2013* lists several calls to action to improve the health and well-being of older adults:

- Developing a new Healthy Brain Initiative Road Map
- Addressing aging and health issues among the lesbian, gay, bisexual, and transgender (LGBT) community
- Using data on physically unhealthy days to guide interventions
- Addressing mental distress among older adults
- Monitoring vaccination rates for shingles (CDC, 2013)

With MCC, these older adults will access—if their socioeconomic status permits—an acute care system. How will the needs of these aging adults influence our healthcare delivery system?

Healthy People 2020

Healthy People 2020 provides science-based, 10-year national objectives for improving the health of all Americans (http://www.healthypeople.gov). With the 2020 document, there is a renewed focus on identifying, measuring, tracking, and reducing health disparities through a determinants-of-health approach. The mission of *Healthy People 2020* is fivefold:

- Identify nationwide health improvement priorities.

- Increase public awareness and understanding of the determinants of health, disease, and disability and the opportunities for progress.
- Provide measurable objectives and goals that are applicable at the national, state, and local levels.
- Engage multiple sectors to take actions to strengthen policies and improve practices that are driven by the best available evidence and knowledge.
- Identify critical research, evaluation, and data collection needs.

The topic areas and objectives of *Healthy People 2020* are based on four overarching goals: (1) attain high-quality, longer lives free of preventable disease, disability, injury, and premature death; (2) achieve health equity, eliminate disparities, and improve the health of all groups; (3) create social and physical environments that promote good health for all; and (4) promote quality of life, healthy development, and healthy behaviors across all life stages. Topic areas of *Healthy People 2020* are listed in **Table 1-1**. Many of the topics relate to chronic disease or prevention of chronic disease.

Table 1-1 TOPICS OF *HEALTHY PEOPLE 2020*

Access to health services	Human immunodeficiency virus (HIV) infection
Adolescent health	Immunization and infectious diseases
Arthritis, osteoporosis, and chronic back conditions	Injury and violence prevention
Blood disorders and blood safety	Lesbian, gay, bisexual, and transgender health
Cancer	Maternal, infant, and child health
Chronic kidney disease	Medical product safety
Dementias, including Alzheimer's disease	Mental health and mental disorders
Diabetes	Nutrition and weight status
Disability and health	Occupational safety and health
Early and middle childhood	Older adults
Educational and community-based programs	Oral health
Environmental health	Physical activity
Family planning	Preparedness
Food safety	Public health infrastructure
Genomics	Respiratory diseases
Global health	Sexually transmitted diseases
Health communication and health information technology	Sleep health
Healthcare-associated infections	Social determinants of health
Health-related quality of life and well-being	Substance abuse
Hearing and other sensory or communication disorders	Tobacco use
Heart disease and stroke	Vision

Source: *Healthy People 2020*. Topics and objectives index. Retrieved from http://healthypeople.gov/2020/topicsobjectives2020/default.aspx.

National Healthcare Quality Report

The National Healthcare Quality Report (U.S. Department of Health and Human Services [USDHHS], 2013) is an indicator of how we, as a country, are doing with quality of care and health disparities. The statistics on quality and access to care are vitally important to individuals across this country. Late identification of persons with chronic disease, due to access issues, leads to poor outcomes, more complications for the individual, and greater healthcare expenditures. These individuals may be young, middle-aged, or older, but their outcomes are similar. As chronic disease requires long-term care, the need for quality care and continued access to that care is essential. Prevention is the key to many chronic conditions, but if there is little quality care and poor access, health outcomes tend to be poor.

Since 2003, the Agency for Healthcare Research and Quality (AHRQ) has reported on progress and opportunities for improving healthcare quality and reducing healthcare disparities. As in prior years, the findings from the National Healthcare Quality Report (NHQR) and the National Healthcare Disparities Report (NHDR) have been integrated into a single report to reinforce the need to consider concurrently the quality of health and disparities across populations when assessing the healthcare system. The 2013 annual report addresses three questions:

- What is the status of healthcare quality and disparities in the United States?
- How have healthcare quality and disparities changed over time?
- Where is the greatest need to improve healthcare quality and reduce disparities? (USDHHS, 2013, p. 1).

Three themes have emerged from this report that emphasize the need to accelerate progress if this country is to achieve higher quality and more equitable health care in the near future:

- Healthcare quality and access are suboptimal in the United States, especially for minority and low-income groups.
- Overall quality is improving, access is getting worse, and disparities are not changing
- Urgent attention is warranted to ensure continued improvements in the following areas:
  - Quality of diabetes care, maternal and child health care, and adverse events
  - Disparities in cancer care
  - Quality of care among states in the South (USDHHS, 2013, p. 2)

Compared with the 2009 report, whose findings were presented in the previous edition of this text, there has been little change in the themes noted over the 4-year period. What follows are selected examples of the health disparities present in the United States today and the limited access that minority or disadvantaged people have to health care.

- Disparities in quality of care are common.
  - Blacks received worse care than whites, and Hispanics received worse care than non-Hispanic whites for approximately 40% of quality measures.
  - Poor and low-income people received worse care than high-income people for 60% of quality measures; middle-income people received worse care for more than half of the measures (USDHHS, 2013, p. 3).
- Disparities in access are also common, especially among American Indians, Alaska Natives, Hispanics, and poor people.
  - Hispanics had worse access to care than non-Hispanic whites for about 70% of measures.
  - Poor people had worse access to care than high-income people for all measures, low-income people had worse access to care for more than 80% of measures,

and middle-income people had worse access to care for 70% of measures (USDHHS, 2013, p. 4).

The National Healthcare Quality Report is plagued by the same problem every year—namely, the data on underserved populations are often incomplete. Some data sources do not collect information to identify specific groups; other sources collect the information, but the numbers in each group are too small for reliable estimates (USDHHS, 2013, p. 9). Obtaining reliable data has been included as a priority in the *HHS Action Plan to Reduce Racial and Ethnic Health Disparities* (National Partnership for Action to End Health Disparities, 2011).

The NHQR has identified some issues that demonstrate *worsening quality of care*, which may lead to chronic physical or mental conditions:

- Children ages 19–35 months who receive three or more doses of *Haemophilus influenzae* type B vaccine
- Maternal deaths per 100,000 live births
- Adults age 40 and older with diagnosed diabetes who had their feet checked for sores or irritation in the calendar year
- Postoperative pulmonary embolism or deep vein thrombosis per 1,000 surgical admissions, age 18 and older
- Admissions for asthma per 100,000 population, age 65 and older
- Adults age 40 and older with diagnosed diabetes who received two or more hemoglobin A_{1c} measurements in the calendar year
- Suicide deaths per 100,000 population
- Women ages 21–65 who received a Pap smear in the last 3 years
- Admissions with Stage III or IV pressure ulcers per 1,000 medical and surgical admissions of length of stay of 5 or more days
- Admissions of patients with diabetes with short-term complications per 100,000

population, age 18 and older (USDHHS, 2013, p. 13)

Finally, the NHQR reports *disparities that are worsening over time*:

- Advanced-stage invasive breast cancer incidence per 100,000 women age 40 and older
- Maternal deaths per 100,000 live births
- Adjusted incidence of end-stage renal disease due to diabetes per 1 million population
- Hospice patients who received the right amount of help for feelings of anxiety or sadness
- Adults ages 18–64 at high risk (e.g., because of chronic obstructive pulmonary disease [COPD]) who have ever received pneumococcal vaccination
- Hospital patients with heart failure and left ventricular systolic dysfunction who were prescribed an angiotensin-converting enzyme (ACE) inhibitor or angiotensin-receptor blocker (ARB) at discharge
- Adults age 50 and older who ever received a colonoscopy, sigmoidoscopy, or proctoscopy
- Home healthcare patients who have less shortness of breath
- Adults age 40 and older with a diagnosis of diabetes who received more than 2 hemoglobin A_{1c} measurements in the calendar year
- Hospital patients with heart attack who received fibrinolytic medication within 30 minutes of arrival (USDHHS, 2013, p. 14)

The Healthcare Consumer

The influx of baby boomers into organizations such as AARP has distinctly affected the activities of that organization and other similar types of organizations. In addition, the new group of seniors is the most ethnically and racially diverse of any previous generation. Members of this well-educated, consumer-driven generation want information about their conditions and all treatment options. They question their health-care professionals and do not blindly accept healthcare advice and treatment options. These consumers want the ability to say "yes" or "no" to treatment options.

William Frist, a heart and lung transplant surgeon and former U.S. Senate Majority Leader and senator from Tennessee, has spoken about two influences on health care today—namely, the rapid ascent of the newly empowered consumer with knowledge that can affect his or her health and the advances in information technology (IT) (Frist, 2014). Neither of these were significant drivers of health care even 3 years ago; Frist, however, believes that the "empowered consumer and rapidly advancing health IT will channel our chaotic, fragmented, and wasteful health care sector toward a more seamless, transparent, accountable and efficient system" (p. 191).

The biggest driver of health status is individual health behavior. Only 10–15% of an individual's health status is attributable to the healthcare service he or she receives (Schroder, 2007). The rest is determined by behavior; genetics; and social determinants, including living conditions, access to food, and education status (Frist, 2014). The number of individuals with chronic disease is climbing, but to avert those conditions for millions of others who are at risk, society must make healthy choices easy for individuals to embrace in their daily lives.

Financial Impact

Total U.S. healthcare spending increased by 3.7% to $2.8 trillion or $8,915 per person in 2012 as compared with data from 2011 (Martin, Hartman, Whittle, Catlin & National Health Expenditure Accounts Team, 2014). Growth has remained fairly stable since 2009, primarily due to the impact of the economic recession (p. 67).

In 2012, the U.S. gross domestic product (GDP) grew almost 1 percentage point faster than the country's health spending did. As a result, the share of the U.S. economy devoted to health care in 2012 was 17.3% as compared

with 17.2% in 2011, and considerably smaller than the high of 17.6% of the GDP in 2009. Martin and colleagues (2014) note several important findings:

- Personal healthcare spending (healthcare goods and services) accounted for 85% of the overall national health spending, increasing 3.9% in 2012. The recession contributed to slower growth in private health insurance spending and out-of-pocket spending by consumers.
- The increase in personal healthcare spending in 2012 was influenced primarily by hospital services, for which spending increased 4.9% in 2012 as compared with 3.5% in 2011.
- Spending for physician and clinical services increased 4.6% in 2012, up from a 4.1% increase in 2011. The faster growth in these services was driven primarily by increases in the volume and intensity of services provided.
- Partially offsetting the increased growth in hospital care and clinician services was slower growth in spending for prescription drugs and nursing home care. The rate of growth for nursing home spending slowed to 1.6% as compared with 4.3% in 2011; this drop is partly attributable to Medicare's reduced payments for skilled nursing facilities that sought to adjust for the large increase in payments that occurred in 2011. Total retail prescription drug spending growth slowed in 2012, increasing by only 0.4%, compared with 2.5% in 2011. This reduced growth rate was driven largely by a decrease in the overall prices paid for retail prescription drugs as numerous brand-name drugs lost their patent protection (e.g., Lipitor, Plavix, and Singulair) (Martin et al., 2014, pp. 67–72).

In the United States in 2008, the top 10 costliest medical conditions, in rank order, were the same for both men and women age 18 years and older: (1) heart disease, (2) cancer, (3) mental disorders, (4) trauma-related disorders, (5) osteoarthritis, (6) asthma, (7) hypertension, (8) diabetes, (9) back problems, and (10) hyperlipidemia (Soni, 2011). However, the highest per-person mean expenditures were in cancer for both men and women—$4,873 and $4,484, respectively. These data indicate that chronic disease is the nation's greatest healthcare problem and the number one driver of health care today. With the aging population and the advanced technologies that assist clients in living longer lives, these costs will only increase.

Recent data from the National Health Interview Survey (NHIS) from 2012 found that one in four families experienced a financial burden in paying for medical care. One in 10 persons in a family was unable to pay anything toward their health care (Cohen & Kirzinger, 2014). Additionally, one in three families with children experienced a financial burden from medical care.

The Organization for Economic Cooperation and Development (OECD) annually tracks and reports on more than 1,200 health system measures across 30 industrialized countries. The United States continues to differ markedly from other countries examined in the OECD report. In 2011, the annual health expenditure per capita (incorporating both public and private expenditures) for an individual in the United States was $8,508 (the 2012 amount was $8,915, as mentioned earlier). This number is significantly higher than that for Norway ($5,669), ranked number 2, and Switzerland ($5,643), ranked number 3 (OECD, 2013). Americans spent more than twice as much on health care as relatively rich countries such as France and Sweden. In fact, the United States spent more than two-and-one-half times the amount that the average OECD country spent on health care, which was $3,339(adjusted for purchasing power parity).

Compared with other OECD countries, the United States has fewer physicians per capita (2.5 per 1,000 population compared with the OECD average of 3.2), more nurses (11.1 per 1,000 population compared with the OECD average

of 8.7), and fewer hospital beds (3.1 per 1,000 population compared with the OECD average of 4.8). This decline in U.S. hospital beds coincides with the reduction in the length of stays in hospitals and an increase in day surgeries.

While life expectancy at birth in the United States was 1½ years greater than the OECD average in 1960, it is now, at 78.7 years, almost 1½ years less than the OECD average of 80.1 years. Switzerland, Japan, Italy, and Spain are the OECD countries with the highest life expectancies, exceeding 82 years (OECD, 2013). Certainly one health risk factor—obesity—has affected any increase in life expectancy. The obesity rate among adults in the United States was 36.5% in 2011, up from 15% in 1978. This is the highest rate among all OECD countries. The average obesity rate for the 15 OECD countries for which data were available was 22.8%.

One positive note is that smoking in the United States has decreased significantly. This rate in the United States decreased from 33.5% in 1980 to 14.8% in 2011. Only Sweden and Iceland have lower rates of smoking.

Interventions

Chronic disease is an issue that is all encompassing, such that interventions from many sources are needed to make a difference. Professional education, evidence-based practice, and legislation affect any potential interventions. Lastly, paradigms from the Centers for Disease Control and Prevention, the Institute of Medicine, and the World Health Organization address chronic disease and ways to mitigate its impact.

Professional Education

One of the challenges in chronic disease care and management is educating healthcare professionals about providing care tailored to those with chronic disease. The differences are vast between caring for a person with an acute illness on a short-term basis and caring for a person with a chronic condition over the long haul.

WHO developed a document outlining the steps to prepare a healthcare workforce for the 21st century that can appropriately care for individuals with chronic conditions. The WHO document calls for a transformation of healthcare training to better meet the needs of individuals with chronic conditions. This document, *Preparing a Healthcare Workforce for the 21st Century: The Challenge of Chronic Conditions* (WHO, 2005), has the support of the World Medical Association, the International Council of Nurses, the International Pharmaceutical Federation, the European Respiratory Society, and the International Alliance of Patients' Organizations.

The competencies delineated by WHO (2005) were identified through a process that included an extensive document/literature review and international expert agreement (p. 14). All competencies were based on addressing the needs of patients with chronic conditions and their family members from a longitudinal perspective, and focused on two types of "prevention" strategies: (1) initial prevention of the chronic disease and (2) prevention of complications from the condition (p. 18). The five competencies include patient-centered care, partnering, quality improvement, information and communication technology, and public health perspective (**Table 1-2**). At first glance, the competencies might not seem unique. However, in an acute care–oriented healthcare delivery system, these concepts are not as prominent. Clients move in and out of the care system quickly, and there is less need for implementation of these concepts.

Evidence-Based Practice

The evidence-based practice movement had its beginnings in the 1970s with Dr. Archie Cochrane, a British epidemiologist. In 1971, Cochrane published a book that criticized physicians for not conducting rigorous reviews of evidence to ensure that they were making appropriate treatment decisions. Cochrane was

Table 1-2 WHO Core Competencies

Patient-Centered Care
Interviewing and communicating effectively
Assisting changes in health-related behaviors
Supporting self-management
Using a proactive approach

Partnering
Partnering with patients
Partnering with other providers
Partnering with communities

Quality Improvement
Measuring care delivery and outcomes
Learning and adapting to change
Translating evidence into practice

Information and Communication Technology
Designing and using patient registries
Using computer technologies
Communicating with partners

Public Health Perspective
Providing population-based care
Systems thinking
Working across the care continuum
Working in primary healthcare–led systems

Reproduced, with the permission of the publisher, from *Preparing a health care workforce for the 21st century: The challenge of chronic conditions.* Geneva, World Health Organization, 2005 (p. 20).

a proponent of randomized clinical trials, and in his exemplar case noted that thousands of low-birth-weight premature infants died needlessly. At the same time there were several randomized controlled trials (RCTs) that had been conducted on the use of corticosteroid therapy to halt premature labor in pregnant women, but the data had never been reviewed or analyzed. After review, these studies demonstrated that this therapy was effective in halting premature labor and thus reducing infant deaths due to prematurity. Cochrane died in 1988, but as a result of his influence and call for systematic review of the literature, the Cochrane Collaboration was launched in Oxford, England, in 1993. The Cochrane Collaboration has 52 review groups composed of individuals around the world who share an interest in developing and maintaining systematic reviews in particular areas (Chan, 2013). The Cochrane Collaboration also hosts the Cochrane Library, which is a sophisticated collection of databases containing current, high-quality research that supports practice.

As healthcare professionals examine the evidence to improve the care of their clients, there are a number of sources for reference. The following agencies and organizations are some of the resources available:

- Agency for Healthcare Research and Quality (AHRQ) (www.ahrq.gov)
- *Clinical Evidence* (www.clinicalevidence .com)
- Cochrane Library (www.thecochranelibrary. com)
- Joanna Briggs Institute (www.joannabriggs .org)
- National Guideline Clearinghouse (www .guideline.gov)
- Task Force on Community Preventive Services (www.thecommunityguide.org)
- U.S. Preventive Services Task Force (www .ahrq.gov/clinic/uspstfab.htm)
- Veterans Evidence-Based Research Dissemination Implementation Center (VERDICT): (www.verdict.research.va.gov)

Legislation

On March 21, 2010, President Barack Obama signed legislation to reform the U.S. healthcare delivery system. The Patient Protection and Affordable Care Act (ACA) and the Health Care and Education Reconciliation Act expanded health insurance coverage to individuals who were not previously covered by any health plan through the implementation of individual and employer mandates as well as through expansion of federal and state programs such as Medicare and Medicaid. According to the Congressional Budget Office (CBO), an estimated 32 million additional

individuals will be covered by 2019 (Albright et al., 2010). Some components of the law address individuals with chronic illness:

- A Patient's Bill of Rights was established.
- High-risk insurance pools were created to make insurance available to individuals with preexisting health conditions until healthcare coverage exchanges are operational in 2014.
- Insurers are no longer able to exclude children with preexisting conditions from being covered under their parents' insurance.
- Insurers are not able to rescind policies to avoid paying medical bills when a person becomes ill.
- Lifetime limits on coverage are prohibited.
- Children are able to stay covered under their parents' insurance plan until age 26.
- Funding for scholarships and loan repayments for primary care practitioners working with underserved populations was expanded.
- Insurers will no longer be able to refuse to sell or renew policies because of an individual's health status, and will no longer be able to exclude coverage for an individual of any age because of a preexisting condition (effective 2014).
- Insurers can no longer charge higher rates because of an individual's health status or gender (effective 2014).
- Health plans will be prohibited from imposing any annual limits on coverage (effective 2014).
- Health plans will no longer be able to charge copayments and deductibles for recommended preventive care (effective 2014).
- Health insurance exchanges will open in each state, allowing individuals and small employers to shop for health insurance policies (effective 2014).
- Tax credits are available to those whose income is above Medicaid eligibility and

below 400% of the poverty level and do not receive acceptable coverage. Additionally, Medicaid eligibility will increase to 133% of the poverty level for all non-elderly individuals ("The Affordable Care Act: One Year Later," 2011).

Instead of creating a new healthcare financing system, in the same way that Medicare and Medicaid were created in the 1960s, the ACA attempted to build on the current system (Jost, 2014). Although building on "what was" was intended to make it easier for implementation, it actually made it much harder. Also, the roll-out of the federal marketplace for healthcare policies on October 1, 2013, was a disaster. Multiple technical and political failures became apparent in the design of the defective, nonfunctional healthcare.gov website. In going forward, one of the challenges of the ACA will be ensuring that its benefits become apparent quickly and dramatically enough to offset the problems (Jost, 2014, p. 10). The ACA does address the real problem of millions of uninsured Americans, and if it succeeds, it will be considered successful; however, it is still too early to know the full impact of the ACA.

CDC's National Center for Chronic Disease Prevention and Health Promotion

According to the CDC (2009), the key chronic diseases in the United States are the following:

- Heart disease and stroke are the first and third leading causes of death, respectively, accounting for more than 30% of all U.S. deaths each year.
- Cancer, the second leading cause of death, claims more than 500,000 lives each year.
- Diabetes is the leading cause of kidney failure, nontraumatic lower-extremity amputations, and new cases of blindness each year among U.S. adults aged 20–74 years.

- Arthritis, the most common cause of disability, limits activity for 19 million U.S. adults.
- Obesity has become a major health concern for people of all ages. One in every 3 adults and nearly 1 in every 5 young people aged 6–19 are obese.

The National Center for Chronic Disease Prevention and Health Promotion (NCCDPHP) is at the forefront of the nation's efforts to promote health and well-being through prevention and control of chronic disease. The NCCDPHP provides leadership to achieve three primary goals:

- Prevent, delay, detect, and control chronic diseases
- Contribute to chronic disease research and apply that research to implement practice and effective intervention strategies
- Achieve equity in health by eliminating racial and ethnic disparities and achieving optimal health for all Americans (CDC, 2009)

The interventions of the NCCDPHP are critical in supporting the nation's public health infrastructure as it works with healthcare providers, public health professionals, educators, and policy makers. To achieve optimal health for all, NCCDPHP's work on the social determinants of health extends beyond the scope of traditional public health practice to include collaboration in education, housing, transportation, justice, labor, and other sectors. The NCCDPHP supports the following activities to prevent and control diseases:

- *Surveillance and applied research*: Measuring and monitoring trends in the burden of chronic disease and associated risk factors. The NCCDPHP supports several surveillance systems including, but not limited to, the Behavioral Risk Factor Surveillance System (BRFSS), Youth Tobacco Survey, Pregnancy Risk

Assessment Monitoring System, and National Program of Cancer Registries. The NCCDPHP has a network of more than 30 academic centers that conduct research to address health problems identified by communities.

- *Promotion of policy, environmental and systems changes at the state and community levels*: As an example, for the past four decades the Office on Smoking and Health has reviewed research and provided 30 scientific reports on health and the use of tobacco.
- *Health communications*: Includes paid advertising, media advocacy, public relations, and health promotion activities.
- *Healthcare system linkages*: Include working with the healthcare system through provision of services such as mammography and tobacco cessation counseling for underserved populations; and working on issues of access to care, planned care, self-management, patient navigation, and quality prevention services (CDC, 2009).

Institute of Medicine

Living Well with Chronic Illness: A Call for Public Health Action (2012) is a report from a committee of the IOM. The IOM contends that better efforts need to be made to maintain or enhance quality of life for individuals and families living with chronic illness. The report (in book form) describes nine exemplar diseases, health conditions, and impairments that have significant implications for the United States' health and economy; impact quality of life and functional status; cut across many illnesses and complications, and/or increase risks for multiple chronic conditions; and impact the community, families, and caregivers of those with chronic disease (p. xvi). These conditions are arthritis, cancer survivorship, chronic pain, dementia, depression, type 2 diabetes, post-traumatic disabling conditions, schizophrenia, and vision and hearing loss. The IOM report notes that identifying these

conditions in this way does not mean that they are more burdensome or important than others, but rather that each illustrates a key functionality or part of a chronic condition. In fact, the authors of this report were advised to not focus on the common high-mortality diseases, but to consider conditions that have the potential to cause or actually do cause functional limitations and/or disabilities (p. 23).

The IOM considers chronic disease to be a public health problem as well as a clinical problem. Using that lens to view the problem means that a population health perspective is necessary to develop interventions and policies. Thus, the best framework to approach chronic disease is an integrated one. The IOM committee adopted the concept of "living well," as proposed by Lorig and colleagues (2006), to reflect the best achievable state of health that encompasses all dimensions of physical, mental, and social well-being (p. 32). The concept of living well, integrated within a broader population health framework, is intended to promote a more holistic perspective beyond the traditional focus on other goals such as primary prevention or expansion of life expectancy (p. 33). **Figure 1-1** depicts the framework proposed by the IOM.

The work of this IOM committee is vast and its findings have been compiled in a book with more than 300 pages. The IOM committee's 17 recommendations addressed 7 questions from the statement of task. Questions included:

- Which chronic diseases should be the focus of public health efforts to reduce disability and improve functioning and quality of life (p. 10)?
- Which populations need to be the focus of interventions to reduce the consequences of chronic disease, including the burden of disability, loss of productivity and functioning, healthcare costs, and reduced quality of life (p. 11)?
- What is the role of primary prevention (for those at highest risk), secondary prevention,

Figure 1-1 Integrated framework for living well with chronic illness.

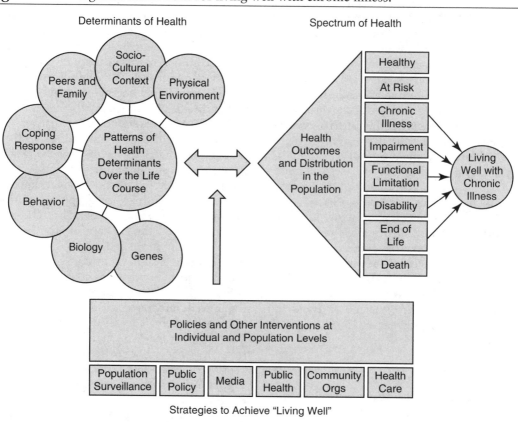

From: Institute of Medicine (2012). *Living well with chronic illness: A call for public health action.* Washington, DC: National Academies Press, p. 32.

and tertiary prevention of chronic disease in reducing or minimizing life impacts (p. 12)?

- Which consequences of chronic diseases are most important to the nation's health and economic well-being (p. 13)?
- Which policy priorities could advance efforts to improve life impacts of chronic disease (p. 14)?
- Which population-based interventions can help achieve outcomes that maintain or improve quality of life, functioning, and disability?

- What is the evidence on the effectiveness of interventions on these outcomes?
- To what extent do the interventions that address these outcomes also affect clinical outcomes?
- To what extent can policy, environmental, and systems change achieve these outcomes (p. 15)?

- How can public health surveillance be used to inform public policy decisions to minimize adverse life impacts (p. 18)?

A number of the recommendations involve the current and future work of the CDC. Many of the recommendations focus on research that needs to be completed to recognize if any of our current models of care for those persons with chronic illness make a difference in quality of life. The recommendations are without priority order or measured ranking, as all are thought to be important strategies and steps to undergird public health action to enable individuals to live well with chronic illness (p. 8). All recommendations, as noted earlier, are based on a public health model.

World Health Organization

WHO has updated its plan for prevention and control of noncommunicable diseases (NCD), the term the organization uses for chronic diseases. The plan, titled the *WHO Global Action Plan for Prevention and Control of NCDs 2013–2020*, provides a road map and a menu of policy options for all WHO member states and other stakeholders, as they take coordinated and coherent action, at all levels, local to global, to attain the nine voluntary global targets. For example, one of those targets is a 25% relative reduction in premature mortality from cardiovascular diseases, cancer, diabetes, or chronic respiratory diseases by 2025.

WHO's vision for the plan is to have a world free of the avoidable burden of noncommunicable diseases, with a goal of reducing the preventable and avoidable burden of morbidity, mortality, and disability due to noncommunicable diseases by means of multisectoral collaboration and cooperation at national, regional, and global levels. The ideal is for populations to reach the highest attainable standards of health and productivity at every age and for those diseases to no longer be a barrier to well-being or socioeconomic development.

The focus of this action plan includes four NCDs—cardiovascular diseases, cancer, chronic respiratory diseases, and diabetes (which collectively make the largest contribution to morbidity and mortality due to NCDs)—and four shared behavioral risk factors—tobacco use, unhealthy diet, physical inactivity, and harmful use of alcohol. WHO recognizes that the conditions in which people live and work and their lifestyles influence their health and quality of life (WHO, 2013b).

The overarching principles and approaches advocated within the plan include the following: (1) a human rights approach; (2) an equity-based approach; (3) national action, international cooperation, and solidarity; (4) multisectoral action; (5) life-course approach; (6) empowerment of people and communities; (7) evidence-based strategies; (8) universal health coverage; and (9) management of real, perceived, and potential conflicts of interest (WHO, 2013b)

Summary

The United States touts itself as having the most sophisticated and technologically advanced health care in the world. Such health care should produce optimal patient outcomes rivaled by none. With U.S. healthcare expenditures now accounting for 17.2% of the country's GDP, it is clear that sophisticated health care comes at a price. Currently the United States spends $8,915 per capita to provide this care—yet outcomes are not optimal and quality care and access to care lag far behind those found in other industrialized nations. When compared with the OECD countries, the United States ranks below the median on most core measures while having the most expensive health care in the world. Life expectancy for U.S. citizens now ranks in the bottom quartile of the 30 countries in the OECD. How can we explain that? What can be done to improve care?

STUDY QUESTIONS

1. Summarize the epidemiology of chronic disease in the United States and globally today.
2. Which factors and influences have led to the increased incidence of chronic disease in the United States and globally?
3. How can we better educate healthcare professionals to care for those with chronic disease? To care for older adults with chronic disease?
4. Compare and contrast chronic disease and chronic illness.
5. Which actions should the United States take to decrease healthcare disparities?

References

Administration on Aging (AOA). (2012). *A profile of older Americans: 2012*. Washington, DC: U.S. Department of Health and Human Services.

The Affordable Care Act: One year later. (2011). http://www.healthcare.gov/law/introduction/index.html

Albright, H. W., Moreno, M., Feeley, T. W., Walters, R., Samuels, M., Pereira, A., & Burke, T. W. (2010). The implications of the 2010 Patient Protection and Affordable Care Act and the Health Care and Education Reconciliation Act on Cancer Care Delivery. *Cancer, 117*(8), 1564–1174.

American Diabetes Association. (2013). The cost of diabetes. *Diabetes Statistics*. http://www.diabetes.org/advocacy/news-events/cost-of-diabetes.html

American Heart Association (2014). Heart disease and stroke statistics – 2014 update, Executive Summary. http://newsroom.heart.org/news/heart-disease-and-stroke-continue-to-threaten-u-s-health

Bloom, D. E., Cafiero, E., Jane-Llopis, S., Abrahams-Gessel, I., Bloom, L. R., Fathima, S., … Weinstein, C. (2011). *The global economic burden of non-communicable diseases*. Geneva, Switzerland: World Economic Forum.

Centers for Disease Control and Prevention (CDC). (2009). Chronic diseases: The power to prevent, the call to control: At a glance 2009. http://www.cdc.gov/chronicdisease/resources/publications/aag/chronic.htm

Centers for Disease Control and Prevention (CDC). (2013). *The state of aging and health in America 2013*. Atlanta, GA: CDC, U.S. Department of Health and Human Services.

Chan, R. (2013). Evidence-based cancer nursing: Cancer nursing and the Cochrane Collaboration. *Cancer Nursing, 36*(1), 1–2. doi: 10.1097/NCC.0b013e3182578a14

Cochrane, A. L. (1971). *Effectiveness and efficiency: Random reflections on health services*. London, UK: Nuffield Provincial Hospitals Trust.

Cohen, R. A., & Kirzinger, W. K. (2014). *Financial burden of medical care: A family perspective*. NCHS Data Brief, no. 142. Hyattsville, MD: National Center for Health Statistics.

Emanuel, E. (1982). We are all chronic patients. *Journal of Chronic Diseases, 35*, 501–502.

Erdem, E. (2014). Prevalence of chronic conditions among Medicare Part A beneficiaries in 2008 and 2010: Are Medicare beneficiaries getting sicker? *Preventing Chronic Disease, 11*,130118. doi: http://dx.doi.org/10.58888/pcd11.1310118

Frist, W. H. (2014). Connected health and the rise of the patient-consumer. *Health Affairs, 33*(2), 191–193. doi: 10.1377/hlthaff.2013.1464

Harris, R. E. (2013). *Epidemiology of chronic disease: Global perspectives*. Burlington, MA: Jones & Bartlett Learning.

Healthy People 2020. (2013). Topics and objectives. http://healthypeople.gov/2020/topicsobjectives2020/default.aspx

Hsi, S. D. (2004). *Closing the chart: A dying physician examines family, faith and medicine*. Albuquerque, NM: University of New Mexico Press.

Institute of Medicine (IOM). (2012). *Living well with chronic illness: A call for public health action*. Washington, DC: National Academies Press.

Jost, T. S. (2014). Implementing health reform: Four years later. *Health Affairs, 33*(1), 7–10. doi: 10.1377/hlthaff.2013.1355

Lorig, K., Holman, H. R., Sobel, D., Laurent, D., Gonzalez, V., & Minor, M. (2006) *Living a healthy life with chronic conditions* (3rd ed.) Boulder, CO: Bull.

Martin, A., Hartman, M., Whittle, L., Catlin, A., & National Health Expenditure Accounts Team. (2014). National health spending in 2012: Rate of health spending growth remained low for the fourth consecutive year. *Health Affairs, 33*(1), 67–77. doi: 10.1377/hlthaff.2013.1254

Mayo, L. (Ed.). (1956). *Guides to action on chronic illness.* Commission on Chronic Illness. New York, NY: National Health Council.

National Cancer Institute. (2011). The cost of cancer. http://www.cancer.gov/aboutnci/servingpeople/understanding-burden/costofcancer

National Health Council. (2013). About chronic diseases. http://www.who.int/nmh/publications/ncd_report2010/en/

National Partnership for Action to End Health Disparities. (2011). HHS action plan to reduce racial and ethnic health disparities. http://www.minorityhealth.hhs.gov/npa/templates/content.aspx?lvl=1&lvlid=33&ID=285

Organization for Economic Cooperation and Development (OECD). (2013). OECD health data 2013: How does the United State compare? http://www.oecd.org/unitedstates/Briefing-Note-USA-2013.pdf

Schroder, S. A. (2007). We can do better: Improving the health of the American people. *New England Journal of Medicine, 357,* 1221–1228.

Soni, A. (2011). *Top 10 most costly conditions among men and women, 2008: Estimates for the U.S. civilian noninstitutionalized adult population, age 18 and older.* Statistical Brief #331. Rockville, MD: Agency for Healthcare Research and Quality. http://www.meps.ahrq.gov/mepsweb/data_files/publications/st331/stat331.shtml

U.S. Department of Health and Human Services (USDHHS). (2013). *2012 National Healthcare Quality Report.* Rockville, MD: Agency for Healthcare Research and Quality.

World Health Organization (WHO). (2005). *Preparing a health care workforce for the 21st century: The challenge of chronic conditions.* Geneva, Switzerland: Author.

World Health Organization (WHO). (2013a). Chronic diseases and health promotion. http://www.who.int/chp/en/

World Health Organization (WHO). (2013b). *Global action plan for prevention and control of noncommunicable diseases 2013-2020.* Geneva. Switzerland: Author.

Chapter 2

The Illness Experience

Pamala D. Larsen

Introduction

Patients enter a healthcare system with symptoms, which are then diagnosed based on pathological findings, and as such are treated and/or cured with medical treatment. For acute disease, this is the pattern. Any interest in the patient's illness experience with an acute event (e.g., appendicitis, tonsillitis, or a fractured leg) is minimal. An individual may be concerned that the tonsillitis will return, the fractured leg may not heal normally, or an adverse event may be associated with the appendectomy, but typically these concerns pass quickly. The United States' acute care–focused healthcare system responds to the pathology with the goal that the individual will recover fully from the condition and return to prior behaviors and roles.

But what happens when the recovery is incomplete or the illness continues and becomes chronic in nature? The individual and family may need to modify previous behaviors and roles to accommodate the chronic condition. The illness experience—that is, the lived experience of the individual and family with chronic disease—includes their perceptions of and beliefs about the condition; their responses to the illness, physically, psychologically, socially, and emotionally; and health and/or illness behaviors associated with the experience.

Illness perceptions are the foundation of understanding individual and family health and illness behavior. Perceptions are subjective and unique. These perceptions may be as narrow as an individual symptom within a disease or as general as an overall perception of a disease (e.g., cancer). As might be expected, the individual with a chronic disease may have different perceptions of the condition than do family members.

The very act of diagnosing a condition as an illness has consequences far beyond the pathology involved. Freidson's classic work from 1970 discussed the meanings an individual and family ascribe to disease. The individual and family have their own unique meanings and perceptions of the condition, and ultimately their own unique illness behaviors.

This chapter provides an overview of the illness experience, including perceptions and behavior demonstrated by individuals and families with chronic disease. It presents a sociological view of the disease as experienced by the patient and family, rather than a medical view. This chapter is not meant to be a comprehensive review of the entire body of knowledge regarding the illness experience, most of which resides within the discipline of psychology, which is vast.

This chapter also follows the illness experience of Jenny, the wife of a 63-year-old man diagnosed with Stage IIIB esophageal cancer, as she and her husband experience cancer.

Cancer. It's esophageal cancer, Stage IIIB. There's been no mistake. The pathology report has not been confused with someone else's. Randy has cancer. We sit quietly in the oncologist's office, Randy, son Brett, and I. No one says a word. There are no words to speak, no questions that we need answered now. We are stunned. We had a normal life before ... before cancer.

Larsen, 2013, p. xv

Impact of Chronic Illness on the Patient and Family

The Lived Experience

Bury's classic work describes the effect that chronic illness has on a patient and family. He describes chronic illness as a biographical disruption. In his words:

Chronic illness ... is precisely that kind of experience where the structures of everyday life and the forms of knowledge which underpin them are disrupted. Chronic illness involves a recognition of the worlds of pain and suffering, possibly even of death, which are normally only seen as distant possibilities or the plight of others. In addition it brings individuals, their families, and wider social networks face to face with the character of their relationships in stark form disrupting normal rules of reciprocity and mutual support. (Bury, 1982, p. 169)

The lived experience includes the patient's and family's illness perceptions and behaviors, but there is much more to the experience. *It is what the patient and family are experiencing at that point and place in time and their interpretation of the experience.* It could be loneliness, stigma, loss, powerlessness, and a myriad of other feelings and beliefs as well as physical symptoms. The lived experience of the individual with chronic illness cannot be measured by an instrument. The patient and family are living on a roller coaster, never knowing when the "next shoe" will drop. Is this a new symptom or an exacerbation of the illness? Is this a normal event due to the treatment? It is often said that a chronic illness should not become an individual's life, that the

patient is more than his or her illness. On any given day while managing a chronic illness, however, it is the illness that is in charge and not the patient. Day after day, nausea, pain, "feeling bad," or fatigue may become the patient's life. It's always something.

Can something go right just once? Can Randy's potassium level be normal just once? Can he not have five straight days of IV fluids and electrolytes as an outpatient? Today he needs blood as well. Oh yes, and the chemo port has to be removed because that's where the infection is. I'm mad, I'm tired. How do people do this? Every day is different, so you can't plan on anything because it always changes. How do people work? How do they care for their families with cancer always in the forefront?

—Jenny

Most chronic illness research is grounded in empirical, analytical methodology that examines relationships between variables; identifies social determinants of health or illness, and uses instruments that measure self-concept; quality of life, hope, illness perceptions, illness behavior, and so forth. However, if we, as healthcare professionals, reduce patients with chronic illness to a "statistically significant result" or a p value or a Pearson's r, we are doing patients and their families a disservice. Such studies reduce patients to an aggregate so that we can say most patients' and families' illness perceptions or behaviors are normal or adaptive or maladaptive. But consciously or unconsciously, we know, in our relationships with patients and families, that chronic illness is much more than numbers.

Illness Perceptions

Each individual has a different perception of an event, an object, or something that happens to them. It may be minor, such as a football game score, a new neighbor, or the elementary school your child attends. If 10 people were asked their perceptions of those minor events or objects, chances are that each will have a different response or perception. The situation is similar with chronic illness. With illness and the accompanying symptoms and treatment, each individual forms his or her own perception of what is going on.

Patients and their families do not develop their own illness beliefs and perceptions within a vacuum, but rather are molded by everyday social interactions, past experiences, sociodemographic factors, and culture. How one behaves due to an illness, implements coping strategies, and generally responds to the illness is based on one's perceptions. These perceptions may be irrational, they may be invalid, or they may stray far from reality. Right or wrong, these perceptions form the basis of patients' and families' behavior when confronted with a chronic illness.

Illness perception research has been dominated by the use of Levanthal's common sense model of self-regulation (Benyamini, 2011; Leventhal et al., 2012). Leventhal and colleagues base their research on psychological theory. They argue that there is both a cognitive representation and an emotional representation of illness (Rudell, Bhui, & Priebe, 2009).

The literature uses two terms: *illness representations* and *illness perceptions*. Both refer to how the patient (and family) views the illness and the events surrounding it. Illness representations belong to individuals, are interpreted by individuals, and may not conform to scientific beliefs. In a majority of studies, illness representations are measured by the Illness Perception Questionnaire, the Illness Perception Questionnaire—Revised, or the Brief Illness Perception Questionnaire. Each of these questionnaires assesses the cognitive and emotional responses to illness (www.uib.no/ipq/). For purposes of this chapter, the terms "illness representations" and "illness perceptions" are used interchangeably.

Patients and families build mental models to make sense of an event (Petrie & Weinman, 2006). Thus, when an individual and family face a health threat, a model of that event is developed. Patients can then visualize the threat and become active problem solvers. Encompassed within those models are their perceptions of the diagnosis, the illness experience,

the treatment, and the consequences, which in turn forecast how they may behave or respond to the crisis. Often these models may not make sense to outsiders, including healthcare professionals, and sometimes the models may be based on inaccurate information. Each model is dynamic, changing as new data from healthcare professionals, the patient's own experiences, and other sources become known to the patient and family and are incorporated into the model. The individual's common-sense representation or model of a health threat is also updated and enriched by actions that promote health, detect risk, and prevent illness (Leventhal, Leventhal, & Breland, 2011). As might be expected, illness perceptions are related to an improvement or worsening of patients' emotional well-being, usually as a result of a change in health status (Fischer et al., 2013).

Why are illness perceptions of interest to healthcare professionals? The primary reason is that perceptions directly influence the emotional—and often the physical—response that patients and families have to illness. A patient's perception may lead to adherence or nonadherence to treatment or abnormal or normal illness behaviors. Thus, understanding the patient's perception is key in understanding patient and family needs and developing a treatment regimen and/or understanding how a treatment regimen may succeed or fail (Petrie & Weinman, 2006).

Leventhal and colleagues (2012) identify five dimensions that represent a patient's view of their illness:

- Identity of the illness: Connecting the symptoms with the illness and having an understanding of the illness. But what happens if the name or label of the disease is not easily found or the diagnosis does not fit the symptoms?
- Timeline: Duration and progression of the illness. "New" patients might have an acute care framework of the chronic disease while continuing patients would have a chronic view (Benyamini, 2011).

- Causes: Perceived reason for the illness. Most patients form hypotheses about the causes, asking questions such as "Did I not exercise enough?" "Did I smoke too much even though I quit 20 years ago?" "Did the environment contribute to my disease?"
- Consequences: What will be the physical, psychosocial, and economic impact of the illness? This is the patient's overall evaluation of the seriousness of his or her disease?
- Controllability: Can this disease be controlled or cured?

Illness perceptions are part of the self-regulation process that takes place in the face of a health threat. This approach also assumes that people are motivated to avoid and/or treat health threats (Benyamini, 2011).

Leventhal and colleagues' explanation leads one to believe that everything fits neatly into a little box, and there is a linear progression from identity to control or curability. But is it really that simple? Imagine that a chronic disease has affected either you or someone in your family. You may have had some knowledge of the disease prior to diagnosis, but now that the condition is "yours," your perception may change. Plus, you begin to search the Internet, which provides more information than you can possibly absorb. You begin with the idea that this condition is controllable, and perhaps curable, but you find too much online data that tells you otherwise. Thus, your beliefs and perceptions of the situation may change overnight, with your emotional responses and behaviors following suit.

Patients and families with chronic illness need to make sense of their illness. They construct models of the illness to make the illness and life seem logical and rational. Rarely does a diagnosis of a chronic condition make sense to patients, so they create a model, in their minds at least, to try to see some clarity, some rationale, some sense. The model is dynamic throughout the illness, but it is what patients and families with chronic illness "hang their hat on"—it helps them cope.

The journal where I kept track of all of Randy's medical entries, weight, oral intake, tube feedings and medications was quite detailed. I believed if I had all of the details on paper, then perhaps I could make some sense of what was going on. Maybe I could problem solve. Maybe I could figure this out.

—Jenny

The formation of a patient's perception of a chronic illness is a complex, multidimensional process involving much more than the physical symptoms. This complexity makes it difficult for the physician and nurse to treat the patient if their professional perceptions do not match the patient's illness perceptions. A number of studies have documented this lack of congruence; three studies are presented here as examples of current research.

Ninety-nine patients with multiple sclerosis (MS) from six sites in Canada rated their relapse frequency, general health, and quality of life; reviewed descriptions of eight health domains and selected the three most important; and completed a utility assessment. Their neurologists completed the same instruments. Neurologists identified physical function domains as important, while patients placed more emphasis on mental health domains. There was a lack of congruence between neurologist and patient ratings in clinical outcomes (exacerbations or flares), general health, and quality of life. Neurologists significantly *underestimated* the number of flares, as compared with the patients' assessment; considered the patients' health status better than the patients themselves; and rated the patients' quality of life better than the patients did. These results suggest that neurologists have an incomplete understanding of patient perceptions (Kremenchutzky & Walt, 2013).

Perceptions of patients and gastroenterologists were compared in regard to irritable bowel syndrome (IBS) and inflammatory bowel disease (IBD). Physicians and patients had differing views in terms of disease chronicity, personal control, and physical and psychological causes of the illness. The differences in perception may influence the patient–physician relationship and could adversely affect treatment adherence and outcomes (Levy et al., 2014).

A multicenter, observational, cross-sectional, descriptive study of 450 patients with chronic obstructive pulmonary disease (COPD) was conducted to determine the degree of physician–patient concordance in the perception of the severity of symptoms. At an aggregate level, breathlessness/shortness of breath, fatigue/tiredness, and coughing were identified by both physicians and patients as being the most relevant symptoms. However, according to the concordance analysis conducted with each patient and his or her pulmonologist, only 52.8% agreed when identifying the symptom that most affected the life of the patient. Recommendations by the authors suggest that physicians take a closer and more accurate view of the impact of the symptoms of the disease on the patient's life and adapt that perception to the patient's reality as much as possible (Miravitlles, Ferrer, Baro, Lieonart, & Galera, 2013, p. 7).

Illness Behavior

Illness behavior varies greatly according to illness-related, patient-related, and physician-related variables and their complex interactions (Sirri, Fava, & Sonino, 2013). The disease model may be the basis for treatment for patients, but it does not take into account the behavioral responses of the patient and family. The concept of illness behavior provides an explanation for clinical phenomena that do not fit the disease model (Sirri et al., 2013).

The earliest concept of illness behavior was described in a 1929 essay by Henry Sigerist. His essay described the "special position of the sick" (as cited in Young, 2004). Talcott Parsons developed this concept further and described the "sick role" in his 1951 work, *The Social System*. A brief examination of the sick role provides a background to illness behavior.

SICK ROLE

Talcott Parsons viewed health as a functional prerequisite of society. From his point of view, sickness was dysfunctional and was a form of social deviance (Williams, 2005). According to Parsons, sickness was a response that permitted individuals to avoid their social responsibilities. Anyone could take on the role, as the role was achieved through failure to keep well.

According to this definition, the sick role has four major components:

- The person is exempt from normal social roles.
- The person is not responsible for his or her condition.
- The person has the obligation to want to become well.
- The person has the obligation to seek and cooperate with technically competent help (Williams, 2005, p. 124).

DEFINITIONS OF ILLNESS BEHAVIOR

Using Parsons's work as a basis, Mechanic's classic work (1962) proposed the concept of illness behavior as symptoms being perceived, evaluated, and acted (or not acted) upon differently by different persons (p. 189). He believed it was essential to understand the subjective perception of the individual, including that person's norms, values, fears, and expected rewards and punishments, to determine how an individual with illness acts. Mechanic (1995) defined illness behavior as the "varying ways individuals respond to bodily indications, how they monitor internal states, define and interpret symptoms, make attributions, take remedial actions and utilize various sources of formal and informal care" (p. 1208).

A more current definition of illness behavior suggests that illness behavior "includes all of the individual's life which stems from the experience of illness, including changes in functioning and activity, and uptake of health services and other welfare benefits" (Wainwright, 2008, p. 76). Simply put, when an individual defines himself or herself as ill, different behaviors may be displayed. A behavior could be as simple as seeking medical treatment or as complex as the individual's emotional response to the treatment. Some healthcare professionals may view illness behavior as a negative response to the illness. However, the illness behavior might be a health behavior—as, for example, when the individual with lung cancer stops smoking.

Influences on Illness Behavior

Marital status may influence illness behavior. In general, married individuals require fewer services because they are healthier, but utilize other services because they are more attuned to preventive care (Thomas, 2003). Searle, Norman, Thompson, and Vedhara (2007) examined the influence of the illness perceptions of patients' significant others and their impact on patient outcomes and illness perceptions. Differences in illness representations of significant others and patients have been shown to influence psychological adaptation in chronic fatigue syndrome and Addison's disease, for example (cited in Searle et al., 2007).

Gender may influence illness behavior and "help-seeking" behavior in chronic conditions. Sociologic analysis has suggested that women are more likely than men to be sick, and to seek medical help for nonfatal and chronic illness (Bury, 2005, p. 55). Lorber (2000) states that women are not more fragile than men, but are more self-protective of their health status.

Race and ethnicity may play a role in illness perceptions and behaviors. In a study by Hughes, Woodward, and Velez-Ortiz (2013) that included African American, black Caribbean, white, Latino, and Asian older adults, chronic illness, role participation, and socioeconomic factors were related in different ways depending on race or ethnicity. Results indicated that for some racially and ethnically diverse older adults, higher income and education were protective against role disruption.

The authors suggest that interventions should take into account the role of culture (p. 1).

Increasing age often brings chronic conditions and disability. However, older individuals in poor health (as measured by medicine's standard measures) often do not see themselves in this way. What may influence older adults' perceptions of their illness and subsequent behavior may not even be considered by healthcare professionals as relevant. Kelley-Moore, Schumacher, Kahana, and Kahana (2006), for example, identified that cessation of driving and receiving home health care influenced older adults' illness perceptions, causing them to self-identify as disabled.

Using a sample of 300 patients with varying chronic illnesses, one group of researchers (Janowski, Kurpas, Kusz, Mroczek, & Jedynhak, 2013) found differences in the frequency of health behavior that were due to gender, with women demonstrating more healthy habits than men. In addition, older adults performed more health-promoting behaviors than younger adults. Higher education was associated with less frequent health-promoting behaviors, and marital status (e.g., being widowed) was associated with more frequent health-promoting behaviors.

One's education and learning, socialization, and past experience, as defined by one's social and cultural background, mediate illness behavior. Past experiences of observing one's parents being stoic, going to work when they were ill, and avoiding medical help, for example, all influence children's future responses. If children see that "hard work" and not giving in to illness pay off with rewards, they will assimilate those experiences and mirror them in their own lives.

One cannot minimize the impact of past experiences of the individual and family on how they deal with their own chronic illnesses or with chronic illnesses developed by their children, parents, or siblings. Each of those experiences affects how the individual and family perceive their current health challenge.

These experiences could be positive as well as negative. In some cases, a negative healthcare experience with a relatively minor injury/illness could have a stronger influence than a positive experience with serious illness. As healthcare professionals, we should not underestimate the patient's and family's perception of their illness and its effect on physical and psychosocial outcomes.

> *I worry how my adult children will process their 64-year-old father's cancer and now his death. How have they viewed his health experiences? How will they assimilate his death into their lives? This is now one of their "past experiences" with chronic illness. Life expectancy continues to increase, and there are more cancer survivors than ever, but it didn't help their father. Their paternal great-grandfather died of a stroke in his late 80s, their paternal grandfather died of cancer at age 73, and now their father has died of cancer at age 64. These past two deaths do not reflect national statistics. Are they thinking … maybe one of us will die of cancer in our 50s?*

> —Jenny

In a small study examining illness perceptions in patients with critical illness in a medical intensive care unit, as well as their surrogates, it was hypothesized that perceptions would vary by demographic, personal, and clinical measures (Ford, Zapka, Gebregziabher, Yang, & Sterba, 2010). Although patient/surrogate factors, including race, faith, and pre-critical illness quality of life were significant, clinical measures were not. The researchers concluded that clinicians should recognize the variability in illness perceptions and the possible implications for patient/surrogate and healthcare professional communication.

Kaptein, Klok, Moss-Morris, and Brand (2010) reviewed 19 studies that examined how illness perceptions could impact an individual's control of asthma. Using the common sense model of self-regulation as the basis for their analysis, the authors created their own model of how these perceptions affected self-management. The researchers concluded that self-management was determined mainly by behavioral factors and not sociodemographic factors. One of those behavioral factors was illness perceptions. The authors noted that changing a patient's illness perceptions is needed to help the patient and healthcare professional achieve optimal asthma control (Kaptein et al., 2010, p. 199).

ILLNESS PERCEPTIONS/BEHAVIORS AND CHRONIC DISEASE

The literature about the effects of illness perceptions and beliefs on behavior and treatment continues to grow. What follows are some representative studies that demonstrate current and continuing work in this area.

Cardiac Disease Several studies have explored the relationships among quality of life, adherence to and choice of treatment, and illness beliefs/perceptions. Juergens, Seekatz, Moosdorf, Petrie, and Rief (2010) studied 56 patients undergoing coronary artery bypass grafting (CABG). Participants were assessed using the Illness Perception Questionnaire—Revised (IPQ-R) prior to and 3 months postsurgery. The researchers concluded that patients' beliefs before surgery strongly influenced their recovery from surgery. They added that perhaps patients could benefit from some presurgery cognitive interventions to change maladaptive beliefs (p. 553). Similarly, Alsen, Brink, Persson, Brandstrom, and Karlson (2010) found that patients' illness perceptions influenced their health outcomes after myocardial infarction. Broadbent, Ellis, Thomas, Gamble, and Petrie (2009) indicate that a brief in-hospital illness perception intervention changed perceptions and improved rates of return to work in patients with myocardial infarction.

Studies in hypertension have examined the relationships between treatment and illness perceptions. Chen, Tsai, and Chou (2010) tested a hypothetical model of illness perception and adherence to prescribed medications. Using a sample of 355 patients with hypertension, they found that adherence could be enhanced by improving the patient's perception of controllability. Other researchers have argued that illness perceptions/beliefs about hypertension have played a role in the choice of medication for treatment of hypertension (Figueiras et al., 2010).

A study by Pickett, Allen, Franklin, and Peters (2013) examined the relationship between hypertension beliefs and self-care behaviors necessary for blood pressure control. After assessing a sample of 111 community-dwelling African Americans, these researchers reached three conclusions: (1) a number of patients believed that the primary cause of hypertension was stress; (2) patients' attribution of hypertension to stress was negatively associated with keeping doctor appointments; and (3) patients' belief that hypertension is a chronic condition was positively associated with keeping doctor appointments and medication adherence. There was no significant relationship with illness representations and eating a healthy diet, engaging in physical activity, or maintaining a healthy weight. Researchers suggest that healthcare professionals carefully assess patients' beliefs about hypertension as part of an effort to more effectively treat and control blood pressure.

Illness perceptions are important in understanding and predicting outcomes in patients with negative cardiac evaluation. In one study, researchers used the Brief Illness Perception Questionnaire to assess 138 patients before and after a negative cardiac evaluation. Participants in the study included patients with chest pain or palpitations. A stronger correlation between illness perceptions and health at follow-up, compared to before the cardiac evaluation, might explain the tendency for poor outcomes among these patients (Jonsbu, Martinsen, Morken, Moum, & Dammen, 2012).

Breast Cancer   A longitudinal study of women with breast cancer assessed illness perceptions prior to a psychosocial intervention. Study variables were assessed using the Illness Perception Questionnaire, among other instruments. Of the 57 women included in the study, 43% of the variance in distress, at baseline, was explained by the patients' illness perceptions. Illness perceptions were related to an improvement or worsening of a patient's emotional well-being (Fischer et al., 2013).

An international study of breast cancer patients in Japan and the Netherlands demonstrated similarities regarding the effect of illness perceptions and quality of life. Positive illness perceptions were associated with higher quality of life (Kaptein et al., 2013).

Bowel Disease   Three studies typify what is known about illness perceptions and their relationship with psychosocial health in individuals with bowel disease. Eighty-three patients with stomas completed the Brief Illness Perception Questionnaire, the Health Orientation Scale, the Hospital Anxiety and Depression Scale, and the Carver Brief HOPE scale. Health status directly influenced their illness perceptions, which in turn influenced their coping. While depression was influenced by illness perceptions, emotion-focused coping, and maladaptive coping, anxiety was influenced by only illness perceptions and maladaptive coping; this result led the researchers to encourage healthcare practitioners to identify and understand the importance of each patient's illness perceptions (Knowles, Cook, & Tribbick, 2013).

In another study examining illness perceptions, sexual health and satisfaction, and body image in patients with IBD, there was support for the adverse impact of IBD-related illness perceptions on anxiety and depression. Other findings included evidence that illness perceptions affected sexual health and relationships (Knowles, Gass, & Macrae, 2013).

Rochelle and Fidler (2012) investigated illness perceptions in patients with IBD.

Their study demonstrated that patients' psychological status and disease-related variables are important predictors of outcome. The study identified specific illness perceptions of patients with IBD that are strongly associated with quality of life.

Chronic Somatic Disease   Researchers examined the illness perceptions of patients with clinically diagnosed and screen-detected type 2 diabetes and compared those results with their partners. Patients (aged 40–75) and their partners completed the Brief Illness Perception Questionnaire. The route to diagnosis had minimal influence on the patients' illness perceptions; however, partners of patients diagnosed through screening, versus clinical symptomology, had very different illness perceptions as compared with the patient. At three years postdiagnosis, the partners remained overwhelmed with the diagnosis (Woolthuis, deGrauw, Cardol, van Weel, Metsemakers, & Biermans, 2013).

Other researchers believe that beliefs about behavior may be as important as illness perceptions about a disease. In one study, 453 patients with type 2 diabetes were recruited to participate in a randomized trial of blood glucose self-monitoring. The study compared the extent to which self-care behaviors of patients with type 2 diabetes are predicted by patients' beliefs about those behaviors as compared with their illness perceptions. The researchers concluded that beliefs about behaviors are at least as important in predicting health-related behaviors, suggesting that behavior change interventions with patient groups might be more effective if they target beliefs about behavior, rather than beliefs about illness (French, Wade, & Farmer, 2013).

The Legitimization of Chronic Illness

Most chronic diseases, such as cancer, diabetes mellitus types 1 and 2, and chronic obstructive pulmonary disease, have specific diagnostic criteria that verify the disease's presence and, therefore, indicate the appropriate treatment. With some illnesses, when symptoms are not well defined and diagnostic tests may be ambiguous, receiving legitimization from a physician or other healthcare professional may be difficult and frustrating. Patients may begin to "doctor hop," hoping to find someone who can identify their condition. As a result, symptomatic persons may be left to question the truth of their own illness perceptions. How do you build a mental model of your illness (as a basis for problem solving) if healthcare professionals and society in general are skeptical of your symptoms? And if your illness perceptions are askew, what will your behavior be?

When a diagnosis is finally made, the patient frequently shows a somewhat joyous initial response to having a name for the recurrent and troublesome symptoms. This reaction results from the decrease in stress over the unknown. These patients have an enormous stake in how their illnesses are understood by healthcare professionals. Patients seek to achieve the legitimacy necessary to elicit sympathy and avoid stigma, and to protect their own self-concept (Mechanic, 1995).

Fibromyalgia (FM) is a chronic syndrome generally characterized by pain and fatigue, but often includes other less obscure symptoms, making the disease difficult to diagnose. A growing body of evidence now points toward a neurobiological basis for the disease (McLean & Clauw, 2005). However, this knowledge has been poorly communicated to healthcare professionals. Often patients are not diagnosed accurately, if at all, leading patients to have no legitimatization of their condition. A qualitative study by McMahon, Murray, Sanderson, and Daiches (2012) reveals the illness experience of such individuals. This experience is divided into five phases: (1) making sense of FM (when I was younger, I didn't have any problems at all); (2) onset and diagnosis (you just feel like you're constantly complaining); (3) invasion of FM (you're just trapped, trapped in this body);

(4) coping with FM (you try to do things in a pattern it will obey); and (5) ongoing struggle (I refuse to give in to it) (pp. 1361–1363). The women in this study had established identities prior to becoming ill, but now they had to "rewrite" their stories and accept a new identity.

Larun and Malterud (2007) examined 20 qualitative studies in a meta-ethnography about the illness experiences of individuals with chronic fatigue syndrome (CFS) to summarize their illness experiences as well as their physicians' perspectives. Across studies, patients spoke of being "controlled and betrayed by their bodies" (pp. 22–23). Although physical activities were mostly curtailed, individuals spoke of mental fatigue that affected memory and concentration, they described difficulty with following conversations, and several patients felt that their learning abilities had decreased (p. 24). One of the themes that emerged was telling stories about *bodies that no longer held the capacity for social involvement.* For some individuals, the most distressing part of the illness was the negative responses from their family members, their colleagues in the workplace, and their physicians, who *questioned the legitimacy of their illness behavior* because of their dynamic symptoms of CFS (p. 25). Thus, their physicians' beliefs about CFS influenced the patients' perceptions of the disease and, therefore, their illness experience. To summarize, the researchers' analysis determined that patients' sense of identity becomes more or less invalid and that a change in identity of the individuals was experienced.

Professional Responses to Illness Behavior and Roles

Healthcare professionals expect patients entering the acute care setting to conform to sick role behaviors at least initially. Most people entering the hospital for the first time are quickly socialized into the healthcare system and are expected to cooperate with treatment, recover, and return home to their normal roles.

Professional expectations and patient responses are in line with social expectations and fit with the traditional medical model of illness as acute and curable. Healthcare professionals "like" patients who are compliant and cooperative and do not question their care. When patients are less cooperative, staff may consider them problematic or nonadherent.

When individuals with chronic illness are hospitalized, they view the situation quite differently than do the healthcare professionals with whom they interact. Patients with multiple chronic conditions may focus on maintaining stability of their chronic conditions so as to prevent unnecessary symptoms, whereas their healthcare professionals are more likely to focus on managing the current acute disorder. In addition, patients who have had multiple prior admissions are more likely to use their hospital savvy to gain what they want or need from the system. They have learned the formal and informal hospital "rules." They have also learned which nurses and nursing assistants provide the best care and which do not. For instance, if the patient is assigned a certain nurse who has not met the needs of the patient in the past, the family may become more vigilant and more visible during the hospital stay, or refuse to have that nurse care for the patient.

When Randy was in ICU during the summer of 2011 when everything fell apart, I became acquainted with several family members of other patients in ICU. We were often in the family lounges together, in the cafeteria, or just talking in the hall. ICU is a lonely place for family members. I hope that nurses who work there realize that. One person I remember distinctly was a mother of a 20-year-old college student who had a traumatic brain injury. The prognosis was vague. The mother had flown in from Florida, had no social support, and was unfamiliar with Colorado, our town, and the hospital. She had asked me a previous time if this was a "good" hospital. I overheard a conversation between one of the nurses and this mother, and the nurse being abrupt with her, telling the mother to be patient, that the doctor had other patients to see, and he would contact her when he could ... all spoken in a stern and lecturing voice. I was shocked at this nurse's behavior. Did she not realize what this mother was going through? Was she not aware of the illness experience of this mother? I went directly to the patient care coordinator of the ICU and asked that Randy never be assigned this nurse. The nurse's behavior was unacceptable, and I did not want her to care for my husband.

—Jenny

In the setting of chronic illness, multiple contacts with the healthcare system may have caused a loss of the "blind faith" that the individual once had in the system. Patients with chronic illness seek a different kind of relationship with healthcare professionals, one where there is "give and take" and one that empowers the patient. The extent to which a patient with chronic illness is included in the formulation of his or her treatment plan likely influences the success of the plan. Although assuming sick role dependency may be adaptive behavior in acute illness, where medical expertise offers hope of a cure, the same is not true in chronic illness. Individuals with chronic illness are the "experts" in their illnesses and should have the ultimate authority in managing those illnesses over time.

Post esophagectomy, Randy had a swallowing evaluation that showed that he was aspirating slightly. So his diet was changed from a clear liquid to a full liquid/thickened liquid diet. Then a cardiovascular surgeon taking call for his doctor ordered a soft diet. I told the nurses that his diet wasn't right, that his surgeon had said he would be on liquids for close to a month. The dietitian came up as well, and I explained it again. But no one listened to either Randy or me. So much for what the patient thinks. So he had roast beef. Randy's surgeon made rounds

late in the evening and asked Randy what he had had for dinner. He told him roast beef, which obviously wasn't the right answer. So it's back to liquids again.

—Jenny

Lack of Role Norms for Individuals with Chronic Illness

Chronic illnesses require that a variety of tasks be completed to meet the requirements of the medical regimen. However, there is a lack of norms for those with chronic illness. What is expected of a patient recovering from cancer surgery? An exacerbation of rheumatoid arthritis? A flare-up of inflammatory bowel disease? Are sick-role behaviors discouraged or not? These individuals enter into and remain in a type of impaired, "at-risk" role. Implicit behaviors for this role are not well defined, leading to role ambiguity. Given this lack of norms, influences on the patient include the degree of disability (with different attributes of disability producing different consequences), visibility of the disability (the less visible the disability, the more normal the response), self-acceptance of the disability (resulting in others reciprocating with acceptance), and societal views of the disabled as either economically dependent or productive. Without role definition, whether disability is present or not, individuals are unable to achieve maximum levels of functioning. They may alter their previous definitions of self to one with limitations, and look to what the future may impose on them.

It is Sunday morning and I am waiting in the OR waiting room. Randy was taken to the OR at 9 a.m. His chemo port will go into his left chest area. There is some question about what kind of tube will be used for the jejunostomy insertion due to his contact allergy to rubber. Although this cancer journey began a month ago, this is the first outward evidence that anything is wrong.

—Jenny

The illness experience of the patient and family continues to mystify healthcare professionals. The literature about the relationship(s) is vast and continues to grow, indicating the importance of these concepts in developing a treatment plan and patient adherence to the plan. What is clear in these studies is that seeing the illness through the lenses of the patient and family is critical in supporting them throughout the experience and improving patient outcomes, both physically and psychosocially.

The current research is almost entirely from the discipline of psychology, and the majority of this research comes from Europe, Canada, and Australia, rather than the United States. Few studies have been nurse-led. Nevertheless, the healthcare professional who has the best opportunity to support the patient and family during the illness experience is the professional nurse. It is the nurse who has the opportunity to "know" the family and understand their beliefs, perceptions, and behaviors. As a discipline, nursing needs to recognize the importance of its role and appreciate how a nurse's insight into the patient and family can support both the physical plan of care and the psychosocial plan of care. It is time for nursing to be a player in this care.

Interventions

There is no "magic" list of interventions to assist and support patients and their families during the illness experience. The current healthcare system—with its acute care focus, fix-and-cure model, and medication for each symptom—does not fit with caring for individuals on a long-term basis. These patients do not need their illness behavior "fixed" or "cured," but instead need a healthcare professional who listens and understands the illness experience.

Understanding illness roles and behaviors in planning interventions allows the healthcare professional to maximize the value of the time spent with the patient. One such intervention, patient and family education, could be improved by integrating knowledge of the

patient's perceptions and roles. The patient who is still in a highly dependent phase cannot benefit from education. As nurses, we often think patient education is the key to everything, but the timing of that education is critical. As improvement in physical status occurs, emphasis on the desire to return to normal roles creates motivation to learn about the condition and appropriate care to maximize health. As the patient moves into the "at-risk" role and becomes aware of the necessity to maximize his or her remaining potential, education provides a highly successful tool both in the hospital and at home. What follows are interventions that *assist and support* patients and families.

Frameworks and Models for Practice

A review of the literature does not reveal any new frameworks for caring for those with chronic illness. However, numerous frameworks exist on self-care and self-management, transitions of care for older adults, and successful aging, along with a smaller number of frameworks that are specific to one chronic disease (e.g., heart failure, type 2 diabetes, and chronic kidney disease). Some of these frameworks are evidence-based, while others are based on anecdotal experiences.

Evidence-based frameworks are critical given the increasing effects that chronic illnesses are having in the healthcare system. Additionally, not all healthcare professionals have the skills to care for individuals with chronic illness. Meeting the psychosocial needs of patients with chronic illness, by itself, is an enormous task. Caring for a patient with chronic illness requires a framework or model for practice that differs from that for caring for a patient with an acute, episodic disease. The frameworks that follow are examples and are not intended to be all-inclusive.

These frameworks and models should not be confused with the disease management models or self-management models discussed elsewhere in this text. Disease management models address the physical symptoms of a condition. Some of those models assign an algorithm to the condition where patients receive certain "care" when their blood work is at an inappropriate level or their symptoms "measure" a certain degree of seriousness. These models manage the disease, but not the illness. Illness frameworks and models address the illness experience of the individual and family that occurs as a result of changing health status.

CHRONIC ILLNESS AND QUALITY OF LIFE

Strauss and colleagues (Strauss & Glaser, 1975; Strauss et al., 1984) published a rudimentary framework that addressed the issues and concerns of individuals with chronic illness. Although simple, this framework was an early attempt to examine the illness experience of the individual and family as opposed to the disease. If healthcare professionals could better understand the illness experience of patients and families, perhaps more appropriate care could be provided. Basic to this care was understanding some of the key problems of chronic illness:

- Prevention of medical crises and their management if they occur
- Controlling symptoms
- Carrying out of prescribed medical regimens
- Prevention of, or living with, social isolation
- Adjustment to changes in the disease
- Attempts to normalize interactions and lifestyle
- Funding—finding the necessary money
- Confronting attendant psychological, marital, and familial problems (Strauss et al., 1984, p. 16)

After identifying the key problems of the individual and family with chronic illness, Strauss and colleagues (1984) suggested basic problem-solving strategies, family and organizational arrangements, and then reevaluation of the consequences of those arrangements. Although this framework is not new, the basic tasks of living with a chronic illness, as presented by Strauss et al., remain salient today.

THE TRAJECTORY FRAMEWORK

From the early work of Strauss and colleagues, the trajectory framework was further refined in the 1980s. Corbin and Strauss (1992) developed this framework so that nurses could (1) gain insight into the chronic illness experience of the patient; (2) integrate existing literature about chronicity into their practice; and (3) provide direction for building nursing models that guide practice, teaching, research, and policy making (p. 10).

A trajectory is defined as the course of an illness over time, plus the actions of clients, families, and healthcare professionals to manage that course (Corbin, 1998, p. 3). The illness trajectory is set in motion by pathophysiology and changes in health status, but patients, families, and healthcare professionals can use strategies to shape the course of dying and, therefore, the illness trajectory (Corbin & Strauss, 1992). Even if the disease is the same, each individual's illness trajectory is different and takes into account the uniqueness of that person (Jablonski, 2004).

Within the model, the term *phase* indicates one of the different stages of the chronic illness experience for the client. There are nine phases in the trajectory model, and although it could be conceived as a continuum, it is not linear. Clients may move through these phases in a linear fashion, regress to a former phase, or plateau for an extended period. In addition, having more than one chronic disease influences movement along the trajectory. The nine phases are as follows: (1) pretrajectory phase or the so-called prevention phase; (2) trajectory phase, where diagnosis may occur; (3) stable phase, where symptoms are controlled and managed; (4) unstable phase, which may bring the inability to control symptoms; (5) acute phase, having unrelieved symptoms or complications; (6) crisis phase requiring emergency treatment; (7) comeback phase, indicating a gradual return to an acceptable way of life; (8) downward phase, characterized by progressive deterioration; and (9) dying phase (Corbin, 2001, pp. 4–5).

Shifting Perspectives Model of Chronic Illness

The shifting perspectives model of chronic illness resulted from the work of Thorne and Paterson (1998), who analyzed 292 qualitative studies of chronic physical illness that were published from 1980 to 1996. Of these, 158 studies became a part of a meta-analysis in which patient roles in chronic illness were described. The work of Thorne and Paterson reflects the "insider" perspective of chronic illness as opposed to the "outsider" view, the more traditional view. This change in perspective represents a shift from the traditional approach of patient-as-client to one of client-as-partner in care (p. 173). Results from the meta-analysis also demonstrated a shift away from focusing on loss and burden, and an attempt to view health within illness.

Analysis of these studies led to the development of the shifting perspectives model of chronic illness (Paterson, 2001). The model depicts chronic illness as an ongoing, continually shifting process where people experience a complex dialectic between the world and themselves (p. 23). Paterson's model considers both the "illness" and the "wellness" of the individual (Paterson, 2003). The illness-in-the-foreground perspective focuses on the sickness, loss, and burden of the chronic illness. This is a common reaction experienced by persons recently diagnosed with a chronic disease. The overwhelming consequences of the condition, learning about their illness, considerations of treatment, and long-term effects contribute to putting the illness in the foreground. As such, the disease becomes the individual's identity.

With the wellness-in-the-foreground perspective, the "self" is the source of identity rather than the disease (Paterson, 2001, p. 23). The individual is in control and not the disease. It does not mean, though, that the individual is physically well, cured, or even in remission of the disease symptoms. Instead, the shift occurs in the individual's thinking, allowing that

person to turn his or her focus away from the disease. However, any threat that cannot be controlled will transition the individual back to the illness-in-the-foreground perspective. Threats include disease progression and lack of ability to self-manage the disease, stigma, and interactions with others (Paterson, 2001).

Lastly, neither the illness perspective nor the wellness perspective is right or wrong. Instead, each merely reflects the individual's unique needs, health status, and focus at the time (Paterson, 2001).

In a similar vein, Whittemore and Dixon (2008) describe the process of integration in chronic illness. Integration is a process undertaken by an individual to achieve a sense of balance in self-managing a chronic illness and living a personally meaningful life (p. 177). In some ways, these authors' work builds on that of Paterson and further refines individual components of integration. Whittemore and Dixon's work refers to "living an illness and living a life."

Motivational Interviewing

Part of supporting and assisting patients and their families through chronic illness is accurately assessing the needs of the patient and family. Typically, motivational interviewing is intended to help a patient become unstuck and to begin the process of changing a behavior (Arechiga, 2010, p. 147). Motivational interviewing is not a set of techniques, but rather a way of being with people. It relies on four main principles: (1) roll with resistance while resisting the "righting reflex"; (2) understand the patient's own motivations to develop discrepancy; (3) express empathy; and (4) enhance self-efficacy to empower the patient (p. 147).

Motivational interviewing is a strategy to better understand a patient's illness perceptions and, in turn, his or her behavior. Additionally, anytime that a healthcare professional can enhance a patient's self-efficacy, that encourages

Evidence-Based Practice Box

Heart failure is a common cause of hospitalizations and readmissions in older adults. This condition affects quality of life by reducing the patient's independence and ability to perform activities of daily living. Jeon and colleagues reviewed qualitative studies that described the illness experience. Thirty studies met the authors' criteria for review. The articles were summarized and entered into QSR NVivo7 for data analysis.

Three overall concepts were identified from the data: (1) impact of congestive heart failure (CHF) on everyday life; (2) common patterns of coping strategies; and (3) factors influencing self-care. Impact of CHF on everyday life included social isolation (identified in 20 of the studies), living in fear, and loss of control. Subcategories of coping strategies included sharing experiences and being flexible to changing circumstances. Lastly, factors influencing self-care included knowledge, availability of and access to health services, continuity and quality of care of health services, comorbidity, and personal relationships. Review of the literature validated the common elements of individuals' experience with CHF as well as providing data for potential interventions.

Source: Jeon, Y, Kraus, S. G., Jowsey, T., and Glasgow, N. J. (2010). The experience of living with chronic heart failure: A narrative review of qualitative studies. *BMC Health Services Research,* 10–77. doi:10.1186/1472-6963-10–77.

the patient's full participation in developing and adhering to a treatment plan.

Other Interventions

A meta-analysis of 25 qualitative studies examining couple-oriented interventions evaluated the impact of the marital relationship on health as well as the negative impact of illness on the partner (Martire, Schulz, Helgeson, Small, & Saghafi, 2010). Couple-oriented interventions involving education, social support, and counseling demonstrated minimal effects. One finding in the study suggested that these interventions could be strengthened by better targeting of partners' influence on patient health behaviors (p. 325).

A psycho-educational group intervention was used with 57 women with breast cancer. Study variables included illness perceptions, coping, and distress. At baseline, 43% of the variance in distress at baseline was explained by the patients' illness perceptions. At the end of the 1-year intervention, the intensity of general distress and breast cancer–related emotions had decreased significantly. The intervention consisted of nine 2- to 2½-hour meetings with a social worker and a nurse practitioner (Fischer et al., 2013).

Hope can be seen as a psychosocial resource to deal with chronic illness. One group of researchers examined studies of hope published between 1980 and 2010 (Duggleby et al., 2012). Criteria for inclusion in the study were qualitative studies of the hope experience of persons 60 years and older with a chronic illness. Twenty studies were included in the meta-synthesis. The researchers concluded that the concept of hope may differ for older adults versus younger adults in its interaction with suffering. Resources for hope are both internal and external, and finding meaning and positive reappraisal are important strategies to help older adults with chronic illness maintain hope.

Researchers sought to evaluate the changes and impact of illness perceptions during a three-session cognitive-behavioral therapy (CBT) intervention with patients with noncardiac chest pain or benign palpitations. If perceptions affect behavior and, in turn, influence patient outcomes, an intervention that changes perceptions would be promising for those with chronic disease. The results from this randomized clinical trial indicated that illness perceptions, as measured with the Brief Illness Perceptions Questionnaire, may mediate the short- and long-term treatment effects of a three-session CBT program (Jonsbu, Martinsen, Morken, Moum, & Dammen, 2013).

The Women to Women project has been instrumental in helping women with chronic illness in rural states manage their illnesses. Through a computer intervention model that provides education, facilitates support groups, and fosters self-care, women have successfully managed their illness responses (Weinert, Cudney, Comstock, & Bansal, 2011).

Embuldeniya and colleagues (2013) analyzed 25 articles to identify the perceived impact and experience of participating in peer support interventions for individuals with chronic disease. Most studies were unrelated to specific diseases. A key motivation for participants' interest in peer support was social isolation. Once the peer support groups ended, perceived outcomes across the studies included finding meaning; empowerment; and changed outlook, knowledge, and behavior.

INTERNET-BASED INTERVENTIONS

The Pew Foundation conducted a telephone survey in both English and Spanish of 2,253 respondents to determine how the Internet was used by persons with chronic disease (Fox & Purcell, 2010). From the data, the authors concluded:

- Adults living with chronic disease are disproportionately offline in an online world. Individuals with chronic disease generally stay in the shallow end of the online activities pool. They are less likely than Internet users who report no chronic conditions to bank online, look for information, use a social network site, or get financial information online (p. 13).
- The Internet access gap creates an online health information gap.
- Health professionals dominate the information mix.
- The social life of chronic disease information is robust (blogging and online health

discussions). Holding all other variables constant, living with chronic disease increases the probability that individuals will blog or participate in online health discussions.
- The impact of online health information may be muted among people living with chronic disease.
- The Internet is like a secret weapon—if someone has access to it (Fox & Purcell, 2010, pp. 2–4).

While social media hold great promise for the future in chronic disease management, little evidence supports the contention that participation in such forums improves patient outcomes. Merolli, Gray, and Martin-Sanchez (2013) conducted a comprehensive review of the literature to determine which resources exist on the Internet for those persons with chronic illness. Nineteen studies met the criteria for the review, with 12 studies being designated predecessors and 7 studies satisfying the criteria of social media/Web 2.0 platforms. Predecessors included discussion forums, bulletin boards, and chat tools. Social media included Facebook, blogging, custom systems (e.g., the Chronic Pain Management System), and virtual worlds (e.g., Second Life).

Although the review produced a limited amount of scientific data, it did identify significant gaps. Generally, studies looked at psychosocial outcomes versus physical health outcomes. The data suggested that social media increased support, information gathering, and empowerment, and improved disease-specific knowledge. At present, the literature primarily focuses on the predecessor group, online support groups, and discussion forums, as opposed to social media, such as blogs, wikis, virtual worlds, and social network sites (p. 10).

Patient-initiated blogging has become a popular means to describe one's illness experience and communicate with others facing similar experiences. Although blogging is a communication tool, perhaps there is more significance to it than merely its communication role. Perhaps it may be psychosocially beneficial to share personal experiences with others, or to become aware that your experiences as a patient with chronic illness are similar to others' experiences. The mere act of writing down experiences may also be a type of "therapy," or emotional catharsis, for the individual. If individuals can write down what is happening to them, perhaps they can more easily "see' their experience and be able to problem-solve issues.

In a nurse-led study, 16 Internet illness blogs were analyzed. Participants were women, ages 20 to 39, who had been diagnosed with cancer. Four dimensions of problems were identified across the blogs: (1) pain and fatigue; (2) insurance and financial barriers; (3) concerns related to fertility; and (4) symptoms of post-traumatic stress and anxiety (Keim-Malpass et al., 2013). The authors concluded that such narratives might provide a foundation for nursing-based interventions versus medicine-based interventions.

> *This is our story, Randy's and mine. Even though he has been gone for many months now, it is still our story, not mine. And this journal encourages me to tell it. I have found much comfort in expressing my thoughts, ugly as they might be. I can't explain why it helps, and I don't even try anymore. People ask me why I would want to publish this journal containing my personal thoughts. I hope, by doing so, that someone else may be helped by reading them. Perhaps others have similar thoughts and are afraid to express them.*
>
> —Jenny

RESEARCH

Do we understand and can we place in an appropriate context the meaning of illness for patients? Why do some individuals ignore symptoms and refuse to seek medical advice, while others with the same condition seek immediate care and relief from their "social roles" at the slightest symptom? A relatively minor symptom in one individual causes great distress, whereas more serious health conditions in others cause little concern.

Mechanic (1986, 1995) asks a question that remains pertinent today: What are the processes or factors that cause individuals exposed to similar stressors to respond differently and present unique illness behaviors? There is much variation in how individuals perceive their health status, seek or do not seek medical care, and function in their social and work roles. What influences these differences?

Mechanic also poses another question: What can healthcare professionals do to modify inaccurate illness perceptions of patients and thus influence behavior and health outcomes? In nursing, much time is spent on patient education, but apparently that is not the answer— perhaps because of a timing issue. A growing body of evidence demonstrates that patients who hold more negative views of illness (e.g., poor illness perceptions) have poorer outcomes. Chronic illness is the condition as the patient and family experience it. What can we do to make a difference in the lives of our patients and their families?

Outcomes

The illness experience is unique for every patient and family. Many variables influence it, as described in this chapter, but there may be other influences that psychosocial scientists have not yet identified. The illness behavior that exists during a chronic illness is not deviant, nor does it need to be "fixed." Rather, it is a response to an illness perception. Healthcare professionals need to support patients and families and more fully understand the lived experience of their illness. As healthcare professionals, we are efficient and effective in working within the disease model. However, the patient and family are in the illness mode as well as the disease mode. Caring for a patient and family with chronic illness requires the art of nursing to be placed front and center, versus the science of nursing. Using the art of nursing is critical in establishing relationships with patients and understanding the illness experience.

CASE STUDY 2-1

John is a 30-year-old man with inflammatory bowel disease (IBD). He has had IBD since he was 15 years old. Recently, his physical health problems became severe enough that he had an ileostomy 2 months ago. He is an "expert" patient, having been in and out of your hospital for years. Apparently his perception of his condition was that the ileostomy would "fix" his problems and he could have a normal life. Although his health should improve, right now he is back on your unit "running" his care. He is extremely angry that he is not well. Additionally, he has little social support.

Discussion Questions

1. Discussing his illness perceptions with John is a delicate subject, but one that needs to be tackled. How would you approach the subject with him? What common ground can you find to begin the conversation?
2. Relationships may or may not be hard to form with patients with chronic illness. It appears that John's relationship with the staff members on your unit is tenuous at best. How do you use the "art" of nursing to work more collaboratively with John?
3. What framework or model might be used as a basis for this patient's psychosocial care?

CASE STUDY 2-2

Kathryn is a 75-year-old woman who was in apparent good health until a routine colonoscopy revealed a Stage III carcinoma in her colon. She and her husband of 50 years are very close, and since the diagnosis, they are refusing to see most visitors, including their children and grandchildren. They both seem depressed and cry a lot.

Discussion Questions

1. Should you intervene? Why or why not?
2. If you intervene, how do you sort out this couple's perceptions and beliefs about Kathryn's condition? As a nurse, you assume that this is the couple's reaction/behavior to the diagnosis, but is it?
3. Describe how you might use motivational interviewing with this couple.

STUDY QUESTIONS

1. Dealing with "expert" patients can be difficult, and many patients with chronic illness are "expert" patients. Often your own "power" as a healthcare professional is threatened. How do you deal with "expert" patients and make it a collaborative relationship?
2. There are no norms for individuals with chronic illness. What does this mean and how does it apply to the patients you care for?
3. Differentiate between health and illness behavior, and give examples of each for someone with end-stage heart failure, Parkinson's disease, or breast cancer.
4. How do healthcare professionals influence the illness perceptions and behavior of patients and families in both positive ways and negative ways?
5. Reflect on your own health and illness experiences. What influences your own perceptions and behaviors?

References

Alsen, P., Brink, E., Persson, L, Brandstrom, Y., & Karlson, B. W. (2010). Illness perceptions after myocardial infarction: Relations to fatigue, emotional distress, and health-related quality of life. *Journal of Cardiovascular Nursing, 25*(2), E1–E10.

Arechiga, A. (2010) Facilitating health behavior change. In D. Wedding & M. L. Stuber (Eds.), *Behavior and medicine* (pp. 145–152). Cambridge, MA: Hogrefe.

Benyamini, Y. (2011). Health and illness perceptions. In H. S. Friedman (Ed.), *The Oxford handbook of health psychology* (pp. 280–293). Oxford, UK: Oxford University Press.

Broadbent, E., Ellis, C. J., Thomas, J., Gamble, G., & Petrie, K. J. (2009). Further development of an illness perception intervention for myocardial infarction patients: A randomized controlled trial. *Journal of Psychosomatic Research, 67,* 17–23.

Bury, M. (1982). Chronic illness as biographical disruption. *Sociology of Health and Illness, 4,* 167–182.

Bury, M. (2005). *Health and illness.* Cambridge, UK: Polity Press.

Chen, S. L., Tsai, J. C., & Chou, K. R. (2010). Illness perceptions and adherence to therapeutic regimens among patients with hypertension: A structural modeling approach. *International Journal of Nursing Studies, 8*(2), 235–245.

Corbin, J. (1998). The Corbin & Strauss chronic illness trajectory model: An update. *Scholarly Inquiry for Nursing Practice, 12*(1), 33–41.

Corbin, J. (2001). Introduction and overview: Chronic illness and nursing. In R. Hyman & J. Corbin (Eds.), *Chronic illness: Research and theory for nursing practice* (pp. 1–15). New York, NY: Springer.

Corbin, J., & Strauss, A. (1992). A nursing model for chronic illness management based upon the trajectory framework. In P. Woog (Ed.), *The chronic illness trajectory framework: The Corbin and Strauss nursing model* (pp. 9–28). New York, NY: Springer.

Duggleby, W., Hicks, D., Nekolaichuk, C., Holstslander, L., Williams, A., Chambers, T., & Eby, J. (2012). Hope, older adults, and chronic illness: A metasynthesis of qualitative research. *Journal of Advanced Nursing, 68*(6), 1211–1223. doi: 10.1111/j.1365-2648.2011.05919.x

Embuldeniya, G., Beinot, P., Bell, E., Bell, M., Nyhof-Young, J., Sale, J. E. M., & Britten, N. (2013). The experience and impact of chronic disease peer support interventions: A qualitative synthesis. *Patient Education and Counseling, 92,* 3–12.

Figueiras, M., Marcelino, D., Claudino, A., Cortes, M., Maroco, J., & Weinman, J. (2010). Patients' illness schemata of hypertension: The role of beliefs for the choice of treatment. *Psychology and Health, 25*(4), 507–517.

Fischer, M. J., Wiesenhaan, M. E., Does-den Heijer A., Kleijn, W. C., Nortier, J. W. R., & Kapstein, A. A. (2013). From despair to hope: A longitudinal study of illness perceptions and coping in a psycho-educational group intervention for women with breast cancer. *British Journal of Health Psychology, 18*, 526–545.

Ford, D., Zapka, J., Gebregziabher, M., Yang, C., & Sterba, K. (2010). Factors associated with illness perception among critically ill patients and surrogates. *Chest, 138*, 59–67.

Fox, S., & Purcell, K. (2010) Chronic disease and the Internet. http://pewinternet.org/Reports/2010/Chronic-Disease.aspx

Freidson, E. (1970). *Profession of medicine*. New York, NY: Dodd, Mead.

French, D. P., Wade, A. N., & Farmer, A. J. (2013). Predicting self-care behaviours of patients with type 2 diabetes: The importance of beliefs about behavior, not just beliefs about illness. *Journal of Psychosomatic Research, 74*, 327–333.

Hughes, A. K., Woodward, A., & Velez-Ortiz, D. (2013). Chronic illness intrusion: Role impairment and time out of role in racially and ethnically diverse older adults. *The Gerontologist*. Epub ahead of print. doi: 10.1093/geront/gnt041

The Illness Perception Questionnaire. http://www.uib.no/ipq/

Jablonski, A. (2004). The illness trajectory of end-stage renal disease dialysis patients. *Research and Theory for Nursing Practice: An International Journal, 18*(1), 51–72.

Janowski, K., Kurpas, D., Kusz, J., Mroczek, B., & Jedynak, T. (2013). Health-related behavior, profile of health locus of control and acceptance of illness in patients suffering from chronic somatic diseases. *PLoS One, 8*(5), e63920. doi: 10.1371/journal.pone.0063920

Jeon, Y., Kraus, S. G., Jowsey, T., & Glasgow, N. J. (2010). The experience of living with chronic heart failure: A narrative review of qualitative studies. *BMC Health Services Research, 10*, 77. doi: 10.1186/1472-6963-10-77

Jonsbu, E., Martinsen, E., Morken, G., Moum, T., & Dammen, R. (2012). Illness perception among patients with chest pain and palpitations before and after negative cardiac evaluation. *Biopsychosocial Medicine, 6*, 19. doi: 10.1186/1751-0759-6-19

Jonsbu, E., Martinsen, E. W., Morken, G., Moum, T., & Dammen, T. (2013). Change and impact of illness perceptions among patients with non-cardiac chest pain or benign palpitations following three sessions of CBT. *Behavioural and Cognitive Psychotherapy, 4*, 398–407.

Juergens, M. C., Seekatz, B., Moosdorf, R. G., Petrie, K. J., & Rief, W. (2010). Illness beliefs before cardiac surgery predict disability, quality of life and depression 3 months later. *Journal of Psychosomatic Research, 68*, 553–560.

Kaptein, A. A., Klok, T., Moss-Morris, R., & Brand, P. L. P. (2010). Illness perceptions: Impact on self-management and control in asthma. *Current Opinion in Allergy and Clinical Immunology, 10*, 194–199.

Kaptein, A. A., Yamaoka, K., Snoei, L., van der Kloot, W., Inoue, K., Tabei, T., ... Nortier, H. (2013). Illness perceptions and quality of life in Japanese and Dutch women with breast cancer. *Journal of Psychosocial Oncology, 31*, 81-2013. doi: 10.1080/07347332.2012.741092

Keim-Malpass, J., Baernholdt, M., Erickson, J. M., Ropka, M. E., Schroen, A. T., & Steeves, R. H. (2013). Blogging through cancer: Young women's persistent problems shared online. *Cancer Nursing, 36*(2), 163–172. doi: 10.1097/NCC.0b013e31824eb879

Kelley-Moore, J. A., Schumacher, J. G., Kahana, E., & Kahana, B. (2006). When do older adults become "disabled"? Social and health antecedents of perceived disability in a panel study of the oldest old. *Journal of Health and Social Behavior, 47*, 126–141.

Knowles, S. R., Cook, S. I., & Tribbick, D. (2013). Relationship between health status, illness perceptions, coping strategies and psychological morbidity: A preliminary study with IBD stoma patients. *Journal of Crohn's and Colitis, 7*, 3471–3478.

Knowles, S. R., Gass, C., & Macrae, F. (2013). Illness perceptions in IBD influence psychological status, sexual health and satisfaction, body image and relational functioning: A preliminary exploration using structural equation modeling. *Journal of Crohn's and Colitis, 7*, e344–e350.

Kremenchutzky, M., & Walt, L. (2013). Perceptions of health status in multiple sclerosis patients and their doctors. *Canadian Journal of Neurological Science, 40*, 210–218.

Larsen, P.D. (2013). Finding a way through cancer, dying and widowhood: A memoir. Bloomington, ID: Archway Publishing

Larun, L., & Malterud, K. (2007). Identity and coping experiences in chronic fatigue syndrome: A synthesis of qualitative studies. *Patient Education and Counseling, 69*, 20–28.

Leventhal, H., Bodnar-Deren, S., Breland, J., Hash-Converse, J., Phillips, L., Levanthal, E., & Cameron, L. (2012). Modeling health and illness behavior. In A. Baum, T. Revenson, & J. Singer (Eds.), *Handbook of health psychology* (2nd ed., pp. 3–35). New York, NY: Psychology Press.

Leventhal, H., Leventhal, E. A., & Breland, J. Y. (2011). Cognitive science speaks to the "common-sense" of chronic illness management. *Annals of Behavior Medicine, 41*, 152–163.

Levy, S., Segev, M., Reicher-Atir, R., Steinmetz, A., Horev, N., Niv, Y., ... Dickman, R. (2014). Perceptions of gastroenterologists and patients regarding irritable bowel syndrome and inflammatory bowel disease. *European Journal of Gastroenterology & Hepatology, 26(1)*, 40-6.. doi: 10.1097/ MEG.0b013e328365ac70

Lorber, J. (2000). Gender and health. In P. Brown (Ed.), *Perspectives in medical sociology* (3rd ed., pp. 40–70). Prospect Heights, IL: Waveland Press.

Martire, L. M., Schulz, R., Helgeson, V. S., Small, B. J., & Saghafi, E. M. (2010). Review and meta-analysis of couple-oriented interventions for chronic illness. *Annals of Behavior and Medicine, 40*, 325–342.

McLean, S. A., & Clauw, D. J. (2005). Biomedical models of fibromyalgia. *Disability and Rehabilitation, 27*, 659–665.

McMahon, L., Murray, C., Sanderson, J., & Daiches, A. (2012). "Governed by the pain": Narratives of fibromyalgia. *Disability and Rehabilitation, 34(16)*, 1358–1366.

Mechanic, D. (1962). The concept of illness behavior. *Journal of Chronic Diseases, 15*, 189–194.

Mechanic, D. (1986). The concept of illness behavior: Culture, situation, and personal predisposition. *Psychological Medicine, 16*, 1–7.

Mechanic, D. (1995). Sociological dimensions of illness behavior. *Social Science and Medicine, 41(9)*, 1207–1216.

Merolli, M., Gray, K., & Martin-Sanchez, F. (2013). Health outcomes and related effects of using social media in chronic disease management: A literature review and analysis of affordances. *Journal of Biomedical Informatics.* http://dx.doi.org/10.1016/j. jbi.2013.04.010

Miravitlles, M., Ferrer, J., Baro, E., Lieonart, M., & Galera, J. (2013). Differences between physician and patient in the perception of symptoms and their severity in COPD. *Respiratory Medicine.* http://dx.doi.org/10.1016/j.rmed .2013.06.019

Parsons, T. (1951). *The social system.* New York, NY: Free Press.

Paterson, B. (2001). The shifting perspectives model of chronic illness. *Journal of Nursing Scholarship, 33(1)*, 21–26.

Paterson, B. (2003). The koala has claws: Applications of the shifting perspectives model in research of chronic illness. *Qualitative Health Research, 13(7)*, 987–994.

Petrie, K. J., & Weinman, J. (2006). Why illness perceptions matter. *Clinical Medicine, 6(6)*, 536–539.

Pickett, S., Allen, W., Franklin, M., & Peters, R. (2013). Illness beliefs in African Americans with hypertension. *Western Journal of Nursing Research.* doi: 10.1177/0193945913491837

Rochelle, T. L., & Fidler, H. (2012). The importance of illness perceptions, quality of life and psychological status in patients with ulcerative colitis and Crohn's disease. *Journal of Health Psychology, 18(7)*, 972–983. doi: 10.1077/1359105312459094

Rudell, K., Bhui, K., & Priebe, S. (2009). Concept, development and application of a new mixed method assessment of cultural variations in illness perceptions: Barts explanatory model inventory. *Journal of Health Psychology, 24*, 336–347.

Searle, A., Norman, P., Thompson, R., & Vedhara, K. (2007). Illness representations among patients with type 2 diabetes and their partners: Relationships with self-management behaviors. *Journal of Psychosomatic Research, 63(2)*, 175–184.

Sirri, L., Fava, G. A., & Sonino, N. (2013). The unifying concept of illness behavior. *Psychotherapy and Psychosomatics, 82*, 74–81. doi: 10.1159/000343508

Sontag, S. (1988). *Illness as metaphor.* Toronto, Canada: Collins.

Strauss, A., & Glaser, B. (1975). *Chronic illness and the quality of life.* St. Louis, MO: Mosby.

Strauss, A., Corbin, J., Fagerhaugh, S., Glaser, B., Maines, D., Suczek, B. & Wiener, C.L. (1984). *Chronic illness and the quality of life* (2nd ed.). St. Louis, MO: Mosby.

Thomas, R. (2003). *Society and health: Sociology for health professionals.* New York, NY: Kluwer.

Thorne, S. E., & Paterson, B. (1998). Shifting images of chronic illness. *Image, 30(2)*, 173–178.

Wainwright, D. (2008). Illness behavior and the discourse of health. In D. Wainwright (Ed.), *A sociology of health* (pp. 76–96). London, UK: Sage.

Weinert, C., Cudney, S., Comstock, B., & Bansal, A. (2011). Computer intervention impact on psychosocial adaptation of rural women with chronic conditions. *Nursing Research, 60(2)*, 82–91.

Whittemore, R., & Dixon, J. (2008). Chronic illness: The process of integration. *Journal of Nursing and Healthcare of Chronic Illness* in association with *Journal of Clinical Nursing, 17(7b)*, 177–198. doi: 10.1111/j.1365-2702.2007.02244.x

Williams, S. J. (2005). Parsons revisited: From the sick role to …? *Health, 9*, 123–144.

Woolthuis, E., deGrauw, W., Cardol, M., van Weel, C., Metsemakers, J., & Biermans, M. (2013). Patients' and partners' illness perceptions in screen-detected versus clinically diagnosed type 2 diabetes: Partners matter! *Family Practice, 30(4)*, 418-425. doi: 10.1093/fampra /cmt003

Young, J. T. (2004). Illness behavior: A selective review and synthesis. *Sociology of Health and Illness, 26(1)*, 1–31.

Chapter 3

Psychosocial Adjustment

Pamala D. Larsen

Introduction

In previous editions, this chapter was titled "Adaptation." The literature uses the terms "adaptation" and "adjustment" interchangeably. Although either term could be used, this author prefers the term "adjustment," as the term better describes a process as well as a final outcome. *Adjustment* refers to the changes in life that are made continuously when one has a chronic illness. Adjustment is not static, but dynamic.

What is interesting about the terms "adaptation" and "adjustment" is that psychologists describe these terms as psychological adjustment or adaptation, whereas in nursing the more common phrase is psychosocial adjustment or adaptation. "Psychosocial" is a broader term and takes into account the social environment as well as the psychological state of being, that one cannot be separated from the other. "Psychosocial" is, therefore, a more inclusive term, while "psychological" is one-dimensional. Thus, in the discipline of psychology, studies describe psychological adjustment, while psychosocial adjustment is encountered more frequently in nursing. However, to be true to each author's intent in the studies and articles described in this chapter, whatever term the author has used

in the article—"adjustment" or "adaptation"— will be used to describe the study.

Individuals with chronic illness unconsciously or consciously chart a course to navigate the challenges of a chronic disease. Throughout the course of their illness, they must rely on a healthcare system in which pharmaceuticals and technology are the hallmarks of quality health care. Although a disease focus may be appropriate to meet the physical needs of the individual, particularly in the acute phase, this perspective does not meet the social, psychological, and emotional needs of patients with chronic conditions. In other words, the disease focus of the healthcare system does not and cannot manage the illness experience of the patient and family. This chapter builds on the previous chapter, "The Illness Experience."

Classic work by Visotsky, Hamburg, Goss, and Lebovits (1961), in studying patients with polio, posed an initial question regarding adaptation. The researchers asked their patients how it was possible to deal with this stressor, polio, and which coping behavior(s) assisted them with achieving a successful outcome. Decades later, researchers continue to ask the same question. Although progress in understanding certain components of adjustment has been made, many questions remain unanswered.

Conceptualizing Psychosocial Adjustment

An early description of adjustment (and a continuing one) is the absence of a diagnosed psychological disorder, psychological symptoms, or negative mood in an individual. One example of a diagnosed condition is *trauma- and stressor-related disorder*, defined as the development of clinically significant emotional or behavioral symptoms in response to an identifiable stress or stressor (American Psychological Association, 2013). Even in Visotsky's study with patients with polio in 1961, there was a movement to discount a psychological disorder being necessary in the definition of adjustment. The presence of a psychological disorder is important, but other variables should also be considered in a definition.

Fife (1994) views the construction of meaning as a central aspect of adaptation to serious illness. The concept of meaning commonly refers to the relationship between individuals and their world, as well as to the individuals' unique perceptions of their place within that world (p. 309). In the face of chronic disease, individuals are forced to redefine the meanings they have assumed to be true in their lives.

In a review article on psychological adjustment to chronic disease, deRidder, Geenen, Kuijer, and van Middendorp (2008) identified five elements of successful adjustment: (1) successful performance of adaptive tasks, (2) absence of psychological disorders, (3) presence of low negative affect and high positive affect, (4) adequate function status (e.g., going to work), and (5) satisfaction and well-being in various life domains (p. 264). Some of these elements are easily "measured." For example, absence or presence of a psychological disorder or returning to work can be verified with a degree of certainty. In contrast, other elements cannot be measured objectively.

There is little consistency in the literature in defining adjustment. Each author/researcher defines the term differently based on his or her own theoretical framework or on the specific outcomes that a study measures— for example, quality of life, self-concept, optimism, well-being, and so forth. Perhaps combining deRidder and colleagues' work with some broad thoughts from Hoyt and Stanton (2012) provides a clearer picture of adjustment. These thoughts include the following concepts:

- Adjustment to chronic illness is multidimensional and includes intrapersonal and interpersonal dimensions. Dimensions of adjustment are interrelated.
- Heterogeneity is the rule, not the exception.
- Adjustment involves both positive and negative dimensions.

Chronic Illness Affects Adjustment in Multiple Life Domains and Roles

Caring for patients with chronic illness includes more than addressing the physical domain; it crosses interpersonal, cognitive, emotional, social, and behavioral domains. Psychosocial adjustment of the individual and family is a holistic process, in which each domain of life affects the others. Therefore, a change in one domain affects adjustment in another domain (Hoyt & Stanton, 2012). Cognitive adaptation might include self-reflection. Adaptation in the behavioral domain may include returning to work. Anxiety, in the emotional domain, may affect the ability to socialize in the interpersonal domain or impact blood pressure in the physical domain. Emotional adaptation could be the absence of depression, and interpersonal and social adaptation may be the willingness to be "social" again and resume previous roles.

Heterogeneity Is the Rule, Not the Exception

If 20 women of the same age with the same stage of breast cancer and same prognosis were placed in a room, each individual would adjust, or not adjust, to her chronic condition differently. Some women would be considered "well adjusted," whereas others might be considered maladjusted. The remaining individuals would fall somewhere in the middle. A person's individual determinants and uniqueness affect the ability of that individual to adjust to the illness. Although adjustment commonalities exist among individuals with chronic illness, there is significant variability as well.

Adjustment can *only* be viewed from the perspective of the individual. Physical changes and function may or may not be pertinent to the individual. As the lived experience of illness is different for each individual and family, so is psychosocial adjustment. The process and outcomes differ because of past experiences, age, gender, ethnicity, socioeconomic status, and other variables that science has yet to identify.

Adjustment Involves Positive and Negative Dimensions

Typically, one thinks of psychosocial outcomes of chronic illness as being negative, as evidenced by distress, anxiety, worry, and other negative states. As stated previously, one definition of positive adjustment is the absence of a psychological disorder. However, there may be another positive side of chronic illness.

It is not unusual to hear individuals with chronic illness make comments such as "Having this disease has been the best thing that ever happened to me—it made me wake up and see what was important." There may be positive aspects of chronic disease, but how patients come to view the disease in this way remains a mystery. Current research on benefit-finding, addressed later in this chapter, may be helpful in understanding this phenomenon.

Adjustment is a process that is neither linear nor lockstep, but dynamic. The list of variables that influence this process are numerous and varied. However, an obvious influence on adjustment is a negative change in health status. When such a change occurs, the lived experience

of the individual and family needs to incorporate different data into their mental model of the illness, and progress made in previous steps toward adjustment may disappear.

This chapter provides an overview of psychosocial adjustment in individuals with chronic illness. Given that entire books have been devoted to coping, adaptation, and adjustment, the scope of this chapter is necessarily limited. However, classic sources and models are included, along with interventions for healthcare professionals.

Impact

Influences on Psychosocial Adjustment

The impact of a chronic illness diagnosis, and subsequent treatment, on an individual and family is felt in all dimensions of their lives. However, it may not be the only factor influencing adjustment. That is, other life influences may come into play that may or may not be related to the illness. There may be issues with a child or a grandchild, financial issues (which may or may not be related to the illness), issues related to owning a business, and so forth. Many years ago, this author interviewed a middle-aged woman who had recently become blind. Options were being reviewed for vocational rehabilitation. During the visit, it became evident that the person was not focusing on what we were discussing, and finally she voiced her concerns. Her 16-year-old daughter was currently hospitalized in an inpatient psychiatric facility. As healthcare professionals, we often make the assumption that the patient's illness is the focal point, but perhaps that is not always the case.

Most concepts addressed in the first section of this text deal with psychosocial adjustment. Whether it is powerlessness, uncertainty, intimacy, or social isolation, all of these factors contribute to an individual and family's psychosocial adjustment. However, another factor to consider in adjustment is the type of chronic illness and its prognosis. Is this chronic illness treatable, potentially fatal, curable, life-shortening, or disabling? The psychosocial adjustment in a patient newly diagnosed with type 2 diabetes is vastly different from that in a patient with Stage IV lung cancer. Unfortunately, researchers often group patients with a variety of chronic diseases at different stages of their illness into one sample, perhaps titled "chronic somatic disease," making it impossible to draw legitimate conclusions and make generalizations about their findings.

For an individual with chronic illness, this illness is now a life experience. In contrast, for family members, it will be remembered as a "past experience" at some point in their lives. This experience, with their own corresponding illness perceptions, becomes assimilated into these persons' memory for future reference.

A systematic review of psychosocial factors and adjustment to chronic pain in persons with disabilities identified other variables impacting adjustment (Jensen, Moore, Bockow, Ehde, & Engel, 2011). Criteria for studies to be included in the review were as follows: (1) adults with physical disability who reported having pain, (2) one measure of a psychosocial predictor domain, and (3) one measure of pain or patient functioning.

The review included 29 studies with 5 disability groups, including patients with spinal cord injury (SCI), muscular dystrophy (MD), multiple sclerosis (MS), acquired amputation, and cerebral palsy (CP). The findings indicated that measures of key psychosocial factors were all associated with important pain-related domains across the five different disability groups (p. 155). It was suggested by the results of this review that reasonable goals of treatment might include the following: (1) increase the use of coping strategies such as task persistence, acceptance of disability, behavioral activities, exercise, ignoring pain, and coping self-statements; (2) increase the belief that the patient can control pain and its effects; and (3) help the patient

seek and obtain more general social support (not including support from others with pain). The findings provide support for a comprehensive biopsychosocial model for understanding chronic pain in adults with physical disabilities.

Researchers found a relationship among spirituality, psychosocial adjustment to illness, and health-related quality of life in 253 patients with Stage 4 or 5 chronic kidney disease and dialysis patients (Davison & Jhangri, 2013). Spirituality was measured by the Spiritual Well-Being Scale, which is designed to evaluate both religious and existential constructs of spirituality. Psychosocial adjustment, as measured by the Psychological Adjustment to Illness Scale (PAIS), was highly correlated with health-related quality of life (HRQoL); however, existential well-being (EWB) remained a significant predictor of HRQoL. The authors concluded that spirituality is a unique factor in patients' HRQoL, independent of their psychosocial adjustment (p. 170).

COPING

How does coping "fit" with psychosocial adjustment? Or is it a stand-alone entity? Richard Lazarus's 1966 book, *Psychological Stress and Coping*, was an initial scholarly work that expanded how coping was conceptualized. Coping is a process that unfolds in the context of a situation or condition that is appraised as personally significant, and as taxing or exceeding the individual's resources (Lazarus & Folkman, 1984). The coping process is initiated in response to the individual's appraisal that important goals have been harmed, lost, or threatened (Folkman & Moskowitz, 2004). What we have learned is that coping is a complex, multidimensional process that is sensitive both to the environment and its demands and resources, and to personality traits that influence the appraisal of stress—in this case, chronic illness—and the resources for coping (Folkman & Moskowitz, 2004). Coping is not a stand-alone concept or phenomenon, but rather is embedded in a complex, dynamic process that involves the person, the environment, and the relationship between them.

How coping is related specifically to adjustment has not been clearly described (Sharpe & Curran, 2006, p. 1154). Intellectually, it is believed that coping strategies contribute to adaptation and may be mediators, but most likely interact with other factors in contributing to adaptation (Stanton & Revenson, 2007).

Two current studies are offered as examples of coping and adjustment. The relationship among attachment, coping, and self-regulation theory with adjustment in chronic illness has been studied less than other concepts. Bazzazian and Besharat (2012) explored the possibility that attachment theory could be part of a model of health as a basis for coping and self-regulation theory that would explain measurable individual differences in adjusting to a diagnosis of type 1 diabetes. The aim of the study was to develop a model of adjustment. Three hundred young adults with type 1 diabetes completed the Adult Attachment Inventory, the Brief Illness Perception Questionnaire, the task-oriented subscale of the Coping Inventory for Stressful Situations, and the well-being scale of the Mental Health Inventory. Three attachment styles were found to have a significant effect on task-oriented coping strategies. Notably, positive illness perceptions and more usage of task-oriented coping strategies predicted better adjustment to type 1 diabetes.

To understand relationships among coping style, locus of control, perceived illness intrusiveness, and disease severity, data were analyzed from 227 older veterans with either chronic obstructive pulmonary disease (COPD) or congestive heart failure (CHF). Regression analysis revealed that illness intrusiveness was associated with younger age and greater disease severity, less internal locus of control, and avoidant/emotion-focused coping. Avoidant/emotion-focused coping, but not active coping, mediated the relationship between illness severity and illness intrusiveness (Hundt et al., 2013). The authors suggest that psychological interventions may reduce illness intrusiveness by targeting an avoidant/emotion-focused coping style and associated behaviors.

Benefit-Finding

Traditionally, the negative sequelae that follow a diagnosis of a chronic and/or life-threatening illness have been the focus of healthcare providers. However, current research suggests that many individuals may also experience positive life changes as a response to a serious illness. The concept of positive life changes is not new, but rather dates from Caplan's (1964) work, which discussed the possibility that crises may present opportunities through constructive resolution of greater personality integration and the development of coping capabilities.

This positive life change has been called stress-related growth, benefit-finding, and post-traumatic growth. All three terms are used in the literature to refer to the positive life changes that people make while coping with negative life events (Park, Lechner, Antoni, & Stanton, 2009).

Positive life changes typically occur in the domains of relationships, self-concept, life philosophy, and coping skills (Park, 2009, p. 11). Park defines stress-related growth as the actual or veridical changes that people have made in relation to their experience with an identified stressful or traumatic event (p. 12). Park acknowledges that different types of physical illness raise different challenges and, in fact, likely influence the levels and types of growth possible. Dimensions of illness that may be considered include symptom onset, presumed etiology, threat to life, life disruption, recovery trajectory, chronicity, permanence of change, and life context. Because illnesses differ greatly on these dimensions, generalizations about perceptions of growth in the context of illness may be uninformative and inaccurate (pp. 22–24).

Benefit-finding may be a predictor of concurrent and future adjustment (Pakenham & Cox, 2009). In a study examining data from 388 patients with multiple sclerosis and 232 of their carers, at baseline and 12 months later, seven distinct benefit-finding dimensions emerged: compassion/empathy; spiritual growth; mindfulness; family relations growth; lifestyle gains; personal growth; and new opportunities. The researchers suggested that these dimensions may be specific to MS or may be applicable with other chronic diseases.

A systematic review of the qualitative literature on post-traumatic growth and life threatening illness revealed several common themes: reappraisal of life and priorities, trauma equals development of self, existential reevaluation, and a new awareness of the body (Hefferon, Grealy, & Mutrie, 2009).

Could positive life changes be a component of psychosocial adjustment? Or should they be considered psychosocial adjustment? One could assume that finding benefits from serious illness would contribute to better adjustment to the illness, but research results on this topic are mixed (Carver, Lechner, & Antoni, 2009).

Next, we consider how we, as healthcare professionals, influence the process of psychosocial adjustment in patients and families.

Interventions

Researchers' broad goals are to understand the process of adjustment, predict outcomes, and, by having predictive ability, modify interventions to meet the needs of patients. A framework that meets those goals is preferable for practice; however, a perfect model does not exist. What follows are sample models/frameworks gleaned from the literature. The differences in the frameworks presented here demonstrate the variance in understanding adjustment.

Frameworks for Understanding Adjustment in Chronic Illness

BIOMEDICAL MODEL

Although one might not consider the biomedical model pertinent when discussing psychosocial adjustment, this model is often used in the acute phase of chronic illness. The medical model provides a framework for treating the pathology of illness. In this model, the patient is a complex set of anatomic parts and interrelated body systems. Anatomic, physiologic, and/or biochemical failures translate into disease, thus promoting a disease-oriented approach to care. Pathophysiology, pharmacotherapy, and technology are emphasized and become prominent when intervening in illness and disease, whether acute or chronic. The biomedical paradigm tends to medicalize all human conditions, suggesting that symptoms can be controlled and cured with biomedical strategies. This model reduces the individual to a disease and fails to recognize the human aspects and experiences of the individual who happens to have a chronic illness, while diminishing social and cultural explanation of disease (Mirowsky & Ross, 2002). Physical complaints and signs or symptoms of disease become the hallmarks of interaction and reaction in the healthcare arena. A biological model may cause healthcare professionals to pay too little attention to the patient and his or her social context (Suls, Luger, & Martin, 2010, p. 16).

In this model, the relationship between the healthcare professional and the patient with chronic illness is one of objectivity, biological pathology, diagnosis, and signs and symptoms, all of which require medical interventions. Healthcare professionals tend to shield themselves from the human aspects of chronic illness, while their technical skill sets, techniques, and procedures become the focus of interaction with the patient (Freeth, 2007). Power and expertise are held exclusively by the healthcare system. The individual with chronic illness may become disempowered to engage in healthcare decisions and rely solely on the healthcare professional.

The biomedical model is insufficient in providing holistic health care to individuals and families with chronic illness (Waisbond, 2007), as it fails to acknowledge the illness experience. Specifically, this model does not acknowledge the person with the chronic condition, who holds knowledge and expertise about the factors that influence his or her physical symptoms of chronic disease—in other words, the expert patient. For example, at the end of the month, Mrs. Jones becomes anxious that she will not have enough money to purchase prescriptions for her hypertension. Although she has adequate funds, Mrs. Jones's stress and worry exacerbate her hypertension. At her doctor's appointment, Mrs. Jones does not inform her physician that the probable cause of her elevated blood pressure is related to her stress about money. The physician responds to Mrs. Jones's hypertension with a change of medication to manage her symptoms. This kind of quantification of all signs and symptoms of disease fails to address the total illness experience of the individual.

Despite the limitations of the biomedical model in adjustment, it is the foundation of evidence-based practice and provides the gold standard for treatment and intervention. This model provides measurable goals for treatment and patient outcomes relative to morbidity and mortality.

CHRONIC CARE MODEL

The chronic care model (CCM) first appeared in the literature in 1998 (Wagner, 1998) and was later refined by Wagner and colleagues (2001). Subsequent research into interventions with chronic illness has resulted in best practices and a national program for improving chronic illness care (Robert Wood Johnson Foundation, 2006–2011).

A key component of the CCM is patient self-management to address deficiencies in the medical model of the healthcare system in managing chronic conditions. Within this model, six major elements interact to produce high-quality care and evidence-based interventions for persons with chronic conditions in health systems at the community, organization, practice, and individual levels: (1) the healthcare system or healthcare organization; (2) clinical information systems; (3) decision support; (4) delivery system design; (5) self-management support; and (6) community, including organizations and resources for patients with chronic illness (Wagner et al., 2001).

The CCM has been widely adopted as an approach to ambulatory care. It has guided national quality improvement initiatives and been an integral part of patient-centered medical home models (Coleman, Austin, Brach, & Wagner, 2009). However, this model focuses on the mortality and morbidity of the patient and family, not the illness experience. In other words, $HgbA_{1c}$ levels, blood pressure readings, medication adherence, appropriate results from pulmonary function tests, and so forth are objective measures, thereby identifying the CCM as a biomedical model.

Two recent systematic reviews of the CCM and chronic illness further describe this model's use and impact. In a review focusing on individuals living with HIV, two of the components of the model, decision support (DS) and clinical information systems (CIS), were assessed for their effectiveness in improving care by changing healthcare professional behavior. Overall, DS and CIS interventions may modestly improve care for individuals living with HIV; nevertheless, the researchers found that the interventions have a greater impact on process measures than on patient outcome measures (Pasricha et al. 2012, p. 127).

Other work with the CCM has involved individuals with diabetes who were being treated in primary care settings (Stellefson, Dipnarine, & Stopka, 2013). This systematic review, unfortunately, identified only nine randomized clinical trials (RCTs). The review concluded that the CCM is effective in improving the health of individuals with diabetes who receive care in a primary care setting. Positive clinical indicators, such as improved $HgbA_{1c}$ levels, have been cited as indicators of the model's success. However, process outcomes (e.g., self-efficacy for disease management and clinical decision making, perceived social support, knowledge of diabetes self-care practices) were not addressed in the studies included in this review.

COMMON SENSE MODEL OF SELF-REGULATION

The common sense model of self-regulation (CSM) (Leventhal et al., 2012), based on biomedical and cognitive models, has become the preferred model in psychological adaptation studies. This model proposes that the patient's illness beliefs and representations of that illness influence adaptation to the illness and health outcomes. According to the CSM, patients develop cognitive and emotional representations of their condition to "make sense" or find meaning in the illness. Leventhal and colleagues identify five dimensions that represent a patient's view of his or her illness:

- Identity of the illness: Connecting the symptoms with the illness and having an understanding of the illness.
- Timeline: Duration and progression of the illness.
- Causes: Perceived reason for the illness.
- Consequences: What will be the physical, psychosocial, and economic impact of the illness?
- Controllability: Can this disease be controlled? Cured?

After identification of these dimensions, Leventhal and colleagues posit that the information gathered from these dimensions becomes the patient's illness perceptions and these, in turn, guide coping and ultimately affect outcomes through the choice of actions arising from these illness perceptions (Benyamini, 2011, p. 293). There is significant evidence that an adaptive perception of a curable/controllable illness is related to better health and functioning (Hagger & Orbell, 2003).

The common sense model has been used extensively as a framework in research in chronic illness. Examples of its application follow:

- The importance of illness perceptions in end-stage renal disease: Associations with psychosocial and clinical outcomes (Chilcot, 2012).

- Explanation of outcomes after mild traumatic brain injury: The contribution of injury belief and Leventhal's common sense model (Snell, Hay-Smith, Surgenor, & Siegert, 2013).
- Predicting self-care behaviours of patients with type 2 diabetes: The importance of beliefs about behavior, not just beliefs about illness (French, Wade, & Farmer, 2013).
- Can the common sense model predict adherence in chronically ill patients: A meta-analysis (Brandes & Mullan, 2013).
- Using the common sense model of self-regulation to review the effects of self-monitoring of blood glucose on glycemic control for non-insulin treated adults with type 2 diabetes (Breland, McAndrew, Burns, Leventhal, & Leventhal, 2013).

BIOPSYCHOSOCIAL MODEL

Engle (1977, 1980) conceived a model that integrates biological, psychological, and social processes in physical illness and health, medical diagnosis, medical treatment, and recovery (Suls et al., 2010, p. 18). This model is not dominated by a single domain, but instead uses a multilevel approach to diagnose, explain, and treat any medical issue. Engle's goal was to understand the full complement of influences at multiple levels of analysis. The interaction of the domains means that a change in one domain results in changes in other domains. Further, it suggests that any interventions involving all of the domains will fare better than a treatment grounded in one domain (Suls et al., 2010). Challenges exist for interdisciplinary research, however, and research that acknowledges all domains continues to be difficult (Suls, Krantz, & Williams, 2013).

Examples of Interventions to Assist and Support the Patient

The literature provides an abundance of descriptive studies defining and measuring adaptation and coping, but few interventional studies exist. It appears that coping and adjustment can, in some way, be measured by specific concepts (e.g. well-being, hope, lack of a psychological disorder), but we are unable to conceptualize those findings into clear interventions or ways healthcare professionals can assist patients with psychosocial adjustment. The distinct attributes of each individual and his or her family make generalizations of interventions difficult.

SELF-MANAGEMENT

Self-management has long been used as an intervention in a number of the concepts that this text addresses, such as uncertainty, powerlessness, adherence, and quality of life. By managing their own care, patients feel that they have more control over their chronic illness and, therefore, often experience a better quality of life. Due to the importance of self-management, an entire chapter in this text has been devoted to the subject. Thus, the present chapter will address this concept only briefly.

Swendeman, Ingram, and Rotheram-Borus (2009) identify three broad categories in chronic disease self-management: physical health, psychological functioning, and social relationships. Elements related to physical health are knowledge and behavior to maintain health status, whereas elements related to psychological functioning include self-efficacy and empowerment as well as emotional status and shifts in identity. Social relationship elements relate to collaborative partnerships with healthcare professionals, family members, and social support.

Self-management programs based on enhancing self-efficacy have proved highly successful in reducing symptoms and encouraging behavior change in many chronic illnesses. Self-efficacy may be considered a personal context variable; thus, it may be a determinant in the appraisal of the illness, the coping strategies used by the individual, and the outcome (physical, emotional, and social adjustment). Although self-efficacy is specific to the task and situation, programs that encourage development of self-efficacy can influence adaptation.

To accomplish self-management, individuals with chronic illness need to apply the following skills: problem solving, decision making, resource utilization, forming partnerships with healthcare professionals, and taking action (Lorig & Holman, 2003). McCorkle and colleagues (2011) present a literature review of the scientific advances in self-management in cancer in the treatment, post-treatment, and end-of-life phases of the cancer continuum. Their review uses terms such as "illness self-management," "self-care," "psycho-educational interventions," and "cognitive-behavioral interventions." Oftentimes studies using cognitive-behavioral interventions are not included in such reviews. For example, in this chapter, this author has chosen to separate out psychologically based strategies.

McCorkle and colleagues identified 16 interventional studies that met their criteria for inclusion in the review. Studies were clustered by interventions during the treatment, post-treatment, and end-of-life phases, with the majority of the studies occurring during treatment. Programs included educational programs, nurse coaching, uncertainty management, monitoring, counseling, skills training, information, and general knowledge about the disease and treatment. There was no standardized "intervention" for self-management. What became apparent was that the 16 studies were time limited; specifically, treatment interventions ranged from 4 to 20 weeks long, post-treatment interventions were 8 to 10 weeks long, and interventions in the end-of-life studies were offered until death. The treatment studies demonstrated decreased psychosocial concerns, less distress, better health-related quality of life, and better psychological adjustment (McCorkle et al., 2011); however, only short-term outcomes were measured, not long-term outcomes.

Lastly, self-management programs have often been coordinated by lay leaders. A Cochrane review identified 17 randomized clinical trials

(RCTs) involving 7,442 participants. Although the interventions shared similar structures and components, the studies demonstrated heterogeneity in conditions studied, outcomes collected, and effects (Foster, Taylor, Eldridge, Ramsay, & Griffiths, 2007). Foster and colleagues concluded that such programs may lead to small, short-term improvements in participants' self-efficacy, self-rated health, cognitive symptom management, and frequency of aerobic exercise. Nevertheless, there is no evidence to suggest that such programs improve psychological health, symptoms, or health-related quality of life, or that they significantly alter healthcare use.

MOTIVATIONAL INTERVIEWING

When Miller and Rollnick (1991) originally developed motivational interviewing (MI), their intent was that counselors who worked with clients with drug and alcohol problems would benefit the most from application of this intervention. After the success of their 1991 book, it became apparent that MI could be used with others who struggle with ambivalence about change. Rollnick, Miller, and Butler (2008) define motivational interviewing as a refined form of the familiar process of guiding (p. ix.).

Rollnick et al. (2008) further describe MI:

> MI is not a technique for tricking people into doing what they do not want to do. Rather, it is a skillful clinical style for eliciting from patients their own good motivations for making behavior changes in the interest of their health. It involves guiding more than directing, dancing rather than wrestling, listening at least as much as telling. The overall "spirit" has been described as collaborative, evocative, and honoring of patient autonomy. (Rollnick et al., 2008, p. 6)

Dart (2011) describes the four main principles of MI as follows: (1) express empathy, (2) support self-efficacy, (3) develop discrepancy, and (4) roll with resistance. Therapeutic communication is important in each and every interaction with the patient. MI is a form of communication that allows patient involvement, respect for each patient as an individual with his or her own agenda, and acceptance of a patient's choices (p. 13).

A search of the *Cochrane Library of Systematic Reviews* does not reveal a review dealing with motivational interviewing and chronic illness. A total of 11 proposed or completed studies about chronic illness and motivational interviewing were listed in the Cochrane Central Register of Controlled Trials from 2005 to the present. Results from the completed studies were mixed. The Health Aging Project (HAP) tested nurse coaching as an intervention to support healthy behavior change in older adults. Nurses were trained in motivational interviewing. The coaching took place on the phone and via email to discuss health behaviors. The intervention group had significantly less illness intrusiveness and health distress than the control group at 6 months, but it is not known whether these outcomes resulted from actual behavior change (Bennett et al., 2005).

Sixty older adults with chronic heart failure were randomly assigned to an interview group (the MI group) or a control group to examine whether a physical activity intervention based on motivational interviewing would improve quality of life in these patients. Over the 5 months of the study, there was a general trend toward improvements in self-efficacy and motivation scores (Brodie, Inoue, & Shaw, 2008).

Solomon and colleagues (2012) examined the effectiveness of a telephone-based counseling program based on motivational interviewing to improve adherence to a medication regimen for osteoporosis. The study, which had a sample size of 2,087, did not reveal any statistically significant improvement in the experimental group in regard to adherence to their medication regime.

PEER AND SOCIAL SUPPORT

As common as self-help and self-support groups are for those with chronic illness, one would expect the research literature to be clear as to their value. Unfortunately, that is not the case. Anecdotal articles exist, but there are few research-based articles. In addition, research commonly looks at support groups for a short period—6, 10, 12, and 15 weeks—whereas a chronic illness could be present for 30, 40, or 50 years.

Stanton and Revenson (2007) suggest that healthcare professionals can improve the interpersonal context of patients by teaching them to develop and maintain social ties, recognize and accept others' help and emotional encouragement, or change their appraisals of the support they are receiving. Psychosocial interventions should be directed toward individual-level change and may include cognitive-behavioral, educational, and interpersonal support components. Support groups may provide emotional support as well as an educational focus. The education is expected to strengthen the individual's sense of control over the disease, reduce feelings of confusion, and enhance decision making (p. 221). The peer support provides emotional support, thereby enhancing self-esteem, minimizing aloneness, and reinforcing coping strategies.

Dibb and Yardley (2006) investigated the role that social comparison might play in adaptation using a self-help group as the context. Social comparison proposes that individuals with similar problems compare each other's health statuses. Often this comparison occurs within self-help groups, which are composed of individuals with similar health issues. It has been suggested that downward comparison, when a comparison is made with a person who is doing less well, initiates positive affect by increasing self-esteem. Conversely, upward comparison with a person doing better may result in hope (Dibb & Yardley, 2006, p. 1603). Findings from this study, which involved 301 clients with Ménière's disease, demonstrated that the strongest and most consistent effect of social comparison was that positively interpreted downward comparisons were associated

with better functional and goal-directed quality of life (p. 1610).

According to the social-cognitive processing model, the expression of one's thoughts and feelings about cancer—that is, "social sharing"—in a supportive way may facilitate psychological adjustment (Boinon et al., 2014). Studies have emphasized the links between positive social support and patients' psychological adjustment, but have devoted less attention to the effects of negative support. In Boinon and colleagues' study, women with breast cancer were surveyed at two points in time, after their surgery and after their adjuvant therapy. Results were consistent with this social environment–oriented approach and demonstrated that repressing one's desire to talk about the experience of the disease after surgery is associated with an increase in psychological distress at the end of treatment. However, there was no beneficial effect of social sharing concerning the disease or of perceived emotional support on psychological adjustment. The researchers concluded that healthcare professionals should develop specific interventions to address the negative reactions of the social network and the way these are perceived and processed by patients. There should be encouragement to strengthen links with "well-meaning" family members and friends and focus on maintaining the feeling of social integration (Boinon et al., 2014).

Parry and Watt-Watson (2010) conducted a systematic review of peer support interventions for individuals with heart disease. Peer support—a specific type of social support that includes appraisal as well as informational and emotional support—has been shown to be an effective intervention for individuals with other chronic illnesses. Only six RCTs, with a total of 1,452 participants, could be identified for the 2010 review. The results suggested that peer support may improve self-efficacy in individuals with heart disease and post-coronary artery bypass graft (CABG) surgery, and may have a beneficial effect on the health and well-being of individuals with heart disease who are recovering from a myocardial infarction (MI) and are post-CABG surgery. However, the authors note that there was little standardization of the training of the peer support persons or standardization of the peer support intervention, and interventions and outcomes were not theoretically or conceptually justified.

The role of social support in diabetes management is not well understood. Strom and Egede (2012) suggest that social support is a multifaceted experience that involves volunteer associations and formal and informal relationships with others. Social support is a perception that one is accepted, cared for, and provided with assistance from certain individuals or a specific group, or the realization of actual support received from another (p. 770). Strom and Egede's review concluded that higher levels of social support influence more positive outcomes in participants; however, these authors note that because most of the studies reviewed were cross-sectional studies, causality cannot be inferred concerning social support and its impact on diabetes management (p. 780).

In addition to face-to-face social/peer support groups, chronic disease social groups commonly appear on Facebook and Twitter. One group of researchers looked at both Facebook and Twitter to characterize groups concerning colorectal cancer, breast cancer, and diabetes (De la Torre-Diez, Diaz-Pernas, & Anton-Rodriguez, 2012). There were 216 breast cancer groups, 171 colorectal cancer groups, and 527 diabetes groups on the two platforms. Although all disease groups addressed prevention and research, the social value of the groups to patients with chronic disease was most significant.

Psychologically Based Strategies

Pakenham (2007) highlights the need for practitioners to facilitate patients' cognitive processing of the implications and meaning of their illness. A blend of cognitive-restructuring strategies, patient-centered approaches, and existential approaches may be helpful to the patient and family.

Cognitive-behavioral strategies can be used to teach coping skills to patients with chronic illness (Folkman & Moskowitz, 2004). Sharpe and Curran (2006) have also encouraged the use of cognitive-behavioral therapy (CBT). Such programs include strategies with the aim of facilitating a realistic, but optimistic attitude toward illness and/or facilitating more adaptive coping strategies. Programs typically include education about the illness, goal setting and pacing, relaxation strategies and attention diversion skills, cognitive therapy, communication skills, and management of high-risk situations (such as exacerbations of the illness).

McAndrew and colleagues (2008) developed two interventions based on the common sense model of self-regulation. The first intervention is a bottom-up concrete/behavioral approach that has been used with patients with diabetes. The approach begins with a focus on behavior to create an overarching view of diabetes as a chronic condition that requires constant self-regulation. The second intervention is conceived as a top-down or abstract/cognitive strategy that provides patients with asthma with a conceptual framework that focuses on asthma being present even when it is asymptomatic (p. 197). The authors suggest that patients may benefit from starting with one strategy or the other. However, it is expected that successful interventions will combine both approaches.

Three Cochrane Collaboration reviews are relevant to patients with chronic illness and the use of psychologically based strategies. Depression is common in patients with incurable cancer. When studies that used psychotherapy in patients with concomitant incurable cancer and depression were reviewed, the evidence supported psychotherapy as being useful in treating depressive states in patients with advanced cancer. However, there is no evidence to support the effectiveness of psychotherapy in patients with clinically diagnosed depression (Akechi, Okuyama, Onishi, Morita, & Furukawa, 2008).

Nineteen studies comparing psychosocial interventions versus usual care in a sample of 3,204 men with prostate cancer were reviewed. The review demonstrated that psychosocial interventions may have small, short-term beneficial effects on certain domains of well-being, such as the physical component of general health-related quality of life and cancer-related quality of life, when compared with usual care. However, the review failed to demonstrate a statistically significant effect on other domains, such as symptom-related quality of life, self-efficacy, uncertainty, distress, and depression (Parahoo et al., 2013).

Lastly, a review of psychological interventions for women with metastatic breast cancer and their effect on psychosocial and survival outcomes was conducted. Psychologically based interventions appear to be effective in improving survival at 12 months, but not at longer-term follow-up. These interventions are effective in reducing psychological symptoms only in some women with metastatic breast cancer (Mustafa, Carson-Stevens, Gillespie, & Edwards, 2013). The reviewers caution that there is a relative lack of data in this field, and that a number of the RCTs reviewed had reporting or methodological weaknesses.

COMPLEMENTARY AND ALTERNATIVE THERAPY

Examples of different techniques that may be used in patients with chronic illness are included in the "Complementary and Alternative Therapies" chapter.

TECHNOLOGY

Perhaps the most well-known computer intervention involving women with chronic illness is the Women to Women (WTW) project developed by Clarann Weinert. This project was launched in 1995 and included three phases over a period of years. The last phase of the project was a two-group study design with 309 middle-aged, rural

women with chronic conditions. Women were randomized into either the experimental group, which received the computer-based intervention, or the control group, which did not receive the intervention. Data were collected at baseline, at the end of the intervention, and 6 months following the project. Positive and negative psychosocial variables of interest to the researchers were social support, self-esteem, acceptance of illness, stress, depression, and loneliness (Weinert, Cudney, Comstock, & Bansal, 2011).

The 11-week computer intervention gave women 24-hour access to a peer-led virtual support group as well as a series of self-study health teaching units on web skills and the five skills of self-management (problem solving, decision making, resource utilization, forming partnerships with healthcare professionals, and taking action). The skills of self-management were derived from Lorig and Holman's work (2003). At all three data collection points, the number of women participating was 250, indicating an 80.9% retention rate. Five of the six psychosocial outcomes were statistically significant at 6 months. The experimental group had higher scores on self-esteem and acceptance of illness and lower scores on depression, loneliness, and stress than did the control group. Although shortly after the intervention higher scores in social support were noted, that result was not maintained at 6 months. Although this computer intervention was successful, the authors caution that the results represent just one piece of the complex adaptation process as experienced by rural women living with chronic conditions (Weinert et al., 2011, p. 89).

As early as 2005, the Cochrane Collaboration published a review of interactive health communication applications (IHCA) for people with chronic disease. IHCAs were defined as computer-based, usually web-based, information packages for patients that combine health information with at least one of the following: social support, decision support, or behavior change support. To assess the effects of IHCAs for individuals with chronic disease, 24 RCTs with 3,739 participants were included in the review. The IHCAs appeared to have largely positive effects on users, such as users becoming more knowledgeable and feeling better socially supported, and may have improved users' behavioral and clinical outcomes compared to nonusers (Murray, Burns, See Tai, Lai, & Nazareth, 2005).

In 2013, the Cochrane Collaboration published two intervention reviews regarding technology and chronic disease. Pak et al. (2013) assessed the effects on health status and health-related quality of life of computer-based diabetes self-management interventions for adults with type 2 diabetes. The 16 RCTs included in this review demonstrated a wide range of interventions, including clinic-based interventions, Internet-based interventions that could be used from home, and mobile phone-based interventions. The researchers concluded that computer-based self-management interventions to manage type 2 diabetes appear to have a small beneficial effect on blood glucose, and that effect was larger in the mobile phone subgroup. In contrast, no evidence supported benefits in other biological outcomes or any cognitive, behavioral, or emotional outcomes.

A review of smartphone and tablet self-management applications for asthma was also conducted. Marcano Belisario, Huckvale, Greenfield, Car, and Gunn (2013) identified only two RCTs, with a total of 408 participants, dealing with this topic. Due to the small number, a narrative synthesis approach was used with the data. Currently, there is not enough evidence to recommend the use of smartphone and tablet computer applications for the delivery of asthma self-management programs.

OTHER INTERVENTIONS TO ASSIST AND SUPPORT THE PATIENT

Hope can be a psychosocial resource for older adults who are dealing with a chronic illness. A meta-analysis of qualitative research on the hope experience from 1980 to 2010 concluded

that older adults may experience hope differently than younger adults. Resources for hope are both internal and external. Finding meaning and positive reappraisal are important to help older adults maintain hope (Duggleby et al., 2012, p. 1211).

The *Healthy People* documents have fueled interest in health promotion and wellness. Interestingly, an increasing number of studies have focused on the use of wellness interventions in chronic illness. Unfortunately, a consensus definition of a wellness intervention does not exist, as each researcher has used different actions as wellness interventions. Stuifbergen and colleagues (2010) conducted a review of studies that included patients with chronic illness and wellness interventions; 190 studies from 1990 to 2007 met the criteria for inclusion in the review. Most of these studies explored a wellness intervention with a sample of individuals with a single chronic illness (e.g., stroke, cancer, heart failure). Of the 190 studies, 89.5% reported positive effects from their wellness intervention, although the intervention and measurement of outcomes varied greatly (p. 133). Interventions ranged from 1 week of health education and coaching for older adults with cardiac conditions to 6 months of swimming for persons with asthma. Similarly, the outcome measurements varied from using standardized tools like the SF-36 or biological measures to self-reports of mobility, ADLs, and other outcomes. Although the immediate positive effects of interventions were encouraging, there was little, if any, follow-up with patients at a later date (p. 139).

Fife (1994) views the construction of meaning as a central aspect of adaptation to serious illness. Patients and families are challenged by a diagnosis of chronic illness and wonder what the "meaning of all of this" is. Searching for meaning has been a component of several psychological adaptation theories (Lee, Cohen, Edgar, Laizner, & Gagnon, 2006). Lee and colleagues designed a RCT using a meaning-making coping process as the intervention. Seventy-four patients with breast and colorectal cancer were included in the sample. The experimental group received up to four sessions that explored the meaning of their emotional responses and their cognitive appraisal of the experience. Each face-to-face session of up to 120 minutes took place at either the patient's home or the clinic (the patient's choice as to location). The meaning-making intervention involved tasks that patients needed to complete during the sessions: (1) acknowledge the present, (2) contemplate the past, and (3) commit to the present, for the future. Outcome measures were based on the Rosenberg Self-Esteem Scale, the Life Orientation Test—Revised, and the Generalized Self-Efficacy Scale. Statistically significant improvements in self-esteem, optimism, and self-efficacy were found for the experimental group as compared to the control group.

Outcomes

The obvious outcome for an individual with chronic illness would be psychosocial adjustment, with each patient and family appropriately "adjusting" to the roller coaster of challenges that occur on a regular basis. But how should psychosocial adjustment be measured, and might it look different for each individual and family? And again, what about individuals with a terminal chronic illness? Can those individuals experience psychosocial adjustment? There are no answers, just questions.

Has our family adjusted to the fact that my husband, the father of our three children, a grandfather to 12, a brother and a son, has a cancer that is not going to be cured? It's now down to a clinical trial or hospice. Have we "adjusted" to that fact or is adjustment even possible? We are all physically and emotionally exhausted. We just "are," and that is all. The end is near and it's not what any of us thought *could happen 18 months ago. Where did those 18 months go? Did we try to "live" during that time, or were we always responding to the next emergency or complication? I look back at my journal and note the many ups and downs, the days of despair, the days of hope. Regrets, yes; "what ifs," always; "should haves," of course. The life of a patient and family with chronic illness and now that illness is ending with death. I didn't know it was like this.*

—Jenny

Evidence-Based Practice Box

Women with chronic illness in rural parts of the western United States confront multiple challenges, ranging from access to health care to social support. Weinert, Cudney, and Spring designed and implemented a three-phase, computer-based intervention to provide support and health information to middle-aged women with chronic illness. These women all lived in rural areas of the intermountain West. Women to Women (WTW) Phase One included 308 women who participated in either an intervention group or a control group. The intervention group experienced gains in their social support as measured by the Personal Resource Questionnaire-85.

In Phase Two, the overall goal for a revised and more sophisticated telehealth intervention was to enhance the potential for rural chronically ill women to better adapt to their chronic illnesses. During Phase Two, 233 women participated in one of three groups: intense intervention, less-intense intervention, or control. The WTW project targeted psychosocial concepts, such as social support, self-efficacy, self-esteem, empowerment, depression, loneliness, and stress, as indicators of psychosocial adaptation. The intervention had a positive influence on the chosen indicators of adaptation to chronic illness.

Phase Three of the project design includes two groups: a computer intervention group and

(continues)

a control group. Eight cohorts of 40 women (20 intervention and 20 control) are participating. The intervention group participates in an 11-week, computer-based intervention in which they have access 24 hours/day to self-study health teaching units, peer-led virtual support groups, and the Internet. Adaptation variables are measured at baseline, in week 12, and in week 24.

From their work, the authors have created a WTW conceptual model for adaptation to chronic illness. The central theme of the model is that the process of psychosocial adaptation to chronic illness is key to developing self-management skills and achieving an acceptable quality of life.

Source: Weinart, C., Cudney, S., & Spring, A. (2008). Evolution of a conceptual model for adaptation to chronic illness. *Journal of Nursing Scholarship,* 40(4), 364–372

CASE STUDY 3-1

Alice is a 39-year-old mother of two who was recently diagnosed with Stage III breast cancer. She has been married for 15 years to her high school sweetheart. During a breast self-examination in the shower, Alice discovered the lump. Her lumpectomy is complete and she begins chemotherapy next week. She is angry that she has cancer and seems to be taking it out on everyone involved with her care, as well as her husband and children. You are her chemo nurse in the oncology office.

Discussion Questions

1. The goal of psychosocial adjustment at this point in Alice's care does not seem possible. How would you develop trust and a relationship with her?
2. Which small steps could you take that will diffuse Alice's anger and deflect it from her family?
3. How would you assess Alice's psychosocial needs?

CASE STUDY 3-2

Bob, age 59, was diagnosed with multiple sclerosis when he was 35. Until recently, he was able to ambulate with a cane. Following his last exacerbation, during which he was hospitalized briefly, it appears that he will need a walker instead. This has been a real blow to Bob's pride and he rarely uses the walker, preferring to use his cane instead. However, with his cane, he is a definite fall risk. He runs a small business and wonders what his employees and customers will think.

Discussion Questions

1. This is another change, and a downward one, for Bob. He was comfortable with the cane and appeared to be psychosocially adjusted, as evidenced by his optimism, well-being, and self-concept. Now it appears that his adjustment has been derailed. As his usual nurse in the MS clinic at a medical center, how can you intervene to assist Bob?
2. Which framework of practice would be most appropriate to use in working with Bob?

STUDY QUESTIONS

1. Why is adjustment to chronic illness important to the patient and family with chronic illness? Why is it important to the healthcare professional?
2. Describe how different personal resources can affect adjustment.
3. Compare and contrast the key concepts of the frameworks discussed in this chapter. Although these models have been developed by psychologists, what could nursing bring to these models that could be applied to patients and their families?
4. Describe, from your perspective, the role of social support in adjustment, whether it be "perceived" social support or "real" social support.
5. Develop a generic teaching plan that addresses psychosocial adjustment to chronic illness. What are key points that could then be individualized to each patient?

References

Akechi, T., Okuyama, T., Onishi, J., Morita, T., & Furukawa, T. A. (2008). Psychotherapy for depression among incurable cancer patients. *Cochrane Database of Systematic Reviews 2008*, *2*, CD005537. doi: 10.1002/14651858.CD005537.pub2

American Psychological Association. (2013). *Diagnostic and statistical manual of mental disorders V (DSM-V)*. New York, NY: Author.

Bazzazian, S., & Besharat, M. A. (2012). An explanatory model of adjustment to type 1 diabetes based on attachment, coping, and self-regulation theories. *Psychology, Health & Medicine*, *17*(1), 47–58. http://dx.doi.org/10.1080/13548506.2011.575168

Bennett, J. A., Perrin, N. A., Hanson, G., Bennett, D., Gaynor, W., Flaherty-Robb, M., ... Potempa, K. (2005). Health aging demonstration project: Nurse coaching for behavior change in older adults. *Research in Nursing and Health*, *28*(3), 187–197.

Benyamini, Y. (2011). Health and illness perceptions. In H. S. Friedman (Ed.), *The Oxford handbook of health psychology* (pp. 280–293). Oxford, UK: Oxford University Press.

Boinon, D., Sultan, S., Charles, C., Stulz, A., Guillemeau, C., Delaloge, S., & Dauchy, S. (2014). Changes in psychological adjustment over the course of treatment for breast cancer: The predictive role of social sharing and social support. *Psycho-Oncology*, *23*(3), 291-8. doi: 10.1002/pon.3420

Brandes, K., & Mullan, B. (2013). Can the common-sense model predict adherence in critically ill patients: A meta-analysis. *Health Psychology Review*. doi: 10.1080/17437199.2013.820986

Breland, J., McAndrew, L. M., Burns, E., Leventhal, E., & Leventhal, H. (2013). Using the common sense model of self-regulation to review the effects of self-monitoring of blood glucose on glycemic control for non-insulin treated adults with type 2 diabetes. *Diabetes Educator*, *39*(4), 541–559. doi: 10.1177/0145721713400079

Brodie, D. A., Inoue, A., & Shaw, D. G. (2008). Motivational interviewing to change quality of life for people with chronic heart failure: A randomized controlled trial. *International Journal of Nursing Studies*, *45*(4), 489–500.

Caplan, G. (1964). *Principles of preventive psychiatry*. New York, NY: Basic Books.

Carver, C. S., Lechner, S. C., & Antoni, M. H. (2009). Challenges in studying positive change after adversity: Illustrations from research on breast cancer. In C. L. Park, S. C. Lechner, M. H. Antoni, & A. L. Stanton (Eds.), *Medical illness and positive life change: Can crisis lead to personal transformation* (pp. 51–62). Washington, DC: American Psychological Association.

Chilcot, J. (2012). The importance of illness perception in end-stage renal disease: Associations with psychosocial and clinical outcomes. *Seminars in Dialysis*, *25*(1), 59–64.

Coleman, K., Austin, B. T., Brach, C., & Wagner, E. H. (2009) Evidence on the chronic care model in the new millennium. *Health Affairs*, *28*(1), 75–85.

Dart, M. (2011). *Motivational interviewing in nursing practice: Empowering the patient*. Sudbury, MA: Jones and Bartlett.

Davison, S. N., & Jhangri, G. S. (2013). The relationship between spirituality, psychosocial adjustment to illness, and health-related quality of life in patients with advanced kidney disease. *Journal of Pain and Symptom Management, 45*(2), 170–178. http://dx.doi.org/10.1016/j.jpainsymman.2012.02.019

De la Torre-Diez, I., Diaz-Pernas, F. J., & Anton-Rodriguez, M. (2012). A content analysis of chronic diseases social groups on Facebook and Twitter. *Telemedicine and e-Health, 18*(6), 404–408.

deRidder, D., Geenen, R., Kuijer, R., & van Middendorp, H. (2008). Psychological adjustment to chronic disease. *Lancet, 372*, 246–254.

Dibb, B., & Yardley, L. (2006). How does social comparison within a self-help group influence adjustment to chronic illness? A longitudinal study. *Social Science & Medicine, 63*, 1602–1613.

Duggleby, W., Hicks, D., Nekolaichuk, C., Holstslander, L., Williams, A., Chambers, T., & Eby, J. (2012). Hope, older adults, and chronic illness: A metasynthesis of qualitative research. *Journal of Advanced Nursing, 68*(6), 1211–1223. doi: 10.1111/j.1365-2648.2011.05919.x

Engle, G. (1977). The need for a new medical model: A challenge for biomedicine. *Science, 196*, 129–136.

Engle, G. (1980). The clinical application of the biopsychosocial model. *American Journal of Psychiatry, 137*, 535–544.

Fife, B. (1994). The conceptualization of meaning in illness. *Social Science & Medicine, 38*(2), 309–316.

Folkman, S., & Moskowitz, J. T. (2004). Coping: Pitfalls and promise. *Annual Review of Psychology, 55*, 45–774.

Foster, G., Taylor, S. J. C., Eldridge, S., Ramsay, J., & Griffiths C. J. (2007). Self-management programmes by lay leaders for people with chronic conditions. *Cochrane Database of Systematic Reviews 2007, 4*, CD005108. doi: 10.1002/14651858.CD005108.pub2

Freeth, R. (2007). Working within the medical model. *Healthcare Counseling & Psychotherapy Journal, 7*(4), 3–7.

French, D. P., Wade, A. N., & Farmer, A. J. (2013). Predicting self-care behavior of patients with type 2 diabetes: The importance of beliefs about behavior, not just beliefs about illness. *Journal of Psychosomatic Research, 74*(4), 327–333.

Hagger, M. S., & Orbell, S. (2003). A meta-analytic review of the common-sense model of illness representations. *Psychology and Health, 18*, 141–184.

Hefferon, K., Grealy, M., & Mutrie, N. (2009). Post-traumatic growth and life threatening physical illness: A systematic review of the qualitative literature. *British Journal of Health Psychology, 14*, 343–378. doi: 10.1348/135910708X332936

Hoyt, M. A., & Stanton, A. L. (2012). Adjustment to chronic illness. In A. Baum, T. A. Revenson, & J. Singer (Eds.), *Handbook of health psychology* (2nd ed., pp. 219–246). New York, NY: Psychology Press.

Hundt, N. E., Bensadon, B. A., Stanley, M. A., Petersen, N. J., Kunik, M. E., Kauth, M. R., & Cully, J. A. (2013). Coping mediates the relationship between disease severity and illness intrusiveness among chronically ill patients. *Journal of Health Psychology, 0*(0), 1–10. doi: 10.1177/1359105313509845

Jensen, M. P., Moore, M. R., Bockow, T. R., Ehde, D. M., & Engel, J. M. (2011). Psychosocial factors and adjustment to chronic pain in persons with physical disabilities: A systematic review. *Archives of Physical Medicine and Rehabilitation, 92*, 146–160. doi: 10.1016/j.apmr.2010.09.021

Lazarus, R. S. (1966). *Psychological stress and the coping process*. New York, NY: McGraw-Hill.

Lazarus, R. S., & Folkman, S. (1984). *Stress, appraisal and coping*. New York, NY: Springer.

Lee, V., Cohen, S. R., Edgar, L., Laizner, A. M., & Gagnon, A. J. (2006). Meaning-making intervention during breast or colorectal cancer treatment improves self-esteem, optimism, and self-efficacy. *Social Science & Medicine, 62*, 3133–3145. doi: 10.1016/j.socscimed.2005.11.041

Leventhal, H., Bodnar-Deren, S., Breland, J., Hash-Converse, J., Phillips, L., Leventhal, E., & Cameron, L. (2012). Modeling health and illness behavior. In A. Baum, T. Revenson, & J. Singer (Eds.), *Handbook of health psychology* (2nd ed., pp. 3–35). New York, NY: Psychology Press.

Lorig, K., & Holman, H. (2003). Self-management education: History, definition, outcomes, and mechanisms. *Annals of Behavioral Medicine, 26*(1), 1–7.

Marcano Belisario, J. S., Huckvale, K., Greenfield, G., Car, J., & Gunn, L. H. (2013). Smartphone and tablet self-management apps for asthma (intervention review). *Cochran Database of Systematic Reviews, 11*, CD010013. doi: 10.1002/14651858.CD010013.pub2

McAndrew, L. M., Musumeci-Szabo, T. J., Mora, P. A., Vileikyte, L….. Leventhal, H. (2008). Using the common sense model to design interventions for the prevention and management of chronic illness threats: From description to process. *British Journal of Health Psychology, 13*, 195–204.

McCorkle, R., Ercolano, S., Lazenby, M., Schulman-Green, D., Schilling, L. S., Lorig, K., & Wagner, E. H. (2011). Self-management: Enabling and empowering patients living with cancer as a chronic illness. *CA: A Cancer Journal for Clinicians, 61*(1), 50–62.

Miller, W. R., & Rollnick, S. (1991). *Motivational interviewing: Preparing people to change addictive behavior.* New York, NY: Guilford Press.

Mirowsky, J., & Ross, C. (2002). Measurement for a human science. *Journal of Health and Social Behavior, 43*, 152–170.

Murray, E., Burns, J., See Tai, S., Lai, R., & Nazareth, I. (2005). Interactive health communication applications for people with chronic disease (intervention review). *Cochrane Database of Systematic Reviews 2005, 4*, CD004274. doi: 10.1002/14651858.CD004274.pub5

Mustafa, M., Carson-Stevens, A., Gillespie, D., & Edwards, A. G. K. (2013). Psychological interventions for women with metastatic breast cancer. *Cochrane Database of Systematic Reviews 2013, 6*, CD004253. doi: 10.1002/14651858.CD004253.pub4

Pak, K., Eastwood, S. V., Michie, S., Farmer, A. J., Barnar, M. L., Peacock, R., ... Murray, E. (2013). Computer-based diabetes self-management interventions for adults with type 2 diabetes mellitus. *Cochrane Database of Systematic Reviews 2013, 3*, CD008776. doi: 10.1002/14651858.CD008776.pub2

Pakenham, K. I. (2007). Making sense of multiple sclerosis. *Rehabilitation Psychology, 52*(4), 380–389.

Pakenham, K. I., & Cox, S. (2009). The dimensional structure of benefit finding in multiple sclerosis and relations with positive and negative adjustment: A longitudinal study. *Psychology and Health, 24*(4), 373–393. doi: 10.1080/08870440701832592

Parahoo, K., McDonough, S., McCaughan, E., Noyes, J., Semple, C., Halstead, E. J., ... Dahm, P. (2013). Psychosocial interventions for men with prostate cancer. *Cochrane Database of Systematic Reviews 2013, 12*, CD008529. doi: 10.1002/14651858.CD008529.pub3

Park, C. L. (2009). Overview of theoretical perspectives. In C. L. Park, S. C. Lechner, M. H. Antoni, & M. L. Stanton (Eds.). *Medical illness and positive life change: Can crisis lead to personal transformation* (pp. 11–30). Washington, DC: American Psychological Association.

Park, C. L., Lechner, S. C., Antoni, M. H., & Stanton, M. L. (Eds.). (2009). *Medical illness and positive life change: Can crisis lead to personal transformation.* Washington, DC: American Psychological Association.

Parry, M., & Watt-Watson, J. (2010). Peer support intervention trials for individuals with heart disease: A systematic review. *European Journal of Cardiovascular Nursing, 9*, 57–67. doi: 10.1016/j.ejcnurse.2009.10.002

Pasricha, A., Deinstadt, R., Moher, D., Killoran, A., Rourke, S., & Kendall, C. (2012). Chronic care model decision support and clinical information systems interventions for people living with HIV: A systematic review. *Journal of General Internal Medicine 28*(1), 127–135.

Robert Wood Johnson Foundation. (2006–2011). Improving chronic illness care. http://www.improvingchroniccare.org/index.php?p=About_US&s=6

Rollnick, S., Miller, W. R., & Butler, C. C. (2008). *Motivational interviewing in health care: Helping patients change behavior.* New York, NY: Guilford Press

Sharpe, L., & Curran, L. (2006). Understanding the process of adjustment to illness. *Social Science & Medicine, 62*, 1153–1166.

Snell, D. L., Hay-Smith, E. J. C., Surgenor, L. J., & Siegert, R. J. (2013). Explanation of outcomes after mild traumatic brain injury: The contribution of injury belief and Leventhal's common sense model. *Neuropsychological Rehabilitation: An International Journal, 23*(3), 333–362. doi: 10.1080.09658521 1.2012.758419

Solomon, D. H., Iversen, M. D., Avorn, J., Gleeson, T., Brookhart, M. A., Patrick, A. R., ... Katz, J. N. (2012). Osteoporosis telephonic intervention to improve medication regimen adherence: A large pragmatic randomized controlled trial. *Archives of Internal Medicine, 172*(6), 477–483.

Stanton, A. L., & Revenson, T. A. (2007). Adjustment to chronic disease: Progress and promise in research. In H. S. Friedman & R. C. Silver (Eds.), *Foundations of health psychology* (pp. 203–233). New York, NY: Oxford University Press.

Stellefson, M., Dipnarine, K., & Stopka, C. (2013). The chronic care model and diabetes management in U.S. primary care settings: A systematic review. *Preventing Chronic Disease, 10*, 120180. doi: http://dx.doi.org/10.5888/pcd10.120180.

Strom, J. L., & Egede, L. E. (2012). The impact of social support on outcomes in adult patients with type 2 diabetes: A systematic review. *Current Diabetes Reports, 12*, 769–781.

Stuifbergen, A. K., Morris, M., Jung, J. H., Pierini, D., & Morgan, S. (2010). Benefits of wellness interventions for persons with chronic and disabling conditions: A review of the evidence. *Disability and Health Journal, 3*, 133–145. doi: 10.1016/j.dhjo.2009.10.007

Suls, J. M., Krantz, D. S., & Williams, G. C. (2013). Three strategies for bridging different levels of analysis and embracing the biopsychosocial model. *Health Psychology, 32*(5), 597–601.

Suls, J. M., Luger, T., & Martin, R. (2010). The biopsychosocial model and the use of theory in health psychology. In J. M. Suls, K. W. Davidson, & R. M. Kaplan (Eds.), *Handbook of health psychology and behavioral medicine* (pp. 15–27). New York, NY: Guilford Press

Swendeman, D., Ingram, B. L., & Rotheram-Borus, M. J. (2009). Common elements in self-management of HIV and other chronic Illnesses: An integrative framework. *AIDS Care, 21*(10), 1321–1334.

Visotsky, H. M., Hamburg, D. A., Goss, M. E., & Lebovits, B. Z. (1961). Coping behavior under extreme stress: Observations of patients with severe poliomyelitis. *Archives of General Psychiatry, 5*, 27–52.

Wagner, E. H. (1998). Chronic disease management: What will it take to improve care for chronic illness? *Effective Clinical Practice, 1*, 2–4.

Wagner, E. H., Austin, B. T., Davis, C., Hindmarch, M., Schafer, J., & Bonomi, A. (2001). Improving chronic illness care: Translating evidence into action. *Health Affairs, 20*(6), 64–78.

Waisbond, S. (2007). Beyond the medical-informational model: Recasting the role of communication in tuberculosis control. *Social Science & Medicine, 65*(10), 2130–2134.

Weinert, C., Cudney, S., Comstock, B., & Bansal, A. (2011). Computer intervention impact on psychosocial adaptation of rural women with chronic conditions. *Nursing Research, 60*(2), 82–91. doi: 10.1097/NNR.0b013e3181ffbcf2

Weinert, C., Cudney, S., & Spring, A. (2008). Evolution of a conceptual model for adaptation to chronic illness. *Journal of Nursing Scholarship, 40*(4), 364–372.

Wise, M., & Marchand, L. (2013). Living fully in the shadow of mortal time: Psychosocial assets in advanced cancer. *Journal of Palliative Care, 29*(2), 76–82.

Zautra, A. J., Hall, J. S., & Murray, K. E. (2010). Resilience: A new definition of health for people and communities. In J. W. Reich, A. J. Zautra, & J. S. Hall (Eds.), *Handbook of adult resilience* (pp. 3–29). New York, NY: Guilford Press.

Chapter 4

Loss

Pamala D. Larsen

It (chronic illness) is a world unto itself, and we who find ourselves there discover that the usual resources for coping are sorely tried. We long to hear from someone who speaks from within personal experience and describes what it is really like to have cancer, to lose a leg, to become blind, or to feel the mind spinning out of control. We long to hear from someone who admits that even enormous love from others does not ease the essential loneliness of illness. We want to hear not clichés but an acknowledgment that illness is not simply an opportunity for personal growth but a soul-wrenching encounter with loss, limitation, and the reality of death. We want to hear from someone who does not go gently into that dark night.

Conway, K, 2007, *Illness and the limits of expression*, p. 2

This chapter examines concepts of loss that are only briefly covered in other chapters. Although they do not merit a stand-alone chapter, these concepts are of critical importance to the patient, family, and healthcare professional. For the losses described in this chapter, there are no simple interventions, nursing or otherwise. Perhaps, this author suggests, mindful presence and listening are the two most important strategies that a healthcare professional might provide for a patient and family in any stage of a chronic illness.

As a person ages, he or she experiences other losses along the way that are distinct from chronic illness, but further compound the losses from chronic illness. Losses such as the death of friends and family members are powerful reminders of the fragility of life. This author remembers her grandparents at ages 89 and 93 with tears in their eyes, talking about their long-dead friends and relatives, and lives that were no more.

When young, that person sees himself or herself as immortal, and thoughts of loss are far, far away. The young individual's world revolves around self. Chronic disease happens to older adults, not us. Moreover, it is not until we have more life experiences that other thoughts enter our minds.

Having a chronic illness means more than "learning to live with it." Life becomes a struggle to maintain control over the defining images of self and one's life. Meanings of self and illness change as the disease progresses or recedes. Experiencing chronic illness may result in an individual's self-concept being tied to the past, present, or future. Time plays a central, albeit hidden, role in shaping self-concept (Charmaz, 1991, p. 229). Life may be going smoothly, but getting "bad news" may catapult one into a crisis. An exacerbation turns a "good day" into a "bad one" and creates a new, distinct reality with its own rules, rhythm, and tempo (p. 4).

63

How can we "help" the patient and family through their lived experience of chronic illness? Certainly, the desire to help is there; after all, nursing is a helping profession—and isn't that what nurses are supposed to do? But is it really that simple? Perhaps the best we can do for the patient and family is to "be there" with them and listen—not talk, but listen, hold their hand, and be mindfully attentive.

Introduction

Everyone loves the story of an individual who triumphs over an illness, is saved from the throes of death, and returns to a normal life. The media delight in telling such stories. Just think about the aftermath of the bombing at the 2013 Boston Marathon. Stories poured forth in the print media and on television about those who had triumphed over their injuries. Losing limbs was a common injury in the bombing attack, and this author remembers a national talk show that featured six or seven young women who had each lost at least one limb. The program described how they had risen above despair and triumphed over their injuries. These stories were meant to offer hope and provide inspiration to those with a chronic injury or disease. "Yes, it can be done" is what these individuals were telling others.

For many, these stories of triumph are inspirational, and the individuals serve as role models for others. Others, however, continue struggling to come to terms with their disease, their losses, their limitations, or even an early death. These individuals feel themselves unraveling, losing control, falling apart, or fearing that they are losing their mind. The stories of triumph gloss over the details of the beginning and continuing difficulties with the chronic condition. Voices of triumph dispel other thoughts.

As a culture, we hide suffering. By keeping the ill, elderly, disabled, and dying out of view, we manage to keep the story of the damaged body, physical weakness, or limitation at arm's length (Conway, 2007, p. 18). We put a positive spin on everything. We endlessly celebrate "survivors," but ignore the contributions of those who did not survive. In the play *Wit*, by Margaret Edson, the primary character is a professor of English literature who is hospitalized for terminal ovarian cancer.

The play opens with the main character saying to the audience, "Hi, how are you feeling today? Great. That's just great." Mimicking the greeting of those who enter her room all day, she alerts the audience to the absurdity of this question, with its call for cheeriness in her dire situation. She goes on to say, "I have been asked, 'How are you feeling today' while I was throwing up into a plastic washbasin. I have been asked as I was emerging from a four hour operation with a tube in every orifice, 'How are you feeling today.'" Finally, she states, "I am waiting for the moment when someone asks me this question and I am dead." (Cited in Conway, 2007, pp. 9–10)

Does this excerpt sound familiar? Would it be something that you would ask a patient? Is that how we, as professional caregivers, act and are perceived by others?

Randy's nurse enters his room. How is Randy doing, the nurse asks. Doesn't he see Randy throwing up green bile crap continuously in the emesis basin? Doesn't he remember that 15 minutes ago when he was in the room, he asked the same question while Randy vomited? Why do I have to answer a stupid, rhetorical question for my husband? Why doesn't this nurse "get" what is going on?

—Jenny

We find it difficult as professional caregivers to comfort those who are suffering. We ask inappropriate questions because we do not know what else to do. We think we have to talk, that silence is not welcome. We are uncomfortable. We want triumph over disease, not suffering.

In *The Illness Narratives*, Kleinman (1988) writes about an experience with a young child.

He relates a story from his early days as a medical student, trying to comfort a 7-year-old girl with severe burns. The daily removal of dressings and dead tissue brought continual screaming from the child. Kleinman tried desperately to distract the child, but nothing worked. One day during a dressing change, he did something completely different. He asked her directly, "Describe what you are going through to me; tell me what is going on in your mind while this happens, what are you feeling." The screaming stopped, and the child began to talk (p. x).

Self

Bury's (1982) classic work on chronic illness as a biographical disruption is a seminal article in medical sociology. Bury's contention was that illness, and especially chronic illness, is the kind of experience where the structures of everyday life and the forms of knowledge that underpin them are disrupted; it involves a recognition of the worlds of pain and suffering, and brings individuals, their families, and wider social networks face to face with the character of their relationships in stark form, disrupting normal rules of reciprocity and mutual support (Bury, 1982, p. 169). Bury refers to the biographical disruption as a one-time event; however, in chronic illness, many events disrupt one's life.

Charmaz (1991) built on the work of Bury by calling chronic illness an interruption. Having a chronic illness means more than "learning to live with it"; it means struggling to maintain control over the defining images of self and one's life (p. 13). Charmaz (1983) coined the phrase "loss of self" with her research in the 1980s, interviewing individuals with chronic illness through a symbolic interactionist perspective. The chronic condition(s) and the illness experience are influences on loss of self. Charmaz (1983) describes the illness experiences of patients as living a restricted life, experiencing social isolation, being discredited, and burdening others. Slowly, the individual with chronic illness feels his or her self-image disappear; this loss of self occurs without the development of an equally valued new one (p. 168).

In a later study of 40 men with chronic illness, Charmaz (1994) describes different identity dilemmas than she observed with women. Charmaz sees these men as "preserving self." As men come to terms with illness and disability, they preserve self by limiting the effects of illness in their lives. They intensify control over their lives. Many assume that they can recapture their past self, and they try to do so. They may devote vast amounts of energy to keeping their illness contained and the disability invisible to maintain their masculinity. At the same time, they often maintain another identity at home—thus creating the duality of a public identity and a private identity in an attempt to preserve self (Charmaz, 1994, p. 282).

Larsson and Grassman (2012) tested concepts from both Bury's and Charmaz's work as they tried to determine, in their qualitative study of adults who had been visually impaired for a significant number of years, whether a biographical disruption was a one-time event, whether it occurs repeatedly, or whether chronic illness may be accepted as a biographically anticipated "normal illness," particularly for those who have experienced a chronic condition for a long period of time (Williams, 2000). Larsson and Grassman's conclusion was that biographical disruptions occur repeatedly over the lifespan in individuals with chronic illness and disabilities and that illness changes do not necessarily have to be wholly unexpected to be experienced as disruptive (p. 1167).

In a qualitative study of Chinese immigrant women in Canada, Anderson (1991) describes how women diagnosed with type 1 diabetes have a devalued self, not only from the disease itself but also because of the experience of being marginalized in a foreign country where they do not speak the language. In a phenomenon similar to the "loss of self" described by Charmaz, these women need to reconstruct a new self.

According to Anderson, influencing this devalued self were the women's interactions with healthcare professionals, which were frequently negative in nature, adding to their stress.

Similarly, eight older women with a chronic disease were asked to describe the meaning of living with a long-term illness. Five themes emerged: loss and uncertainty, learning one's capacity and living accordingly, maintaining fellowship and belonging, having a source of strength, and building anew. However, clearly the guiding premise of each woman was that chronic illness brought about reassessment and formation of a new understanding of self, and a sense of being revalued by the world (Lundman & Jansson, 2007).

Time

Often patients and families compartmentalize their lives, perhaps as a way to view the illness in another context. The idea is to separate the illness from one's other life—that is, the former life, the normal life. There may be no particular reason why, but mostly the patient and family want to distance themselves from the illness experience. One begins to refer to the chronic illness as "before" and "after"—for example, before the cancer was diagnosed and after the diagnosis. All life events are focused on "before" and "after," by saying, for instance, "it was the Christmas after he was diagnosed" or "preschool graduation was before she was diagnosed." Patients and families want to clearly delineate which part of life–that is, which time—is being referred to. For others, this separation later becomes "before death" and "after death." It is the survivors' way of measuring time. There are two separate and distinct parts of one's life, "before" and "after": "before," when life was normal, and now "after," when one has to seek a new normal.

Author Randy Shilts also referred to the AIDS epidemic as "before" and "after." The epidemic would cleave lives into two. "Before" meant innocence (Shilts, 1987, p. 12).

Work

American culture often defines and identifies individuals based on their occupation. At a social gathering, you are asked, "What do you do for a living? Where do you work?" Such inquiries are an easy way to start a conversation between strangers. With disability and chronic disease, however, there are no easy answers to those questions. You stammer and stutter and finally say, "I retired early because of my COPD." Work occupies a central place in the lives of most people, and most adults experience this part of their lives through paid employment. Paid employment gives us social identity.

It is difficult to know how many individuals with chronic disease or injury have to leave employment every year. Nearly all people whose work lives are affected by a serious illness—whether acute, chronic, or terminal—face common issues: the centrality of work in their lives; the uncertainty of how illness will affect their future and how to negotiate the necessary steps, which involve disclosing their illness; and deciding whether to stay at work, take a leave of absence, or leave completely (Walker, 2010, p. 630). Leaving work because of the onset or progression of a chronic illness has an enormous impact on a person's life. Apart from the obvious effect on income, some of this importance may be explained through the changed identity that results from the end of an individual's work life. When a person retires, it is presumed that his or her social identity changes. However, leaving a job because of illness is an involuntary action and is often accompanied by an unwanted social identity (p. 633).

With respect to employment status, adults younger than 65 years of age with a history of cancer plus heart disease are less likely to be employed in the past 12 months compared with individuals without a history of cancer or heart disease. Statistics are similar for adults with diabetes (Dowling et al., 2013). Consistent with other studies, Dowling and colleagues observed that employment, lost productivity, and burden of illness varied substantially across subgroups of cancer survivors. As might be expected, survivors who had cancers associated with short survival, or who had multiple cancers, consistently experienced the highest levels of burden compared with individuals with other single-site cancers (p. 3397).

Touch

The sense of touch provides a powerful means of eliciting and modulating human emotion. We use touch to share our feelings with others and to enhance the meaning of other forms of verbal and nonverbal communication (Gallace & Spence, 2010, p. 247). In premature infants, research supports the use of touch as a nursing intervention to stimulate an infant's neurologic system. Some touch may be associated with procedures, while other touch is comforting in nature (Smith, 2012). Similarly, there is research that supports the use of "gentle human touch" as an intervention with premature infants to reduce the physiologic effects of pain, increased respiratory rate, increased heart rate, and crying during heel stick procedures (Herrington & Chiodo, 2014).

Although various definitions of touch exist, Estabrooks's (1989) identification of the three types of touch best describes the touch related to nursing. These three types of touch include caring touch, protective touch, and task touch. For the purposes of this chapter, the focus is on caring touch, which implies an emotional and physically robust nurse's capacity to care about others, with or without reciprocal response from the client receiving touch (Bush, 2001). Research points to the fact that the experience of touch is laden with psychosocial as well as physiological implications (p. 257).

There is little discussion about the need for touch in those who are ill, disabled, or elderly. Interestingly, though, touch deprivation is particularly profound among older adults, with that group of individuals being the most likely to receive only minimal amounts of touch (as cited in Bush, 2001). Older adults with multiple comorbidities, families who live far away, and friends who have died or who can no longer visit due to their own health issues have little caring touch in their lives when they need it the most. Task touch remains, but the intent of task touch and that of caring touch are far different. Now that the older adult's body aches and is "full" of chronic illness, there may be no caring touch or someone to sit quietly at a bedside with mindful presence and hold hands, gently. Also, sometimes the body aches too much because of disease, and caring touch becomes difficult, if not impossible.

> *I want so badly to hug Randy, but even when I am careful, he winces with pain. The cancer has taken over his body and everything hurts and aches. I gently try to massage his back with lotion, but it is difficult because his ribs are so exposed. I long to touch him, and I know that he longs to be touched, his eyes tell me that, but it is painful, so I hold his hands gently instead.*
>
> —Jenny

Death

There are times in chronic illness when an individual feels a sense of alienation from the body, perhaps because intellectually he or she is trying to protect his- or herself from an awareness of loss (Conway, 2007, p. 50). Physical damage may restrict a person's functioning, dominate his or her thoughts, and profoundly alter the experience of loss. Conway refers to this condition as the damaged self.

When a person is actually near death, it becomes impossible to preserve the self. The self is reduced, or perhaps gives way to a dying body. "The human form had seemed to pulsate, like a fist opening and closing, moving back and forth from strength to weakness.... the way the body would open as if into a palm, vulnerable, extended, and then reform into the fist in search of survival. Then, at some point, the fist would not reform itself, and the pulsating would stop. There is no self, only the body gasping out its last breath" (as cited in Conway, 2007, pp. 54–55).

There is little focus in this text on death from chronic illness; however, it is a reality for many patients and families. Death of a loved one frequently means the loss of an attachment figure, a person to whom one has had and still has a deeply significant emotional bond (Stroebe, 2011, p. 149). Tie and Poulsen (2013) view terminal illness as a threat to attachment bonds. Given the demands on both the healthy and sick partner dealing with a terminal illness, there is a high potential for adjustment injury.

Randy started to withdraw from me in July of 2011. The long weeks in the hospital, the code blue, the ARDS, the everything, took a great deal from him. Perhaps he could already foresee the future and know that his time was shorter than either of us expected. I don't know. And it is only now, looking back nearly two years after his death, that I can clearly see his withdrawal and the change in his demeanor. He wasn't the same anymore.

—Jenny

Permanent separation brings with it a myriad of reactions, such as despair, loneliness, hurt, and anger. The "why" questions come fast and furious. Why him or her? Why now? Why was Joe down the street cured of his disease and my spouse was not? Why did I not get a chance to say goodbye? Why did she have to suffer so much and then die? And then comes the fairness issue—"It's not fair." And then you realize, again, that life is not fair and never has been.

The day we knew would come came yesterday. The pain in Randy's chest is more cancer. There are only two choices: a clinical trial or hospice. It was Randy's decision that he not be in a clinical trial, saying that he knew the results would help someone, but he was tired and didn't want to do this anymore. (Larsen, 2013, p. 42)

The experience of dying involves the ultimate confrontation with the limits of language. How does a person describe this experience—dying from a chronic condition? How does a person describe the suffering he or she might have? When death is expected and the physical pain is not severe, then individuals can think and perhaps describe their feelings of dying. However, for many, the pain may be intense even with medication, or perhaps medication is given for sedation and, with decreased cognitive function, speech becomes difficult.

Our cemetery plots are purchased. I had visited the cemetery a couple of weeks ago by myself, but I needed to make a final decision, and Randy wanted to go with me this time. I hate the names that cemeteries give certain areas. The Garden of Tranquility. We both have little twenty-by-twenty plots for our ashes.... With esophageal cancer you know that death is a common outcome, but somehow you think you'll be different. You'll win the fight against cancer; you will be the miracle. But it turns out it isn't you. Maybe it's someone else, or no one. (Larsen, 2013, p. 49)

Klass, Silverman, and Nickman (1996) describe the importance of continuing the relationship with a deceased loved one as the more heavily weighted work in grief and challenges the age-old concept that disengaging from the loved one is a function of grief and mourning. If freed from a prior relationship with a deceased loved one, it is thought, then the survivor would be free and able to engage in new relationships.

However, Klass and colleagues (1996) view a continuing relationship with the deceased as a resource for enriching functioning in the present. The relationship with the deceased may help the bereaved prepare for or enrich any new relationships in which the survivor becomes involved (as cited in Walter & McCoyd, 2009, p. 329). The relationship with the deceased is still there, but evolves into a different relationship over time.

It has been two years since Randy's death from cancer, {and a} marriage that spanned 43 years plus the four years prior to that when we were a couple. I look back and can't believe that so much time has passed since his death. What have I been doing? I look at my journal to see where I've "been." Frankly, sometimes I don't remember. I've finally established a "new" normal that doesn't include Randy. "Randy thoughts" continue, but it is harder now to imagine him being with me. I see that as a blessing in disguise. And now, I've met someone else whom I care for deeply. Pretty amazing at age 66, but it has happened. So how do Randy and my "significant other" both share time with me, and what about the guilt I feel knowing that I have found someone else? It's difficult at best, but I know that Randy will always be a part of my new life, a ghost from the past, the father of my three children and grandfather to 12. He is always with me, and I will love him forever, but in a different way than I have in the past. A new normal awaits me if I allow it to happen.

—Jenny

Pruchno, Cartwright, and Wilson-Genderson (2009) developed two alternative hypotheses to explain how mental health fares in the transition from caregiving to widowhood. The first hypothesis, based on stress and coping theory, posits that people who experience greater strain while the spouse is alive will experience greater difficulty following the death. The second hypothesis suggests that greater strain during caregiving will result in better post-death outcomes, as the survivor experiences a sense of relief when the partner dies (p. 808).

In Pruchno and colleagues' study, the variable of interest was the quality of the marital relationship prior to death, expressed as "marital closeness" in this study. In a longitudinal, prospective study that included 315 couples in which one partner was experiencing end-stage renal disease (ESRD), individuals reporting closer predeath marital relationships (marital closeness) experienced more intense grief and less relief following the death of their spouse (p. 815).

Chronic Sorrow

The concept of chronic sorrow was first described by Olshansky in 1962 when he was working with parents of children with mental challenges. His conclusion was that chronic sorrow was a natural response to a tragedy instead of becoming neurotic (p. 193). The essence of chronic sorrow is a painful discrepancy between what is perceived as reality and what continues to be dreamed of (Roose, 2002). The loss is a living loss; it is about living with the realization that the loss cannot be removed and requires energy for adaptation (p. 26).

Two studies discuss the existence of chronic sorrow in individuals with chronic illness. Sixty-one patients with multiple sclerosis were interviewed about chronic sorrow and also screened for depression. Of the 61 patients, 38 met the criteria for chronic sorrow. The participants in the study described feeling sorrow, fear, anger, and anxiety. Frustration and sadness were constantly present or were periodically overwhelming (Isaksson, Gunnarsson, & Ahlstrom, 2007, p. 318). The researchers identified seven themes: loss of hope, loss of control over the body, loss of integrity and dignity, loss of a healthy identity, loss of faith that life is just, loss of social relations, and loss of freedom (Isaksson et al., 2007). Implications for healthcare professionals include providing psychological support for these individuals. But how does one provide the appropriate help when the patient perceives such significant losses? Is it even realistic to think that healthcare professionals can do so?

Ahlstrom (2007) interviewed 30 working-age adults with an average disease duration of 18 years. Of these adults, 16 experienced chronic sorrow, defined as recurring losses. The losses in this study were consistent with the findings of other studies on chronic sorrow, even though the group was heterogeneous regarding diagnosis.

Responses to Loss

Transcending Loss

Charmaz (1991) discussed transcendence of loss in her book *Good Days, Bad Days: The Self in Chronic Illness and Time*. Both loss and transcendence emerge from the experience of illness and the different meanings that patients and families assign to those terms. Transcendence of self encompasses more than one's body and much more than an illness. Thus, illness does not fill or flood the self, even though it may fill and flood the illness experience. Transcendence implies self-acceptance, rather than any acceptance of illness cloaked in stigmatized images and expectations of resignation (p. 258). However, neither loss nor transcendence is a static point in time of an illness. Individuals experience both, albeit at different times in their illness.

Although grief is a natural reaction to the loss of anything perceived as having value, grief research has primarily focused on death and bereavement (Brion, Menke, & Kimball, 2013). Brion and colleagues, for example, studied persons who were newly diagnosed with HIV and were experiencing the diagnosis as a traumatic loss and the grief that accompanies that loss.

Perhaps there is a middle path between coping methods that overemphasize active confrontation of negative emotions and those that reinforce avoidance. The middle path is *self-compassion*. Neff (2003) identified three dimensions of self-compassion: (1) self-kindness rather than self-judgment, (2) recognition of shared humanity rather than isolation, and (3) mindfulness (holding painful thoughts and feelings in balanced awareness rather than over-identifying with or avoiding them). Brion et al. (2013) suggest that grief work and the development of

self-compassion may help individuals transcend the negative self-judgments, shame, and self-blame associated with HIV-related grief and stigma. This *transcendence* may allow an individual to turn from unhealthy coping behaviors and engage more fully with treatment (p. 515).

Creation of a New Identity

Individuals with chronic disease often create a new identity that includes the losses associated with their disease. Individuals may regulate a more positive self-image if they reformulate their "new and revised" self-concept so that it is compatible with the limitations of the illness (Gois et al., 2012, p. S34). Restructuring of self to maintain self-integrity and self-regulation is a systematic human tendency to preserve stable and positive self-views when a self-devaluation threat (e.g., chronic disease) occurs.

Creating a new identity is anxiety producing and uncomfortable. It is not that the individual wants to change identities, but rather chronic illness, like a thief in the night, has taken away part of one's self. The old life had a somewhat predictable routine that may have included work, family, social events, volunteer activities, and other events. Now the routine includes a medical regimen that is time intensive and may be painful. Doctor appointments invade private time. With chronic illness, both physical and psychosocial losses occur. The new life is no longer "your" life, so the individual looks for other ways to reinvent the self. Honest questions to oneself may include: Do I still have value? Can I still make a difference in some way? Do others still value me? How do I turn lemons into lemonade?

Readers will notice that this chapter does not offer up any interventions to help an individual create a new identity. For each of us, losses of chronic illness may affect us differently and, in turn, the ways in which we approach creation of a new identity are different. This is similar to the grief experienced after death of a loved one. There is no path through grief, and each of us has to find our own way. Perhaps we wend our way with the help of professional guidance, supportive friends, new activities in one's life, and so forth—but the fact remains that grief is a solitary journey.

The Process of Integration

Whittemore and Dixon (2008) refer to a process of integration that occurs in individuals with chronic illness. Integration represents the process undertaken by an individual to achieve a sense of balance in self-managing a chronic illness and living a personally meaningful life (p. 177). Results from past theoretical and empirical work (Fleury, 1991; Hernandez, 1995; Medich, Stuart, & Chase, 1997; Whittemore Chase, Mandle, & Roy, 2002) suggest that the process of integration may be an important aspect of adjusting to and living with the losses of chronic illness.

The process of integration is complex and multifactorial, as suggested by a qualitative study that interviewed 26 individuals, each with several chronic illnesses. Each individual had a variety of physical losses. Whittemore and Dixon (2008) refer to the phases of integration experienced by the study participants as "shifting sands," "staying afloat," "weathering the storms," "rescuing oneself," and "navigating life" (p. 181).

Role of Resilience

Throughout the literature, hardiness and resilience are suggested to influence individuals' ability to cope with loss. One thinks of the "hardy," stoic farmer or rancher as someone with resilience. Wise and Marchand (2013), however, write about the psychosocial assets of the resilient person with advanced cancer. Examples of personal assets from their study include positive relationships, purpose in life, faith, and mastery, all of which contribute to living fully in mortal time.

Does resilience exist before the illness, or is it an outcome of the adjustment process after loss? Past research has studied human resilience as a dynamic process used to successfully adapt to an adversity. However, Zautra, Hall, and Murray (2010) argue that resilience is best defined as an outcome of successful adaptation to adversity (p. 4).

Part of resilience may include positive reframing for those facing chronic illness. Perhaps because older adults have more life experiences, this group may fare better in the face of chronic illness. Older adults' more frequent life experiences with stressors and adversity, relative to the quantity of these experiences for younger adults, perhaps make them more prepared to handle a stressor such as chronic illness. As an example, a person may view a wheelchair, cane, or walker as a symbol of deterioration of the body; however, with positive reframing, the walker may be labeled as helpful to enable mobility and maintain one's independence. Another example of reframing is to view oneself as a survivor and not a victim (Rybarczyk, Emery, Guequierre, Shamaskin, & Behel, 2012).

Mindful Presence

Many times when caring for someone with chronic illness, whether as a professional caregiver or a family caregiver, there seems to be little, from a physical perspective, that one can do for the person. Palliative care strategies may be used to address the symptomology present, albeit not as successfully as one would like at times, but there are not any answers—nothing that you can do to quiet the patient or loved one and make him or her "feel better." In this scenario, mindful presence may be what you have to offer as a caregiver.

As caregivers, we believe we should be "doing" something, and if not "doing," then talking to the patient and family. Listening is often given little consideration. To truly listen to the patient, one needs a mindful presence. Mindfulness conveys acceptance, patience, trust (in one's own intuition), nonjudging, nonstriving, letting go, and a beginner's mind, seeing everything as if for the first time. Personal preference and critical thought are suspended when one is mindful (Wittenberg-Lyles, Goldsmith, Ferrell, & Ragan, 2013). "Presence is a useful summary of this account as it conveys both present time and person present, a 'now' and an awareness attentive in it. Presence requires practice and emphasizes personal experience. You have to be there" (Childs, 2007, p. 369). Mindful presence involves a nurse being non-verbally present for a patient and family while also being attentive, in the moment, nonjudgmental, and empathic (Wittenberg-Lyles et al., 2013, p. 95). The nurse is completely dedicated to the circumstances he or she finds in the here and now, and values "being" over "doing," in the belief that compassionately bearing witness to a patient's and family's suffering may be the greatest gift a caregiver can give (p. 106).

Outcomes

In the face of loss, expectations might include being positive, developing a "new" normal, creating a new identity, and feeling valued. However, for those who have experienced a chronic illness and the losses accompanying it, such expectations may be lofty or not realistic. Outcomes may also be different among individuals experiencing a terminal chronic illness versus a non-life-threatening chronic illness. As such, the outcomes and expectations vary greatly among patients and families.

I remember writing about Randy's cancer diagnosis in our Christmas letter of 2010, saying that we were up to the challenge of cancer. That we could do it. Even now 2 years after his death, I still believe that we gave it our "all" for the 18 months of his illness. Yes, we did it.

—Jenny

Evidence-Based Practice Box

Olshansky (1962) described chronic sorrow as the reactions of parents who had children with mental disabilities. However, in the last 20 years, the term "chronic sorrow" has been used in the context of adults with chronic conditions who suffer a variety of losses during their illness. The aims of Ahlstrom's (2007) study were twofold: (1) to describe the losses of persons who were severely afflicted with chronic illness and, therefore, may experience chronic sorrow; and (2) to identify meaningful underlying patterns related to these losses in the form of chronic sorrow through an abductive approach to analysis. Thirty persons of working age with an average disease duration of 18 years were interviewed twice. The average age of the participants was 51 years, and all had a need for personal assistance over the last 3 months because of their physical disability. The inductive findings demonstrated that all of these individuals had experienced repeated physical, emotional, and social losses. Most common were loss of bodily function, loss of relationships, loss of autonomous life, and loss of life imagined. The deductive findings of the study suggested that chronic sorrow exists in the study population.

Source: Ahlstrom, G. (2007). Experiences of loss and chronic sorrow in persons with severe chronic illness. *Journal of Nursing and Healthcare of Chronic Illness* in association with the *Journal of Clinical Nursing, 16,* 3a, 76–83.

STUDY QUESTIONS

1. Describe your thoughts about the chapter-opening quote from Conway.
2. Reflect on your experiences of caring for someone who has a chronic illness with a terminal prognosis. How does this chapter provide insight into that person's behavior and your own behavior?
3. Mindful presence is an underutilized strategy of healthcare professionals. Describe how it could enhance your practice.

References

Ahlstrom, G. (2007). Experiences of loss and chronic sorrow in persons with severe chronic illness. *Journal of Nursing and Healthcare of Chronic Illness* in association with the *Journal of Clinical Nursing, 16*(3a), 76–83. doi: 10.1111/j.1365-2702.2006.01580.x

Anderson, J. M. (1991). Immigrant women speak of chronic illness: The social construction of the devalued self. *Journal of Advanced Nursing, 16,* 710–717.

Brion, J. M., Menke, E. M., & Kimball, C. (2013). Grief and HIV medication adherence: The work of transcending loss. *Journal of Loss and Trauma, 18,* 499–520. doi: 10.1080/15325024.2012.719341

Bury, M. (1982). Chronic illness as biographical disruption. *Sociology of Health and Illness, 4*(2), 167–182.

Bush, E. (2001). The use of human touch to improve the well-being of older adults: A holistic nursing intervention. *Journal of Holistic Nursing, 19,* 256–270. doi: 10.1177/089801010101900306

Charmaz, K. (1983). Loss of self: A fundamental form of suffering in the chronically ill. *Sociology of Health and Illness, 5*(2) 168–195.

Charmaz, K. (1991). *Good days, bad days: The self in chronic illness and time.* New Brunswick, NJ: Rutgers University Press.

Charmaz, K. (1994). Identity dilemmas of chronically ill men. *Sociological Quarterly, 35*(2), 269–288.

Childs, D. (2007). Mindfulness and the psychology of presence. *Psychology and Psychotherapy: Theory, Research and Practice, 80,* 367–376.

Conway, K. (2007). *Illness and the limits of expression.* Ann Arbor, MI: University of Michigan Press.

Dowling, E. C., Chawla, N., Forsythe, L. P., deMoor, J., McNeel, T., Rozjabek, H. M., ... Yabroff, K. R. (2013). Lost productivity and burden of illness in cancer survivors with and without other conditions. *Cancer, 119*(18), 3393-401. doi: 10.1002/cncr.28214

Estabrooks, C. A. (1989). Touch: A nursing strategy in the intensive care unit. *Heart & Lung, 18,* 392–401.

Fleury, J. (1991). Empowering potential: A theory of wellness motivation. *Nursing Research, 40,* 286–291.

Gallace, A., & Spence, C. (2008). The science of interpersonal touch: An overview. *Neuroscience and Biobehavioral Reviews, 34,* 246–259. doi: 10.1016/j.neubiorev.2008.10.004

Gois, C. J., Ferro, A.C., Santos, A.L., Sousa, F.P., Quaklin, S.R., do Carmo, I. & Barbosa, A.F. (2012). Psychological adjustment to diabetes mellitus: Highlighting self- integration and self-regulation. *Acta Diabetologica, 49*(suppl 1), S33–S40.

Hernandez, C. A. (1995). Integration: The experience of living with insulin (type 1) diabetes mellitus. *Canadian Journal of Nursing Research, 28,* 337–356.

Herrington, C. J., & Chiodo, L. M. (2014). Human touch effectively and safely reduces pain in the newborn intensive care unit. *Pain Management Nursing, 15*(1), 107–115.

Isaksson, A-K., Gunnarsson, L-G., & Ahlstrom, G. (2007). The presence and meaning of chronic sorrow in patients with multiple sclerosis. *Journal of Clinical Nursing, 16*(11c), 315–324. doi: 10.1111/j.1365-2702.2007.01995.x

Klass, D., Silverman, P. R., & Nickman, S. L. (Eds.). (1996). *Continuing bonds: New understandings of grief.* Washington, DC: Taylor & Francis

Kleinman, A. (1988). *The illness narratives: Suffering, healing and the human condition.* New York, NY: Basic Books.

Larsen, P. D. (2013). *Finding a way through cancer, dying and widowhood: A memoir.* Bloomington, ID: Archway Publishing.

Larsson, A. T., & Grassman, E. J. (2012). Bodily changes among people living with physical impairments and chronic illnesses: Biographical disruption or normal illness? *Sociology of Health & Illness, 34*(8), 1156–1169. doi: 10.1111/j.11467-9566.2012.01460.x

Lundman, B., & Jansson, L. (2007). The meaning of living with a long-term disease: To revalue and be revalued. *Journal of Clinical Nursing, 16*(7b), 109–115. doi: 10.1111/j1365-2702.2007.01802.x

Medich, C. J., Stuart, E., & Chase, S. K. (1997). Healing through integration: Promoting wellness in cardiac rehabilitation. *Journal of Cardiovascular Nursing, 11,* 66–79.

Neff, K. D. (2003). Self-compassion: An alternative conceptualization of a healthy attitude toward oneself. *Self and Identity, 2,* 85–101.

Olshansky, S. (1962). Chronic sorrow: A response to having a mentally defective child. *Social Casework, 43,* 190–193.

Pruchno, R. A., Cartwright, F. P., & Wilson-Genderson, M. (2009). Effects of marital closeness on the transition from caregiving to widowhood. *Aging and Mental Health, 13*(6), 808–817.

Roose, S. (2002). *Chronic sorrow: A living loss.* New York, NY: Brunner-Routledge.

Rybarczyk, B., Emery, E. E., Guequierre, L. L., Shamaskin, A., & Behel, J. (2012). The role of resilience in chronic illness and disability in older adults.

Annual Review of Gerontology and Geriatrics, 2012, 173–187.

Shilts, R. (1987). *And the band played on: Politics, people and the AIDS epidemic.* New York, NY: St. Martin's Press.

Smith, J. R. (2012). Comforting touch in the very pre-term hospitalized infant. *Advances in Neonatal Care, 12*(6), 349–365.

Stroebe, M. S. (2011). Grief and bereavement. In S. Folkman (Ed.), *The Oxford handbook of stress, health and coping* (pp. 148–172). London, UK: Oxford University Press.

Tie, S., & Poulsen, S. (2013). Emotionally focused couple therapy with couples facing terminal illness. *Contemporary Family Therapy, 35,* 556–567.

Walker, C. (2010). Ruptured identities: Leaving work because of chronic illness. *International Journal of Health Services, 40*(4), 620–643.

Walter, C. A., & McCoyd, J. L. M. (2009). *Grief and loss across the lifespan: A biopsychosocial perspective.* New York, NY: Springer.

Whittemore, R., Chase, S. A., Mandle, C. L., & Roy, C. (2002). Lifestyle change in type 2 diabetes: A process model. *Nursing Research, 51,* 18–25.

Whittemore, R., & Dixon, J. (2008). Chronic illness: The process of integration. *Journal of Nursing and Healthcare of Chronic Illness* in association with *Journal of Clinical Nursing, 17*(7b), 177–187.

Williams, S. J. (2000). Chronic illness as biographical disruption or biographical disruption as chronic illness? *Sociology of Health and Illness, 22*(1), 40–67.

Wise, M., & Marchand, L. (2013). Living fully in the shadow of mortal time: Psychosocial assets in advanced cancer. *Journal of Palliative Care, 29*(2), 76–82.

Wittenberg-Lyles, E., Goldsmith, J., Ferrell, B., & Ragan, S. L. (2013). *Communication in palliative nursing.* New York, NY: Oxford University Press.

Zautra, A. J., Hall, J. S., & Murray, K. E. (2010). Resilience: A new definition of health for people and communities. In J. W. Reich, A. J. Zautra, & J. S. Hall (Eds.), *Handbook of adult resilience* (pp. 3–29). New York, NY: Guilford Press.

Chapter 5

Spirituality

Rebecca Carron

Finding spiritual meaning {in a chronic illness} is welcoming my lungs into the wholeness of my individual. My lungs are not "the other," but all is part of the whole. Spiritual meaning is about accepting and loving myself as a whole individual. It's honoring the self and body. Life is a journey.

—Mary, living with pulmonary hypertension

Introduction

An individual living with chronic illness experiences many complex emotional feelings that may include frustration, depression, or anger (Lorig et al., 2012). These feelings can lead an individual to feel overwhelmed with the self-management tasks and skills he or she needs to learn to effectively manage the condition. Spirituality is one source of comfort and support that can help an individual cope with the stress and anxiety of chronic illness (Lorig et al., 2012). People can use spirituality to find meaning in chronic illness, which in turn may help them interpret their illness in a positive manner (Lorig et al., 2012).

Consideration of spirituality as a supportive intervention in chronic illness leads to many questions. What are the spiritual care needs of individuals with chronic illness? What is known about nurses and spiritual nursing care? How can nurses meet the spiritual needs of their patients with chronic illness? This chapter addresses these questions and identifies the role of spiritualty in the management of chronic illness. Nursing and healthcare organizations mandate integration of spiritual needs in care plans. The *Code of Ethics for*

Nurses with Interpretive Statements by the American Nurses Association (2001), for example, includes statements concerning spiritual care needs. For instance, Provision 1.2 of the *Code of Ethics* requires that an individual's "value system and religious beliefs should be considered in planning health care with and for each individual" (p. 7). The Joint Commission (2013) states that an individual has the right not to be discriminated against due to religion or culture.

National surveys indicate that spiritual beliefs are important to Americans. A national Gallup poll conducted in May 2011 of 1,108 adults aged 18 and older found that 92% of Americans believed in God (Gallup, 2014). In November 1944, by comparison, the same Gallup poll reported that 96% of Americans believed in God; in August 1967, it found that 98% of respondents believed in God. These surveys suggest that more than 90% of Americans continue to believe in God.

Spiritual beliefs are of particular importance to older Americans, who are most likely to be affected by chronic illness. When the Pew Research Center's (2012) Religion & Public Life Project examined the number of people identifying with a religion, it found that while 32% of people aged 18–29 did not claim any affiliation with a religion, 90% of people aged 65 and older were affiliated with a religion. Among the 46 million unaffiliated adults, 68% believed in God, and 37% stated that they were "spiritual" but not "religious."

Spirituality can be an important source of support in chronic illness. A study of the use of complementary and alternative medicine (CAM) in U.S. adults, using data from the 2002 National Health Interview Survey (NHIS), found that 43% of adults used prayer for health purposes (Barnes, Powell-Griner, McFann, & Nahin, 2004). The five most commonly used CAM therapies were prayer for one's health (43.0%), intercessory prayer (24.4%), natural products (18.9%), deep breathing exercises (11.6%), and participation in a prayer group (9.6%). Conditions treated with CAM included chronic pain, anxiety, and depression. Women, black adults, and Asian adults were most likely to use CAM therapy that included prayer for health reasons. Rates of using mind–body therapies that included prayer for health ranged from 56.3% to 66% in people aged 60–85 and older. Excluding prayer, usage rates of mind–body therapies in older adults ranged from 6.4% in the 85 years and older age group to 14.4% in the 60-69 age group, suggesting a high use of prayer in the oldest age group with the highest rate of chronic illness (i.e., older adults).

Information on the use of prayer as a health intervention is important for healthcare professionals. Put simply, healthcare professionals need to have more knowledge regarding the importance of spirituality to their patients. Unfortunately, the 2007 NHIS survey did not include prayer as a CAM therapy (Barnes, Bloom, & Nahin, 2008). To read more about those spiritual practices that were considered unconventional healing practices, please refer to Kaptchuk and Eisenberg (2001).

Bell and colleagues (2006) analyzed CAM use based on the 2002 NHIS data among people with and without self-reported diabetes—one of the leading chronic conditions in the United States. Their sample included 2,479 people with diabetes and 28,526 people without diabetes. Overall, CAM use rates were significantly higher among people with diabetes (72.8%; $p < 0.0001$) than among persons without diabetes (61.2%). Prayer—that is, self-prayer, other prayer, or prayer groups—was more frequently used as a health intervention by people with diabetes than by people without diabetes.

Holistic nursing care includes care of an individual's body, mind, and spirit. While a cure is usually not possible for persons living with a chronic illness, opportunities for healing, growth, and wholeness are available (Mariano, 2009). Spirituality involves multiple ways of knowing, including cognitive, experiential, intuitive, aesthetic, and an inner sense or knowing (Burkhardt & Nagai-Jacobson, 2009). Spiritual practices can help individuals find purpose and meaning, as well as connection with others and the transcendent, within their illness experience (Burkhardt & Nagai-Jacobson, 2009).

Spirituality and Health

Research suggests a strong link between spirituality and health. However, spirituality can have both positive and negative effects on health. Schnall et al. (2010) examined relationships between religiosity and cardiovascular outcomes in a sample of 92,395 women aged 50–79 years who were enrolled in the Women's Health Initiative Observational Study. Their results indicated that religious affiliation, frequency of religious service attendance, and drawing strength and comfort from religion were linked to decreased all-cause mortality. The risk reduction ranged from 10% to 20%. The results also indicated that religiosity did not protect against coronary heart disease (CHD) events. The authors suggested that the decrease in all-cause mortality was not related to a decrease in CHD events, and that other unknown variables could be involved. The mechanism by which spirituality affects health is unclear.

A study of religion/spirituality in people with chronic pain revealed some interesting relationships between religiosity/spirituality and pain. Rippentrop, Altmaier, Chen, Found, and Keffala (2005) examined religiosity/spirituality in a sample of 122 individuals (54 males, 68 females) with chronic musculoskeletal pain; the individuals had an average age of 52.7 years. The results indicated that private religious practices such as prayer and meditation were related to poorer physical health. Rippentrop et al. (2005) suggested that people with the worst physical health might rely more on spiritual practices for comfort. Lack of forgiveness was related to more pain problems. Daily spiritual experiences, forgiveness, and support from a faith community were associated with better mental health, but religiosity/spirituality was not directly related to pain levels. This study again demonstrates that spirituality can affect health, but the mechanism of action is not well understood.

Several other explanations have been proposed for the beneficial relationship between spirituality and health. McCullough, Hoyt, Larson, Koenig, and Thoresen (2000) conducted a meta-analysis of 42 research studies involving 125,826 participants; their review focused on the relationship between religious involvement and all-cause mortality. The meta-analysis found religious involvement to be associated with lower all-cause mortality (odds ratio: 1.29). Powell, Shahabi, and Thoresen (2003) reviewed studies involving spirituality and religion on health outcomes. They reported evidence that suggested religion or spirituality was protective against cardiovascular disease, probably due to the relationship between spirituality and a healthy lifestyle. Religious attendance also protected against mortality; however, a healthy lifestyle did not entirely account for the beneficial effect. Perhaps religion and spirituality promote development of social supports, resulting in better health (Hill & Pargament, 2003). Attachment to God may also result in

lower levels of physiological stress and loneliness. Finally, use of spirituality as a coping tool may promote better health (Hill & Pargament, 2003).

In addition to positive effects, religious and spiritual beliefs can have detrimental effects on people's lives and health. Psychotic disorders can contain delusions or fixed beliefs that involve religious themes (American Psychiatric Association, 2013). In 2002, Andrea Yates drowned her five children due to religious convictions about Satan, herself, and her children (CNN.com/US, 2007). Yates was subsequently diagnosed with severe depression with schizophrenic symptoms. Cases have been reported of people who performed eye enucleations after reading Matthew 5:29–30; these Bible verses instruct an individual to pluck out an eye if it provokes sin (Koenig, King, & Carson, 2012). The New Testament's Book of Revelation was part of the philosophical background and motives for Charles Manson and his "Family," who murdered actress Sharon Tate and six other people in California in 1969 (Bugliosi, 1975).

More knowledge is needed about the type of faith healing that occurs at religious shrines such as that located in Lourdes, France (Koenig et al., 2012). In *The Nun's Story* (Hulme, 1956), Sister William remarked to Sister Luke that the real cure of Lourdes was the peace and happiness of faith that came from the pilgrimage.

Knowledge regarding attitudes of healthcare professionals toward the effects of spirituality on health is also important for the provision of spiritual health care. Many nurses believe in the beneficial effects of spirituality for individuals. Grant (2004) surveyed 299 nurses at a southwestern U.S. university teaching hospital. The results indicated that 100% of the nurses believed that spirituality could provide individuals with inner peace, as well as strength to cope (98%), physical relaxation (97%), self-awareness (96%), and a greater sense of connection to others (94%). The study also found that nurses who regarded themselves as spiritual generally thought that spirituality could help individuals.

A nurse's own spiritual background can affect spiritual care. In a qualitative study of spiritual care offered by nurse practitioners (NPs) in primary healthcare settings, Carron and Cumbie (2011) found that participants often spoke about the relationship between the spirituality of the NP and using spirituality in practice. Statements by participants included the following:

> *If you have a firm religious belief or you feel comfortable with your own spirituality, then it is going to be easier for you to bring that up to a patient, a friend, whoever. But if you're not even comfortable with your own concept of a higher power ... I think that would be more difficult to relate with anyone else. (p. 557)*

Spirituality and religion are coping strategies that can help patients and families manage the stress of illness (Glanz & Schwartz, 2008). As noted in the previous chapter, chronic illness can result in many losses, including loss of health, independence, vigor, ability to work, social relationships, and unmet goals and challenges (Koenig et al., 2012). In their seminal work *Stress, Appraisal, and Coping*, Lazarus and Folkman (1984) stated that psychological stress was "a particular relationship between the individual and the environment that is appraised by the individual as taxing or exceeding his or her resources and endangering his or her well-being" (p. 19). Thus, some individuals might find a particular incident stressful, while other individuals might view the same incident as nonstressful. The difference lies in the person's appraisal or significance of what is happening to him or her (Lazarus & Folkman, 1984). Existential beliefs, such as in God or the order of the universe, can help people find meaning and maintain hope in stressful events (Glanz & Schwartz, 2008; Lazarus & Folkman, 1984).

Use of spirituality can lead to either adaptive or maladaptive coping. Lazarus and Folkman (1984) noted that beliefs such as in God can sustain people and help them cope with very challenging situations—a response known as adaptive coping. Conversely, spiritual maladaptive coping can occur when an individual thinks that a stressful situation or illness is punishment from a punitive God (Lazarus & Folkman, 1984).

A study by Thuné-Boyle, Stygall, Keshtgar, Davidson, and Newman (2012) exemplifies the research suggesting maladaptive religious/spiritual coping in women with a new diagnosis of breast cancer. In this study, a sample of 155 women in the United Kingdom, with a mean age of 55.7 years, 44.8% married, and 72.1% believing in the existence of God, completed several spiritual measures including a religious coping tool. The authors found that negative religious coping, such as feeling punished or abandoned by God, was significantly associated with anxiety and depression, which could in turn affect the woman's adjustment to her diagnosis. Thuné-Boyle et al. suggested that a spiritual assessment could help identify areas of spiritual distress that might represent barriers to illness adjustment.

Positive religious coping, however, was demonstrated in a study of individuals with advanced cancer in the United States. Tarakeshwar et al. (2006) examined religious coping in a sample of 170 individuals with advanced cancer, defined by distant metastasis and failure of first-line chemotherapy. The mean age of the sample was 57.46 years with 77.6% of the sample having health insurance. Religion was important or somewhat important to 85.9% of the study participants. Assessment of several spiritual measures indicated that use of positive religious coping was related to better quality of life. However, positive religious coping was also associated with more physical symptoms. The authors noted that while religious coping can influence quality of life, individuals with better quality of life might also use more religious resources to cope with their illness.

Also, people with more physical symptoms might use religious coping for support and strength. The study further suggested that use of negative religious coping was associated with decreased quality of life. Finally, the authors suggested that a spiritual assessment with a few questions could help ascertain the importance of religion to individuals, the influence of religion on coping and understanding of their illness, and whether the individual's religious needs were met.

In summary, spirituality influences health through mechanisms that are positive and life-giving, but also in very negative ways. It is essential for healthcare professionals to assess the coping skills and effects of spiritual views of patients, caregivers, and families living with chronic illness.

Historical Perspectives of Spirituality in Chronic Illness

Nursing and spirituality have a long history of interrelationship. Florence Nightingale, for example, clearly viewed nursing from a spiritual perspective. At age 16, she experienced a call from God to His service, although the nature of the service was not specified (Macrae, 2001). In a small work entitled "Una and the Lion," Nightingale wrote that nursing was concerned with caring for the "living body—the temple of God's spirit" (Nightingale, 1868/2010, p. 6). In *Notes on Nursing* (1860/1969), she stated that the purpose of nursing was "to put the patient in the best position for nature (i.e., God) to act upon him" (p. 133).

Spirituality has been integrated into health care since the earliest known times. Shamanism is practiced by all indigenous groups worldwide and involves working with the forces of nature and spirits who can bring illness or death (Barnum, 2003). In medieval times, health care was often provided within monasteries (Barnum, 2011). In the United States, many early schools of nursing were affiliated with a religious institution (O'Brien, 2014).

During the latter part of the 20th century, nursing practice began to incorporate more scientific knowledge as the basis of patient care (O'Brien, 2014). Specifically, nursing adopted the biopsychosocial model of health care and eliminated the emphasis on spirituality and spiritual nursing practices (Barnum, 2011). More recently, shifts regarding spirituality in health care have again occurred, with spirituality drawing renewed attention (Barnum, 2011; O'Brien, 2014). In 1961, the inaugural edition of the *Journal of Religion and Health* appeared. The editor, George Christian Anderson (1961), stated that understanding and a multidisciplinary approach to health care was needed; no single group possessed the whole truth. Anderson recognized that a person's philosophy of life contributed to total health; consequently, the interaction among social, psychological, organic, and spiritual factors needed further examination and understanding.

In the 1990s, more research studies examining the relationships among spirituality, religion, and health were published. This trend has continued to grow with the establishment of spiritual institutions such as the Center for Spirituality, Theology, and Health at Duke University (http://www.spiritualityandhealth.duke.edu/). The Center, founded in 1998, promotes dialogue among researchers, clinicians, theologians, and others interested in the connection between spirituality and health.

Many national health organizations that deal with chronic illness have made information about spirituality and health available on their websites. For example, information on the role of spirituality as a support resource can be found on the following websites: National Center for Complementary and Alternative Medicine (NCCAM; http://nccam.nih.gov.), Centers for Disease Control and Prevention (CDC; http://www.cdc.gov), American Heart Association (http://www.heart.org), and American Cancer Society (http://www.cancer.org).

Definitions

To provide effective spiritual care to people with chronic illness, it is important to distinguish between terms used in the literature such as *spiritual* or *spirituality* and *religion* or *religiosity*. These terms can be difficult to define due to the wide variety of religious and spiritual practices, as well as the evolving meaning of the terms over time.

The term *religion* is derived from the Latin word *religare*, meaning "to tie back or restrain" (*Merriam-Webster Online Dictionary*, 2014). Religion can be practiced in a community or alone, but it generally includes shared beliefs and practices (Burkhardt & Nagai-Jacobson, 2009). Religion usually concerns the relationship between an individual and the transcendent, whether this is God, Allah, Buddha, Dao, a higher power, or ultimate truth or reality. The term "religion" can also be accompanied by negative connotations, including issues related to rigidity, hypocrisy, and church–state separation (Koenig et al., 2012).

Spirituality is more difficult to define due to the lack of accepted characteristics and its evolving nature (Koenig et al., 2012). The word *spirit* is derived from the Latin word *spiritus*, meaning "breath" (*Merriam-Webster Online Dictionary*, 2014). Many people express their spirituality within the structure of their religious denomination (Burkhardt & Nagai-Jacobson, 2009). Chittister (2001) identified a clear distinction between religion and spirituality: "religion is about ritual, about morals, about systems of thought ... spirituality is about coming to consciousness of the sacred ... It is in that consciousness that an individual comes to wholeness" (p. 16). Burkhardt and Nagai-Jacobson (2009) wrote, "Spirituality is the essence of who we are and how."

Chittister (2001) states:

> The truly spiritual individual ... knows that spirituality is concerned with how to live a full life, not an empty one. Real spirituality is life illumined by a compelling search for wholeness. It is contemplation in the eye of chaos. It is life lived to the full ... spirituality ... is the individual search for the divine within us all. (pp. 13–14, 61)

Spirituality is defined by *Merriam-Webster Online Dictionary* (2014) as being concerned with spirit, sacred matters, religious values, or the supernatural. O'Brien (2014) conceptualized spirituality as having two dimensions: (1) a spiritual connection with God or the transcendent and (2) a religious component consisting of an individual's faith practices, which might or might not be based in an organized religious tradition. Religion and spirituality both share a belief in the transcendent, but spirituality often involves a path of discovery, questioning, belief, devotion, and surrender that goes beyond organized religion (Koenig et al., 2012). In contrast, secularists, agnostics, and atheists do not acknowledge a connection with the transcendent (Koenig et al., 2012).

Spiritual well-being is another commonly encountered term in spirituality research and practice. This term is not found in *Merriam-Webster's* online dictionary (2014). Rather, spiritual well-being is defined by common threads in the literature that include connection to God or a higher power (religious well-being) and having a purpose and meaning in life (existential well-being) (Ellison, 1983).

The Functional Assessment of Chronic Illness Therapy—Spiritual Well-Being Scale (FACIT-Sp), a commonly used spiritual assessment tool, measures spiritual well-being with two subscales that reflect this view (Peterman, Fitchett, Brady, Hernandez, & Cella, 2002). The first subscale is labeled "meaning and peace" and measures meaning, peace, and purpose in life. The second subscale, labeled "faith," measures the relationship between spiritual/religious beliefs and illness. In a similar manner, the *Nursing Interventions Classification* (NIC) describes spiritual well-being as a "process of developing/unfolding of mystery through harmonious interconnectedness that springs from inner strengths" (Dochterman & Bulechek, 2004, p. 881).

The terms *spirituality* and *healing* are related. The words *heal*, *whole*, and *holy* stem from the same Old English word *hal*, meaning "whole" (Burkhardt & Nagai-Jacobson, 2009; *Merriam-Webster Online Dictionary*, 2014). Burkhardt and Nagai-Jacobson (2009) wrote:

> *{B}y its nature, healing is a spiritual process that attends to the wholeness of a person. The work of healing requires recognition of the spiritual dimension of each person, including the healer, and awareness that spirituality permeates every encounter. (p. 623)*

In summary, healthcare professionals need to understand the common links between religion and spirituality. It is an oversimplification of the differences between terms to label "religion" as based on the practices and beliefs of a particular organization and "spirituality" as more individual. A fundamental link between religion and spirituality is that both involve the sacred as expressed through God, the transcendent, or one's interpretation of the ultimate. The search for the sacred in life is the journey and destination of many people (Hill & Pargament, 2003).

Spiritual Context in Nursing Theories

Many nursing theories have a spiritual context. Interventions and programs to influence health behavior, such as lifestyle changes, are most effective when they are based on a theory of health behavior (Glanz, Rimer, & Viswanath, 2008). Theories help explain human behavior that may be facilitating or blocking chronic illness management. A *theory* can be defined as a "set of interrelated concepts, definitions, and propositions that present a *systematic* view of events or situations by specifying relations among variables, in order to *explain* or *predict* the events or situations" (Glanz et al., 2008, p. 26). Nursing theories address areas of interest and are "patterns that guide the thinking about, being, and doing of nursing" (Smith & Parker, 2010, p. 8).

While it is not the goal of this chapter to review the spiritual context of every nursing theory, a few examples are presented here to emphasize the relevance of spiritualty to nursing theory and nursing care. Although Florence Nightingale is not considered a nursing theorist according to modern standards, her vision of nursing continues to influence modern nursing (Dunphy, 2010). Spirituality played a major role in Nightingale's individual development and her views on health and nursing (Dossey, 2000). Specifically, she equated service to God with care of humanity (Calabria & Macrae, 1994). According to Nightingale, scientific truths were God's laws, and by discovering these laws of truth in areas such as sanitation, health could be promoted (Calabria & Macrae, 1994; Dunphy, 2010).

Watson's theory of human caring (2008) was based on the concept of caring science, which Watson proposed was the "essence of nursing and the foundational disciplinary core of the profession" (p. 17). She described caring as including spiritual ways of knowing and being. Many of the 10 core *Caritas Processes* in her theory, for example, integrate caring with honoring belief systems, connection to an individual's spirit, creation of a healing environment, and openness to the spiritual dimension of the human experience of life and death. Watson built on Nightingale's ideas that the body is often able to heal itself if placed in the right environment. A *Caritas* nurse incorporates an individual's spiritual beliefs to promote healing, strength, and wholeness.

The Roy adaptation model assumed that people find support in each other, the community, and a supreme power (Roy, 2009). According to this model, a supreme power or God is manifested in the diversity of the world. Roy's nursing model focuses on the role of nurses in helping people to adapt to changing circumstances. Roy (2009) believed that knowledge about an individual's spirituality helps one understand that individual's values and beliefs. These beliefs and values, in turn, influence an individual's response to environmental factors.

In particular, spirituality helps to define an individual's concept of self, which could influence health behavior.

In a similar manner, other nursing theories also emphasize the role of an individual's spirituality in shaping attitudes and responses to illness. The Neuman systems model, for example, focuses on the role of an individual's spirituality in shaping an individual's response to environmental stressors with lines of defense and resistance (Aylward, 2010). Leininger's theory of culture care diversity and universality also includes the importance of religious and spiritual factors that can affect the cultural response of people to illness (Leininger & McFarland, 2010). Rogers's theory of the science of unitary human beings, however, does not include a specific spiritual component. Rogers believed that people were unified human energy fields that could not be subdivided into systems such as a spiritual system (Butcher & Malinski, 2010). In contrast, Cowling (2004), in his description of unitary appreciative inquiry that built on Rogers's science of unitary human beings, included the value of physical, mental, and spiritual data to explain the "wholeness of human existence" (p. 279) and create the "inherent pattern of unity that is human life and the fullness of human experience" (p. 279).

O'Brien (2014) developed a conceptual model for a middle-range theory of spiritual well-being in illness (**Figure 5-1**). O'Brien believed that

Figure 5-1 A conceptual model of spiritual well-being in illness.

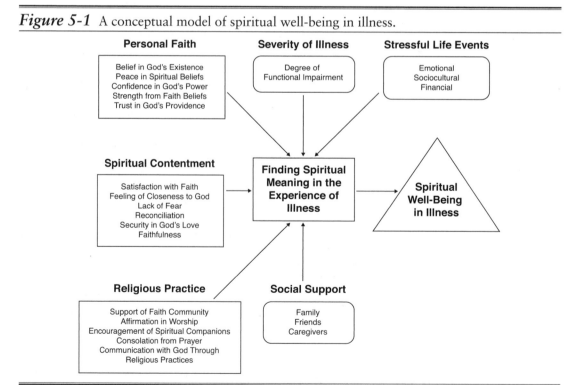

Source: O'Brien, M. E. (2014). *Spirituality in nursing: Standing on holy ground* (5th ed.). Burlington, MA: Jones & Bartlett Learning.

people have a spiritual nature, in addition to their physical and psychosocial nature, that is capable of transcending or accepting illness or disability. O'Brien's theory emphasizes the ability to find spiritual meaning in the experience of illness, which in turn could lead to spiritual well-being. According to this theory, several factors affect an individual's ability to find spiritual meaning in illness, including individual faith, spiritual contentment, and religious practices. Mediating factors in the relationships may include severity of illness, social support, and stressful life events.

The quality of an individual's faith may influence an individual's ability to find spiritual meaning and well-being in illness (O'Brien, 2014). For example, some people might consider illness to be a punishment from God for a past transgression. Other people might be fearful of God's judgment or anger rather than trusting in God's love for them. Nurses have the opportunity to intervene and support an individual with spiritual distress through referrals, encouragement of spiritual practices used in the past, and guidance and advocacy for the ill individual (O'Brien, 2014).

Carron and Cumbie (2011) developed a conceptual model for the implementation of spiritual care by nurse practitioners/advanced practice nurses (NPs/APNs) in adult primary care settings (**Figure 5-2**). Their model emphasizes the nurse–patient relationship. As the NP and patient develop a relationship, the NP conducts a spiritual assessment of the patient's spiritual supports. Based on this patient assessment and the NP/APN's own spiritual knowledge and

Figure 5-2 Nursing model for the implementation of spiritual care by APNs.

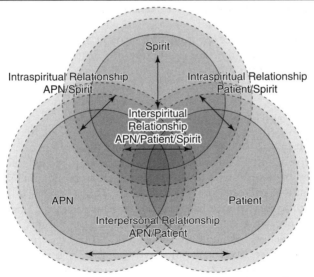

An Evolving Dynamic Relationship Between APN/Patient/Spirit

Source: Carron, R., & Cumbie, S. A. (2011). Development of a conceptual nursing model for the implementation of spiritual care in adult primary healthcare setting by nurse practitioners. *Journal of the American Academy of Nurse Practitioners, 23*(10), 552–560. doi: 10.1111/j.1745-7599.2011.00633.x © 2011 American Academy of Nurse Practitioners.

background, the practitioner develops and integrates spiritual interventions into the relationship with the patient to help the patient manage life challenges. The three interconnecting circles in Carron and Cumbie's model (see Figure 5-2) represent the NP/APN, patient, and spirit. The circles are dotted to reflect an evolving dynamic between these three entities.

Nursing theory influences all levels of care in chronic illness management, including nursing care, education, administration, and knowledge development, as well as providing structure for nursing practice, research, and scholarship (Smith & Parker, 2010). Nursing theories support the concept that an individual is a holistic combination of body, mind, and sprit. Nurses caring for people with chronic illness need to be familiar with the various nursing theories and their use in providing optimal nursing care for people living with chronic illness.

Issues

A discussion of spirituality and health includes many complex issues. Some of these issues, such as the positive and negative aspects of spirituality for health, have been discussed in earlier sections of this chapter. Other significant issues in spirituality and health include measurement and outcomes.

A primary concern in spirituality research is measurement. What is being measured, and are these appropriate items to be measuring? For example, it is relatively easy to measure the number and frequency of people who attend a faith-based service on a regular or intermittent basis. It is not quite so easy to measure the effects of prayer for an individual, commonly known as intercessory prayer. Which outcomes should be measured? Pain relief? Spiritual well-being? Complication rate after surgery?

Benson et al. (2006) measured the effects of certainty and uncertainty of receiving intercessory prayer with three groups of patients undergoing cardiac bypass (CABG) surgery. The first group (Group 1) of randomly assigned patients received intercessory prayer after being told they might or might not receive intercessory prayer. The second group (Group 2) did not receive intercessory prayer after being told they might or might not receive intercessory prayer. The third group of patients (Group 3) received intercessory prayer after being told they would receive intercessory prayer. Primary outcomes of the study included postoperative complications within 30 days of the CABG procedure; secondary outcomes were major events and 30-day mortality. The results indicated postoperative complications occurred in 52% of Group 1, 51% of Group 2, and 59% of Group 3. Major events and 30-day mortality were similar across the three groups. Intercessory prayer was provided for 14 days beginning the night before each participant's surgery. The intercessory prayers included the phrase for a successful surgery, with a quick recovery and no complications. Benson and colleagues (2006) concluded that intercessory prayer did not affect the chances of experiencing a complication-free recovery, and the certainty of receiving intercessory prayer resulted in a higher incidence of complications. Benson et al. (2006) also noted that the increase in complications in Group 3 could have been due to chance.

The Benson et al. (2006) study illustrates the difficulty associated with measurement in spiritual studies. Carron, Hart, and Naumann (2006) questioned the role of prayer as a primary medical treatment as in the Benson study. Carron et al. proposed that the purpose of prayer was to support the inner spiritual life of an individual; thus, prayer could serve as an adjunct coping resource in a challenging life situation such as CABG surgery. For example, Dunn and Horgas (2000) reported that 96% of a sample of 50 community-dwelling elders used prayer as a coping resource for stress. In the Benson et al. (2006) study, it appeared to be difficult to control the prayer intervention, as almost all participants in all three groups believed that friends, relatives, and their religious communities would be praying for them. Benson et al. also noted that the participants could have also been praying for themselves, and non-study prayer could not be controlled.

A Cochrane review examined the role of intercessory prayer (Roberts, Ahmed, Hall, & Davison, 2009). Ten intercessory prayer studies with 7,646 patients were analyzed for outcomes including death, clinical state, rehospitalization, quality of life, and satisfaction with treatment. The authors concluded that, based on the evidence, a recommendation could not be made either for or against the use of intercessory prayer, because the majority of studies did not support a positive effect from intercessory prayer. This review again illustrates the complexity of conducting spiritual studies, particularly in regard to measured outcomes.

Another issue in spirituality measurement is the challenge of measuring spiritual care provided by nurses. What is nursing spiritual care, and what should be measured? Hubbell, Woodward, Barksdale-Brown, and Parker (2006) examined the spiritual care practices of a sample of 65 nurse practitioners in North Carolina. To assess use of spiritual care by NPs in their practice, the NPs completed a modified Nurse Practitioner Spiritual Perspective Survey (NPSCPS) questionnaire based on the Oncology Nurse Spiritual Care Perspective Scale (Taylor, Highfield, & Amenta, 1994). The results indicated that 73% of the participants only rarely or occasionally provided spiritual care to their patients. The most commonly reported spiritual activities were referral to clergy (54%), encouraging a patient to pray (46%), and talking about a spiritual topic with a patient (39%). Notably, NPs defined spiritual care as listening, talking, holding hands, using music, and caring—a range that may not have been fully captured by the NPSCPS.

Other issues with spiritual care include the definition of spiritual care. Carron and Cumbie (2011) found that older patients equated spiritual care with a kind and caring attitude on the part of the nurse. However, a nurse practitioner who was interviewed for the study believed that a kind and caring attitude was part of nursing and that spiritual care depended on your definition. Spiritual care is not standardized, and while nurses believe in the value of spiritual care, they are uncertain when and how to implement spiritual interventions (Grant, 2004). Nursing needs to develop a consensus on the meaning of spiritual care and the manner in which it is to be implemented (Grant, 2004).

Spiritual Assessment

A spiritual assessment can provide clues regarding the influence of a person's spiritual views on his or her health. Healthcare professionals often establish long-term relationships with individuals and families living with chronic illness. A spiritual assessment can be helpful in developing spiritual care interventions.

Prior to conducting a spiritual assessment, Anandarajah and Hight (2001) described several prerequisite factors that could enhance a spiritual assessment—namely, spiritual self-understanding and self-care, relationship, and timing. First, a healthcare professional needs to acknowledge his or her own spiritual background to understand another individual's values and beliefs. Healthcare professionals also need to take the time to care for themselves so that they will have the energy to give to others. Spiritual self-care measures may include time with family and friends, contemplation, community service, or religious/spiritual practices.

The second prerequisite for spiritual assessment is establishment of a strong relationship with the individual (Anandarajah & Hight, 2001). A patient might feel more open to spiritual discussion if that individual already has a trusting relationship with the healthcare professional.

The last prerequisite for spiritual assessment is appropriate timing of the spiritual discussion (Anandarajah & Hight, 2001). Spiritual discussions could be appropriate especially when discussing a new diagnosis of a chronic illness, ongoing chronic illness or chronic pain, advance directives, or terminal care planning.

Table 5-1 The HOPE Questions for a Formal Spiritual Assessment in a Medical Interview

H: Sources of hope, meaning, comfort, strength, peace, love, and connection

O: Organized religion

P: Personal spirituality and practices

E: Effects on medical care and end-of-life issues

Source: Anandarajah, G. & Hight, E. (2001). Spirituality and medical practice: Using the HOPE questions as a practical tool for spiritual assessment. *American Family Physician, 63*(1), 81–89.

Table 5-2 B-E-L-I-E-F Mnemonic

B: Belief system (involvement in spiritual or religious group)

E: Ethics or values (important values or ethics)

L: Lifestyle (spiritual rituals, dietary restrictions)

I: Involvement in a spiritual community (participation in spiritual community activities)

E: Education (spiritual instruction, involvement in religious schools)

F: Future events (immunization, birth control, abortion, blood transfusions, death)

Reprinted from Journal of Pediatric Health Care, 14(5), McEvoy, M. An added dimension to the pediatric health maintenance visit: The spiritual history, Pages 216-220, Copyright 2000, with permission from Elsevier.

A spiritual assessment can be either formal or informal. An informal spiritual assessment involves listening to the patient for spiritual clues regarding his or her spiritual care needs (Anandarajah & Hight, 2001). These spiritual clues could include conversation focused on topics such as a search for meaning, fear of the unknown, hope and hopelessness, or isolation (Anandarajah & Hight, 2001).

The HOPE spiritual assessment was developed for healthcare professionals in a routine clinic environment (Anandarajah & Hight, 2001). This assessment focuses on open-ended questions built around the mnemonic of HOPE (**Table 5-1**).

McEvoy (2000) developed the B-E-L-I-E-F mnemonic to aid in spiritual assessment in a pediatric setting. However, this mnemonic is also applicable in adult settings (**Table 5-2**).

Several types of follow up to a spiritual assessment are possible (Anandarajah & Hight, 2001). Sometimes, only the presence of the healthcare professional is needed. Other suggested actions include incorporating spirituality into a patient's preventive care (e.g., prayer or walks in nature), using spirituality as an adjunct therapy (e.g., saying the rosary during a treatment), or modifying treatment based on a patient's spiritual preferences, particularly in regard to end-of-life issues (Anandarajah & Hight, 2001).

In the spiritual care research of Carron and Cumbie (2011), a study participant offered an example of a simple spiritual assessment, based on the relationship between the nurse and individual. An intervention was derived from the following assessment:

If you let that individual really know you're concerned about that condition, whether it's a cold or it's a lifetime thing or whether it is terminal, that individual is going to feel it {Relationship}. When that individual feels it, it's awfully easy then; that individual becomes open to you. You view the opening ... you can't just come across bluntly, but you can maybe, at some time or the other, ask them if they believe in God or if, you don't want to say "God," you might say "a higher being" to open the door {Assessment, knowledge of own spiritual base}. A lot of times that's all it takes and then they will usually come back with, "Yes, I believe." But then also, you can go further and say, "There is hope; no matter in what you're dealing with, there's hope" {Intervention based on relationship and assessment}. (p. 557)

Table 5-3 General Spirituality Measures

- The Spiritual Perspective Scale (Reed, 1986)
- Spirituality Assessment Scale (Howden, 1992)
- The Spirituality Scale (Delaney, 2005)
- The Ironson-Woods Spirituality/Religiousness Index (short form) (Ironson et al., 2002)

Table 5-4 Spiritual Well-Being Measures

- The Functional Assessment of Chronic Illness Therapy—Spiritual Well-Being Scale (FACIT-Sp) (Peterman et al., 2002)
- The Spiritual Well-Being Scale (SWBS) (Ellison, 1983)
- JAREL Spiritual Well-Being Scale (Hungelmann, Kenkel-Rossi, Klassen, & Stollenwerk, 1989)
- The Spirituality Index of Well-Being (SIWB) (Daaleman & Frey, 2004)

As these examples demonstrate, a spiritual assessment can be performed in a clinical setting. Begin with one question from the HOPE or B-E-L-I-E-F tool, for example, and then expand or branch out with your own ideas to find the center of strength and connection for an individual and/or family.

Spirituality Measures and Tools

Several tools are available to measure levels of spirituality in people. These spiritual measurement tools are especially useful in spiritual research, but can also be used in a clinical setting. Monod et al. (2011) conducted a systematic review of spirituality instruments and measures. Their literature search found 35 spiritual instruments that assessed spirituality in adults. Instruments that focused exclusively on religiosity were excluded. The instruments were classified as general spirituality ($N = 22$), spiritual well-being ($N = 5$), spiritual coping ($N = 4$), and spiritual needs ($N = 4$). Examples of the spiritual measures identified by Monod et al. (2011) are included in **Tables 5-3, 5-4, 5-5, and 5-6**. These measurement scales were validated in many populations, including patients with breast cancer, arthritis pain, alcoholism, substance abuse, acute or chronic disease, psychiatric problems, cancer, and HIV/AIDS; felony offenders; and geriatric outpatients (Monod et al., 2011). Consequently, many of the tools are applicable to chronic illness. The reader is encouraged to read more about the specific tools of interest, for which literature can be located by

Table 5-5 Spiritual Coping Measures

- A Semi-Structured Clinical Interview for Assessment of Spirituality and Religious Coping for Use in Psychiatric Research: Interview Based (Mohr, Gillieron, Borras, Brandt, & Huguelet, 2007)
- The Spiritual Strategies Scale (Nelson-Becker, 2005)

Table 5-6 Spiritual Needs Measures

- Spiritual Needs Inventory (Hermann, 2006)
- The Spiritual Interests Related to Illness Tool (Spirit) (Taylor, 2006)

name or author. Spirituality tools can be used to further assess the relationships between spirituality or spiritual well-being and outcomes such as quality of life (Monod et al., 2011).

The Spiritual Well-Being Scale (SWBS) and the Functional Assessment of Chronic

Illness Therapy—Spiritual Well-Being Scale (FACIT-Sp) are among the most commonly identified spiritual measurement tools used in research (Monod et al., 2011). The SWBS, which was developed in 1982 by Paloutzian and Ellison, is one of the oldest spiritual measurement tools. This self-report scale measures spiritual well-being with two subscales: (1) religious well-being or relationship to God and (2) existential well-being, which is a measure of finding purpose and satisfaction with life. The SWBS has been criticized for its emphasis on a more evangelical Protestant perspective of spiritual well-being due to questions focusing on an individual's relationship with God (Peterman et al., 2002).

Peterman et al. (2002) developed the FACIT-Sp in response to a need for a measure of spiritual well-being in chronic or life-threatening illness that broadly interprets spirituality. These authors noted that their scale was designed for people who considered themselves spiritual, but not religious. The tool consists of two subscales: (1) faith and (2) meaning/peace. There are no references in the scale to God or the use of a specific religious practice such as prayer. Instead, the FACIT-Sp focuses on spiritual well-being as a search for meaning, peace, and purpose in life, as well as the relationship between illness and an individual's spiritual beliefs. The FACIT-Sp includes statements about the value of faith or spiritual beliefs, purposefulness of life, having a sense of peace, and knowing that everything will happen for the best within the illness experience.

All of these spirituality instruments and measures have limitations. Monod et al. (2011) identified limited data on the psychometric properties of most of the reviewed instruments. Also, test–retest reliability data were limited for the instruments. In addition, Monod et al. (2011) noted that while some scales measure spiritual well-being, there is a lack of scales that measure spiritual distress; as these authors noted, the absence of spiritual well-being is not necessarily equivalent to spiritual distress.

In conclusion, the range of spiritual instruments indicates the interest in measures of spirituality and health.

Nursing Spiritual Interventions

Spiritual care interventions in chronic illness are based on knowledge gained through theory, historical perspectives, assessment, and measurement. O'Brien (2014) proposed a theology of caring to ground spiritual nursing care and interventions. According to this author, the essential components of spiritual care are *being*, *listening*, and *touch*. These actions between a nurse and individual can reflect the spiritual dimension of the nurse–patient relationship. The nurse could be present with an individual, actively listening, and then responding to thoughts of the individual with either physical or verbal touch through a word of support or comfort (O'Brien, 2014).

Knowledge is needed regarding spiritual care interventions by nurses and nurse practitioners. Grant (2004) examined the spiritual practices of 299 nurses in a southwestern U.S. state teaching university hospital. The five spiritual therapies most commonly used by nurses were holding a patient's hand (92%), listening (92%), laughter (84%), prayer (71%), and being present with a patient (62%). Spiritual counseling ranked 11th on the list (29%), and scripture reading was 12th (26%). The spiritual interventions used least often were biofeedback (8%), acupuncture (7%), chanting (4%), fasting (4%), and repatterning (2%). The study also indicated situations in which nurses thought spiritual interventions could be beneficial. The five most frequently cited situations were a patient explicitly requesting spiritual support (98%), a patient who is about to die (96%), grieving (93%), a patient or family who receives bad news (93%), and crying (86%). Other situations where spiritual interventions could be useful, according to the nurses, included a patient who often prays or seems close to God (81%), a patient who is a member of a church (71%), a patient who is alienated from friends and family (67%), a patient who is angry at God (65%), and a patient who is experiencing physical pain (46%). Based on his study, Grant (2004) reported that nurses believed spirituality could be beneficial, but the results also suggested nurses were unsure which spiritual therapies to use and when to use them. Grant (2004) suggested more research was needed in spiritual nursing care.

Quinn Griffin and colleagues (2008) examined spiritual practices among 84 individuals with and without heart failure. The authors designed a religious and spiritual interventions checklist for the study. The heart failure group consisted of 30 men and 14 women, and the non-heart failure group consisted of 7 men and 33 women. The participants were older than age 65, with the majority between 65 and 75 years of age. The results indicated that participating in family activities, helping others, and recalling positive thoughts were the religious and spiritual interventions used the most both by the total sample and by each subgroup. Praying alone and going to a house of worship or quiet place were also used by a majority of the participants in both groups. This study further adds to the body of knowledge regarding spiritual practices of older adults, many of whom live with chronic illnesses.

Carron and Cumbie (2011) identified spiritual nursing care perceptions of older adults (aged 65 or older) (N = 5) in their study of spirituality in primary care. The older adults stated that spiritual care by nurses included a kind and caring attitude on the part of nurses. One adult participant stated: "If you're kind and considerate and helping an individual, what more spiritual could you be?" (p. 555). Another adult participant supported this view with his remarks:

It's the sense of caring and sense of being welcome; what that does is cause a patient to feel better about the environment, feel better about himself, and help with the potential practices

that are going to take place. Now all of that … will find {its way} into the spirit and improve spiritual well-being, I believe. And I believe that a smile costs nothing. (pp. 555–556)

All of these studies confirm Grant's (2004) assertion that research needs to clarify which spiritual care interventions are appropriate and when they should be used in practice. In addition, the development of tools to measure nurses' spiritual and/or religious care interventions and intentions are needed. In other words, are nurses measuring what needs to be measured?

The time needed to implement spiritual interventions in practice by clinicians is also a critical factor in their development and use. A 2011 randomized controlled trial (RCT) examined the effectiveness of a home-based video and workbook encouraging spiritual coping in helping a sample of older adults manage chronic illness (McCauley, Haaz, Tarpley, Koenig, & Bartlett, 2011). A sample of 100 adults, of whom 62% were female, with an average of three chronic illnesses, was randomized into two groups. The most common chronic illnesses were hypertension (74%), arthritis (54.5%), diabetes (41.4%), and heart disease (27.3%). The spiritual intervention video consisted of stories of spiritual coping told by adults from various spiritual backgrounds. The workbook supplemented the video themes of (1) trusting in the care of a higher being, (2) cleaning "house" of destructive habits, (3) giving thanks for life's blessings, (4) helping others or finding life's purpose, and (5) asking for help or social and spiritual support. The control group received an educational intervention focused on standard care educational themes, including weight, diet, smoking, blood pressure, and activity. The results indicated that energy levels increased significantly in the spiritual intervention group and decreased in the educational intervention group. The researchers concluded that their spiritual intervention was not offensive, required no additional clinical time, and produced increased energy in the patients. The authors noted that fatigue can be an indicator of depression. They also recommended incorporating a spiritual history into the patient assessment and further suggested that patients explore how to incorporate their beliefs into their healthcare management.

Nursing interventions can also involve care of the inner spirit of the individual being cared for, as well as the healer or nurse. Nurses need to be aware that each individual manifests his or her own spirituality in unique ways (Burkhardt & Nagai-Jacobson, 2009). Interventions tending to the spirit can include touch, such as holding hands; supporting significant individual relationships through family, friends, spiritual groups, pictures, artwork, or pet visits; and supporting spiritual rituals such as prayer, meditation, mindfulness, presence, and awareness (Burkhardt & Nagai-Jacobson, 2009).

Spiritual interventions do not have to be difficult, be time consuming, or involve a particular religious domain. As an example, Treolar (2000) described the use of a spiritual intervention in an individual encounter with a patient suffering from metastatic lung cancer. Treolar noticed a Bible in the room and asked the woman if she had a religious faith that was important to her. Faith was important to the woman, but the hospital chaplain had not been to see her. Treolar offered to pray with the woman, and she accepted. Treolar wrote, "I began to pray for comfort and strength for her and her family, for wisdom for her and the health care staff, and for future decisions about treatment" (p. 283). According to Treolar, the intervention took 5 minutes during an IV infusion. This author concluded that "spiritual care can be integrated into everyday interactions with patients, providing that one is sensitive to spiritual cues" (p. 284).

Spirituality and Research

Research suggests that an individual's spirituality influences health outcomes in the face of many chronic illnesses. Spirituality has been evaluated from multiple perspectives in the literature. This section addresses the role of spirituality research and provides examples of spirituality as a health outcome in well-being and several chronic illnesses.

WELL-BEING

Well-being relates to life satisfaction, happiness, hopefulness, and morale, as well as finding purpose and meaning in life (Koenig et al., 2012). Self-rated health is a strong predictor of well-being, according to recent research. Religion and spirituality can influence well-being through direct effects such as beliefs and activities or indirectly through psychosocial effects. In a review of 224 quantitative studies, Koenig et al. (2012) reported that 78% found a positive relationship between religion and well-being.

For example, the positive effects of spirituality and well-being were demonstrated in a forgiveness study. Krause and Ellison (2003) examined forgiveness and psychological well-being in a nationwide sample of 1,316 people (51% white and 49% black) with an average age of 74.5 years. The results indicated that forgiveness of others was associated with increased psychological well-being compared to being less willing to forgive others. Receiving forgiveness from God was also important in well-being, but not as important as forgiving others. However, the authors suggested that receiving forgiveness from God could enable the participants to forgive others. Forgiveness was also associated with fewer depressive symptoms and greater life satisfaction. The authors suggested that forgiveness was important in maintaining social relationships. These results are similar to those in Grant's (2004) study, which found that 93% of nurses believed that spirituality could help with the forgiveness of others.

HUMAN IMMUNODEFICIENCY VIRUS/ACQUIRED IMMUNODEFICIENCY SYNDROME

Research suggests spirituality is supportive to people living with human immunodeficiency virus (HIV)/acquired immunodeficiency syndrome (AIDS). An illness such as HIV/AIDS can lead individuals and their families/significant others to question the meaning and purpose of life as well as their relationship to God or others (Cotton et al.,

2006). One study examined the role of spirituality in 450 individuals—86% male, 55% minorities, mean age 43.3 years—with a mean length of HIV diagnosis of 8.4 years. Factors associated with increased spirituality and religion included religious affiliation, African American ethnicity, lower alcohol use, higher self-esteem, greater optimism, higher life satisfaction, and lower overall functioning. On the meaning/peace and faith subscales of the FACIT-Sp (Expanded Version), 94% of the participants found some sense of purpose in their life, 88% found some comfort in their faith, and 75% reported a stronger faith as a result of their illness. Clinical parameters such as viral counts were not generally associated with spirituality. The participants also used positive coping strategies such as seeking a connection to God more often than negative coping strategies such as feeling abandoned by God.

Scarinci, Quinn Griffin, Grogoriu, and Fitzpatrick (2009) examined spiritual well-being and spiritual practices in a sample of 83 HIV-infected women (62.7% African American, 75.9% single, and 86.7% Christian). The average time since HIV diagnosis was 10.88 years. The most commonly used spiritual practices included praying alone (51.81%), helping others (37.35%), and exercise (36.14%). The women also had a high level of spiritual well-being that was related to spiritual practices. The authors suggested their results continued to support the positive link between spirituality and health.

HEART FAILURE

Spirituality can help in the management of chronic heart failure. Heart failure affects 5.1 million individuals in the United States (CDC, 2013). Bekelman et al. (2007) examined the relationships between spiritual well-being and depression in 60 people aged 60 and older with New York Heart Association Class II–IV heart failure. The mean age of the study participants was 75 years, and 22% of the sample was female. Spiritual well-being was measured with the FACIT-Sp (Peterman et al., 2002)

and depression with the Geriatric Depression Scale—Short Form (GDS-SF) (Yesavage & Sheikh, 1986). The meaning/peace subscale of the FACIT- Sp was significantly associated with lower depression scores ($r_2 = -.57$, $p < .001$). The faith subscale of the FACIT-Sp was also significantly associated with lower depression scores ($r_2 = -.38$, $p < .01$). The results suggested that increased levels of spiritual well-being could help mitigate the depression that often accompanies chronic heart failure as well as improve quality of life. Bekelman et al. (2007) also suggested having a sense of meaning and peace in one's life could help the individual transcend the limitations and challenges associated with chronic illness.

DEPRESSION

Many studies have explored the link between depression and spirituality. Koenig et al. (2012) examined 124 studies of depression and spirituality. They reported that 65% of these studies noted inverse relationships between religion and depression. Examples of research focusing on depression and spirituality in chronic illness are described in this section.

Payman and Ryburn (2010) found that intrinsic religiosity significantly predicted depression scores at 24 months follow-up in 94 patients (71% women, mean age 76 years) diagnosed with geriatric major depression. "Intrinsic religiosity" referred to motivation from religious beliefs. The authors proposed that persons with a high level of intrinsic religiosity might hide depression because their spiritual beliefs would encourage them to appear to be happy. Conversely, people with religious beliefs might be more truthful in responses, so the results might, in fact, be accurate. Regardless of the mechanism involved, the authors recommended that use of religion be considered to support older adults as they encountered the losses associated with aging.

The second research study is an example where an investigation into spirituality and depression showed mixed results. Baetz, Bowen, Jones, and

Koru-Sengul (2006) analyzed data from the 2002 Canadian Community Health Survey of approximately 37,000 community-dwelling Canadians aged 15 and older to examine relationships between spirituality and psychiatric disorders; their goal was to determine if spirituality had a protective effect. Participants in the survey were asked if spiritual values were important in their lives, and if spiritual values provided a sense of meaning, strength, and understanding in life. Frequency of worship was also assessed. More-frequent worship attendance was associated with less risk for depression and other psychiatric conditions (adjusted odds ratio: 0.87–0.93; 95% confidence interval: 0.82–0.97). In this study, higher spiritual values were associated with greater risk for depression, mania, and social phobia (adjusted odds ratio: 1.06–1.21; 95% confidence interval: 0.99–1.32). The authors suggested that worship attendance might be protective against depressive and other related disorders, while people with depression might attend services less often due to fatigue and the low energy associated with depressive disorders. The authors suggested that the association of high levels of spiritual values with depression and other psychiatric disorders might be the result of depression, mania, or social phobia leading people to seek answers through spiritual values of meaning, strength, and understanding. Spiritual values might also help people grow and learn from their psychiatric illnesses.

Rye et al. (2005) examined the effects of forgiveness in relation to depression in divorced adults. The sample was composed of 149 people, of whom 75% were women, with a mean age of 45 years. The participants had been divorced a mean of 1.08 years. The subjects were divided into three groups, with one group receiving instruction on a secular forgiveness intervention, one group being given a religious intervention, and a third control group having no intervention. The secular and religious interventions both consisted of eight group sessions discussing the themes of processing and coping with negative feelings, learning about forgiveness, and moving toward forgiveness. However, the leader of the religious intervention group encouraged its members to use their religious beliefs as support in working out forgiveness. Non-denominational scriptural texts were used to support forgiveness. The control or comparison group was provided with information about community sources for divorce support. The results on forgiveness, depression, and anger scales indicated that both the secular and religious interventions helped the participants develop forgiveness toward their former spouses. Members of the secular intervention group decreased their depressive symptoms over time compared to the control group, although trait anger was not affected by the intervention. The religious intervention group showed no treatment effects on depression or trait anger compared to the control group. The authors suggested that some of the participants in the secular group could have been using some type of individual religious forgiveness practice, or religion might not be important to some people in forgiveness.

Koenig et al. (2012) suggest that the lack of treatment effects in some studies involving spirituality and depression could be the result of the study design, scoring error, or measurement tools that are not able to adequately measure the topic of interest. In addition, failure to account for confounding factors might affect the outcomes. Finally, these authors suggest that more information is needed on the effects of spirituality and depression, including factors such as the type of depression, the kind of religion or spirituality used in the study, and the characteristics of the individual or situation used in the study.

Type 2 Diabetes Mellitus

The prevalence of type 2 diabetes mellitus (T2DM) is increasing in the United States. The CDC (2011) reported that 25.8 million people—8.3% of the U.S. population—had diabetes in 2010, with T2DM accounting for 90% to 95% of all cases of diabetes. Self-management practices, such as diet, exercise, and blood glucose monitoring, are important to help control the condition and avoid complications of T2DM (CDC, 2011).

Spirituality can be a valuable coping resource for people living with T2DM. Utz et al. (2006) examined self-management practices among 73 African Americans living with type 2 diabetes. The sample consisted of 42 women and 31 men, with a mean age of 59.8 years. Spirituality was a source of support for many of the participants, although some participants stated that spirituality did not have a role in their self-management practices. Spiritual practices that supported diabetes self-management included prayer for support and strength to care for self, prayer for help with coping with the illness, and social support through church activities. The study participants also believed that God gave knowledge to the healthcare professionals who cared for them. Utz et al. (2006) suggested that healthcare professionals be supportive of individuals who use spiritual support for coping with their illness.

Similarly, Polzer and Miles (2007) found that spirituality was an important factor that influenced self-management in a sample of 29 African American men and women with T2DM aged 40–75. Grounded theory was used to analyze participant interviews. The results indicated that participants' relationship with God was expressed through three themes of relationship and responsibility. In the first theme, God was in the background with a supporting role in T2DM self-management; the individuals' spirituality taught them that they should care for themselves out of respect for God's gift of being created in the divine image. The second theme of relationship and responsibility revealed God to be in the forefront and the individual with T2DM in the background. Participants who believed in this type of God relationship saw God as in charge. They believed that if God disapproved of their self-management program, there could be consequences for the individual with T2DM. In the third thematic group, God was seen as healer. Participants in this group believed that God could heal them; as a result, T2DM self-management was not necessary. Polzer and Miles (2007) noted there were only two participants in the third group,

so only tentative conclusions could be drawn. These authors suggested that a spiritual assessment could help identify people living with T2DM who could benefit from incorporation of spiritual beliefs and practices into their T2DM plan of care.

Evidence-Based Practice Box

Harvey and Cook (2010) examined the role of spirituality in self-management practices in a sample of 41 African American and non-Hispanic white women. The average age of the women was 72.9 years, and chronic illnesses in the sample of women included heart disease and hypertension (48.8%), arthritis (24.4%), diabetes and complications from diabetes such as dialysis (14.6%), and other chronic illnesses (12.2%). Qualitative interviews were conducted with the women, and the results were analyzed using grounded theory from a symbolic interactionism framework. The women were asked to define spirituality and to describe the role of spirituality in their self-management practices. The results showed that most of the women defined spirituality as a connection to a higher power (i.e., God) and connection with others. The women relied on God for guidance, and they often spoke to God during their day. The women's spirituality gave them a sense of purpose and meaning in life.

Four themes emerged regarding the role of spirituality in self-management practices: (1) God's involvement in illness management (God was in charge of their health and the women trusted God with the outcomes); (2) prayer as mediator (women petitioned God to help with management or to ease symptoms); (3) spirituality as a coping mechanism (connection with God helped the women cope with stress, pain, and helplessness); and (4) combining conventional and spiritual practices (the women believed God and self-management/medicine worked together to maintain health). The authors reported that the

(continues)

women's spirituality supported their self-management practices on a daily basis. Also, the women noted they had a responsible role to play in their self-management—for example, taking their medicine. The evidence from this study indicated that more research needs to look at cultural and spiritual implications for self-management programs among the elderly living with chronic illness.

Source: Harvey, I. S., & Cook, L. (2010). Exploring the role of spirituality in self-management practices among older African-American and non-Hispanic White women with chronic conditions. *Chronic Illness,* 6, 111-124. doi: 10.1177/1742395309350228

CAREGIVERS

No discussion of spirituality outcomes would be complete without mentioning the role of spiritual support for caregivers of people with chronic illness. When concern focuses on only the individual with chronic illness, the needs of the caregiver—usually a family member—can often be overlooked.

Yeh and Bull (2009) examined the role of spiritual well-being and mental health in a convenience sample of 50 family caregivers of older people with heart failure. The caregivers had a mean age of 60.3 years and were 70% female and 30% men. Family caregivers represented 98% of the caregivers. The mean age of the patients with heart failure was 76.47 years, and 79% were women. The tool used for measuring spiritual well-being was the JAREL Spiritual Well-Being Scale (Hungelmann, Kenkel-Rossi, Klassen, & Stollenwerk, 1996). Coping strategies of caregivers were measured with the Carers' Assessments of Managing Index (CAMI) (Nolan, Keady, & Grant, 1995). The mental health of the caregivers was measured with the Symptom Questionnaire (Kellner, 1987).

The results of this study indicated high levels of spiritual well-being among the caregivers on the three subscales of faith/belief, life/self-responsibility, and life satisfaction/self-actualization. The caregivers also had high levels of coping skills on the three subscales of problem solving and coping, alternative perception of events, and dealing with stress symptoms. The mean scores on the Symptom Questionnaire revealed that the caregivers were moderately anxious, although scores for depression, somatic symptoms, and hostility were in the normal range. However, some caregivers scored in the severe range of anxiety (28%), had above-average scores for depression (22%), and evidenced increased somatic symptoms (16%). Spiritual well-being demonstrated a significant inverse relationship with mental health scores ($r = -.055$, $p = 0.000$). The total coping scores also had a significant inverse relationship with the total negative mental health scores ($r = -0.44$, $p = 0.001$).

In conclusion, higher levels of spiritual well-being were associated with better caregiver mental health in the Yeh and Bull (2009) study. The coping strategies of problem solving and reappraisal of events were also associated with better mental health of caregivers. This study suggested that attending to the spiritual needs of caregivers was important in helping them cope with the burden of chronic illness.

Illness Narratives and Chronic Illness

Illness narratives provide another lens through which to view the effects of spirituality on chronic illness. Molzahn et al. (2012) used narrative inquiry from a social constructionist perspective to understand how individuals living with serious illness "story and re-story their lives, and how they story health, healing, living, and dying over time" (p. 2349). The sample consisted of 32 participants (18 men, 14 women) with an age range of 37–83 years. Chronic illnesses in the sample included cancer (10 people), end-stage renal disease (14), and HIV/AIDS (8). Four spiritual themes emerged from the study: (1) reflecting on spirituality, religion, and personal beliefs; (2) crafting beliefs for their own lives; (3) finding meaning; and (4) transcending beyond words. The authors found that the participants discussed spirituality from a broad perspective that included developing their own belief systems with a "self-defining spirituality" (p. 2354). Molzahn et al. (2012) concluded:

> *Rather than believing that they understand all religious or spiritual perspectives, health professionals may find that careful listening and engaging in thoughtful discussion about important life questions and beliefs will enhance spiritual holistic care. (p. 2354)*

Outcomes

Spirituality can be an important adjunct therapy in caring for persons with chronic illness. Research has demonstrated the positive effects of spirituality on health. However, as with all treatments, spirituality can also have negative effects on health depending on the individual's perspective of spiritual issues. Healthcare professionals need to complete a spiritual assessment prior to suggesting incorporating spiritual practices into a treatment program, to help avoid negative consequences. Use of spiritual practices as a treatment modality could be integrated into care with the cooperation of the individual.

The current state of the science in regard to spirituality demonstrates that more research needs to be conducted, particularly in the areas of assessment, implementation, and outcomes. Healthcare professionals also need to assess their own thoughts and beliefs regarding the use of spiritual practices in conjunction with conventional allopathic medicine.

Chronic illness is increasing in the United States. Older Americans, in particular, are susceptible to one or more chronic, lifelong illnesses. Assessing the spiritual needs of people living with chronic illness will help healthcare professionals use an individual's spiritual beliefs as a powerful, supportive, coping tool (**Table 5-7**). The strength that comes from faith may enable people with chronic illness to find purpose and meaning within the lived experience of their illness.

Table 5-7 CLINICAL GUIDELINES INCORPORATING SPIRITUAL CARE

Occupational Therapy Practice Guidelines for Adults with Alzheimer's Disease and Related Disorders

Schaber, P. (2010). *Occupational therapy practice guidelines for adults with Alzheimer's disease and related disorders.* Bethesda, MD: American Occupational Therapy Association. http://www.guideline.gov/content.aspx?id=16321&search=spiritual+care

Clinical Practice Guidelines for Quality Palliative Care

National Consensus Project for Quality Palliative Care. (2009). *Clinical practice guidelines for quality palliative care* (2nd ed.). Pittsburgh, PA: Author. http://www.guideline.gov/content.aspx?id=14423&search=spiritual+care

Assessment and Management of Chronic Pain

Institute for Clinical Systems Improvement (ICSI). (2011). *Assessment and management of chronic pain.* Bloomington, MN: Author. http://www.guideline.gov/content.aspx?id=36064&search=spiritual+care

End-of-Life Care During the last Days and Hours

Registered Nurses' Association of Ontario (RNAO). (2011). *End-of-life care during the last days and hours.* Toronto, ON: Author. http://www.guideline.gov/content.aspx?id=34759&search=spiritual+care

Department of Defense Clinical Practice Guideline for Management of Major Depressive Disorder

Department of Veteran Affairs, Department of Defense. (2009). *VA/DoD clinical practice guideline for management of major depressive disorder (MDD).* Washington, DC: Author. http://www.guideline.gov/content.aspx?id=15675&search=spiritual+care

CASE STUDY 5-1

Miranda is a 54-year-old black female who presents for a 3-month check-up for her type 2 diabetes. She was diagnosed 6 months ago in the busy family practice clinic where you work as an RN. Miranda is currently working on lifestyle changes, is taking metformin, and is engaging in daily self-management practices of glucose testing and foot care. She does not smoke. Her latest hemoglobin A_{1c} level is 7.2, which is a decrease from her last 3-month check of 7.6. While you are checking her in and getting her weight and vital signs, Miranda mentions how difficult her diabetes is for her to manage at home. She mentions that she prays for help from God.

Discussion Questions

1. Miranda mentioned that she is having difficulty managing her diabetes. She also introduced the role of spirituality in her diabetes care. How would you respond to the clinical cues she provided?
2. How could spirituality be incorporated into her plan of care?
3. Would you feel comfortable discussing spiritual care interventions with Miranda? Why or why not?

CASE STUDY 5-2

John Simpson is a 76-year-old white male who presents for his annual physical in your cardiology clinic. You work in the clinic as an RN. The last time you saw John was 6 months ago, when he came in for a check-up for his heart failure. He was diagnosed with heart failure 1 year ago and is on multiple oral medications. You know from reading the newspaper that John's wife died 2 months ago. The clinic sent John a sympathy card, which you signed. While talking with John, he mentions how lonely he is since his wife died. He said his wife used to attend church services on a regular basis, but he seldom went with her. He looks at you and asks if he might find support for his loneliness and difficult heart failure regimen at church.

Discussion Questions

1. How would you respond to John?
2. Which spiritual assessment questions would be appropriate to ask John?
3. Houses of worship often have an active social agenda for members, sometimes including nursing activities. How would involvement in church activities help John's loneliness and heart failure?

STUDY QUESTIONS

1. Why has current research in spirituality increased?
2. How would you differentiate between the terms *spirituality* and *religiosity*?
3. What are issues that complicate spirituality research?
4. Which factors should be evaluated in spiritual care research?
5. What is the role of spirituality in the management of an individual with a chronic illness?
6. Is a spiritual assessment an important part of management of a chronic illness management? Why or why not?
7. What are some nursing spiritual interventions to use in chronic illness management?
8. How does spirituality affect healthcare outcomes in chronic illness? Explain.
9. Which questions would you ask patients to elicit stories about the role of spirituality in their lives?
10. Is spirituality incorporated into your work? Explain.

References

American Nurses Association. (2001). *Code of ethics for nurses with interpretive statements*. Washington, DC: Author.

American Psychiatric Association. (2013). *Diagnostic and statistical manual of mental disorders (DSM-V)* (5th ed.). Arlington, VA: Author

Anandarajah, G., & Hight, E. (2001). Spirituality and medical practice: Using the HOPE questions as a practical tool for spiritual assessment. *American Family Physician, 63*(1), 81–89.

Anderson, G. C. (1961). Editorial. *Journal of Religion and Health, 1*(1), 9–11.

Aylward, P. D. (2010). Betty Neuman's system's model. In M. E. Parker & M. C. Smith (Eds.), *Nursing theories and nursing practice* (3rd ed., pp. 182–201). Philadelphia, PA: F. A. Davis.

Baetz, M., Bowen, R., Jones, G., & Koru-Sengul, T. (2006). How spiritual values and worship attendance relate to psychiatric disorders in the Canadian population. *Canadian Journal of Psychiatry, 51*(10), 654–661.

Barnes, P. M., Bloom, B. & Nahin, R. L. (2008). *Complementary and alternative medicine use among adults and children: United States, 2007. National Health Statistics Reports,* no 12. Hyattsville, MD: National Center for Health Statistics.

Barnes, P. M., Powell-Griner, E., McFann, K., & Nahin, R. L. (2004). *Complementary and alternative medicine use among adults: United States, 2002.* Advance data from *Vital and Health Statistics,* no 343. Hyattsville, MD: National Center for Health Statistics.

Barnum, B. S. (2003). *Spirituality in nursing: From traditional to new age* (2nd ed.). New York, NY: Springer.

Barnum, B. S. (2011). *Spirituality in nursing: The challenges of complexity* (3rd ed.). New York, NY: Springer.

Bekelman, D. B., Dy, S. M., Becker, D. M., Wittstein, I. S., Hendricks, D. E., Yamashita, T. E., … Gottlieb, S.H. (2007). Spiritual well-being and depression in patients with heart failure. *Society of General Internal Medicine, 22,* 470–477. doi: 10.1007/s11606-006-0044-9

Bell, R. A., Suerken, C. K., Grzywacz, J. G., Lang, W., Quandt, S. A., & Arcury, T. A. (2006). Complementary and alternative medicine use among adults with diabetes in the United States. *Alternative Therapies, 12*(5), 16–22.

Benson, H., Dusek, J., Sherwood, J. B., Lam, P., Bethea, C. F., Carpenter, W., … Hibberd, P.L. (2006). Study of the Therapeutic Effects of Intercessory Prayer (STEP) in cardiac bypass patients: A multicenter randomized trial of uncertainty and certainty of receiving intercessory prayer. *American Heart Journal, 151,* 934–942.

Bugliosi, V. (with Gentry, C.). (1975). *Helter skelter.* New York, NY: Bantam Books.

Burkhardt, M. A., & Nagai-Jacobson, M. G. (2009). Spirituality and health. In B. M. Dossey & L. Keegan (Eds.), *Holistic nursing: A handbook for practice* (5th ed., pp. 617–645). Sudbury, MA: Jones and Bartlett.

Butcher, H. K., & Malinski, V. M. (2010). Martha E. Rogers' science of unitary human beings. In M. E. Parker & M. C. Smith (Eds.), *Nursing theories and nursing practice* (3rd ed., p. 253–276). Philadelphia, PA: F. A. Davis.

Calabria, M. D., & Macrae, J. A. (Eds.). (1994). *Suggestions for thought by Florence Nightingale*. Philadelphia, PA: University of Pennsylvania Press.

Carron, R., & Cumbie, S. A. (2011). Development of a conceptual nursing model for the implementation of spiritual care in adult primary healthcare setting by nurse practitioners. *Journal of the American Academy of Nurse Practitioners, 23*(10), 552–560. doi: 10.1111/j.1745-7599.2011.00633.x

Carron, R., Hart, A. M., & Naumann, R. (2006). Response to "Study of the Therapeutic Effects of Intercessory Prayer (STEP) in cardiac bypass patients: A multicenter randomized trial of uncertainty and certainty of receiving intercessory prayer by Benson, H. et al. [Letter to the editor] [Electronic version]. *American Heart Journal, 152*(6), e63.

Centers for Disease Control and Prevention (CDC). (2011). *National diabetes fact sheet: National estimates and general information on diabetes and prediabetes in the United States, 2011*. Atlanta, GA: U.S. Department of Health and Human Services, Centers for Disease Control and Prevention. http://www.cdc.gov/diabetes/pubs/pdf/ndfs_2011.pdf

Centers for Disease Control and Prevention (CDC). (2013). Heart failure fact sheet. http://www.cdc.gov/dhdsp/data_statistics/fact_sheets/fs_heart_failure.htm

Chittister, J. (2001). *Illuminated life: Monastic wisdom for seekers of light*. Maryknoll, NY: Orbis Books.

CNN.com/US. (2007). Andrea Yates case: Yates found not guilty by reason of insanity. http://www.cnn.com/2007/US/law/12/11/court.archive.yates8/index

Cotton, S., Puchalski, C. M., Sherman, S. N., Mrus, J. M., Peterman, A. H., Feinberg, J., … Tsevat, J. (2006). Spirituality in patients with HIV/AIDS. *Journal of General Internal Medicine, 21*, S5–S13. doi: 10.1111/j.1525-1497/2006.0642.x

Cowling, W. R. III. (2004). Unitary appreciative inquiry. In P. G. Reed, N. C. Shearer, & L. H. Nicoll (Eds.), *Perspectives on nursing theory* (pp. 271–284). Philadelphia, PA: Lippincott Williams & Wilkins.

Daaleman, T. P., & Frey, B. B. (2004). The Spirituality Index of Well-Being: A new instrument for health-related quality-of-life research. *Annals of Family Medicine, 2*(5), 499–503. doi: 10.1370./afm.89

Delaney, C. (2005). The Spirituality Scale: Development and psychometric testing of a holistic instrument to assess the human spiritual dimension. *Journal of Holistic Nursing, 23*, 145–167, doi: 10.1177/0898010105276180

Dochterman, J. M., & Bulechek, G. M. (2004). *Nursing interventions classification (NIC)* (4th ed.). St. Louis, MO: Mosby.

Dossey, B. M. (2000). *Florence Nightingale: Mystic, visionary, healer*. Springhouse, PA: Springhouse.

Dunn, K. S., & Horgas, A. L. (2000). The prevalence of prayer as a spiritual self-care modality in elders. *Journal of Holistic Nursing, 18*(4), 337–351.

Dunphy, L. H. (2010). Florence Nightingale's legacy of caring and its applications. In M. E. Parker & M. C. Smith (Eds.), *Nursing theories and nursing practice* (3rd ed., pp. 35–53). Philadelphia, PA: F. A. Davis.

Ellison, C. W. (1983). Spiritual well-being: Conceptualization and measurement. *Journal of Psychology and Theology, 11*(4), 330–340.

Gallup. (2014). More than 9 in 10 Americans continue to believe in God. http://www.gallup.com/poll/147887/americans-continue-believe-god

Glanz, K., Rimer, B. K., & Viswanath, K. (Eds.). (2008). *Health behavior and health education: Theory, research, and practice* (4th ed.) San Francisco, CA: Jossey-Bass.

Glanz, K., & Schwartz, M.D. (2008). Stress, coping, and health behavior. In K. Glanz, B. K. Rimer, & K. Viswanath (Eds.), *Health behavior and health education: Theory, research, and practice* (4th ed., pp. 211–236). San Francisco, CA: Jossey-Bass.

Grant, D. (2004). Spiritual interventions: How, when, and why nurses use them. *Holistic Nursing Practice, 18*(1), 36–41.

Hermann, C. (2006). Development and testing of the spiritual needs inventory for patients near the end of life. *Oncology Nursing Forum, 33*(4), 737–744.

Hill, P. C., & Pargament, K. I. (2003). Advances in the conceptualization and measurement of religion and spirituality. *American Psychologist, 58*(1), 64–74. doi: 10.1037/0003-066X.58.1.64

Howden, J. W. (1992). *Development and psychometric characteristics of the Spirituality Assessment Scale*. Unpublished doctoral dissertation, Texas Women's University.

Hubbell, S. L., Woodward, E. K., Barksdale-Brown, D. J., & Parker, J. S. (2006). Spiritual care practices of nurse practitioners in federally designated nonmetropolitan areas of North Carolina. *Journal of the American Academy of Nurse Practitioners, 18*(8), 379–385. doi: 10.1111/j.1745-7599.2006.00151.x

Hulme, K. (1956). *The nun's story*. Boston, MA: Little, Brown.

Hungelmann, J., Kenkel-Rossi, E., Klassen, L., & Stollenwerk, R. (1989). Development of the JAREL spiritual well-being scale. In R. M. Carrol-Johnson (Ed.), *Classification of nursing diagnosis: Proceedings of the*

8th Conference, North American Diagnosis Association (pp. 393–398). Philadelphia, PA: J. B. Lippincott.

Hungelmann, J., Kenkel-Rossi, E., Klassen, L., & Stollenwerk, R. (1996). Focus on spiritual well-being: Harmonious interconnectedness of mind–body–spirit: Use of the JAREL spiritual well-being scale. *Geriatric Nursing, 17,* 262–266.

Ironson, G., Solomon, G. F., Balbin, E. G., O'Cleirigh, C., George, A., Kumar, M., ... Woods, T.E. (2002). The Ironson-Woods Spirituality/Religiousness Index is associated with long survival, health behaviors, less distress, and low cortisol in people with HIV/AIDS. *Annals of Behavioral Medicine, 24*(1), 34–48.

Joint Commission. (2013). Speak up: Know your rights [Brochure]. http:www.jointcommission.org/Speak_Up_Know_Your_Rights/

Kaptchuk, T. J., & Eisenberg, D. M. (2001). Varieties of healing.2: A taxonomy of unconventional healing practices. *Annals of Internal Medicine, 135*(3), 196–204.

Kellner, R. (1987). A symptoms questionnaire. *Journal of Clinical Psychiatry, 48,* 268–274.

Koenig, H. G., King, D. E., & Carson, V. B. (2012). *Handbook of religion and health* (2nd ed.). New York, NY: Oxford University Press.

Krause, N., & Ellison, C. G. (2003). Forgiveness by God, forgiveness of others, and psychological well-being in late life. *Journal for the Scientific Study of Religion, 42*(1), 77–93.

Lazarus, R. S., & Folkman, S. (1984). *Stress, appraisal, and coping.* New York, NY: Springer.

Leininger, M. M., & McFarland, M. R. (2010). Madeleine Leininger's theory of culture care diversity and universality. In M. E. Parker & M. C. Smith (Eds.), *Nursing theories and nursing practice* (3rd ed., pp. 317–336). Philadelphia, PA: F. A. Davis.

Lorig, K., Holman, H., Sobel, D., Laurent, D., González, V., & Minor, M. (2012). *Living a healthy life with chronic conditions* (4th ed.). Boulder, CO: Bull.

Macrae, J. A. (2001). *Nursing as a spiritual practice.* New York, NY: Springer.

Mariano, C. (2009). Holistic nursing: Scope and standards of practice. In B. M. Dossey & L. Keegan (Eds.), *Holistic nursing: A handbook for practice* (5th ed., pp. 47–73). Sudbury, MA: Jones and Bartlett.

McCauley, J., Haaz, S., Tarpley, M. J., Koenig, H. G., & Bartlett, S. J. (2011). A randomized controlled trial to assess effectiveness of a spiritual-based intervention to help chronically ill adults. *International Journal of Psychiatry in Medicine, 41*(1), 91–105. doi: 10.2190/PM.41.1.h

McCullough, M. E., Hoyt, W. T., Larson, D. B., Koenig, H. G., & Thoresen, C. (2000). Religious involvement and mortality: A meta-analytic review. *Health Psychology, 19*(3), 211–222.

McEvoy, M. (2000). An added dimension to the pediatric health maintenance visit: The spiritual history. *Journal of Pediatric Health Care, 14,* 216–220. doi: 10.1067.mph.2000104608

Merriam-Webster online dictionary and thesaurus. (2014). http://www.merriam-webster.com

Mohr, S., Gillieron, C., Borras, L., Brandt, P. Y., & Huguelet, P. (2007). The assessment of spirituality and religiousness in schizophrenia. *Journal of Mental and Nervous Disorders, 195*(3), 247–253.

Molzahn, A., Shields, L., Bruce, A., Stajduhar, K., Makaroff, K. S., Beuthin, R., ... Shermak, S. (2012). People living with serious illness: Stories of spirituality. *Journal of Clinical Nursing, 21,* 2347–2356. doi: 10.1111/j.1365-2702.2012.04196.x

Monod, S., Brennan, M., Rochat, E., Martin, E., Rochat, S., & Büla, C. J. (2011). *Journal of General Internal Medicine, 26*(11), 1345–1347. doi: 10.1007/s11606-011-1769-7

Nelson-Becker, H. (2005). Development of a spiritual support scale for use with older adults. *Journal of Human Behavior in the Social Environment, 11,* 195–212.

Nightingale, F. (1860/1969). *Notes on nursing: What it is and what it is not.* New York, NY: Dover.

Nightingale, F. (1868/2010). *Una and the lion.* Nabu Press through Amazon.com (http://www.amazon.com).

Nolan, M., Keady, J., & Grant, G. (1995). CAMI: A basis for assessment and support with family carers. *British Journal of Nursing, 4,* 822–826.

O'Brien, M. E. (2014). *Spirituality in nursing: Standing on holy ground* (5th ed.). Burlington, MA: Jones & Bartlett Learning.

Paloutzian, R. F., & Ellison, C. W. (1982). Loneliness, spiritual well-being and quality of life. In L. A. Peplau & D. Perlman (Eds.), *Loneliness: A sourcebook of current theory, research and therapy* (pp. 224–237). New York, NY: Wiley-Interscience.

Payman, V., & Ryburn, B. (2010). Religiousness and recovery from inpatient geriatric depression: Findings from the PEJAMA Study. *Australian and New Zealand Journal of Psychiatry, 44,* 560–567.

Peterman, A. H., Fitchett, G., Brady, M. J., Hernandez, L., & Cella, D. (2002). Measuring spiritual well-being in people with cancer: The Functional Assessment of Chronic Illness Therapy—Spiritual Well-Being

Scale (FACIT-Sp). *Annals of Behavioral Medicine, 24*(1), 49–58.

Pew Research Center. (2012). "Nones" on the rise. http://www.pewforum.org/2012/10/09/ones-on-the-rise/

Polzer, R. L., & Miles, M. S. (2007). Spirituality in African Americans with diabetes: Self-management through a relationship with God. *Qualitative Health Research, 17*(2), 176–188.

Powell, L. H., Shahabi, L., & Thoresen, C. (2003). Religion and spirituality: Linkages to physical health. *American Psychologist, 58*(1), 36–52.

Quinn Griffin, M. T., Salman, A., Lee, Y., Seo, Y., & Fitzpatrick, J. J. (2008). A beginning look at the spiritual practices of older adults. *Journal of Christian Nursing, 25*(2), 100–102.

Reed, P. G. (1986). Religiousness among terminally ill and healthy adults. *Research in Nursing and Health, 9,* 35–41.

Rippentrop, A. E., Altmaier, E. M., Chen, J. J., Found, E. M., & Keffala, V. J. (2005). The relationship between religion/spirituality and physical health, mental health, and pain in a chronic pain population. *Pain, 116,* 311–321. doi: 10.1016/j.pain.2005.05.008

Roberts, L., Ahmed, I., Hall, S., & Davison, A. (2009). Intercessory prayer for the alleviation of ill health (review). *Cochrane Database of Systematic Reviews 2009, 2,* CD000368. doi: 10.1002/1465/1858.CD000368. pub3

Roy, C. (2009). *The Roy adaptation model* (3rd ed.). Upper Saddle River, NJ: Pearson Education.

Rye, M. S., Pargament, K. I., Pan, W., Yingling, D. W., Shogren, K. A., & Ito, M. (2005). Can group interventions facilitate forgiveness of an ex-spouse? A randomized control trial. *Journal of Consulting and Clinical Psychology, 73*(5), 880–892. doi: 10.1037/0022-006X.73.5.880

Scarinci, E. G., Quinn Griffin, M. T., Grogoriu, A., & Fitzpatrick, J. J. (2009). Spiritual well-being, and spiritual practices in HIV-infected women: A preliminary study. *Journal of the Association of Nurses in AIDS Care, 20*(1), 69–76.

Schnall, E., Wassertheil-Smoller, S., Swencionis, C., Zemon, V., Tinker, L., O'Sullivan, M. J., . .Goodwin, M. (2010). The relationship between religion and cardiovascular outcomes and all-cause mortality in the women's health initiative observational study. *Psychology and Health, 25*(2), 249–263. doi: 10.1080/08870440802311322

Smith, M. C., & Parker, M.E. (2010). Nursing theory and the discipline of nursing. In M. E. Parker & M.C. Smith (Eds.), *Nursing theories and nursing practice* (3rd ed., pp. 3–15). Philadelphia, PA: F. A. Davis.

Tarakeshwar, N., Vanderwerker, L. C., Paulk, E., Pearce, M. J., Kasl, S., & Prigerson, H. G. (2006). Religious coping is associated with the quality of life of patients with advanced cancer. *Journal of Palliative Medicine, 9*(3), 646–657.

Taylor, E. J. (2006). Prevalence and associated factors of spiritual needs among patients with cancer and family caregivers. *Oncology Nursing Forum, 33*(4), 729–735.

Taylor, E. J., Highfield, M., & Amenta, M. (1994). Attitudes and beliefs regarding spiritual care: A survey of cancer nurses. *Cancer Nursing, 17*(6), 479–487.

Thuné-Boyle, I. C. V., Stygall, J., Keshtgar, M. R. S., Davidson, T. I., & Newman, S. P. (2013). Religious/spiritual coping resources and their relationship with adjustment in patients newly diagnosed with breast cancer in the UK. *Psycho-Oncology, 22,* 646–658. doi: 10.1002/pon.3048

Treolar, L. L. (2000). Integration of spirituality into health care practice by nurse practitioners. *Journal of the American Academy of Nurse Practitioners, 12*(7), 280–285.

Utz, S. W., Steeves, R. H., Wenzel, J., Hinton, I., Jones, R. A., Andrews, D., ... Oliver, M.N. (2006). "Working hard with it": Self-management of type 2 diabetes by rural African Americans. *Family & Community Health, 29*(3), 195–205.

Watson, J. (2008). *Nursing: The philosophy and science of caring* (rev. ed.). Boulder, CO: University of Colorado Press.

Yeh, P., & Bull, M. (2009). Influences of spiritual well-being and coping on mental health of family caregivers for elders. *Research in Gerontological Nursing, 2*(3), 173–180.

Yesavage, J. A., & Sheikh, J. I. (1986). Geriatric Depression Scale (GDS): Recent evidence and development of a shorter version. *Clinical Gerontology, 6,* 165–173.

Chapter 6

Social Isolation

Nicholas R. Nicholson, Jr.

Introduction

The idea that human beings are social beings is a concept that is hardly debatable. However, the impact of social isolation on humans, their families, and their communities is an idea that is relatively new in the scientific literature. The need to view the health and well-being of human beings in a holistic manner is more important now than ever. Increased focus on the intersection of physical, psychological, and social health is critically important in the increasingly complex world of managing chronic illness. According to the World Health Organization (WHO), health is defined as "a state of complete physical, mental and social well-being and not merely the absence of disease or infirmity" (WHO, 2003).

As the nature of chronic illness changes and becomes increasingly complex to manage, the ability to maintain social health is paramount. An individual's ability to socialize, or lack thereof, is an important predictor of numerous negative health outcomes. A person who is socially isolated, especially an older adult (age 65 and older), is at an increased risk of social isolation and its harsh consequences. There has been a fair amount of conceptual ambiguity related to what social isolation is and is not; therefore, it is important that the theoretical underpinnings be outlined and clearly defined. As healthcare professionals, it is important that we understand the psychosocial construct of social isolation, as it will influence how the individual who stands before you responds to every aspect of your carefully planned care.

The existence of social isolation increases our awareness of the need for humans to associate with each other in an authentic intimate relationship, whether characterized by caring or some other emotion, such as anger. When we speak of social isolation, we think first of the affected person; then almost immediately we consider that individual's relationships. This chapter demonstrates that, as a process, social isolation is a prominent feature in a variety of illnesses and disabilities across the life cycle.

The Nature of Social Isolation

Known aspects of social isolation are identified in this chapter, as well as related concepts that are important to consider in any discussion of social isolation. These related concepts comprise negative social network members and their potential impact on individuals. Additionally, it is important to present social isolation in relation to similar states of human apartness, including aloneness, loneliness, and solitude.

NEGATIVE SOCIAL NETWORK MEMBERS

Social relationships have the potential to exert both health-promoting and health-damaging effects in older persons (Seeman, 2000). It is widely assumed that for each additional social network member, there is a dose-response in the amount of benefit that member provides to the individual. This is often the case, but not always. Some social network members may actually be considered negative, in the sense that they constantly take away time and draw effort from the individual, as opposed to helping. In healthy relationships, there should be a certain amount of give and take. However, negative social network members are *takers* and do not give, such that their net sum is detrimental.

The quality of the social network members includes individuals who provide both positive and negative influences on the (older) adult. Increased disability is the result of individuals who have negative social network influences or negative social exchanges (Mavandadi, Rook, & Newsom, 2007). High-quality social network members, in contrast, may provide regular caring behaviors. Additional examples include those persons who provide goods and services to ease various burdens of the individuals. The existence of few strong bonds (Berkman, Glass, Brissette, & Seeman, 2000) and the extent and relative quality of social networks (Mistry, Rosansky, McGuire, McDermott, Jarvik, & UPBEAT Collaborative Group, 2001) are influential to the development of social isolation.

SOCIAL ISOLATION VERSUS SIMILAR STATES OF HUMAN APARTNESS

In the past, social isolation has been treated as a distinct phenomenon, or it has been combined or equated with other states relating to human apartness. The literature is replete with a variety of definitions of social isolation, many of which are interrelated, synonymous, or confused with other distinct but related phenomena. In the spirit of conceptual clarity, several concepts that often overlap in the literature are described here.

Social Isolation Versus Aloneness Referring to aloneness, Killeen (1998) stated "Someone

alone is obviously by themselves, and therefore they might be lonely, but this might not be the case at all" (p. 764). This concept can be seen as either a positive or negative experience depending on the individual's perspective. Being alone implies that there is control or choice involved with the decision to get away from others (Killeen, 1998). In absolute terms, alone can be thought of as being by oneself by choice (or not) and is not subjective in nature. A concept analysis examining aloneness in reference to chronic illness found that the attributes of aloneness change depending on which stage of treatment the individual is in (Pierce, Wilkinson, & Anderson, 2003).

The feelings attributed to aloneness can change from vulnerability, fearfulness, helplessness, loss of control of self, and identity confusion to include self-reliance, hope, resourcefulness, self-determination, and self-reflection (Pierce et al., 2003). This reflects the dual nature of the concept, where it can be positive and evident of self-healing or negative and symptomatic of losing control. Clearly, the experience of the objective aloneness of the individual and its associated circumstances can have a serious impact on the feeling of being alone. This feeling may be associated with deficits in social support networks, diminished participation in these networks or in social relationships, or feelings of rejection or withdrawal.

Social Isolation Versus Loneliness According to Hagerty, Lynch-Sauer, Patusky, Bouwseema, and Collier (1992), loneliness "implies a need for another person or group that has been disrupted and is discussed in the context of absence or loss" (p. 175). Feelings of incongruity between the desired and achieved levels of social contact are the hallmark signs of loneliness (Perlman, 1987; Walton, Shultz, Beck, & Walls, 1991). There is a negative connotation assigned to loneliness, suggesting that the desired interaction is unreachable. An example of this is that "the lonely experience is a sense of utter aloneness as well as aimlessness and boredom" (Younger, 1995, p. 58). It is clear that there is a negative subjective feeling when an individual experiences loneliness. A study performing a factor analysis of the concepts of loneliness, social support, and social networks showed that these three constructs are not different from one another, but it is recommended that these concepts be measured separately (Lubben & Gironda, 1996).

Social Isolation Versus Solitude As valuable as life may be when we engage in a variety of relationships, time reserved for solitude is also necessary as we seek rest or contemplative opportunity in *our own space*. The weaving together of individual possibilities for social engagement or solitude develops a certain uniqueness and texture in personal and community relationships. These distinctive personal configurations of engagement and disengagement have consequences for our work and social lives. It is critical, therefore, that healthcare professionals understand the value and distinctness of solitude from social isolation. Deliberate apartness—often described as solitude—is a distancing from one's social network, but this state is typically accompanied by positive feelings and is often voluntarily initiated.

The notion that social isolation can be positive, beneficial, and in some cases sought after by individuals is a misconception. Social isolation, as defined in this chapter, is a negative experience that comprises an experience based on unmet needs or feelings related to social relationships. Individuals do not seek social isolation to feel better or to experience something positive. Again, conceptual ambiguity may be at play in these instances, which in turn highlights the need to be clear with constructs and concepts. Individuals whose social network consists of one or more individuals who are considered negative social network members may find benefit

by seeking solitude. Individuals who feel obligated to certain social network members may need time away to rest. Solitude may offer time to recharge oneself physically and emotionally and allow an individual to continue with these relationships. Individuals do not self-isolate.

SOCIAL ISOLATION AND CHRONIC ILLNESS

Chronic illness is multidimensional, and persons with chronic illness and their social networks must assume a variety of tasks: managing treatment regimens, controlling symptoms, preventing and managing crises, reordering time, managing the illness trajectory, dealing with healthcare professionals, normalizing life, preserving a reasonable self-image, keeping emotional balance, managing social isolation, funding the costs of health care, and preparing for an uncertain future (Strauss, Corbin, Fagerhaugh, Glaser, Maines, & Suczek, 1984). As persons with chronic illnesses struggle to understand the failure of their body and maintain personal and social identities, they may become fatigued, become sicker, or lose hope more readily. Should this happen, they may more easily withdraw from their social networks. Individuals who have four or more chronic illnesses have been shown to be at increased risk for social isolation (Havens & Hall, 2001).

Social network members may find it difficult, depending on their level of commitment, to continue support during exacerbations of other comorbid conditions. This may be especially true during older adulthood, when each individual is dealing with his or her own comorbidities and may find it increasingly difficult to help others. These individuals, therefore, may look for increased support to meet their own needs.

Like many chronic psychological illnesses such as depression, social isolation is a phenomenon that may require an ongoing, lifelong effort to integrate individuals socially. Based on what is known about social isolation, there is no single solution that will "cure" isolates. Rather, interventions that have shown promise in mitigating social isolation consist of group behavioral therapies that focus on teaching life/social skills to help individuals reintegrate socially (Cattan, White, Bond, & Learmouth, 2005; Dickens et al., 2011).

Nearly all of the numerous negative health outcomes of social isolation can be categorized as chronic illnesses. Coronary heart disease (CHD) (Boden-Albala, Litwak, Elkind, Rundek, & Sacco, 2005), decreased cognition (Beland, Zunzunegui, Alvarado, Otero, & Del Ser, 2005), dementia (Fratiglioni, Paillard-Borg, & Winblad, 2004), mood disorder (Golden et al., 2009), inactivity (Eng, Rimm, Fitzmaurice, & Kawachi, 2002; Shankar, McMunn, Banks, & Steptoe, 2011), smoking (Shankar et al., 2011), poor nutrition (Locher, Ritchie, Roth, Baker, Bodner, & Allman, 2005), and increased falls (Faulkner, Cauley, Zmuda, Griffin, & Nevitt, 2003) are all comorbidities that are chronic in nature. Each of these conditions also requires a complex treatment regimen for its management.

From Ambiguity to Clarity: The Evolution of Social Isolation

Lack of contact with one's social network members has been suggested as a psychosocial phenomenon that is responsible for a wide variety of important aspects of diminished human health (Cobb, 1979). This modern notion—namely, that social relationships may be a critical aspect of the health and well-being of individuals—was demonstrated clearly in Berkman and Syme's (1979) seminal work, which identified increased mortality in those persons with lower levels of social networks. Since the publication of these authors' work, myriad replication studies have reaffirmed the general finding that social networks are an important aspect of health. It is difficult to ignore nearly 35 years of research suggesting the importance of having human beings connect with one another and the health benefits of such relationship, in addition to the health risks associated with a lack of such connection.

Through evolution of this line of thinking, the literature suggests that the label given to a lack of social networks—that is, *social isolation*—is no longer an adequate representation of this construct. Social isolation has morphed from a label simply indicating a small number of social network members to a more robust construct. This construct now encompasses social networks as well as the connection to those networks (Cornwell & Waite, 2009; Nicholson, 2009). With the literature moving toward a recognition that social isolation is a complex construct including both subjective and objective components, the focus can move from a state of conceptual ambiguity to an assessment of the best ways of measurement and beyond. First, however, we discuss the definition of social isolation.

Social Isolation Defined

Social isolation is the distancing of an individual, psychologically and/or physically, from his or her network of desired or needed relationships with other persons. Therefore, social isolation is a loss of place within one's group(s). This isolation may be voluntary or involuntary. In cognitively intact persons, social isolation can be identified as such by the isolate. Specifically defined, social isolation is "a state in which the individual lacks a sense of belonging socially, lacks engagement with others, has a minimal number of social contacts and they are deficient in fulfilling and quality relationships" (Nicholson, 2009, p. 1346). Social isolation can be described as the merging of both subjective and objective aspects of an individual's health. Being socially isolated is an all-encompassing state that is the result of not only a deficit in the number of social contacts one has, but also a deficiency in the perceived quality of these connections. This definition accounts for both the individual's perceived experience (subjective aspect) and the actual number of social contacts (objective aspect).

Typology of Social Contact

Social contact is an important component of social isolation, but not the entire piece. As stated earlier, the definition of social isolation includes the objective number of social contacts. The number of social contacts is often called one's social network. An individual's social network provides many important positive benefits, including different types of support. Wenger's classic (1991) research has demonstrated that individuals have five distinct types of social networks in their lives: (1) the local family-dependent support network; (2) the locally integrated support network; (3) the local self-contained support network; (4) the wider community-focused support network; and (5) the private restricted support network (**Table 6-1**).

Understanding that individuals have different types of social support networks provides insight into tailoring interventions aimed at maximizing the benefits of these social support networks. If one could obtain information about the types of social networks to which individuals belong, it would be possible to focus on increasing involvement with these social support networks. By better elucidating the problem of social isolation through an increased understanding of social network types (a portion of social isolation), it may become easier to connect with clients and understand their complex chronic health issues as they relate to the social environment.

INCIDENCE AND PREVALENCE

Prevalence of social isolation in community-living adults has a wide range, with a high end of 49.8% and a low end of 2% (Dickens, Richards, Greaves, & Campbell, 2011; Greaves & Farbus, 2006; Ibrahim, Abolfathi Momtaz, & Hamid, 2013; Nicholson, Molony, Fennie, Shellman, & McCorkle, 2010; Smith & Hirdes, 2009; Victor, Bond, & Bowling, 2003; Victor, Scambler, & Bond, 2009). The incidence of social isolation is 4.5 cases of social isolation per 100 person-years (Nicholson et al., 2010).

SOCIAL ISOLATION AND OLDER ADULTS

Older age, with its many losses of physical and psychological health, social roles, mobility, economic status, and physical living arrangements, can contribute to decreasing social networks and increasing isolation (Howat, Iredell, Grenade,

---

Table 6-1 WENGER'S TYPOLOGY OF SOCIAL NETWORKS

- **The local family-dependent support network** is primarily focused on local family contact with few, if any, peripheral friends or neighbors. Most of the support is provided by relatives.
- **The locally integrated support network** is based on close relationships with family, friends, and neighbors. Individuals who fit this category typically are in the same location for an extended period of time.
- **The local self-contained support network** is highlighted by a lack of close-knit relationships and infrequent contact with at least one family member of the social network. Individuals who fit this category are typically childless, so they may have increased reliance on neighbors. These networks tend to be smaller.
- **The wider community-focused support network** is typically a network where individuals are active despite geographical distances with family. It may be common for this individual to have a lack of close family. Networks tend to be fairly large and are often associated with those who have retired and migrated elsewhere.
- **The private restricted support network** is characterized by a lack of local family members (except a spouse or partner). Contact with neighbors is uncommon, as is involvement with community organizations. This network type includes independent couples and those living alone. Networks tend to be small. and these individuals may be in need of support and outreach.

Sources: Wenger, 1984, 1991, 1997; Wenger & Burholt, 2004; Wenger, Davies, Shahtahmasebi, & Scott, 1996.

Nedwetzky, & Collins, 2004; Victor et al., 2002). This factor will become even more of an issue in the future, as the number of older adults is expected to increase arithmetically and proportionately in the next two decades. Older adults currently make up 12.9% of the overall U.S. population (Fowles & Greenberg, 2009).

Social isolation has been linked with functional disability. One definition of functional disability is "the degree of difficulty or inability to independently perform basic activities of daily living (ADLs) or other tasks essential for independent living" (Mendes de Leon, Gold, Glass, Kaplan, & George, 2001, p. S179). Consequently, functional disability may impact social networks by preventing older adults from seeking engagement with other members. Network size and social interaction are significantly associated with functional disability risk (Mendes de Leon et al., 2001). Older adults who are more socially engaged report less functional disability (odds ratio [OR] = 0.84; 95% CI: 0.75–0.95) (Mendes de Leon, Glass, & Berkman, 2003).

Social isolation has been shown to be a serious health risk for older adults (Findlay, 2003; Findlay & Cartwright, 2002), with studies indicating a relationship between all-cause mortality (Ceria, Masaki, Rodriguez, Chen, Yano, & Curb, 2001), coronary disease (Eng et al., 2002), and cognitive impairments (Barnes, Mendes de Leon, Wilson, Bienias, & Evans, 2004; Beland et al., 2005; Holtzman, Rebok, Saczynski, Kouzis, Wilcox Doyle, & Eaton, 2004; Zunzunegui, Alvarado, Del Ser, & Otero, 2003).

In a contradictory finding, older adults with extensive social networks were protected against dementia (Fratiglioni et al., 2004; Seidler, Bernhardt, Nienhaus, & Frolich, 2003; Wang, Karp, Winblad, & Fratiglioni, 2002). Also, as described earlier, although low social engagement may not be a form of social isolation per se, it is a psychological isolator and, therefore, a risk factor in social isolation (Howat et al., 2004). For example, depressive symptoms in older adults were shown to be decreased by

social integration (Ramos & Wilmoth, 2003). Isolated older adults have increased risk for coronary heart disease (Eng et al., 2002), and death related to congestive heart failure appears to be predicted by social isolation (Murberg, 2004). Similarly, post-stroke outcomes—for example, additional strokes, myocardial infarction, or death—may be predicted by pre-stroke isolation (Boden-Albala et al., 2005).

Isolated women before a diagnosis of breast cancer, when compared with socially integrated women, have been found to have a 66% increase in all-cause mortality (Kroenke, Kubzansky, Schernhammer, Holmes, & Kawachi, 2006). Quality of life among breast cancer survivors is affected negatively by social isolation (Michael, Berkman, Colditz, Holmes, & Kawachi, 2002). Finally, and perhaps most relevant to health and cost outcomes, socially isolated older adults have been found to be four to five times more likely to be rehospitalized within a year from their previous hospitalization (Giuli, Spazzafumo, Sinolla, Abbatecola, Lattanzio, & Postacchini, 2012; Mistry et al., 2001).

Although much of the current research in social isolation with older adults has focused on community-living adults, one growing segment of study is assisted-living arrangements, one of the fastest-growing segments of senior housing (Hawes, Phillips, Rose, Holan, & Sherman, 2003). In assisted-living settings, where there are many internal (to the setting) social networks, positive reports of life satisfaction, quality of life, and perception of home have been noted (Street, Burge, Quadagno, & Barrett, 2007). Assisted living has the potential to focus on health promotion and function maintenance, such as the identification of social isolation and appropriate interventions (Resnick, 2007).

Strictly speaking, social isolation is not confined to a place. The individual who is socially isolated is not necessarily homebound or placebound, although that is typically the case. That being said, environments that are removed from the majority of the community (such as rural locations) or those not conducive to safety (such as high-crime areas) can contribute to social isolation (Klinenberg, 2001).

Social isolation as a function of location has been demonstrated, particularly for the older adult in urbanized settings, in a number of countries other than the United States (Klinenberg, 2001). In these cases, older adults cannot leave their homes because of lack of transportation or fear of assault, so they may increasingly isolate themselves from others. This situation is intensified by distrust, low socioeconomic status, or locale, and it is worse if the older adult has a chronic illness compounding his or her constraints. Driving cessation may be an eventual reality as one ages. Limited or no driving restricts activities outside the home (Marottoli, Mendes de Leon, Glass, Williams, Cooney, & Berkman, 2000), thereby limiting interactions with others for the older adult.

RISK FACTORS AND PREDICTORS OF SOCIAL ISOLATION

In recent years, the literature on social isolation has shed light on this phenomenon's antecedents. A true understanding of what leads to social isolation allows for more upstream thinking, which focuses on prevention rather than reaction to the condition. Once the negative health outcomes of social isolation are present, an individual's health status becomes markedly worse. Risk factors associated with social isolation are described according to categories outlined by Howat et al. (2004): (1) physical, (2) psychological, (3) economic, (4) work/family changes, and (5) environmental. In addition to these five categories, a *demographic factors* category is added here.

Physical Factors It has been suggested that individuals who are overweight may be socially isolated due to an increased level of self-consciousness toward socialization activities (Nicholson & Shellman, 2013). Christakis and Fowler (2007) have demonstrated that weight gain includes a social component. Specifically, weight gain in one person is associated with weight gain in that individual's social network of friends, siblings, and spouses.

An increased number of health problems is also associated with becoming socially isolated (Havens, Hall, Sylvestre, & Jivan, 2004). Havens et al. (2004) suggest that older adults with four or more chronic illnesses are at increased risk for social isolation. Inability to maintain physical functioning is likewise associated with social isolation (Sawada, Shinohara, Sugisawa, & Anme, 2011). Older adults who are socially isolated report more functional disability when compared to those who are socially integrated (Mendes de Leon et al., 2003).

Individuals who engaged in risky health behavioral activities such as smoking appear to be more likely to be socially isolated (Pantell, Rehkopf, Jutte, Syme, Balmes, & Adler, 2013). Nicholson, Dixon, and McCorkle (2014) report that smoking was predictive of future social isolation over a 12-year period. Christakis and Fowler (2008) have identified a phenomenon in which individuals who smoke tend to cluster together in the same small social network. Also, those who smoke have been found to be at the periphery of societal networks, in general, as smokers continue to be marginalized within many societies.

The way that individuals see and rate their own health has been demonstrated to be predictive of social isolation (Ibrahim et al., 2013; Wilson, Harris, Hollis, & Mohankumar, 2011). Persons who see their health as poor or rate their health that way are much more likely to become socially isolated over time (Nicholson et al., 2014).

Sleep and personal care habits are an important part of the health and well-being of human beings throughout the lifespan. When the sleep cycle is disturbed, a number of consequences may follow. Individuals who are tired during the day are less likely to engage with their social networks and, therefore, are at increased risk of social isolation (Lee, Tsai, Ouyang, Yang, Yang, & Hwang, 2013). Lack of rest is a precursor to a cascade in which less social engagement leads to social isolation.

As a person maneuvers through the typical day-to-day routine of social activities, the importance of free movement, seeing, and hearing may not be considered. In relation to the social aspect of health, these sensory functions are critically important. Impairment of mobility, vision, or hearing has been shown to lead to social isolation (Wenger & Burholt, 2004).

Psychological Factors   There are numerous psychological predictors of social isolation. According to Blazer (2005), depression has a "clear, but not obvious relationship" with social isolation (p. 497). This statement exemplifies the complexity of these closely related concepts. Social workers, who are in a good position to understand these concepts, identify depression as a key component of social isolation (McCrae et al., 2005). Those who are in a depressed state have been found to be at significant risk for social isolation (Iliffe, Kharicha, Harari, Swift, Gillmann, & Stuck, 2007). New research suggests that persons with depressive symptoms are nearly twice as likely (OR = 1.8) to become socially isolated as compared to those individuals without depressive symptoms (Nicholson et al., 2014). Persons who have a diagnosis of personality disorder or have been institutionalized in a psychiatric facility are also more likely to become socially isolated (Smith & Hirdes, 2009).

Religious engagement is an important aspect of predicting social isolation. Original measures of social networking used church membership as part of the scoring to determine if an individual was socially isolated (Berkman & Syme, 1979). Lack of religious engagement or infrequent participation in religious activities has been shown to predict social isolation (Nicholson et al., 2014; Pantell et al., 2013).

Economic Factors   Changes in socioeconomic status, such as changes in employment status or retirement, have been correlated with social isolation. The lack of employment of both caregiver

and care recipient can have an adverse effect on health. Retirement is a life-changing event for older adults and tends to be a source of stress. Some older adults retire willingly, whereas others are pressured to leave their jobs to make way for newer, younger employees. There is a close association between small social networks and early retirement (Elovainio et al., 2003). Individuals who have close social network ties to individuals at work may be at increased risk of social isolation due to the sudden decrease in access to these individuals through typical day-to-day interactions. Income and social status are important variables in determining the risk of becoming socially isolated (Wilson et al., 2011). Constrained finances (Iliffe et al., 2007) and low income (Bassuk, Glass, & Berkman, 1999) have been shown to have a strong correlation with social isolation.

Lower income status, especially when coupled with less education, negatively influences health status and is associated with both a limiting social network and greater loneliness, which in turn impacts health status and social isolation. In addition to problems of employment potential, economic and social concerns may arise over the costs incurred by health care, employment discrimination, subsequent inability to secure insurance, and loss of potential friendship networks at work—all of which are factors in increasing social isolation or reducing social interactions. In fact, economic stresses exaggerate the costs of chronic illness.

Work/Family Changes   A life event such as the death of a relative, friend, or close neighbor has been shown to increase social isolation among older adults (Wenger & Burholt, 2004). Death of that individual within their social network is likely to prevent an individual from engaging in the social network. Not socializing has been found to lead to and be a part of being socially isolated (Longman, Passey, Sinder, & Morgan, 2013). Individuals who are married or even widowed are less likely to become socially isolated (Smith & Hirdes, 2009). When a person is isolated from family, that individual is more likely to become socially isolated (Longman et al., 2013).

Environmental Factors   Factors related to the environment have been shown to be predictive of social isolation. Individuals who live in urban housing as opposed to rural housing have been found to be more likely to become socially isolated (Ibrahim et al., 2013). Additionally, according to Ibrahim and colleagues (2013), lack of home ownership may be predictive of social isolation. Living alone produces a home environment that leads to fewer social networks, an important component of social isolation (Havens et al., 2004; Iliffe et al., 2007; Wenger & Burholt, 2004).

Demographic Factors   Men are more likely to become socially isolated than women (Iliffe et al., 2007). Older age also increases the risk for social isolation (Havens & Hall, 2001; Iliffe et al., 2007). Some research suggests that race and/or ethnicity may lead to social isolation (Ajrouch, Antonucci, & Janevic, 2001; Ibrahim et al., 2013). Less education has been shown to be related to social isolation (Iliffe et al., 2007).

Consequences of Social Isolation

Over the past 35 years, substantial research has been undertaken by numerous researchers from a multitude of disciplines that demonstrates how social isolation results in negative health outcomes. The psychosocial phenomenon of social isolation is generally accepted to be an important risk factor that should be considered during interviews with clients in the healthcare environment as well as when working with individuals living in the community. These negative health consequences of social isolation are organized into four categories according to the Berkman et al. (2000) framework: (1) physiological, (2) psychological, (3) health behavioral, and (4) other.

Consequences to Self

PHYSIOLOGICAL CONSEQUENCES

A great deal of this literature focuses on all-cause mortality as the ultimate negative health outcome of being socially isolated (Eng et al., 2002; Giles, Glonek, Luszcz, & Andrews, 2005; Pantell et al., 2013). Coronary heart disease and its resultant mortality are easily identified in the literature (Boden-Albala et al., 2005). Overall well-being has been found to be diminished in individuals who are socially isolated (Golden et al., 2009).

PSYCHOLOGICAL CONSEQUENCES

Diminished psychological and cognitive well-being has been shown to be an outcome of being socially isolated. Cognitive decline occurs when individuals do not participate in social activities (Beland et al., 2005). Death by suicide is a risk for socially isolated individuals (Eng et al., 2002). Poorer cognitive function (Shankar, Hamar, McMunn, & Steptoe, 2013), as well as increases in dementia (Fratiglioni et al., 2004), may be consequences of social isolation as well. According to Golden and colleagues (2009), mood is negatively impacted by social isolation.

HEALTH BEHAVIORAL CONSEQUENCES

Socially isolated individuals have been found to have multiple health risk behaviors, including higher levels of inactivity and increased rates of smoking (Eng et al., 2002; Shankar et al., 2011). Both smoking and a sedentary lifestyle are associated with well-known health consequences. Additionally, socially isolated individuals have an increased risk for poor nutrition (Locher et al., 2005).

OTHER CONSEQUENCES

Some other negative health outcomes connected with social isolation do not fit within the three categories outlined by Berkman et al. (2000). For example, being socially isolated has been shown to increase risk for rehospitalization (Giuli, Papa, Mocchegiani, & Marcellini, 2012; Mistry et al., 2001) and avoidable admissions (Longman et al., 2013).

Social isolation is a condition that touches on all aspects of an individual's well-being, including physical, psychological, and, of course, social health. Quality of life has been found to be poorer for individuals who are socially isolated (Hawton et al., 2011). Socially isolated individuals also experience an increased number of falls (Faulkner et al., 2003).

Social Isolation and Social Roles

Any weakening or diminishment of relationships or social roles may produce social isolation for individuals or their significant others. Clients who lose family, friends, and associated position and power are inclined toward feelings of rejection, worthlessness, and loss of self-esteem (Ravish, 1985). These feelings become magnified by the client's culture if that culture values community (Litwin & Zoabi, 2003; Siplic & Kadis, 2002). For example, social isolation of both caregiver and care recipient occurred in one case in which a woman's husband had Alzheimer's disease. The couple had been confined for more than two years in an apartment in a large city, from which the confused husband frequently wandered. The woman's comment, "I'm not like a wife and not like a single person either," reflected their dwindling social network and her loss of wifely privileges, but not obligations. This ambiguity is common among many individuals whose spouses are incapacitated. Moreover, after a spouse dies, the widow or widower often grieves as much for the loss of the role of a married person as for the loss of the spouse.

The loss of social roles can occur as a result of illness or disability, social changes throughout the lifespan (e.g., in school groups, with career moves, or in unaccepting communities), marital dissolution (through death or divorce), or secondary to ostracism incurred by membership in a "wrong" group. The loss of social roles and the resultant isolation of the individual have proved useful analytic devices in the examination of issues of the aged, the widowed, and the physically impaired, and in psychopathology.

Social Isolation and Culture

As globalization and sensitivity to U.S. multiculturalism increases, with the concurrent absorption of multiethnic, multilingual, and multireligious individuals into yet other cultures, there is an overlap of these issues within the mainstream healthcare systems. This is especially true of cultural groups whose members have not become assimilated into the dominant culture. Language differences and traditional living arrangements may impede their social adaptation. In addition, many immigrants, especially those with chronic illness, are less able to engage in support networks, given their long working hours, low-paying jobs, lack of health insurance, and changes in family lifestyles and living arrangements.

When reviewing the healthcare literature and its relationship with culture, two overarching issues are noted: (1) the definitions of culture are conceptually broad and/or indistinct, and (2) mainstream healthcare is struggling to integrate these multicultural groups, with varying degrees of success being observed. The former issue needs additional time for the concept of culture to evolve; however, the latter issue is something that should be addressed now. Some questions may arise as to the temporality of culture and race/ethnicity. In other words, do groups of individuals connect culturally because they are of similar race/ethnicity backgrounds, or does the culture drive how individuals see their race/ethnicity? Either way, being of a certain race and/or group has been suggested to lead to social isolation (Ajrouch et al., 2001; Ibrahim et al., 2013). If certain racial/ethnic groups prefer to connect with those with similar interests, there may be fewer opportunities for their members to engage with other individuals, particularly if the racial/ethnic subgroup is small. It is important, given the numerous negative health outcomes from social isolation, that cultural norms and racial/ethnic group be assessed when dealing with individuals with chronic illness. It is through this assessment that a more holistic plan of care can be developed and implementation of that plan can begin.

When one speaks of assessing social isolation among unique ethnic groups, the number, type, and quality of contacts must be considered, especially given the lens through which each individual of that person's culture views the world. It is not only the client's perspective, but also the provider's communication patterns, roles, relationships, and traditions that are important elements to consider in both assessment and intervention. Matching culturally similar providers to clients may be an effective way to meet client needs. At the same time, healthcare educators and service professionals recognize the issues associated with a smaller supply of providers and the greater numbers of clients in a dominant healthcare system coping with multiculturalism.

One approach to assessing social relationships requires the professional to approach each person, regardless of his or her cultural milieu, with respect and dignity, in an explicit good faith effort to inquire about, understand, and be responsive to the client's culture, needs, and person. The healthcare professional must set aside prejudices and stereotypes and use, instead, an authentic sensitive inquiry into the client's beliefs and well-being (Browne, 1997; Treolar, 1999). Through honesty and humility, healthcare professionals have an opportunity to learn about multiculturalism from their clients.

Identifying Social Isolation

The importance of social isolation is becoming more widely recognized as a construct that warrants surveillance in health care, especially critical care (Alspach, 2013). The question becomes how to detect its existence in clients. Arguably, after the concept of social isolation is defined, the next most important step is to determine how to detect this condition in susceptible and vulnerable adults. Through accurate measurement of social isolation, researchers and clinicians will be able to accurately screen/identify those persons with the condition as well as determine whether interventions are effective.

Being able to differentiate between individuals with social isolation and those without social isolation is a critically important part of the process. As noted earlier, individuals who are socially isolated are at risk for numerous negative health outcomes; they need to be accurately identified so preventive measures can be implemented. Preventive measures could include increasing social support systems tailored to the specific area in which the individual has deficiencies (objective versus subjective aspect). Specific interventions that have shown effectiveness in reducing social isolation are discussed in more detail later in this chapter.

When social isolation is suspected, a systematic assessment can help determine potential interventions. The key to assessing social isolation is to observe for three distinct features: (1) negativity, (2) involuntary or other imposed solitude, and (3) declining quality and number of individuals within the isolate's social networks. Social isolation must be distinguished from other conditions such as loneliness or depression, both of which may show similar manifestations in clients. Because social isolation can be destructive, the healthcare professional must be resourceful in assessing which issue predominates (objective versus subjective social isolation) at any particular point in time and focus on that consideration.

When properly conducted, an assessment yields its own suggestions for responsive interventions. For instance, the assessment may indicate that the client is a lifelong isolate; it would then be necessary to evaluate steps tailored to help this individual move toward lessening his or her social isolation. Assessment typically involves the clinical dyad of caregiver and client. It is at this level that assessment is critical to the development of appropriate and effective interventions. Without an adequate and sensitive assessment, interventions are likely to be ineffective or incomplete.

In another example, if the healthcare professional discovers that a support network is lax in calling or contacting a client, the professional can help the client and support network rebuild bridges with each other. Keep in mind that support groups are typically used to meet this need. As an illustration, if the network is overwhelmed, information can be provided about respite programs. Such interventions will help members of the social network maintain the energy levels necessary to help their relative or friend with chronic illness.

As new interventions are created and tested to mitigate social isolation, it is important that measurements are sensitive to change and the overall accuracy is precise. Instruments that purport to measure social isolation must allow for sufficient change in the scoring to reflect a legitimate change (improvement or worsening) of the condition. This sensitivity to change in a measure needs to be accurate, in the sense that if an individual's social isolation status improves, the instrument will show it. Otherwise, a perfectly efficient and effective intervention could be created, yet might not be measured accurately via an instrument.

The major issue in measuring social isolation is that the existing instrumentation does not fully capture the conceptual definition of social isolation. For example, social isolation, as described in this chapter, has no specific instrument of measurement. Some researchers have used instruments that define social isolation as an extreme lack of social networks or support, whereas others use a group of questions that purport to measure this condition. The closely related concept of social networks has two frequently used research measures that may be useful when assessing social isolation. Because there is some conceptual overlap of both constructs—specifically, the number of social contacts—measures used to assess social networks may serve as a useful initial assessment for social isolation.

Several instruments are described in the literature that measure social constructs, including social networks and belongingness, yet none measures social isolation specifically as defined here. The definition of social isolation includes social networks and one's feelings of belonging within these networks. Two measures quantify at least one of these, belongingness or social networks, and are recommended as initial screening tools. These measures are the Lubben Social Network Scale (LSNS-6) for social networks and the Social Connectedness Scale Revised (SCS-R)

(Lee, Draper, & Lee, 2001). The Lubben Social Network Scale (LSNS-18) is an appropriate measure to use with older adults because it is specifically designed for application in that population (Lubben, 2003; Lubben & Gironda, 2003a, 2003b). The LSNS-18 has three subscales consisting of friends, family, and neighbors; each of the subscales includes 6 questions, for a total of 18 items. Out of the 6 questions in each subscale, the first two refer to size, the next two refer to frequency, and the last two refer to interdependent relationships. The total score ranges from 0 to 90. As the LSNS-18 score decreases, the extent to which an individual is socially isolated increases. The LSNS-18 is typically divided into quartiles to indicate those persons with the most limited social networks in relation to those persons with the least limited social networks. Reliability has been demonstrated with a Cronbach's alpha of 0.82 for the total scale 0.82 for the family subscale, 0.87 for the friend subscale, and 0.80 for the neighbor subscale (Lubben & Gironda, 2003a).

The SCS-R was created as an operational measure of the theoretical concept of belongingness (Lee & Robbins, 1995). It measures the amount of interpersonal closeness and the degree of difficulty in maintaining that closeness between people. Having a lack of a sense of belonging is a necessary component to being socially isolated. The SCS-R has a total of 20 items, 10 positively worded and 10 negatively worded. The revised instrument (SCS-R) has been found to be more normally distributed than its predecessor (SCS) (Lee et al., 2001).

There is a need for a psychometrically tested instrument specifically designed to measure social isolation as the construct has evolved. The instruments mentioned in this section are good screening measures, but they have not been subjected to the rigorous testing called for in the literature (Henly, 2013). The importance of theoretically designed and rigorously tested instruments with the most current methodology, such as item response theory, is critical in detecting and differentiating social isolation.

Social Components of Social Isolation

Mere numbers of people surrounding someone do not cure negative social isolation; an individual can be socially isolated even in a crowd if his or her significant social network is lost. This situation is true for members of such groups as those living or working in sheltered-care workshops, residents in long-term care facilities, and people in prisons. What is critical to social isolation is that, because of situations imposed on them, individuals perceive themselves as disconnected from meaningful discourse with people important to them.

Associated with social isolation is reciprocity or mutuality—that is, the amount of give and take that occurs between isolated individuals and their social networks. Throughout the years, much evidence has accumulated indicating that informal networks of social support offer significant emotional assistance, information, and material resources for a number of populations. These support systems appear to foster good health, help maintain appropriate behaviors, and alleviate stress (Cobb, 1979).

The examination of reciprocity in the relationships of social networks focuses not only on social roles and the content of the exchange, but also on the level of agreement between the isolated person and his or her "others" in the network (Randers, Mattiasson, & Olson, 2003). The incongruence between respondents in a social network regarding their exchanges can alert the healthcare professional to the level of emotional or material need or exhaustion that exists in either respondent.

CASE STUDY 6-1

It had been nearly 4 months since Scott left Patti to find his own way. The couple had been together nearly 35 years, but had drifted apart over the last 5 years. Patti was happy being a homemaker and spending her free time with Scott and his friends. However, this left Patti without her own group of friends, as she often ignored her own friends to meet Scott's social needs, and he did not get along with any of Patti's friends. Patti's only living family, her sister, moved across the country about a decade ago for work. She is always so busy that it has been difficult to keep in touch. Patti has gone out a few times with old friends from high school, but they are all married and she just does not feel as if she fits in anymore. Also, since Scott moved out, it has been difficult for Patti to maintain the house, the lawn, snow removal, and even the bills (she is on a fixed income).

Patti has since secured employment as a cashier as a local supermarket. After her second week on the job, she came home to celebrate her birthday with her cats, only to find her heating system was broken. As Patti sits holding her two cats for warmth, she thinks to herself, "I need go somewhere where it's warm, but where? I need to find someone to get this heater fixed, but where do I look? I need someone to listen and give me advice, but who?

Case Study Discussion Questions

1. What are the risk factors that Patti has for social isolation?
2. As her healthcare professional, which area(s) would you focus on first? What is your first step(s)?
3. Which resources would you recommend that Patti access?
4. If Patti's condition persists, which chronic negative health outcomes is Patti at additional risk for?

Interventions

When recommending interventions, it is important to remember that care planning requires healthcare professionals to work with the client to provide the best possible outcomes. Guiding people, rather than forcing them to go along with interventions, necessitates the healthcare professional offer a rationale for the proposed interventions. This method of thinking is similar to the difference between medication and treatment regimens. If individuals are expected to simply comply with the treatment, there is an implication that one must follow the treatment blindly. With adherence, the implication is much different. This perspective implies that the treatment plan is a collaborative team effort and the client is doing his or her part. Among the client's responsibilities are updating aspects of the plan that no longer work well and then sharing this information with the healthcare professional.

Flexibility by the healthcare professional and a desire to tailor interventions may promote a more successful approach in mitigating social isolation. In designing interventions with clients, the healthcare professional must ask if he or she is giving reasonable rationales, assurances, or support. At the same time, the professional should remember that some cultures value the authority and the expertise of other family members over that of the individual. Consequently, the healthcare professional may have to provide a rationale for suggested interventions to the ranking authority within the support group. Frequently, this is a male figure, often older, who is considered most deserving of explanations. Other cultures may be matriarchal, in which case a woman may be the ranking authority.

Because the situation of each person with chronic illness is unique, interventions vary (Holley, 2007). Nonetheless, certain useful techniques and strategies can be generalized.

Basically, these strategies require that a balance of responsibilities be developed between the healthcare professional and the client with the following aims:

- Increasing the moral autonomy or freedom of choice of the isolate
- Increasing social interaction at a level acceptable to the client
- Using repetitive and recognizable strategies that are validated with the client, which correlate to reducing particular isolating behaviors

Another point to remember is that to be most effective, interventions must structure themselves in group formats and should be coupled with an educational or supportive input (Cattan et al., 2005). Keeping or rebuilding social networks and feelings of belonging could be impacted through social media. The social use of media was found primarily among those who were seeking connectedness (Ahn & Shin, 2013) and is on the rise in some countries (White & Selwyn, 2013). Some specific interventions use Internet-based activities with the goal of reducing social isolation through social activities online (Ballantyne, Trenwith, Zubrinich, & Corlis, 2010). These Internet-based interventions have been shown to enhance participation in social activities by persons who may not otherwise have been privy to these activities (Blit-Cohen & Litwin, 2004; Sum, Mathews, Pourghasem, & Hughes, 2009).

The healthcare professional must also take into account the client's type of social network typology (see the earlier discussion of Wenger's 1991 research). The professional can then make contact with the individuals indicated to be most accommodating to the isolate, explain the situation, make future plans to bring them and the isolate together, and assess the outcome afterward. However, it may not always be possible to bring uninterested family members back into the isolate's social network.

CASE STUDY 6-2

The move into assisted living was not a decision made lightly. George and his family had discussed this possibility for nearly 3 months after his wife, Glenda, died suddenly. George grew up in the house where he currently lives, and all of his social connections are nearby, including his friends and neighbors of nearly 50 years. However, George has consistently lost weight, has fallen a few times, and has experienced severe bouts of the "blues" for the past 3 months. Since Glenda's death, George has also had difficulty performing his activities of daily living (ADL). He has a part-time helper whom his son pays to help George a few days a week. George's only living family member, his son Tom, lives in a nearby state. It has become increasingly difficult for Tom to care for George, as Tom's wife is expecting a child soon. Tom wants George to move somewhere safe, where the staff can prevent him from falling and take care of his other medical conditions. Specifically, Tom wants George to move to a facility near him. George reluctantly has agreed to sign the paperwork to sell the house and move to an assisted-living facility near Tom in one month.

Case Study Discussion Questions

1. Often as individuals age, there is a recurring theme of "loss." Which "losses" has George experienced? Which "losses" will George experience in one month?
2. Examining George's risk of social isolation now versus after he moves into the facility, when is George most at risk for social isolation? Why?
3. What are the positives of moving to the assisted-living facility? What are the negatives?

Management of Self: Identity Development

The need for an ongoing identity leads an individual to seek a level where he or she can overcome, avoid, or internalize stigma and, concomitantly, manage the resulting social isolation. Social networks can be affected by stigma. Managing various concerns requires people with chronic illness to develop a new sense of self consistent with their disabilities. This "new" life is intertwined with the lives of members of their social networks, which may now include both healthcare professionals and other persons with chronic illnesses. Lessons must be learned to deal with new body demands and associated behaviors. Consequently, the individual with chronic illness must redevelop an identity with norms different from previous ones.

The willingness to change to different and unknown norms is just a first step—one that often takes great courage and time. For instance, one study indicated that clients with pronounced physical, financial, and medical care problems following head and neck surgery exhibited prolonged social isolation 1 year postsurgery (Krouse, Krouse, & Fabian, 1989). Although no single study has indicated the amount of time necessary to complete such identity transformations, anecdotal information suggests that this period can last several years; indeed, for some, it is a lifelong experience.

Individuals who are homebound due to physical limitations and are socially isolated may benefit from the ubiquity of Internet/web-based interventions. Additionally, individuals who live a great distance from one another will not have to travel to engage their social network members, which may increase the feeling of connectedness and belonging.

Management of Self: Identity Transformation

Clarifying how networks form and function is a significant contribution in managing the client with concomitant chronic illness and social isolation. The perceptive healthcare professional should know that much of the management done by individuals with chronic illness and their networks is not seen or well understood by healthcare professionals today (Corbin & Strauss, 1987). However, one can use Charmaz's (1987) findings as a guide for assessing the likely identity level of the individual when trying to understand potential withdrawal or actual isolation.

Charmaz (1987), using a sample consisting of mostly middle-aged women, developed a framework of hierarchical identity transformations that is useful in diagnosing a chronically ill individual's proclivity toward social networking and in discovering which social network might be most appropriate. This hierarchy of identity takes into account a reconstruction toward a desired future self, based on past and present selves, and reflects the individual's relative difficulty in achieving specific aspirations. Charmaz's analysis progresses toward a "salvaged self" that retains a past identity based on important values or attributes while still acknowledging dependency.

Initially, the individual takes on a supernormal identity, which assumes an ability to retain all previous success values, social acclamation, struggles, and competition. At this identity level, the individual with chronic illness attempts to participate more intensely than an individual in a nonimpaired world despite the limitations of illness. The next identity level that the person moves to is the restored self, with the expectation of eventually returning to the previous self, despite the chronic illness or its severity. Healthcare professionals might identify this self with the psychological state of denial, but in terms of identity, the individual has simply assumed that there is no discontinuation with a former self. At the third level, the contingent personal identity, the individual defines the self in terms of potential risk and failure, indicating the individual still has not come to terms with a future self but has begun to realize that the supernormal identity will no longer be viable. Finally, the level of the salvaged self is reached, whereby the individual attempts to define the self as worthwhile, despite recognizing that the present circumstances invalidate any previous identity (Charmaz, 1987).

Not only does social isolation relate to stigma, but it can also develop as an individual loses hope of sustaining aspirations for a normal or supernormal self, which are now unrealistic. As persons with chronic illness act out regret, disappointment, and anger, their significant others and healthcare professionals may react in kind, perpetuating a downward spiral of loss, anger, and subsequent greater social isolation. The idea of identity hierarchies, therefore, alerts the caregiver to a process in which shifts in identity are expected.

The reactions, health advice, and experiences of individuals with chronic illness must be taken into account in managing that particular identity, as well as the various factors that help shape it. Both the social network and adapted norms now available play a role at each stage in identity transformation. At the supernormal identity level, individuals with chronic illness were in only limited contact with healthcare professionals, but presumably enjoyed greater contact with healthier individuals who acted as their referents (Charmaz, 1987).

Management of Self: Application of Identity and Transformation to Practice

Development and transformation of one's identity are two important theoretical steps that culminate in the most important third step, application to practice. Healthcare professionals spend countless hours with clients who are at various stages of dealing with their own chronic illness. Dealing with chronic illness requires each person to work through the various stages of understanding and managing the illness. Each individual is at a different point in this process at any given moment in time. By helping the individual identify and evolve throughout the chronic illness process, there is an opportunity to increase social integration. The close connection formed during the process of helping the individual become autonomous in the management of himself or herself through identification and transformation can be a tool to improve the person's social health.

In one study, through a close connection formed over weeks and months spent working with the same client, nursing students were able to form a close bond with older adults who were socially isolated (Nicholson & Shellman, 2013). This close bond enabled students to implement several strategies to help older adults become more socially integrated. The resulting increase in social integration reflected the time spent building a trusting relationship, which could then be used to support the older adults in trying other measures to reduce their social isolation. Self-management strategies such as taking the lead on creating a social calendar and following up with old friends and family members were especially effective tools. The older adults were empowered through the intervention process to take the lead, while the students moved from a doer role to a facilitator role to a supportive role over time.

Respite for Caregivers

The need for respite has been cited as one of the greatest necessities for isolated older adults with illness and their caregivers, many of whom are themselves older adults. The purpose of respite is to relieve caregivers for a period of time so that they may engage in activities that help sustain them or their loved ones, the care recipients. Respite involves four elements: (1) purpose, (2) time, (3) activities, and 4) place. The time may be divided into short blocks or last for a longer (but still relatively short-term) period, both of which temporarily relieve the caregiver of responsibility. Activities may be practical, such as grocery shopping; psychological, such as providing time for self-replenishment or recreation; or physical, such as providing time for rest or medical/nursing attention.

Respite may occur in the home or elsewhere, such as senior centers, daycare centers, or long-term care facilities. Senior centers usually accommodate persons who are more independent and flexible, often offering social gathering places and events, meals, and health assessment/exercise/maintenance activities. Daycare centers typically host individuals with more diminished functioning. Other settings, such as long-term care facilities, manage clients with an even greater inability to function.

Respite may be delivered by paid or unpaid persons who may be friends, professionals, family, employees, or neighbors. Although many care recipients welcome relief for their caregiver, some may fear abandonment. The family caregiver and the healthcare professional must work together to assure the care recipient that he or she will not be abandoned (Biordi, 1993). Therefore, the professional has a great deal of latitude in using the four elements to devise interventions tailored to meet the needs of an isolated caregiver and care recipient.

Individuals who are in need of respite care may be at risk for disengaging from a social network member due to the overwhelming burden of caring for that person. Often a loved one or caregiver starts out with a tremendous amount of energy and every intention of being present each step of the way, but gets worn down mentally and physically over time. The loved one may not be seen by the caregiver as a negative social network member, yet the health and well-being of the caregiver may be diminished and the caregiver put at risk of social isolation. Caregivers may be at additional risk of social isolation if they do not feel as if they belong due to being overburdened or having their feelings of love and optimism change to feelings of resentment and obligation. The caregiver is a critically important member of the social network. With a small amount of relief or respite care, caregivers may continue to engage their loved one and their social network and feel loved and supported themselves, thus passing those feelings on to the individual.

Support Groups

Support groups, or even peer counselors (Holley, 2007), have been identified for a wide variety of chronic illnesses and conditions, such as breast cancer (Reach to Recovery), bereavement (Widow to Widow), and alcoholism (Alcoholics Anonymous). These groups or individuals assist those persons with chronic illness or disabilities to cope with their illness and the associated changes in identities and social roles owing to their chronic illness or disability. Such counseling can help enhance one's self-esteem, provide alternative meanings of the illness, suggest ways to cope, assist by identifying specific interventions that have helped others, or offer services or care for either the isolate or the caregiver (Holley, 2007). Almost every large city or county has lists of resources that can be accessed: health departments, social work centers, schools, and libraries. The Internet is also a source of information about support groups and resource listings. Some resources list group entry requirements or qualifications.

Because of their variety and number, support groups are not always available in every community, so healthcare professionals may find themselves in the position of developing a group. Therefore, as part of a community assessment, the healthcare professional should not only note the groups currently available, but also identify someone who might be willing to develop a needed group. In addition, the healthcare professional may have to find a meeting place, refer clients to the group, assist clients in discussing barriers to their care, and, if necessary, develop structured activities (such as exercise regimens for arthritic individuals). In addition, the use of motivational devices, such as pictures, videos, audio recordings, reminiscence therapy, or games, may be helpful in developing discussions. Demonstrations of specific illness-related regimens, such as exercises, clothing aids, or body mechanics, are also useful to support groups. During meetings, professionals should be alert to problems the isolate may have in integrating into groups, such as resistance to meeting new people, low self-esteem, apprehension over participation in new activities, or problems of transportation, access, and inconvenient meeting times.

Social activity groups are one way of integrating isolated institutionalized individuals or of reversing hospital-induced confusion; such groups could be recreational therapy groups or those developed particularly to address a special interest (e.g., parents facing the imminent death of a child). Given the limited financial resources typical of most persons who have chronic illness, support groups without costs to the individual and family with chronic illness are more likely to be welcomed.

COMPUTERS

For many persons, including homebound older adults or people with disabilities, computers have helped offset social isolation and loneliness through features such as access to the Internet, which allows the person to reach family and friends or to find new friends, activities, and other common interests. Computers can also be used to provide fun activities, such as games. In the United States, computers are more widely available than elsewhere, and more so among persons with a higher socioeconomic status and the more highly educated. Increasingly, online groups offer support, such as that described for breast cancer patients (Hoybye, Johansen, & Tjomboj-Thomsen, 2005).

Advances in computer technology have included special attachments, such as cameras, breathing tubes, and special keyboards and font sizes, that can customize computers to meet the needs of the isolated or disabled individual, including persons with visual impairment. In parts of the United States, outreach efforts are increasing, as projects aim to reduce the social isolation of the home-bound by providing computers and Internet access to caregivers and care recipients. The use of information and other communication technologies has been helpful in alleviating barriers to the return to work for persons with spinal cord injuries and the resulting disabilities (Bricout, 2004). Telecommuting enables home-based work, and has proved effective for individuals with mobility or transportation limitations, or those whose illnesses or disabilities necessitate rest periods incompatible with typical work environments. Computers have also been used to relieve isolation or loneliness, and assist in the management of chronic illness and support groups located in rural environments (Clark, 2002; Hill & Weinert, 2004; Johnson & Ashton, 2003; Weinert, Cudney, & Winters, 2005).

Whether connecting via the Internet, using word processing, corresponding via email, taking classes, or joining social networking sites, computers also allow isolates to actively fill many hours of otherwise empty time, bringing a measure of relief to tedium while expanding their intellectual and social lives. The caveat, of course, is that the use of the computer, and especially the Internet, could itself be an isolating factor for many individuals. This creates a danger of virtual reality overrunning actual reality, in which case isolates compound their isolation. Even in the face of these risks, the computer offers many more advantages than disadvantages in terms of overcoming some elements of isolation.

Touch

In cultures where touch is important, families and professionals must learn the use and comfort of touch. American studies indicate that the elderly are the least likely group to be touched, yet they find touch very comforting. Pets may be useful alternatives to human touch and human interaction; pet therapy is increasingly used as an intervention in families, communities, and group settings such as nursing homes (Banks, 1998; Collins, Fitzgerald, Sachs-Ericsson, Scherer, Cooper, & Boninger, 2006). Feeling loved and having it demonstrated through touch can do much to reduce isolation and its often concomitant lowered self-esteem. Because some individuals find touch uncomfortable, professionals must assess (by simply asking or observing flinching, grimacing, or resignation) the family's or isolate's responsiveness to touch.

Outcomes

Social isolation is a chronic psychosocial condition that is always part of the client's underlying illness process. Too often social isolation stays in the background or appears as *background noise* influencing the client's illness trajectory. The trajectory of a socially isolated individual may involve additional support by nurses and other healthcare professionals because the client does not have the essential foundational support in place. This foundational support could be as simple as provision of a ride to and from appointments. Another example may be that an individual feels that he or she does not belong anywhere, which may lead to feelings of pessimism toward treatment and its potential benefits. Optimism in the healthcare arena is important and should not be underestimated.

Nurses and other healthcare professionals are valuable partners in the lives and well-being of individuals who are socially isolated and may be the only glimmer of hope to uncover this phenomenon and assist clients to overcome it. For example, the most socially isolated individuals may also be the most difficult to locate. Often these individuals are in situations where social integration is difficult or impossible. Visiting nurses have a unique opportunity to assess for and uncover social isolation in their homebound clients. All clients must be homebound to receive visiting nursing services, but some are more permanently homebound when compared to others. Long-term homebound clients may be at increased risk of social isolation, especially if they are living in a rural area. These individuals should be assessed and referrals should be implemented.

Implementation of these referrals should set into motion provision of a cascade of resources, including the services of an interprofessional team who is responsible for educating clients as to which resources are available and supporting them as much as possible until they are able to move from identity development to transformation of self-management care. Once that occurs, clients will be better able to take responsibility for their social health. Through careful long-term support and relationship building, the nurse has an opportunity to promote empowerment in the individual. It is through this empowerment that clients will be healed in a truly holistic manner, taking into account their physical, psychological, and social well-being.

Evidence-Based Practice Box

Title: CARELINK study to reduce social isolation using nursing students.

Purpose: To test the effects of a university student model of care intervention offered through the CARELINK program on social isolation.

Methods: A two-group, post-test-only design.

Sample: Community-dwelling older adults ($N = 56$).

Intervention: Nursing students were trained to deliver an empowerment program to older adults living in the community over a 16-week period. Each of the visits used a variety of techniques, including (1) reminiscence; (2) exercise-talk discussions; (3) goal-oriented, social engagement-directed discussions; (4) coaching; and (5) modeling.

Hypothesis: Older adults in the CARELINK program who receive student visits will have significantly less social isolation when compared with those who have not yet had any visits.

Results: Older adults in the comparison group, who had not yet received the CARELINK program, were nearly 12 times more likely to be socially isolated.

Discussion and Implications for Practice: The empowerment intervention offered through the CARELINK program had positive effects on reducing social isolation in older adults. CARELINK provides an uncomplicated and inexpensive intervention to decrease social isolation. For individuals who are homebound or have extreme difficulty due to transportation issues, their social isolation may be reduced through targeted interventions using nursing students. This model can be used as a low-cost intervention by visiting nurses or designated personnel to holistically care for each client through mitigation of social isolation.

Source: Nicholson Jr., N. R., & Shellman, J. (2013). Decreasing social isolation in older adults: Effects of an empowerment intervention offered through the CARELINK program. *Research in Gerontological Nursing, 6*(2), 89–97. doi:10.3928/19404921-20130110-01

References

Ahn, D., & Shin, D. (2013). Is the social use of media for seeking connectedness or for avoiding social isolation? Mechanisms underlying media use and subjective well-being. *Computers in Human Behavior, 29*, 2453–2462.

Ajrouch, K. J., Antonucci, T. C., & Janevic, M. R. (2001). Social networks among blacks and whites: The interaction between race and age. *Journals of Gerontology: Series B, Psychological Sciences and Social Sciences, 56*(2), S112–S118. http://psychsoc.gerontologyjournals.org/cgi/content/full/56/2/S112

Alspach, J. G. (2013). Loneliness and social isolation: Risk factors long overdue for surveillance. *Critical Care Nurse, 33*(6), 8–13. doi: 10.4037/ccn2013377

Ballantyne, A., Trenwith, L., Zubrinich, S., & Corlis, M. (2010). "I feel less lonely": What older people say about participating in a social networking website. *Quality in Ageing and Older Adults, 11*, 25–35.

Banks, M. R. (1998). *The effects of animal-assisted therapy on loneliness in an elderly population in long-term care facilities.* Louisiana State University Health Sciences Center School of Nursing, Baton Rouge, LA.

Barnes, L. L., Mendes de Leon, C. F., Wilson, R. S., Bienias, J. L., & Evans, D. A. (2004). Social resources and cognitive decline in a population of older African Americans and whites. *Neurology, 63*(12), 2322–2326. http://www.neurology.org/cgi/reprint/63/12/2322

Bassuk, S. S., Glass, T. A., & Berkman, L. F. (1999). Social disengagement and incident cognitive decline in community-dwelling elderly persons. *Annals of Internal Medicine, 131*(3), 165–173. doi: 10.1037/0033-2909.104.1.97

Beland, F., Zunzunegui, M. V., Alvarado, B., Otero, A., & Del Ser, T. (2005). Trajectories of cognitive decline +and social relations. *Journals of Gerontology: Series B, Psychological Sciences and Social Sciences, 60*(6), P320–P330. http://psychsoc.gerontologyjournals.org/cgi/reprint/60/6/P320

Berkman, L., Glass, T., Brissette, I., & Seeman, T. E. (2000). From social integration to health: Durkheim in the new millennium. *Social Science & Medicine, 51*(6), 843–857. doi: 10.1016/S0277-9536(00)00065-4

Berkman, L., & Syme, L. (1979). Social networks, host resistance, and mortality: A nine-year follow-up study of alameda county residents. *American Journal of Epidemiology, 109*(2), 186–204. http://aje.oxfordjournals.org/cgi/reprint/109/2/186

Biordi, D. (1993). *In-home care and respite care as self-care.* Unpublished data.

Blazer, D. (2005). Depression and social support in late life: A clear but not obvious relationship. *Aging & Mental Health, 9*(6), 497–499. doi: 10.1080/13607860500294266

Blit-Cohen, E., & Litwin, H. (2004). Elder participation in cyberspace: A qualitative analysis of Israeli retirees. *Journal of Aging Studies, 18*, 385–398.

Boden-Albala, B., Litwak, E., Elkind, M. S., Rundek, T., & Sacco, R. L. (2005). Social isolation and outcomes post stroke. *Neurology, 64*(11), 1888–1892. doi: 10.1212/01.WNL.0000163510.79351.AF

Bricout, J. C. (2004). Using telework to enhance return to work outcomes for individuals with spinal cord injuries. *Neurorehabilitation, 19*(2), 147–159.

Browne, A. J. (1997). The concept analysis of respect applying the hybrid model in cross-cultural settings. *Western Journal of Nursing Research, 19*(6), 762–780.

Cattan, M., White, M., Bond, J., & Learmouth, A. (2005). Preventing social isolation and loneliness among older adults: A systematic review of health promotion interventions. *Aging & Society, 25,* 41.

Ceria, C. D., Masaki, K. H., Rodriguez, B. L., Chen, R., Yano, K., & Curb, J. D. (2001). The relationship of psychosocial factors to total mortality among older Japanese-American men: The Honolulu heart program. *Journal of the American Geriatrics Society, 49*(6), 725–731. http://www3.interscience.wiley.com/cgi-bin/fulltext/118968090/PDFSTART

Charmaz, K. (1987). Struggling for a self: Identity levels of the chronically ill. In J. Roth & P. Conrad (Eds.), *Research in the sociology of health care.* Greenwich, CT: JAI Press.

Christakis, N. A., & Fowler, J. H. (2007). The spread of obesity in a large social network over 32 years. *New England Journal of Medicine, 357*(4), 370–379. doi: 10.1056/NEJMsa066082

Christakis, N. A., & Fowler, J. H. (2008). The collective dynamics of smoking in a large social network. *New England Journal of Medicine, 358*(21), 2249–2258. doi: 10.1056/NEJMsa0706154

Clark, D. J. (2002). Older adults living through and with their computers. *Computers, Informatics, Nursing, 20*(3), 117–124.

Cobb, S. (1979). Social support and health through the life course. In M. W. Riley (Ed.), *Aging from birth to death.* Boulder, CO: Westview Press.

Collins, D., Fitzgerald, S., Sachs-Ericsson, N., Scherer, M., Cooper, R., & Boninger, M. (2006). Psychosocial well-being and community participation of service dog partners. *Disability and Rehabilitation: Assistive Technology, 1*(1–2), 41–48.

Corbin, J., & Strauss, A. (1987). Accompaniments of chronic illness: Changes in body, self, biography, and biographical time. In J. Roth & P. Conrad (Eds.), *Research in the sociology of health care.* Greenwich, CT: JAI Press.

Cornwell, E. Y., & Waite, L. J. (2009). Measuring social isolation among older adults using multiple indicators from the NSHAP study. *Journals of Gerontology: Series B, Psychological Sciences and Social Sciences, 64*(suppl 1), i38–i46. doi: 10.1093/geronb/gbp037

Dickens, A. P., Richards, S. H., Greaves, C. J., & Campbell, J. L. (2011). Interventions targeting social isolation in older people: A systematic review. *BMC Public Health, 11,* 647. doi: 10.1186/1471-2458-11-647

Dickens, A. P., Richards, S. H., Hawton, A., Taylor, R. S., Greaves, C. J., Green, C., ... Campbell, J. L. (2011). An evaluation of the effectiveness of a community mentoring service for socially isolated older people: A controlled trial. *BMC Public Health, 11,* 218-2458-11-218. doi: 10.1186/1471-2458-11-218

Elovainio, M., Kivimaki, M., Vahtera, J., Ojanlatva, A., Korkeila, K., Suominen, S., ... Koskenvuo, M. (2003). Social support, early retirement, and a retirement preference: A study of 10,489 Finnish adults. *Journal of Occupational & Environmental Medicine, 45*(4), 433–439. doi: 10.1097/01.jom.0000058334.05741.7a

Eng, P. M., Rimm, E. B., Fitzmaurice, G., & Kawachi, I. (2002). Social ties and change in social ties in relation to subsequent total and cause-specific mortality and coronary heart disease incidence in men. *American Journal of Epidemiology, 155*(8), 700–709. doi: 10.1093/aje/155.8.700

Faulkner, K. A., Cauley, J. A., Zmuda, J. M., Griffin, J. M., & Nevitt, M. C. (2003). Is social integration associated with the risk of falling in older community-dwelling women? *Journals of Gerontology: Series A, Biological Sciences and Medical Sciences, 58*(10), M954–M959. http://biomed.gerontologyjournals.org/cgi/content/full/58/10/M954

Findlay, R. (2003). Interventions to reduce social isolation amongst older people: Where is the evidence? *Aging & Society, 23,* 647–658. doi: 10.1017/S0144686X03001296

Findlay, R., & Cartwright, C. (2002). *Social isolation and older people: A literature review.* Ministerial Advisory Council on Older People.

Fowles, D., & Greenberg, S. (2009). A profile of older Americans: 2008. http://www.aoa.gov/AoAroot/Aging_Statistics/Profile/2008/index.aspx

Fratiglioni, L., Paillard-Borg, S., & Winblad, B. (2004). An active and socially integrated lifestyle in late life might protect against dementia. *Lancet Neurology, 3*(6), 343–353. doi: 10.1016/S1474-4422(04)00767-7

Giles, L. C., Glonek, G. F., Luszcz, M. A., & Andrews, G. R. (2005). Effect of social networks on 10 year survival in very old Australians: The Australian longitudinal study of aging. *Journal of Epidemiology and Community Health, 59*(7), 574–579.

Giuli, C., Papa, R., Mocchegiani, E., & Marcellini, F. (2012). Predictors of participation in physical activity for community-dwelling elderly Italians. *Archives of Gerontology and Geriatrics, 54*(1), 50–54. doi: 10.1016/j.archger.2011.02.017

Giuli, C., Spazzafumo, L., Sirolla, C., Abbatecola, A. M., Lattanzio, F., & Postacchini, D. (2012). Social isolation risk factors in older hospitalized individuals. *Archives of Gerontology and Geriatrics, 55*(3), 580–585. doi: 10.1016/j.archger.2012.01.011

Golden, J., Conroy, R., Bruce, I., Denihan, A., Greene, E., Kirby, M., & Lawlor, B. (2009). Loneliness, social support networks, mood and wellbeing in a community-dwelling elderly. *International Journal of Geriatric Psychiatry, 24,* 657–781.

Greaves, C. J., & Farbus, L. (2006). Effects of creative and social activity on the health and well-being of socially isolated older people: Outcomes from a multi-method observational study. *Journal of the Royal Society of Health, 126*(3), 134–142.

Hagerty, B., Lynch-Sauer, J., Patusky, K., Bouwsema, M., & Collier, P. (1992). Sense of belonging: A vital mental health concept. *Archives of Psychiatric Nursing, 6*(3), 172–177. doi: 10.1016/0883-9417(92)90028-H

Havens, B., & Hall, M. (2001). Social isolation, loneliness, and the health of older adults in Manitoba, Canada. *Indian Journal of Gerontology, 1*(15), 126–144.

Havens, B., Hall, M., Sylvestre, G., & Jivan, T. (2004). Social isolation and loneliness: Differences between older rural and urban Manitobans. *Canadian Journal on Aging, 23*(2), 129–140. doi: 10.1353/cja.2004.0022

Hawes, C., Phillips, C. D., Rose, M., Holan, S., & Sherman, M. (2003). A national survey of assisted living facilities. *The Gerontologist, 43*(6), 875–882.

Hawton, A., Green, C., Dickens, A., Richards, S., Taylor, R., Edwards, R., ... Campbell, J. (2011). The impact of social isolation on the health status and health-related quality of life of older people. *Qualitative Life Research, 20*, 57–67. doi: 10.1007/s11136-010-9717-2.

Henly, S. (2013). Use progress in psychometrics to advance nursing science: Revisiting factor analysis. *Nursing Research, 62*(3), 147–148.

Hill, W. G., & Weinert, C. (2004). An evaluation of an online intervention to provide social support and health education. *Computers, Informatics, Nursing, 22*(5), 282–288.

Holley, U. A. (2007). Social isolation: A practical guide for nurses assisting clients with chronic illness. *Rehabilitation Nursing, 32*(2), 51–56.

Holtzman, R. E., Rebok, G. W., Saczynski, J. S., Kouzis, A. C., Wilcox Doyle, K., & Eaton, W. W. (2004). Social network characteristics and cognition in middle-aged and older adults. *Journals of Gerontology: Series B, Psychological Sciences and Social Sciences, 59*(6), P278–P284. http://psychsoc.gerontologyjournals.org/cgi/content/full/59/6/P278

Howat, P., Iredell, H., Grenade, L., Nedwetzky, A., & Collins, J. (2004). Reducing social isolation amongst older people implications for health professionals. *Geriaction, 22*(1), 13–20.

Hoybye, M. T., Johansen, C., & Tjomboj-Thomsen, T. (2005). Online interaction: Effects of storytelling in an internet breast cancer support group. *Psychooncology, 14*(3), 211–220.

Ibrahim, R., Abolfathi Momtaz, Y., & Hamid, T. A. (2013). Social isolation in older Malaysians: Prevalence and risk factors. *Psychogeriatrics, 13*(2), 71–79. doi: 10.1111/psyg.12000; 10.1111/psyg.12000

Iliffe, S., Kharicha, K., Harari, D., Swift, C., Gillmann, G., & Stuck, A. E. (2007). Health risk appraisal in older people 2: The implications for clinicians and commissioners of social isolation risk in older people. *British Journal of General Practice, 57*(537), 277–282. http://www.ncbi.nlm.nih.gov/pmc/articles/PMC2043334/?tool=pubmed

Johnson, D., & Ashton, C. (2003). Effects of computer-mediated communication on social support and loneliness for isolated persons with disabilities. *American Journal of Recreational Therapy, 2*(3), 23–32.

Killeen, C. (1998). Loneliness: An epidemic in modern society. *Journal of Advanced Nursing, 28*(4), 762–770. doi: 10.1046/j.1365-2648.1998.00703.x

Klinenberg, E. (2001). Dying alone: The social production of urban isolation. *Ethnography, 2*(4), 501–531.

Kroenke, C. H., Kubzansky, L. D., Schernhammer, E. S., Holmes, M. D., & Kawachi, I. (2006). Social networks, social support, and survival after breast cancer diagnosis. *Journal of Clinical Oncology, 24*(7), 1105–1111. doi: 10.1200/JCO.2005.04.2846

Krouse, J., Krouse, H., & Fabian, R. (1989). Adaptation to surgery for head and neck cancer. *Laryngoscope, 99*, 789–794.

Lee, R., Draper, M., & Lee, S. (2001). Social connectedness, dysfunctional interpersonal behaviors and psychological distress: Testing a mediator model. *Journal of Counseling Psychology, 48*(3), 310–318.

Lee, R., & Robbins, S. B. (1995). Measuring belongingness: The social connectedness and the social assurance scales. *Journal of Counseling Psychology, 42*(2), 232.

Lee, Y. T., Tsai, C. F., Ouyang, W. C., Yang, A. C., Yang, C. H., & Hwang, J. P. (2013). Daytime sleepiness: A risk factor for poor social engagement among the elderly. *Psychogeriatrics, 13*(4), 213–220. doi: 10.1111/psyg.12020

Litwin, H., & Zoabi, S. (2003). Modernization and elder abuse in an Arab-Israeli context. *Research on Aging, 25*(3), 224–246.

Locher, J. L., Ritchie, C. S., Roth, D. L., Baker, P. S., Bodner, E. V., & Allman, R. M. (2005). Social isolation, support, and capital and nutritional risk in an older sample: Ethnic and gender differences. *Social Science & Medicine, 60*(4), 747–761. doi: 10.1016/j.socscimed.2004.06.023

Longman, J., Passey, M., Singer, J., & Morgan, G. (2013). The role of social isolation in frequent and/or avoidable hospitalization: Rural community-based service providers' perspectives. *Australian Health Review, 37*(2), 223–231. doi: 10.1071/AH1215210

Lubben, J. (2003). *An international approach to community health care for older adults.* Philadelphia, PA: Lippincott Williams & Wilkins.

Lubben, J., & Gironda, M. (1996). Assessing social support networks among older people in the United States. In H. Litwin (Ed.), *The social networks of older people: A cross-national analysis* (p. 144). Westport, CT: Praeger.

Lubben, J., & Gironda, M. (2003a). Centrality of social ties to the health and well being of older adults. In B. Berkman & L. Harooytan (Eds.), *Social work and health care in an aging world: Informing education, policy, practice, and research* (pp. 319–350). New York, NY: Springer.

Lubben, J., & Gironda, M. (2003b). Measuring social networks and assessing their benefits. In C. Phillipson, G. Allan, & D. Morgan (Eds.), *Social networks and social exclusion* (pp. 20-49). Hants, UK: Ashgate.

Marottoli, R. A., Mendes de Leon, C. F., Glass, T. A., Williams, C. S., Cooney, L. M. Jr., & Berkman, L. F. (2000). Consequences of driving cessation: Decreased out-of-home activity levels. *Journals of Gerontology: Series B, Psychological Sciences and Social Sciences, 55*(6), S334–S340.

Mavandadi, S., Rook, K. S., & Newsom, J. T. (2007). Positive and negative social exchanges and disability in later life: An investigation of trajectories of change. *Journals of Gerontology: Series B, Psychological Sciences and Social Sciences, 62*(6), S361–S370.

McCrae, N., Murray, J., Banerjee, S., Huxley, P., Bhugra, D., Tylee, A., & Macdonald, A. (2005). "They're all depressed, aren't they?": A qualitative study of social care workers and depression in older adults. *Aging & Mental Health, 9*(6), 508–516. doi: 10.1080/13607860500193765

Mendes de Leon, C. F., Glass, T. A., & Berkman, L. F. (2003). Social engagement and disability in a community population of older adults: The New Haven EPESE. *American Journal of Epidemiology, 157*(7), 633–642. doi: 10.1093/aje/kwg028

Mendes de Leon, C. F., Gold, D., Glass, T., Kaplan, L., & George, L. (2001). Disability as a function of social networks and support in elderly African Americans and Whites: The Duke EPESE 1986–1992. *Journals of Gerontology: Series B, Psychological Sciences and Social Sciences, 56B*(3), S179–S190. http://www.ncbi.nlm.nih.gov/pubmed/11316843

Michael, Y. L., Berkman, L. F., Colditz, G. A., Holmes, M. D., & Kawachi, I. (2002). Social networks and health-related quality of life in breast cancer survivors: A prospective study. *Journal of Psychosomatic Research, 52*(5), 285–293. doi: 10.1016/S0022-3999(01)00270-7

Mistry, R., Rosansky, J., McGuire, J., McDermott, C., Jarvik, L., & UPBEAT Collaborative Group. (2001). Social isolation predicts re-hospitalization in a group of older American veterans enrolled in the UPBEAT program: Unified psychogeriatric biopsychosocial evaluation and treatment. *International Journal of Geriatric Psychiatry, 16*(10), 950–959. doi: 10.1002/gps.447

Murberg, T. A. (2004). Long-term effect of social relationships on mortality in patients with congestive heart failure. *International Journal of Psychiatry in Medicine, 34*(3), 207–217. doi: 10.2190/GKJ2-P8BD-V59X-MJNQ

Nicholson, N. (2009). Social isolation in older adults: An evolutionary concept analysis. *Journal of Advanced Nursing, 65*(6), 1342–1352. doi: 10.1111/j.1365-2648.2008.04959.x

Nicholson, N. R. Jr., Dixon, J. K., & McCorkle, R. (2014). Predictors of diminished levels of social integration in older adults. *Research in Gerontological Nursing, 7*(1), 33–43. doi: 10.3928/19404921-20130918-02

Nicholson, N., Molony, S., Fennie, K., Shellman, J., & McCorkle, R. (2010). *Predictors of social isolation in community living older persons.* Unpublished PhD dissertation, Yale University, New Haven, CT.

Nicholson, N. R. Jr., & Shellman, J. (2013). Decreasing social isolation in older adults: Effects of an empowerment intervention offered through the CARELINK program. *Research in Gerontological Nursing, 6*(2), 89–97. doi: 10.3928/19404921-20130110-01

Pantell, M., Rehkopf, D., Jutte, D., Syme, S. L., Balmes, J., & Adler, N. (2013). Social isolation: A predictor of mortality comparable to traditional clinical risk factors. *American Journal of Public Health, 103*(11), 2056–2062. doi: 10.2105/AJPH.2013.301261; 10.2105/AJPH.2013.301261

Perlman, D. (1987). Further reflections on the present state of loneliness research. *Journal of Social Behavior and Personality, 2*, 17–26.

Pierce, L. L., Wilkinson, L. K., & Anderson, J. (2003). Analysis of the concept of aloneness as applied to older women being treated for depression. *Journal of Gerontological Nursing, 29*(7), 20–25. http://www.ncbi.nlm.nih.gov/pubmed/12874936

Ramos, M., & Wilmoth, J. (2003). Social relationships and depressive symptoms among older adults in southern Brazil. *Journals of Gerontology: Series B, Psychological Sciences and Social Sciences, 58*(4), S253–S261. http://www.ncbi.nlm.nih.gov/pubmed/12878659

Ravish, T. (1985). Prevent isolation before it starts. *Journal of Gerontological Nursing, 11*(10), 10–13.

Resnick, B. (2007). Assisted living: The perfect place for nursing. *Geriatric Nursing, 28*(1), 7–8. doi: 10.1016/j.gerinurse.2006.11.003

Sawada, Y., Shinohara, R., Sugisawa, Y., & Anme, T. (2011). The relation between the maintenance of physical functions and social interaction among community-dwelling elderly people: A six-year follow-up study. *Journal of Physical Therapy Science, 23,* 171–175.

Seeman, T. E. (2000). Health promoting effects of friends and family on health outcomes in older adults. *American Journal of Health Promotion, 14*(6), 362–370. http://www.ncbi.nlm.nih.gov /pubmed/11067571

Seidler, A., Bernhardt, T., Nienhaus, A., & Frolich, L. (2003). Association between the psychosocial network and dementia: A case-control study. *Journal of Psychiatric Research, 37*(2), 89–98. doi: 10.1016/S0022-3956(02)00065-1

Shankar, A., Hamer, M., McMunn, A., & Steptoe, A. (2013). Social isolation and loneliness: Relationships with cognitive function during 4 years of follow-up in the English longitudinal study of ageing. *Psychosomatic Medicine, 75*(2), 161–170. doi: 10.1097/ PSY.0b013e31827f09cd

Shankar, A., McMunn, A., Banks, J., & Steptoe, A. (2011). Loneliness, social isolation, and behavioral and biological health indicators in older adults. *Health Psychology, 30*(4), 377–385. doi: 10.1037/ a0022826

Siplic, F., & Kadis, D. (2002). The psychosocial aspect of aging. *Socialno Delo, 41*(5), 295–300.

Smith, T. F., & Hirdes, J. P. (2009). Predicting social isolation among geriatric psychiatry patients. *International Psychogeriatrics, 21*(1), 50–59. doi: 10.1017/ S1041610208007850

Strauss, A., Corbin, J., Fagerhaugh, S., Glaser, B., Maines, D., & Suczek, B. (1984). *Chronic illness and the quality of life* (2nd ed.). St. Louis, MO: Mosby.

Street, D., Burge, S., Quadagno, J., & Barrett, A. (2007). The salience of social relationships for resident well-being in assisted living. *Journals of Gerontology: Series B, Psychological Sciences and Social Sciences, 62*(2), S129–S134.

Sum, S., Mathews, R., Pourghasem, M., & Hughes, I. (2009). Internet use as a predictor of sense of community in older people. *Cyberpsychological Behavior, 12,* 235–239.

Treolar, L. L. (1999). People with disabilities—the same, but different: Implications for health care practice. *Journal of Transcultural Nursing, 10*(4), 358–364.

Victor, C., Scambler, S., Bond, J., & Bowling, A. (2000). Being alone in later life: Loneliness, social isolation and living alone. *Reviews in Clinical Gerontology, 10,* 407–417. doi: 10.1017/S0959259800104101

Walton, C. G., Shultz, C. M., Beck, C. M., & Walls, R. C. (1991). Psychological correlates of loneliness in the older adult. *Archives of Psychiatric Nursing, 5*(3), 165–170. doi: 10.1016/0883-9417(91)90017-Y

Wang, H. X., Karp, A., Winblad, B., & Fratiglioni, L. (2002). Late-life engagement in social and leisure activities is associated with a decreased risk of dementia: A longitudinal study from the Kungsholmen project. *American Journal of Epidemiology, 155*(12), 1081–1087. doi: 10.1093/aje/155.12.1081

Weinert, C., Cudney, S., & Winters, C. (2005). Social support in cyberspace: The next generation. *Computers, Informatics, Nursing, 23*(1), 7–15.

Wenger, G. C. (1984). *The supportive network: Coping with old age.* London, UK: Allen & Unwin.

Wenger, G. C. (1991). A network typology: From theory to practice. *Journal of Aging Studies, 5*(2), 147–162.

Wenger, G. C. (1997). Social networks and the prediction of elderly people at risk. *Aging and Mental Health, 1*(4), 311. doi: 10.1080/13607869757001

Wenger, G. C., & Burholt, V. (2004). Changes in levels of social isolation and loneliness among older people in a rural area: A twenty-year longitudinal study. *Canadian Journal on Aging, 23*(2), 115–127. doi: 10.1353/ cja.2004.0028

Wenger, G. C., Davies, R., Shahtahmasebi, S., & Scott, A. (1996). Social isolation and loneliness in old age: Review and model refinement. *Aging & Society, 16,* 333–358.

White, P., & Selwyn, N. (2013). Moving on-line? An analysis of patterns of adult internet use in the UK, 2002–2010. *Information, Communication & Society, 16,* 1–27. doi: 10.1080/1369118X.2011.611816

Wilson, D. M., Harris, A., Hollis, V., & Mohankumar, D. (2011). Upstream thinking and health promotion planning for older adults at risk of social isolation. *International Journal of Older People Nursing, 6*(4), 282–288. doi: 10.1111/j.1748-3743.2010.00259.x

World Health Organization (WHO). (2003). Preamble to the constitution of the World Health Organization as adopted by the International Health Conference, New York, 19–22 June, 1946; signed on 22 July 1946 by the representatives of 61 states (official records of the World Health Organization, no. 2, p. 100) and entered into force on 7 April 1948. http://www.who.int/about /definition/en/print.html

Younger, J. B. (1995). The alienation of the sufferer. *Advances in Nursing Science, 17*(4), 53–72. http://www .ncbi.nlm.nih.gov/pubmed/7625781

Zunzunegui, M. V., Alvarado, B. E., Del Ser, T., & Otero, A. (2003). Social networks, social integration, and social engagement determine cognitive decline in community-dwelling Spanish older adults. *Journals of Gerontology: Series B, Psychological Sciences and Social Sciences, 58*(2), S93–S100. http://psychsoc.gerontology-journals.org/cgi/content/full/58/2/S93

Chapter 7

Uncertainty

Faye I. Hummel

Uncertainty built inside me, like a violent thunderstorm on a hot summer day. There was no escape from the uncertainty that rained down on me and drenched me to my very core. The flood of uncertainty eroded my confidence, my hopes, my dreams, my future. The dark cloud of uncertainty shadows me, even on the sunniest of days.

—Sarah, 59-year-old female with breast cancer

Introduction

Uncertainty in chronic illness is inescapable. Chronic illness is marked by unpredictable changes in physical, cognitive, social, psychological, and lifestyle functions. It restricts the terrain of the sufferer to local and familiar territory where that person is least likely to be exposed to the gaze and questions of others (Goffman, 1963). With chronic illness, the timing, duration, and severity of symptoms are erratic. Misgivings about what the affected individual may be able to achieve in the present or in the future persist. Doubt about the success of treatment to slow disease progression and modify the disease course erodes self-confidence and generates stress and worry. Chronic illness brings a prolonged state of impending adversity.

The Greek legend of Damocles's sword illuminates the insidious nature of uncertainty inherent to chronic illness. In this tale, Dionysius was a cruel and unjust ruler with vast power and riches. Yet in spite of his supremacy, Dionysius feared reprisal. One day, Damocles,

a friend, told Dionysius how happy he must be to have such wealth and comforts. Dionysius invited Damocles to take his place for a day. Damocles was treated to every luxury. He was the happiest man in the world—that is, until he noticed he was seated beneath a sharp sword suspended by a single horse hair (*Encyclopedia Britannica*, 2011).

Damocles's sword symbolizes the unpredictability of chronic illness and the precarious nature of everyday life for persons with chronic illness. On any given day, an individual with chronic illness may miss a cherished or important activity, experience loss of autonomy due to limitations and special needs, or do without equipment, treatments, and pharmaceuticals because they are unaffordable. Everyday life can change dramatically and be filled with ambiguity. Uncertainty in chronic illness is a cognitive stressor marked by a loss of control and a perception of doubt. Uncertainty impedes coping and adjustment to chronic illness, increases psychological and emotional distress, and diminishes quality of life.

The Nature of Uncertainty

Persons with chronic illness cannot assign a definite value to objects or events or predict outcomes with accuracy (Bailey et al., 2009). Uncertainty arises when "details of situations are ambiguous, complex, unpredictable, or probabilistic; when information is unavailable or inconsistent; and when people feel insecure in their own state of knowledge or the state of knowledge in general" (Brashers, 2001, p. 478). A person who believes himself or herself to be uncertain *is* uncertain. Further, uncertainty may be experienced in relation to the probability of an event. When the likelihood of an event is 0% or 100%, uncertainty is lowest. Uncertainty is highest when there are multiple alternatives with equal probability of occurring (Brashers, 2001). Attributes of probability, perception, and temporality are present in every situation of uncertainty (McCormick, 2002).

Uncertainty is a hallmark of acute and chronic illness. It is experienced by those persons with chronic illness who may fear or experience rejection and social isolation; some may be concerned with diagnosis and treatment, while others may worry about recurrence of their illness even if their physical health is improving. For example, despite ambiguity about their illness and prognosis, persons with chronic obstructive pulmonary disease (COPD) have been shown to be unwilling to give up hope for continued life, relying on their history of bouncing back from repeated exacerbations of their chronic illness and holding out hope they can do it once again (Lowey, Norton, Quinn, & Quill, 2013).

Sources of Uncertainty

Uncertainty permeates all aspects of one's life across the chronic illness continuum. Illness uncertainty is triggered by four sources:

- Ambiguity about the illness state
- Complexity of the treatment and health-care system
- Inadequate information about the disease and the seriousness of the illness
- Unpredictability about the disease course and the disease trajectory (Mishel, 1988; Mishel & Braden, 1988)

In research conducted with persons with HIV disease, Brashers and colleagues (2003) extended Mishel's (1990) model of uncertainty in illness to include not only medical uncertainty, but also personal and social sources of uncertainty. Sources of medical uncertainty identified by persons with HIV disease included ambiguity with their HIV diagnosis and associated diagnostic tests as well as unpredictability and multiplicity of opportunistic infections. Personal sources of uncertainty were related to the invisibility of their chronic illness, social roles, and precarious financial situations due to the expense of the medications necessary to keep the disease in check (Brashers et al., 2003).

Similarly, Miller (2012) identified personal and social sources of uncertainty, as well as medical sources of uncertainty, that persisted in cancer survivorship. Medical sources of uncertainty related to the diagnosis, treatment, and prognosis of the disease, whereas personal sources of uncertainty related to self-identity and career. Relationship and family consequences of chronic illness were included in the social sources of uncertainty (Miller, 2012).

Martin and colleagues (2010) identified sources of uncertainty across the transplantation trajectory. In their study, 38 individuals who were waiting for or who had received an organ transplant were interviewed. During all phases of the transplant experience, participants reported medical, personal, and social forms of uncertainty. With 244 older African American and Caucasian long-term survivors of breast cancer, Gil and colleagues (2005) found the most important triggers for uncertainty were hearing about someone else's cancer and the person's own new aches and pains.

Theories of Uncertainty

Early work on uncertainty distinguished clinical from functional uncertainty (Davis, 1960).

McIntosh (1974, 1976) took the concept further by examining uncertainty in persons with cancer and other chronic conditions.

Two theories of uncertainty in illness are attributed to Mishel (1988, 1990). Mishel (1988) used Lazarus and Folkman's (1984) stress and coping theory as a basis for her theory of uncertainty. This middle-range theory explains how individuals with illness cognitively process illness-related stimuli to construct meaning for illness events. The first theory of uncertainty in illness (UIT) focused on the diagnostic and treatment phases of an illness or an illness with a poor prognosis. This theory posits uncertainty is present in illness states that are confusing, multifaceted, and unpredictible. Uncertainty, according to this theory, is a cognitive state where the individual is unable to attribute meaning to or interpret an illness event due to a lack of cues, so as to give value to and/or accurately anticipate outcomes (Mishel, 1988). UIT encompasses three major themes: (1) antecedents of uncertainty, (2) appraisal of uncertainty, and (3) coping with uncertainty. The desired outcome is personal control by adaptation (Mishel, 2014).

Mishel subsequently extended her uncertainty theory to chronic illness. Mishel (1990) recognized that those persons with acute illness experienced time-limited uncertainty, whereas those persons with chronic conditions experienced uncertainty throughout their lives. To capture the experience of ongoing uncertainty in chronic illness, she added the concepts of self-organization and probabilistic thinking to UIT in reconceptualizing her uncertainty in illness theory (RUIT). In this way, UIT progressed from predicting, controlling, and eliminating uncertainty to managing and accepting uncertainty as a way of life in chronic illness. The desired health outcome is consciousness expansion (Mishel, 2014). Uncertainty in chronic illness often remains constant, but patients are able to attach meaning to symptoms based on the consistency of their symptom patterns. Event familiarity develops over time through experience (Guadalupe, 2010).

The first major theme of UIT is the antecedents of uncertainty. The primary antecedent of uncertainty is the stimuli frame, which is composed of three components: (1) symptom pattern, (2) event familiarity, and (3) event congruence. Symptom pattern is the consistency of symptoms to form a pattern. Event familiarity is the degree to which a situation is habitual, is repetitive, or contains recognizable cues, as well as time and experience in a healthcare environment (Mishel, 1988, p. 225). Event congruence is the consistency between the expected experience and the actual experience of an illness-related event. Reliable and stable events subsequently facilitate interpretation and understanding. In this way, the stimuli frame has the potential to reduce uncertainty (Mishel, 1988).

In this theory, uncertainty is a cognitive response generated from the ambiguous nature of the illness experience (Mishel, 2014). According to UIT, the stimuli frame is influenced by two variables: cognitive capacity and structure providers. Cognitive capacity refers to the ability of a person to process information. It can be altered or diminished by information overload, a person's inability to process information, or physiologic factors that impair mental ability. Structure providers are the resources used to interpret the stimuli frame. Healthcare professionals are included in this concept. Structure providers can reduce uncertainty by helping to interpret an illness event or to identify symptom patterns, event familiarity, and event congruence for a patient and family. They serve as a credible authority, and provide social support and education. Credible authority is the degree to which a person has trust and confidence in his or her healthcare professional. Social support is the ability of the person to express his or her thoughts and feelings with family and friends and with other individuals who are also experiencing the disease. Education is the knowledge and information needed to gain insight into illness-related events. Together, cognitive capacity and structure providers support the development of a cognitive schema to interpret illness events and, therefore, have the potential to diminish uncertainty (Mishel, 2014).

If one does not have sufficient cues to structure or categorize an illness event, uncertainty arises. Inconsistent symptom patterns, lack of familiarity with healthcare professionals and procedures, and unanticipated illness experiences contribute to this uncertainty. A person's cognitive capacity may be impaired by illness-related factors such as pain or medication, creating difficulty in constructing meaning from the stimuli cues. Uncertainty may lead to psychological distress if coping responses are insufficient to resolve or manage uncertainty. Conversely, receiving assurance from a trusted and competent healthcare professional about some aspect of the individual's chronic condition can diminish uncertainty.

Uncertainty is appraised as neutral until it is assessed to be a danger or an opportunity. Illness events perceived as a danger imply harm. Uncertainty is perceived as a threat to well-being based on previous personal experiences. With perceived harm, coping strategies are implemented to reduce uncertainty. Uncertain events evaluated as opportunities imply a potential for a positive outcome. Judgment of uncertainty as an opportunity is explained as construction of a positive meaning for an event based on one's personal beliefs or purposeful misrepresentation (Mishel, 1990, 2014). In the case of uncertainty as opportunity, strategies to maintain uncertainty are initiated. If coping strategies are effective, adaptation will occur (Mishel, 1988, 2014).

A growing body of evidence has resulted from researchers' use of uncertainty theory as a conceptual framework. Notably, research has explored and elaborated on the major theoretical constructs, resulting in a greater understanding of uncertainty (Mishel, 2014). Uncertainty theory provides a foundation for insight into and understanding of the complexity of chronic illness.

Impact

Uncertainty Is Certain In Chronic Illness

The dynamic nature of chronic illness makes uncertainty a part of life (Mishel, 1999). In acute illness, individuals act to decrease uncertainty, whereas individuals with chronic conditions seek to manage uncertainty. Even though uncertainty is experienced in the present, uncertainty is based on past experiences and assumptions for the future (Penrod, 2001). Embedded within the illness experience are ambiguity, inconsistency, vagueness, unpredictability, unfamiliarity, and the unknown, all of which create uncertainty (Mishel, 1984). Persons with chronic illness may experience situations and symptoms for which they have no experience or knowledge, thus triggering uncertainty. Uncertainty, then, is a psychological state in which individuals initially perceive the situation and subsequently respond relative to how they believe it will impact them. As such, uncertainty is a neutral experience, neither good nor bad (Brashers, 2001; Mishel, 1988). The assessment of uncertainty as beneficial or harmful determines one's affective response to it (Mishel, 1988).

Uncertainty is the inability of an individual to understand the meaning of illness-related events such as disease process or treatment (Mishel, 1988) and that person's perception of ambiguity, complexity, inconsistency, and unpredictability associated with illness and illness-related events (Mishel, 1984, 1990). A vague prognosis, lack of illness-related information, unpredictability of symptoms, and the occurrence of complications may all lead to uncertainty (Mishel, 1984, 1988).

When certainty exists, the future is taken for granted. In contrast, when uncertainty exists, the future becomes the focus, with attempts to capture a clear vision of what is not clear (McCormick, 2002). Persons with chronic conditions do not know how their chronic illness will affect their future. They may feel good one day and incapacitated the next. They may receive inconsistent information from health-care professionals and other sources (e.g., the Internet) about disease management and life-style changes. Uncertainty clouds their ability to determine if aches and pains are associated with an exacerbation of the disease process or are simply a part of everyday living.

Building on Mishel's (1981, 1988, 1990) theoretical work on uncertainty in acute and chronic illnesses, scholars have identified similar experiences of uncertainty in many chronic illnesses. Indeed, uncertainty is a universal phenomenon among chronic illnesses including cancer (Clayton, Mishel, & Belyea, 2006; Sammarco & Konecny, 2010), peritoneal dialysis (Madar & Bar-Tal, 2009), multiple sclerosis (McNulty, Livneh, & Wilson, 2004), chronic pain (Johnson, Zautra, & Davis, 2006), organ transplantation (Lasker, Sogolow, Olenik, Sass, &Weinrieb, 2010; Martin et al., 2010), and HIV/AIDS (Brashers et al., 2003).

Illness uncertainty influences coping with and adapting to chronic illness. In their study, Johnson and colleagues (2006) examined the role of uncertainty in 51 women coping with pain from fibromyalgia. Women experiencing greater pain levels and high illness uncertainty had more difficulty coping with their disease. Similarly, women with endometriosis reported uncertainty and emotional distress in their lives (Lemaire, 2004). Uncertainty is one of the greatest challenges in successfully adapting to chronic illness. Individuals with a variety of chronic illnesses and increased levels of uncertainty experience diminished levels of adjustment (McNulty et al., 2004).

Uncertainty is present across the illness trajectory, during events of diagnosis, treatment, and prognosis (Mishel, 1981, 1984, 1988). A longitudinal study examined uncertainty and anxiety in 127 women with suspected breast cancer during the diagnostic period. The results demonstrated that uncertainty and anxiety were significantly higher before the diagnosis than after the diagnosis. Uncertainty and anxiety were significantly lower among women diagnosed with benign disease than among those women with a malignant diagnosis (Liao, Chen, Chen, & Chen, 2008).

In another study, uncertainty was measured in three groups of adolescents and young adults with cancer at specific times in their cancer experience: newly diagnosed, diagnosed for 1 to 4 years, and diagnosed for 5 or more years. The overall level of uncertainty remained unchanged among the three groups, although differences existed in the specific concerns related to uncertainty (Decker, Haase, & Bell, 2007). In a different study, women who had undergone surgery for ovarian malignancies reported that anxiety and depression played an important role in uncertainty throughout their illness (Schulman-Green, Ercolano, Dowd, Schwartz, & McCorkle, 2008).

Denny (2009), in a qualitative study of 31 women with endometriosis, found uncertainty exists around the diagnosis, the disease course, and the future. In a longitudinal, descriptive study of individuals with an implantable cardioverter-defibrillator, 21 male participants—who were educated, married, and white—demonstrated that uncertainty did not change significantly over time (Mauro, 2010).

Uncertainty is pervasive and can persist for long periods of time, even after life-saving procedures and treatments are complete (Martin et al., 2010; Mauro, 2010). Persson and Hellstrom (2002) reported uncertainty as a theme that emerged from interviews with nine patients after ostomy surgery. Similarly, uncertainty of cancer recurrence was highlighted by persons with colorectal cancer (Simpson & Whyte, 2006). For breast cancer survivors, survivor uncertainty persists long after treatment completion due to fear of recurrence (Dirksen & Erickson, 2002) and erodes quality of life (Sammarco & Konecny, 2008). Among patients with breast cancer, uncertainty affects the illness experience, adaptation, quality of life, and sense of hope (Sammarco, 2001).

From the moment of my diagnosis of breast cancer to this very day, uncertainty persists. First it was doubt about my diagnosis, then my surgery, treatment, and follow-up care. Were my healthcare providers competent? Did I have enough information to make the right decisions? The deaths of two close friends from breast cancer haunted me and heightened my vigilance of and worry about every ache and pain. When I learned another friend with breast cancer was diagnosed with lung cancer, I couldn't help but think the same thing could be happening to me. Had my cancer gone to other places in my body and I just didn't know it yet? I felt vulnerable, as though any day, I would hear more bad news. Sure enough, a suspicious mammogram confirmed my cancer fears. Even though I was relieved to hear the biopsy revealed the new breast tumor was benign, I was once again caught in the web of uncertainty.

Doubt and fear continue to twist my reason and optimism. I simply can't dismiss the ever-present possibility that cancer will return at any time. Uncertainty, a constant reminder there simply is no guarantee with cancer.

—Sarah

Uncertainty appears to decrease with age. That is, older adults report more tolerance of uncertainty compared to their younger counterparts (Basevitz, Pushkar, Chaikelson, Conway, & Dalton, 2008). This finding appears to be prevalent around the world: Older people in Taiwan report less illness uncertainty than when they were younger (Lien, Lin, Kuo, & Chen, 2009). Younger Taiwanese women with breast cancer report higher uncertainty due to concerns with changes in their physical condition, careers, and family roles (Liao et al., 2008).

Other differences in uncertainty have also been noted in the literature. Sammarco and Konecny (2010) reported higher levels of uncertainty in Latina breast cancer survivors compared to Caucasian breast cancer survivors. Additionally, the patient's level of education may affect uncertainty and stress. In one study (Madar & Bar-Tal, 2009), better-educated patients were better able to manage levels/feelings of uncertainty and stress. Perhaps highly educated patients can more easily process information, which in turn decreases uncertainty.

Current research supports a positive association between symptom severity and uncertainty in chronic illness. In persons undergoing home peritoneal dialysis, uncertainty was positively associated with self-rated illness severity (Madar & Bar-Tal, 2009). Kang (2006) reported similar findings with adults diagnosed with atrial fibrillation; those individuals with greater symptom severity perceived more uncertainty. Wolfe-Christensen, Isenberg, Mullins, Carpentier, and Almstrom (2008) found a similar relationship among college students with asthma.

Uncertainty and Social Networks

Illness uncertainty affects the individual with chronic illness as well as those persons within the patient's social network, including caregivers, family members, and friends. Members of a social network of someone with a chronic illness face their own feelings and fears of uncertainty and unpredictability (Donovan-Kicken & Bute, 2008; Mitchell, Courtney, & Coyer, 2003; Northouse et al., 2002) and may experience discomfort and anxiety about how to act and what to say to the person with chronic illness. Adults with a parent with probable Alzheimer's disease report uncertainty about their own predisposition for Alzheimer's disease as well as conflicting caregiver roles and financial responsibilities. Social sources of uncertainty experienced by these families included unpredictability of social reactions and social interactions, including family dynamics (Stone & Jones, 2009).

In a qualitative study investigating the experiences of informal caregivers, including spouses and adult children, of stroke survivors, Greenwood, Mackenzie, Wilson, and Cloud (2009) reported uncertainty as a central theme. Reich, Olmsted, and van Puymbroeck (2006) reported uncertainty significantly impacted the partner relationships of patients with fibromyalgia.

CASE STUDY 7-1

Marilyn, a 24-year-old medical student, lives alone in a one-bedroom apartment. She is an only child and has strong ties with her parents, who live in a nearby state. Marilyn communicates with them frequently and relies on them for social and emotional support.

Marilyn experienced her first seizure at age 10, and was subsequently diagnosed with epilepsy. Despite medications to control her seizure activity, she continued to experience seizure activity throughout her adolescence. She missed classes and social events, but she graduated from high school and college.

Recently Marilyn experienced a grand mal seizure during an evening shift as a medical student in a busy emergency room. She was sent home by her physician supervisor. Her lack of sleep for the past several weeks had left her exhausted, and she was distressed by the rigor of her program. Marilyn was embarrassed, but relieved her colleagues didn't seem to know about or acknowledge the "incident." She had kept her diagnosis of epilepsy a secret. She was worried what people would think and how they might treat her if they knew. Her parents were worried, however, and called daily to provide comfort and support.

Over the next several weeks, Marilyn's seizure activity continued, despite changes in her medications. The new medications made her groggy and dull, and she had difficulty concentrating. She felt sad and depressed. It was after another grand mal seizure during a busy hospital shift that Marilyn was asked by the medical school administration to withdraw from her classes. Marilyn was devastated and overcome with uncertainty. Doubt consumed her every thought: Will my seizures ever be controlled? Can I become a physician? Will I be able to work? Will I ever marry? Can I have children? Will I be able to balance work and everyday life? What is my future? Do I have a future?

Discussion Questions

1. Discuss how uncertainty is manifested for Marilyn.
2. Explore the issue of uncertainty for a chronic illness using the four constructs of uncertainty (ambiguity, complexity, inconsistency, and unpredictability).
3. Design an action plan to assist Marilyn and her family to manage her illness uncertainty and promote quality of life.

Uncertainty as Opportunity

Mishel (1988) proposed a reconceptualization of uncertainty from a deficit to a source of personal growth. Uncertainty outcomes are not always negative. Indeed, uncertainty can be a useful coping mechanism for persons with chronic illness. Sometimes not knowing is better than knowing (Greenwood et al., 2009).

March was our "ignorance is bliss" month. Radiation and chemotherapy were over in February, and although the effects of the treatment had been brutal, we felt that better days surely were coming. Randy's next PET scan wasn't scheduled until mid-April, giving us 6 weeks of respite from treatment, albeit uncertainty as well as respite. However, it served as a healing time for us mentally. The future might be bright or bleak, as we were uncertain what the PET scan would show, but somehow, not knowing was okay. We were able to move cancer to the side for a while.

—Jenny

Uncertainty can provide the opportunity for persons with chronic illness to reevaluate their lives and establish priorities. The literature reflects evidence of positive reappraisal, including increased tolerance and appreciation for others, greater self-acceptance, increased optimism and joy in life (McCormick, 2002), getting a second chance in life, and enjoying the simple pleasures of life. In the case of a potentially negative outcome, uncertainty can be more desirable than certainty. Maintaining a level of uncertainty can help an individual with a chronic illness preserve hope (Brashers, Goldsmith, & Hsieh, 2002; Mishel, 1988).

Uncertainty as Harm

A number of emotional responses to the appraisal of uncertainty as harm may occur. Responses are discussed in this section.

STRESS

Illness uncertainty diminishes one's problem-centered coping and heightens emotion-centered coping. Uncertainty is a significant psychological stressor, particularly in a cultural context that values predictability and control (Mishel, 1990). Those individuals with less tolerance of uncertainty have greater perceptions of stress and poorer emotional well-being (Kurita, Garon, Stanton, & Meyerowitz, 2013). In 44 dyads composed of individuals with Parkinson's disease and their caregivers, uncertainty in illness did not predict distress for persons with the disease; however, uncertainty emerged as a significant predictor of distress for their caregivers. Caregivers reported stress as they faced an uncertain future regarding their caregiver responsibilities and tasks (Sanders-Dewey, Mullins, & Chaney, 2001).

A high degree of uncertainty is related to increased emotional distress, anxiety, and depression (McCormick, 2002). Persons with multiple sclerosis (MS) who reported greater uncertainty about their chronic illness were less hopeful and had more negative moods (Wineman, Schwetz, Zeller, & Cyphert, 2003). Illness uncertainty significantly correlates with negative mood states and affects the perceived symptom severity in persons with primary brain tumors (Lin, Chiang, Acquaye, Vera-Bolanos, Gilbert, & Armstrong, 2013). Higher levels of uncertainty are associated with diminished mood and quality of life in persons with chronic illness (Bailey et al., 2009).

ANXIETY

Chronic illness entails significant changes and need for adjustment, which often leads to feelings of anxiety. Persons with chronic illness are often worried and anxious about how and when their bodies will fail them (Arber & Spencer, 2013). Anxiety can be triggered by experiences of distrust and disbelief from others, a chronic illness that is invisible to others, or an illness that lacks specific diagnostic parameters. For example, in one study, young people with chronic fatigue syndrome or myalagic encephalopathy experienced higher levels of anxiety than healthy controls and young people with other chronic illnesses. Anxiety was conceptualized in this research as unpredictability of the future and a sense of vulnerability (Fisher & Crawley, 2012). In a meta-analysis, 50 research studies were examined to synthesize the state of the science on uncertainty in relation to women undergoing diagnostic evaluation for suspected breast cancer. All of the studies reported patients feeling anxiety that persisted throughout the diagnostic period until the final diagnosis (Montgomery, 2010).

LOSS OF CONTROL

One's perception of self-control impacts illness uncertainty (Mishel, 1997). Failure to control one's body and daily illness symptoms causes uncertainty and unpredictability (Beech, Arber, & Faithfull, 2012). A perceived lack of control emerges when an individual with a chronic condition (1) lacks sufficient information or knowledge about the illness, (2) has unpredictable illness symptoms, and (3) perceives his or her social support and health care to be inadequate. A decline in self-efficacy and sense of mastery may contribute to a lack of confidence in making decisions about treatment and daily activities. To gain a sense of control and regulate uncertainty, persons with chronic conditions may put their lives on hold and delay decisions and treatments. Mishel (1988) hypothesized that persons with a high internal locus of control would be more likely to perceive uncertainty as an opportunity, whereas people with an external locus of control would appraise uncertainty as a threat or danger. If the person's external locus of control is related to a strong belief in a higher power, then uncertainty may not necessarily be viewed as a threat or danger by the individual (McCormick, 2002).

WAITING

Waiting is a hallmark of the healthcare system. Waiting creates a loss of control for those who must wait for treatment decisions, test results, appointments, and so forth. Waiting produces anxiety, depression, panic, and uncertainty (Bailey, Wallace, & Mishel, 2007; Mishel, 1999; Wallace, 2003). Waiting is "a grueling experience of unsure stillness" (Bournes & Mitchell, 2002, p. 62). Among women suspected of having breast cancer, waiting has been described as limbo (Montgomery, 2010). In a qualitative research study with 21 women and 5 men who had been affected by cancer, waiting emerged as a theme. Waiting was described by many of the informants "as the worst part of the cancer experience: waiting for diagnosis, waiting for treatment, waiting for remission, and waiting for relapse" (Mulcahy, Parry, & Glover, 2010, pp. 1065–1066). Waiting became a feature of the cancer experience, exacerbating the constant uncertainty at each stage of the cancer journey—waiting for a diagnosis, waiting for treatment, waiting for good news, waiting for test results, waiting for death.

McCormick, McClement, and Naimark (2005) explored the experience of patients waiting for coronary artery bypass graft (CABG) surgery. Telephone interviews were conducted with 25 participants. The researchers concluded that lengthy waits resulted in significant psychological disturbance, including anxiety and uncertainty about the future. Bailey and colleagues (2009) examined the constructs of ambiguity, complexity, inconsistency, and unpredictability in 126 persons being treated under a watchful-waiting protocol for individuals with chronic hepatitis C. Ambiguity was identified as a primary construct of illness uncertainty and had the strongest relationships with depressive symptoms, quality of life, and fatigue.

Watchful waiting is a protocol often used in chronic conditions. It consists of observation, expectant management, active monitoring, or deferred treatment (Wallace, Bailey, O'Rourke, & Galbraith, 2004). Watchful waiting, however, provokes uncertainty. Without active treatment, many persons with chronic conditions worry how their illness will unfold in the future. For example, the person may wonder, "Is the cancer growing while I wait?" As such, these persons must not only manage their lives with a chronic illness, but deal with uncertainty about disease progression (Bailey et al., 2009).

Wallace (2005) examined the antecedents associated with uncertainty in 19 men with prostate cancer who were undergoing watchful-waiting management. The study results revealed significant relationships among level of education, length of illness, and uncertainty, lending support to Mishel's (1988) uncertainty in illness model and enhancing understanding of the various factors that influence uncertainty.

Lack of Information

Information may either increase or decrease uncertainty. Information about a particular chronic illness may or may not be readily available to patients and their social network, or the information from various sources may be contradictory. Additionally, individuals who seek information may not have the cognitive abilities to comprehend, integrate, and apply that information. Health information can be challenging and difficult to understand. Frequently, it contains medical jargon that is not easily understood. Some individuals with chronic illness may avoid information and bad news about their chronic illness (Arber & Spencer, 2013).

Outcomes in chronic illness are difficult to predict. There are no clear milestones in the chronic illness trajectory due to individual differences and responses to illness and treatment. Due to this unpredictability, it is challenging for the healthcare professional to provide an accurate progression of the disease or a timeline, thus adding to uncertainty.

Patients need healthcare professionals to provide the desired level and amount of information. However, the amount of information needed and wanted by patients varies significantly. Additionally, patients may want information that family members do not, and vice versa. The educational level of the person with chronic illness affects the time needed for that individual to construct meaning and context for the events in chronic illness. Persons with more education, more social support, and more trust in healthcare professionals experience less uncertainty (Mishel, 1988).

Evidence-Based Practice Box

Illness uncertainty continues long after diagnosis and treatment of a chronic illness. A large body of evidence, for example, indicates that prostate cancer affects functional, physical, and psychological well-being, leading to a reduced quality of life. However, the majority of research and interventions for men with prostate cancer have focused only on the affected men. Partners of men with prostate cancer are impacted by the cancer experience as well and report distress and uncertainty about the future.

The CONNECT program—a self-management psychosocial intervention for men with prostate cancer and their partners—was developed and implemented to improve patients' self-efficacy in managing their cancer. The CONNECT program also encouraged couples to develop a team approach to illness management. In a study of this program, the sample included 24 couples assigned to the intervention group, and the same number assigned to the control group. The 9-week CONNECT program consisted of topics such as system management, sexual dysfunction, uncertainty management, positive thinking, and couple communication. The program was delivered in group meetings and one-to-one telephone sessions. Implications for practice include the utility of a protocol that provides a consistent self-management intervention for men with prostate cancer and their partners that ensures quality care and outcomes.

Source: McCaughan, E., Prue, G., McSorley, O., Northouse, L., Schafenacker, A., & Parahoo, K. (2013). A randomized controlled trial of a self-management psychosocial intervention for men with prostate cancer and their partners: A study protocol. *Journal of Advanced Nursing,* 69(11), 2572-2583.

Interventions for Managing Uncertainty

Certainty and predictability of outcomes are valued in Western society. When persons face chronic conditions with uncertain outcomes, they search for a cure (Mishel, 1990). The goal of nursing interventions is to reduce uncertainty in persons with chronic illness and promote self-confidence in their abilities, thereby increasing certainty in their daily lives. A number of approaches may be used to enhance self-confidence and promote certainty. Social support provides a foundation for and enables the person with a chronic illness to rely on others, including family members, friends, or healthcare professionals. Education and information, given at the right time, at the right place, and at the right educational level, are instrumental in promoting certainty. Trust and confidence in one's healthcare professional are essential in managing chronic illness.

Managing uncertainty is a complex and dynamic endeavor that requires thoughtful and vigilant assessment by the healthcare professional. Some patients may embrace uncertainty with no need or want for more information, as more information might bring bad news. Some individuals with chronic illness may embrace a watch-and-wait perspective and remain content with their present knowledge rather than seek information about their future. Whatever the patient's attitude, strategies to maximize perceptions of confidence and control are essential in managing uncertainty. Cognitive, emotive, and behavioral strategies act in concert to affect a patient's perception of uncertainty. First, however, an assessment of the psychological and physical factors that potentially contribute to uncertainty is essential.

Interventions to manage uncertainty include strategies to (1) control emotion, (2) restructure life to incorporate the unpredictability of symptoms and promote normalization of life, and (3) understand the illness to better formulate an illness schema (Mishel, 1999). The strategies for management of illness uncertainty discussed in this section are based on Mishel's (1988) uncertainty theory. (See **Figure 7-1**).

Cognitive Strategies

Uncertainty can be reduced with cognitive strategies that provide and process facts, assist with problem solving, and address knowledge deficits. Illness meaning can be enhanced through personalized plans of care and appropriate educational interventions. Nurses can reduce uncertainty with structural resources that include education, social support, and care from healthcare professionals who are credible sources of confidence and authority (Donovan-Kicken & Bute, 2008; Mishel, 1988, 1999).

COGNITIVE REFRAMING

Cognitive reframing techniques are powerful tools that assist patients in dealing with and managing symptoms, reducing uncertainty, and finding meaning in life. Cognitive reframing seeks to alter one's cognitive schema and identify other ways of interpreting present and future situations and circumstances. In essence, it creates a new perspective on a situation still while acknowledging the reality.

Figure 7-1 Adaptation to Uncertainty

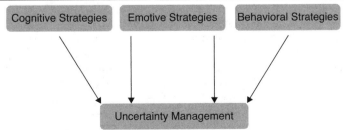

Bailey and colleagues (2004) evaluated the effectiveness of an intervention to help men cognitively reframe and manage the uncertainty of watchful waiting. Those in the intervention group received weekly calls from a nurse, while those in the control group received the usual care. Intervention participants reported greater improvement in their quality of life and their future quality of life compared to the control group.

Nurses can teach patients reframing strategies by helping them examine their expectations and exploring ways to set realistic expectations for themselves. Cognitive reframing requires ongoing attention and repetition, so nurses must provide ongoing encouragement and support for patients to use this technique successfully. Cognitive reframing techniques help persons rethink their perceptions of uncertainty and can impact mood and hopefulness.

KNOWLEDGE

Knowledge is a tool to manage uncertainty. Knowledge is essential in making treatment choices; it is also essential to regain control of one's life. Patients and families have multiple sources of information that they can access—for example, healthcare professionals, credible websites, and other patients. Both objective and subjective sources of information are needed.

Objective information is accessed when healthcare professionals rely on evidence-based literature to provide chronic illness information to patients. They provide the best information and resources within their domain of understanding, that of the "outsider." In addition, technology enables persons with chronic illness to access the same scientific literature that is available to their healthcare professionals.

Subjective information about a chronic illness, in contrast, may come from the perspective of others who are experiencing the same chronic illness and have an "insider's" perspective. The illness experience lies in the purview of the person with the chronic illness. Peers living with the same chronic condition provide a source of information that may or may not be helpful.

Education for patients and their social support network has long been the hallmark of quality health care. Regardless of the inevitability of disease progression and physical or mental decline intrinsic to chronic illness, education is an effective tool that promotes a sense of control. Persons with chronic illness do not equally respond to and have expectations for information to address uncertainty (Brashers & Hogan, 2013). Often, it is difficult to ascertain the amount of information that individuals want or can process. As healthcare professionals, we often provide more information, particularly at the beginning of a diagnosis, than the person with chronic illness and family can absorb. More is not always better. For some individuals, knowledge to reduce uncertainty can increase anxiety and disrupt feelings of hope that the existence of uncertainty offers (Brashers & Hogan, 2013). A thorough assessment of the needs of the individual and family, taking into account their readiness to learn, physical and emotional state, educational background, past life experiences, and cultural beliefs, forms the basis for educational interventions.

The healthcare professional should be aware that for some patients, health information does not decrease uncertainty. Not knowing may be less threatening and less stressful than receiving potentially bad news (Brashers et al., 2002; Brashers, Neidig, & Goldsmith, 2004). For other persons, having adequate information enables them to cope, participate in healthcare decisions, and deal with uncertainty. The premise that individuals with chronic illness and their families desire information is a value of Western healthcare practice. However, for some persons in diverse social groups, healthcare decisions are within the purview of others, whether they are family members, healthcare professionals, or a "higher power."

The literature on treatment decision making suggests that individuals who resist assuming this active role may be overwhelmed, may be misinformed as to the treatment options, and, in general, may lack the capacity to participate. In a qualitative study with five women diagnosed with breast cancer, in-depth interviews revealed patients' ambivalence in making treatment decisions reflected efforts to recast identities and positions of patients and physicians in the cancer care organization. Patients seek not only information but also interpretation of information by their oncologists (Sinding et al., 2010).

Cultural values and beliefs must be considered in education. Persons from family-centered cultures may be reluctant to assume responsibility for seeking information about their chronic disease and treatment and instead rely on family members to take charge. In family-centered cultures, families interact with healthcare professionals to seek information and may handle information in such a manner as to shield the person with the chronic illness from negative information that may result in the loss of hope (Brashers et al., 2002).

Nurses play a pivotal role by providing the right education in the right manner and at the appropriate point in the illness trajectory. Nurses may assist individuals in identifying credible sources of information that match the patient's cognitive processing ability. For many chronic conditions, volunteer agencies serve as resources that provide information and social support. Professional organizations are excellent resources for persons with a chronic condition.

CARE COORDINATION

Healthcare professionals should consider a social–ecological approach to patient/family-centered care management, in which the person with chronic illness and family, the interprofessional care team, and the healthcare organization all communicate and interact to promote certainty. In this model, the care coordinator works with the patient/family to establish realistic goals and gain access to adequate resources for self-care. Knowledge of self-management programs that incorporate information about the chronic disease is essential for the individual and family. Identification of triggers that exacerbate illness symptoms and the activities that help modify and manage those symptoms are important aspects of self-management.

The care coordinator provides connections between patients and providers across the care continuum. This person helps the patient and family navigate the complexities of the healthcare system and manage the logistical details of treatment and changing plans of care (Freeman, 2006).

NORMALIZATION

Normalization is restructuring one's life to incorporate the unpredictability of chronic illness symptom onset, severity, and duration. Part of normalization may be developing a routine. Adapting a routine for each day can provide normalcy to patients, even while understanding that many things may disrupt it. Nevertheless, being able to "fall back" into somewhat of a routine in managing one's care may provide some stability.

A holistic nursing assessment includes how individuals and their families negotiate illness-related disruptions in their daily lives, with particular attention being paid to symptom management. To lessen illness uncertainty, healthcare professionals work with their patients to develop an individualized symptom management plan. A focus on daily routines and expectations reduces uncertainty and diminishes anxiety. Living in the present with a "today focus" rather than a "tomorrow focus" helps reduce uncertainty (Greenwood et al., 2009).

Individuals may need assistance in setting priorities for activities of daily living, applying strategies to diminish illness symptoms such as fatigue or pain, and fostering a plan of care that engenders confidence and normalcy to the highest degree possible. People can cushion the effects of uncertainty by developing a structure or routine that encourages familiar and recognizable patterns of behavior. Routines focus on physiological as well as emotional responses to illness.

SOCIAL SUPPORT

Social support plays an important role in uncertainty and psychosocial adjustment. Such support provides stable relationships where people can openly express emotions and feelings and find reassurance of their humanness and worthiness. Supportive others assist those with chronic conditions to reappraise uncertainty as either opportunity or inconsequential, and to incorporate uncertainty as a normal part of life. Social support directly and indirectly reduces uncertainty (Lien et al., 2009; Mishel, 1988). It facilitates information seeking, decreases avoidance behavior, and encourages reappraisal of uncertainty (Brashers et al., 2004). When persons with chronic illness have the opportunity to discuss and reflect on their illness, they gain insight and clarity about their situation and achieve more certainty (Bar-Tel, Barnoy, & Zisser, 2005). Active and reflective listening by nurses promotes opportunities for persons to reflect on and gain understanding of their illness experience.

Healthcare professionals must be aware of the importance of social support in not only reducing uncertainty, but also enhancing quality of life. In Latina survivors of breast cancer, perceived social support and uncertainty played a pivotal role in these women's ability to manage and maintain quality of life. Perceived social support promoted better quality of life, whereas uncertainty diminished quality of life (Sammarco & Konecny, 2008). In a follow-up study, Sammarco and Konecny (2010) examined the differences between Latina and Caucasian survivors of breast cancer

and their perceived social support, uncertainty, and quality of life. Caucasians reported significantly higher levels of perceived social support and quality of life compared to their Latina counterparts. Healthcare professionals must be aware of these differences and integrate cultural values and demographic differences into their plans of care.

Nurses provide social support through humanistic caring behaviors (Neville, 2003, p. 213). Caring is an intrinsic component of nursing practice and is inherent in the nurse–patient dyad. Through these relationships, the nurse provides stability.

Advice giving is an effective support intervention when the advice is appropriate, relevant, and presented in a positive manner. However, when giving advice to persons with chronic illness, healthcare professionals need to assess whether the individual wants their advice. If the individual is not receptive to advice, then other forms of support, such as active listening or emotional support, may be more appropriate (Thompson & O'Hair, 2008).

The nurse may need to assist the patient in establishing a social network. In addition to family members and friends, nurses and other healthcare professionals are an important source of social support. Brashers and colleagues (2004) examined the effect of social support on management of uncertainty in persons living with HIV or AIDS. They found social support helps people with HIV and AIDS through both information gathering and information avoiding; providing instrumental support, skill development, acceptance, and validation; allowing venting; and encouraging shifts in perspective.

Emotive Strategies

Addressing psychological issues in chronic illness is vital to diminish uncertainty and increase quality of life (Lasker et al., 2010). Emotive interventions can alter feelings of uncertainty.

Management programs that enhance coping and improve overall well-being can be effective in persons with chronic illness (Gil et al., 2006).

ACKNOWLEDGE EMOTIONS

Healthcare professionals must acknowledge and respect the wide range of emotions that persons and their families experience in conjunction with chronic illness. These emotions may span a continuum from fear and despair to hope and determination. All emotions are valid in the illness experience. However, when emotions interfere with one's ability to manage chronic illness and uncertainty, these dysfunctional emotions need to be explored. Persons with chronic illnesses must be given the opportunity to tell their story and voice their volatile emotions in a safe environment. Development of a plan for managing dysfunctional emotive responses to illness uncertainty and referral to resources for psychosocial support are essential.

Uncertainty can be used to move from a perspective of limited choices to that of multiple opportunities (Mishel, 1990). However, the healthcare professional must assess the appropriateness of this strategy for each person with chronic illness and his or her family. The cultural imperative to "think positive" about the outcomes of a chronic illness may leave those who do not believe this feat is possible isolated from the support needed to confront their uncertain future (Willig, 2011). Healthcare professionals must be vigilant to the underlying meaning of language used by persons with chronic conditions. The use of hope language by persons with a chronic illness may be understood by the healthcare professional as optimism, but this interpretation must always be viewed with caution. In one study that sought to evaluate whether hope language truly expresses optimism, interviews were conducted with candidates for epilepsy surgery. Thematic analysis of the data found that only one-third of all hope statements by patients were coded as expressions of optimism, while one-third were not optimistic and included themes of worry and uncertainty. The remaining third had unclear meanings (Patton, Busch, Yee, Kubu, Gonzalez-Martinez, & Ford, 2013).

FORMULATE COGNITIVE SCHEMA

Mishel (1999) suggests forming an illness schema as a management method for uncertainty. Nurses can work with patients to construct personal scenarios of their illness that include the beginning of the illness, the progression of the illness, and the means by which recovery will occur. Such a cognitive schema provides patients with an opportunity to integrate incongruent events into an individualized illness framework that provides meaning and understanding. Promoting self-care behaviors facilitates redefining an uncertain situation into one that is manageable.

DEVELOP TRUST AND CONFIDENCE IN HEALTHCARE PROFESSIONALS

Chronic illness requires attention to issues of life and death, and wellness and illness, as well as daily management of symptoms and treatment. Trust and confidence in healthcare professionals play significant roles in reducing uncertainty in persons with chronic illness (Madar & Bar-Tal, 2009). Patient/family-centered communication should acknowledge and address illness uncertainty. Healthcare professionals can use reflective and summative statements that convey empathy, active listening, and exploration of values and emotions that foster trust and confidence (Johnson & Gustin, 2012). When the cultural norms of the patient differ from the cultural norms of the healthcare professional, uncertainty can develop. To instill trust and confidence, healthcare professionals must incorporate the cultural beliefs and norms of their patients and their families as appropriate (Lor, Khang, Xiong, Moua, & Lawver, 2013).

PROMOTE SPIRITUAL AND PSYCHOLOGICAL
WELL-BEING

Mindfulness is an attribute of consciousness associated with psychological well-being. Brown and Ryan (2003) report a relationship between mindfulness and positive emotional states. Mindfulness-based stress reduction employs techniques that help individuals cope with clinical and nonclinical problems (Grossman, Niemann, Schmidt, & Walach, 2004) and mitigate the negative effects of illness uncertainty. An interventional study of persons with cancer demonstrated that increased mindfulness over time results in decreases in mood disturbances and stress (Brown & Ryan, 2003).

Mindfulness techniques are accessible to everyone and do not require either financial resources or special equipment. Nurses can assist patients in identifying appropriate mindfulness strategies to incorporate into their activities of daily living. These activities focus on outcomes such as acceptance and living in the present, and recognition and acknowledgment of negative thoughts, feelings, or coping difficulties. Mindfulness exercises to reduce the negative effects of uncertainty include meditation, deep breathing exercises, and listening to music. In one study, psychological and spiritual well-being and quality of life increased after implementation of meditation healing exercises in persons with end-stage renal disease; moreover, meditation healing exercises significantly diminished uncertainty (Triamchaisri, Mawn, & Artsanthia, 2013).

Attention to spiritual aspects of well-being is important in addressing issues of uncertainty. In a sample of 50 individuals with multiple sclerosis (MS), researchers examined the contributions of illness uncertainty and spiritual well-being to psychosocial adaptation. Spiritual well-being influenced adaptation to MS and mitigated the impact of uncertainty on adaptation (McNulty et al., 2004).

Behavioral Strategies

Healthcare professionals must be alert to expressions of uncertainty. These expressions can be ascertained in language and in behavior such as withdrawing from self-care activities or social interaction.

MANAGING UNPREDICTABILITY:
ANTICIPATORY GUIDANCE

An understanding of the nature of uncertainty enhances one's ability to describe and explain influences on behavior and anticipate appropriate interventions aimed at improving outcomes (Brashers, 2001). In anticipation of progressive disability, nurses may refer persons to rehabilitative therapies to enhance and prolong independence in their daily activities, occupation, and relationships. In addition, other members of the interprofessional team should be consulted as necessary to help the patient and family deal with financial or vocational issues that may contribute to uncertainty. Individuals with chronic illness may seek advice from others with the same condition to assist them in anticipating an effective way to engage in health promotion and maintenance activities.

A combination of cognitive, emotive, and behavioral approaches to management of uncertainty is essential. Older women who have survived breast cancer, for example, experience ongoing illness uncertainty, fears about cancer recurrence, and symptoms from treatment side effects. In such women, vicarious experiences such as hearing about cancer in a friend, having unfamiliar aches and pains, and media coverage of cancer can trigger feelings of uncertainty. Based on the theory of uncertainty in illness (Mishel, 1988, 1997), an uncertainty management intervention for older long-term survivors of breast cancer was developed. This intervention consisted of cognitive-behavioral messages delivered by audiotapes and a self-help manual. In a study of this intervention, 483 recurrence-free women (342 white and 141 African American women) were randomly assigned to either the intervention or usual care (control) group. Nurses guided women through the intervention during four weekly telephone sessions and focused on one of four skills: relaxation, pleasant imagery, calming self-talk, and distraction. The nurses guided the women through the self-help manual that contained educational material and resources. Results indicated that the intervention group had improvements in cognitive reframing (viewing their situation in a more positive light), cancer knowledge, and a variety of coping skills. At 20 months postintervention, women continued to demonstrate benefits from the intervention in terms of decreased uncertainty and improved personal growth.

Cognitive-behavioral interventions are beneficial to women with chronic illness. These interventions improve knowledge and behavioral skills and help foster a more positive appraisal of the illness. Research in this area supports the importance of nurses in assisting persons with chronic illness to identify appropriate sources of information and in developing behavioral skills (Gil et al., 2006; Gil, Mishel, Germino, Porter, Carlton-LaNey, & Belyea, 2005).

Outcomes

In the face of chronic illness, uncertainty is itself chronic, persisting over the trajectory of the illness. Negative effects of uncertainty can be ameliorated by anticipating and understanding individual and family needs across the disease course. Nurses and other healthcare professionals can work with persons with chronic illness to modify negative outcomes of the illness experience and promote adaptation to and positive perceptions of uncertainty.

Chronic illness management is complex and requires an interprofessional team to address the various physical and psychosocial aspects of the illness. The complexity of the healthcare system can leave persons with a chronic illness confused and wondering who is in charge of their care when they see a different provider at each healthcare visit. This uncertainty fosters insecurity, leads to a perception of lack of control, and inhibits the ability to plan (Arber & Spencer, 2013). To ameliorate these concerns,

healthcare professionals must maintain a willingness to address the physical and psychosocial issues of uncertainty with their patients and their families. Discussions of challenges inherent with illness uncertainty by the healthcare professional, however, are contingent upon the readiness and receptivity of patients and families to discuss the impact of uncertainty in their daily lives.

Nurses can serve as valuable partners to persons and families who have chronic conditions. Nurses should provide guidance and support during illness instability and uncertain experiences. Along with other members of the healthcare team, they can moderate the effects of uncertainty by providing positive communication and essential information in a timely manner. Human behavior and reactions to chronic illness vary widely. Individuals with a chronic illness face complex psychological challenges as they make choices about treatment and management of their condition. Accordingly, uncertainty assessment needs to be a fundamental element of all nursing assessments of persons with chronic illness. Interventions to address the physical and psychosocial dimensions of chronic illness, including, uncertainty must be patient/family-centered. Patient/family-centered care acknowledges the variation in treatment protocols for any given chronic illness and differences that may be inherent in patient/family cultural beliefs and practices regarding treatment and management of chronic illness. Nursing assessments and interventions directed toward reducing uncertainty can promote adjustment to and improve quality of life for those with chronic conditions (Elphee, 2008). Theory-based nursing interventions designed to educate and support persons with chronic illness as they integrate and manage uncertainty across their disease trajectory are essential. Unacknowledged and unaddressed uncertainty can erode quality of life for an individual with a chronic condition as well as for the members of the patient's social network.

CASE STUDY 7-2

Heather is 45 years old, lives in a small rural community, and is married to Bill, her husband of 25 years. She is an optometrist and has a thriving professional practice. She and her husband have three daughters, who are married and live nearby.

During her high school and college years, Heather was on the basketball team. She enjoyed outdoor physical activities and participated in sports with her children. At the age of 37, Heather was diagnosed with rheumatoid arthritis (RA) after a suspicious fracture of her ankle. Heather sought information about her new diagnosis and was able to effectively manage her symptoms.

A few years later, Heather's RA progressed rapidly and management of her symptoms became challenging. She became overwhelmed and uncertain about all aspects of her life. She experienced extreme fatigue and was less able to spend time at her work. Her financial future was uncertain. She was worried about the side effects of the medications, but the new prescriptions were beyond her financial means. She had spontaneous fractures in her feet and joint involvement in her knees that made it difficult to ambulate, much less exercise. She gained weight.

A recent visit to her rheumatologist exacerbated Heather's depression and anguish. He wrote prescriptions for medications and instructed Heather to get a specialized brace to stabilize her knee for ambulation. Heather did not have the financial resources to obtain either the brace or the new medications. The physician addressed her fatigue with veiled accusations that she was simply lazy and needed to exercise and lose weight. Heather is overwhelmed with the management of the emotional, financial, and physical challenges that she is experiencing because of her RA. She is uncertain and she wonders if she will be able to find the needed resources to return to a normal life.

Discussion Questions

1. Identify and discuss the medical, personal, and social sources of uncertainty for Heather in conjunction with RA.
2. Propose appropriate cognitive, emotive, and behavioral strategies to alter Heather's perception of uncertainty.

STUDY QUESTIONS

1. Discuss the medical, personal, and social sources of illness uncertainty.
2. Using Mishel's theory of uncertainty, assess and provide a plan of care to address illness uncertainty with a patient in your practice.
3. How does cognitive reframing assist a patient with illness uncertainty?
4. The primary antecedent of Mishel's theory is the stimuli frame. Describe its components and discuss how each influences illness uncertainty.
5. Discuss the three ways in which uncertainty is appraised by persons with a chronic illness. Based on each of these appraisals, describe appropriate patient and family educational/information strategies.

References

Arber, A., & Spencer, L. (2013). "It's all bad news": The first 3 months following a diagnosis of malignant pleural mesothelioma. *Psycho-Oncology, 22*, 1528–1533.

Bailey, D. E., Landerman, L., Barroso, J., Bixby, P., Mishel, M. H., Muir, A. J., ... Clipp, E.. (2009). Uncertainty, symptoms, and quality of life in persons with chronic hepatitis C. *Psychosomatics, 50*(2), 138–146.

Bailey, D. E., Mishel, M. H., Belyea, M., Stewart, J. L., & Mohler, J. (2004). Uncertainty intervention for watchful waiting in prostate cancer. *Cancer Nursing, 27*(5), 339–346.

Bailey, D. E., Wallace, M., & Mishel, M. H. (2007). Watching, waiting and uncertainty in prostate cancer. *Journal of Clinical Nursing, 16*, 734–741.

Bar-Tel, Y., Barnoy, S., & Zisser, B. (2005). Whose informational needs are considered? A comparison between cancer patients and their spouses' perceptions of their own and their partners' knowledge and informational needs. *Social Science and Medicine, 60*(7), 1459–1465.

Basevitz, P., Pushkar, D., Chaikelson, J., Conway, M., & Dalton, C. (2008). Age-related differences in worry and related processes. *International Journal of Aging and Human Development, 66*(4), 283–305.

Beech, N., Arber, A., & Faithfull, S. (2012). Restoring a sense of wellness following colorectal cancer: A grounded theory. *Journal of Advanced Nursing, 68*, 1134–1144.

Bournes, D. A., & Mitchell, G. J. (2002). Waiting: The experience of persons in a critical care waiting room. *Research in Nursing & Health, 25*, 58–67.

Brashers, D. E. (2001). Communication and uncertainty management. *Journal of Communication, 51*, 477–497.

Brashers, D. E., Goldsmith, D. J., & Hsieh, E. (2002). Information seeking and avoiding in health contexts. *Human Communication Research, 28*, 258–271.

Brashers, D. E. & Hogan, T. P. (2013). The appraisal and management of uncertainty: Implications for information-retrieval systems. *Information Processing and Management, 49*, 1241–1249.

Brashers, D. E., Neidig, J. L., & Goldsmith, D. J. (2004). Social support and the management of uncertainty for people living with HIV or AIDS. *Health Communication, 16*, 305–331.

Brashers, D. E., Neidig, J. L., Russell, J. A., Cardillo, L. W., Haas, S. M., Dobbs, L. K., ... Nemeth, S. (2003). The medical, personal, and social causes of uncertainty in HIV illness. *Issues in Mental Health Nursing, 24*, 497–522.

Brown, K. W., & Ryan, R., M. (2003). The benefits of being present: Mindfulness and its role in psychological well-being. *Journal of Personality and Social Psychology, 84*(4), 822–848.

Clayton, M. F., Mishel, M. H., & Belyea, M. (2006). Testing a model of symptoms, communication, uncertainty and well-being in older breast cancer survivors. *Research in Nursing and Health, 29*, 18–39.

Davis, F. (1960). Uncertainty in medical prognosis clinical and functional. *American Journal of Sociology, 66*, 41–47.

Decker, C. L., Haase, J. E., & Bell, C. J. (2007). Uncertainty in adolescents and young adults with cancer. *Oncology Nursing Forum, 34*(3), 681–688.

Denny, E. (2009). "I never know from one day to another how I will feel": Pain and uncertainty in women with endometriosis. *Qualitative Health Research, 19*(7), 985–995.

Dirksen, S., & Erickson, J. (2002). Well-being in Hispanic and non-Hispanic Caucasian survivors of breast cancer. *Oncology Nursing Forum, 29*, 820–826.

Donovan-Kicken, E., & Bute, J. J. (2008). Uncertainty of social network members in the case of communication-debilitating illness or injury. *Qualitative Health Research, 18*(1), 5–18.

Elphee, E. E. (2008). Understanding the concept of uncertainty in patients with indolent lymphoma. *Oncology Nursing Forum, 35*(3), 449–454.

Encyclopedia Britannica. (2011). Damocles. http://www.britannica.com/EBchecked/topic/150566/Damocles

Fisher, H., & Crawley, E. (2012). Why do young people with CFS/ME feel anxious? A qualitative study. *Clinical Child Psychology and Psychiatry, 18*(4), 556–573.

Freeman, H. P. (2006). Patient navigation: A community centered approach to reducing cancer mortality. *Journal of Cancer Education, 21*(1 suppl), S11–S14.

Gil, K., Mishel, M., Belyea, M., Germino, B., Porter, L., & Clayton, M. (2006). Benefits of the uncertainty management intervention for African American and Caucasian older breast cancer survivors: 20-month outcomes. *International Journal of Behavioral Medicine, 13*, 286–294.

Gil, K. M., Mishel, M. H., Germino, B., Porter, L. S., Carlton-LaNey, I., & Belyea, M. (2005). Uncertainty management intervention for older African American and Caucasian long-term breast cancer survivors. *Journal of Psychosocial Oncology, 23*, 3–21.

Goffman, E. (1963). *Stigma: Notes on the management of spoiled identity*. New York, NY: Simon and Schuster.

Greenwood, N., Mackenzie, A., Wilson, N., & Cloud, G. (2009). Managing uncertainty in life after stroke: A qualitative study of the experiences of established and new informal carers in the first 3 months after discharge. *International Journal of Nursing Studies, 46*, 1122–1133.

Grossman, P., Niemann, L., Schmidt, S., & Walach, H. (2004). Mindfulness-based stress reduction and health benefits: A meta-analysis. *Journal of Psychosomatic Research, 57*(1), 35–43.

Guadalupe, K. (2010). Understanding a meningioma diagnosis using Mishel's theory of uncertainty in illness. *British Journal of Neuroscience Nursing, 6*(2), 77–82.

Johnson, L. M., Zautra, A. J., & Davis, M. C. (2006). The role of illness uncertainty on coping with fibromyalgia symptoms. *Health Psychology, 25*(6), 696–703.

Johnson, R. F., & Gustin, J. (2012). Acute lung injury and acute respiratory distress syndrome requiring tracheal intubation and mechanical ventilation in the intensive care unit: Impact on managing uncertainty for patient-centered communication. *American Journal of Hospice & Palliative Medicine, 30*(6), 569–575.

Kang, Y. (2006). Effect of uncertainty on depression in patients with newly diagnosed atrial fibrillation. *Progress in Cardiovascular Nursing, 21*(2), 83–88.

Kurita, K., Garon, E. B., Stanton, A. L., & Meyerowitz, B. E. (2013). Uncertainty and psychological adjustment in patients with lung cancer. *Psycho-Oncology, 22*, 1396–1401.

Lasker, J. N., Sogolow, E. D., Olenik, J. M., Sass, D. A., & Weinrieb, R. M. (2010). Uncertainty and liver transplantation: Women with primary biliary cirrhosis before and after transplant. *Women & Health, 50*, 359–375.

Lazarus, R., & Folkman, S. (1984) *Stress appraisal and coping*. New York, NY: McGraw-Hill.

Lemaire, G. S. (2004). More than just menstrual cramps: Symptoms and uncertainty among women with endometriosis. *Journal of Obstetric, Gynecologic, and Neonatal Nursing, 33*, 71–79.

Liao, M. N., Chen, M. F., Chen, S. C., & Chen, P. L. (2008). Uncertainty and anxiety during the diagnostic period for women with suspected breast cancer. *Cancer Nursing, 31*(4), 274–283.

Lien, C. Y., Lin, H. R., Kuo, I. T., & Chen, M. L. (2009). Perceived uncertainty, social support and psychological adjustment in older patients with cancer being treated with surgery. *Journal of Clinical Nursing, 18*, 2311–2319.

Lin, L., Chiang, H-H., Acquaye, A. A., Vera-Bolanos, E., Gilbert, M. R., & Armstrong, T. S. (2013). Uncertainty, mood states, and symptom distress in patients with primary brain tumors. *Cancer, 119*, 2796–2806.

Lor, M., Khang, P. Y., Xiong, P., Moua, K. F., & Lawver, D. (2013). Understanding Hmong women's beliefs, feelings, norms, and external conditions about breast and cervical cancer screening. *Public Health Nursing, 30*(5), 420–428.

Lowey, D. E., Norton, S. A., Quinn, J. R., & Quill, R. E. (2013). Living with advanced heart failure or COPD: Experiences and goals of individuals nearing the end of life. *Research in Nursing & Health, 36*, 349–358.

Madar, H., & Bar-Tal, Y. (2009). The experience of uncertainty among patients having peritoneal dialysis. *Journal of Advanced Nursing, 65*(8), 1664–1669.

Martin, S. C., Stone, A. M., Scott, A. M., & Brashers, D. E. (2010). Medical, personal, and social forms of uncertainty across the transplantation trajectory. *Qualitative Health Research, 20*, 182–196.

Mauro, A. M. (2010). Long-term follow-up study of uncertainty and psychosocial adjustment among implantable cardioverter defibrillator recipients. *International Journal of Nursing Studies, 47*(9), 1080–1088.

McCaughan, E., Prue, G., McSorley, O., Northouse, L., Schafenacker, A., & Parahoo, K. (2013). A randomized controlled trial of a self-management psychosocial intervention for men with prostate cancer and their partners: A study protocol. *Journal of Advanced Nursing, 69*(11), 2572–2583.

McCormick, K. M. (2002). A concept analysis of uncertainty in illness. *Journal of Nursing Scholarship, 34*(2), 127–131.

McCormick, K. M., McClement, S., & Naimark, B. J. (2005). A qualitative analysis of the experience of uncertainty while awaiting coronary artery bypass surgery. *Canadian Journal of Cardiovascular Nursing, 15*(1), 10–22.

McIntosh, J. (1974). Processes of communication, information seeking and control associated with cancer: A selective review of the literature. *Social Science and Medicine, 8*, 167–187.

McIntosh, J. (1976). Patients' awareness and desire for information about diagnosed but undisclosed malignant disease. *Lancet, 2*, 300–303.

McNulty, K., Livneh, H., & Wilson, L. M. (2004). Perceived uncertainty, spiritual well-being, and psychosocial adaptation in individuals with multiple sclerosis. *Rehabilitation Psychology, 49*(2), 91–99.

Miller, L. E. (2012). Sources of uncertainty in cancer survivorship. *Journal of Cancer Survivorship, 6*(4), 431–440.

Mishel, M. H. (1981). The measurement of uncertainty in illness. *Nursing Research, 30*(5), 258–263.

Mishel, M. H. (1984). Perceived uncertainty and stress in illness. *Research in Nursing and Health*, 7(3), 163–171.

Mishel, M. H. (1988). Uncertainty in illness. *Image: Journal of Nursing Scholarship*, 20, 225–232.

Mishel, M. H. (1990). Reconceptualization of the uncertainty in illness theory. *Image: Journal of Nursing Scholarship*, 22, 256–262.

Mishel, M. H. (1997). Uncertainty in acute illness. *Annual Review of Nursing Research*, 15, 57–80.

Mishel, M. H. (1999). Uncertainty in chronic illness. *Annual Review of Nursing Research*, 17, 269–294.

Mishel, M. H. (2014). Theories of uncertainty in illness. In M. J. Smith & P.R. Liehr (Eds.), *Middle range theory for nursing* (3rd ed., pp. 53–86). New York, NY: Springer.

Mishel, M. H., & Braden, C. J. (1988). Finding meaning: Antecedents of uncertainty. *Nursing Research*, 37, 98–103.

Mitchell, M. L., Courtney, M., & Coyer, F. (2003). Understanding uncertainty and minimizing families' anxiety at the time of transfer from intensive care. *Nursing and Health Sciences*, 5, 207–217.

Montgomery, M. (2010). Uncertainty during breast diagnostic evaluation: State of the science. *Oncology Nursing Forum*, 37(1), 77–83.

Mulcahy, C. M., Parry, D. C., & Glover, T. D. (2010). The "patient patient": The trauma of waiting and the power of resistance for people living with cancer. *Qualitative Health Research*, 20(8), 1062–1075.

Neville, K. (2003). Uncertainty in illness: An integrative review. *Orthopedic Nursing* 22(3), 206–214.

Northouse, L. L., Mood, D., Kershaw, T., Schafenacker, A., Mellon, S., Walker, J., … Decker, V. (2002). Quality of life of women with recurrent breast cancer and their family members. *Journal of Clinical Oncology*, 20, 4050–4064.

Patton, D. J., Busch, R. M., Yee, K. M., Kubu, C. S., Gonzalez-Martinez, J., & Ford, P. J. (2013). Hope language in patients undergoing epilepsy surgery. *Epilepsy & Behavior*, 29, 90–95.

Penrod, J. (2001). Refinement of the concept of uncertainty. *Journal of Advanced Nursing*, 34, 238–245.

Persson, E., & Hellstrom, A. (2002). Experiences of Swedish men and women 6 to 12 weeks after ostomy surgery. *Journal of Wound, Ostomy and Continence Nursing*, 29(2), 103–108.

Reich, J. W., Olmsted, M. E., & van Puymbroeck, C. M. (2006). Illness uncertainty, partner caregiver burden and support, and relationship satisfaction in fibromyalgia and osteoarthritis patients. *Arthritis & Rheumatism*, 55(1), 86–93.

Sammarco, A. (2001). Perceived social support, uncertainty, and quality of life of younger breast cancer survivors. *Cancer Nursing*, 24(3), 212–219.

Sammarco, A., & Konecny, L. (2008). Quality of life, social support and uncertainty among Latina breast cancer survivors. *Oncology Nursing Forum*, 35, 844–849.

Sammarco, A., & Konecny, L. M. (2010). Quality of life, social support, and uncertainty among Latina and Caucasian breast cancer survivors: A comparative study. *Oncology Nursing Forum*, 37(1), 93–99.

Sanders-Dewey, J. E. J., Mullins, L. L., & Chaney, J. M. (2001). Coping style, perceived uncertainty in illness, and distress in individuals with Parkinson's disease and their caregivers. *Rehabilitation Psychology*, 46, 363–381.

Schulman-Green, D., Ercolano, E., Dowd, M., Schwartz, P., & McCorkle, R. (2008). Quality of life among women after surgery for ovarian cancer. *Palliative Support Care*, 6(3), 239–247.

Simpson, M. F., & Whyte, F. (2006). Patients' experiences of completing treatment for colorectal cancer in a Scottish district general hospital. *European Journal of Cancer Care*, 15(2), 172–182.

Sinding, C., Hudak, P., Wiernikowski, J., Aronson, J., Miller, P., Gould, J., & Fitzpatarick-Lewis, D. (2010). "I like to be an informed person but …": Negotiating responsibility for treatment decisions in cancer care. *Social Science & Medicine*, 71, 1094–1101.

Stone, A. M., & Jones, C. L. (2009). Sources of uncertainty: Experiences of Alzheimer's disease. *Issues in Mental Health Nursing*, 30, 677–686.

Thompson, S., & O'Hair, H. D. (2008). Advice-giving and the management of uncertainty for cancer survivors. *Health Communication*, 23, 340–348.

Triamchaisri, S. K., Mawn, B. E., & Artsanthia, J. (2013). Development of a home-based palliative care model for people living with end-stage renal disease. *Journal of Hospice & Palliative Nursing*, 15(4), E1–E10.

Wallace, M. (2003). Uncertainty and quality of life of older men who undergo watchful waiting for prostate cancer. *Oncology Nursing Forum*, 30, 303–309.

Wallace, M. (2005). Finding more meaning: The antecedents of uncertainty revisited. *Journal of Clinical Nursing*, 14, 863–868.

Wallace, M., Bailey, D., O'Rourke, M., & Galbraith, M. (2004). The watchful waiting management option for older men with prostate cancer: State of the science. *Oncology Nursing Forum*, 31(6), 1057–1064.

Willig, C. (2011). Cancer diagnosis as discursive capture: Phenomenological repercussions of being positioned within dominant constructions of cancer. *Social Science & Medicine, 73*, 897–903.

Wineman, N. M., Schwetz, K. M., Zeller, R., & Cyphert, J. (2003). Longitudinal analysis of illness uncertainty, coping, hopefulness, and mood during participation in a clinical drug trail. *Journal of Neuroscience Nursing, 35*(2), 100–107.

Wolfe-Christensen, C., Isenberg, J. C., Mullins, L. L., Carpentier, M. Y., & Almstrom, C. (2008). Objective versus subjective ratings of asthma severity: Differential predictors of illness uncertainty and psychological distress in college students with asthma. *Children's Health Care, 37*, 183–195.

Chapter 8

Quality of Life

Cheryl Gies

Introduction

In the stirring autobiography, *Closing the Chart: A Dying Physician Examines Family, Faith and Medicine,* 40-year-old son, brother, husband, father, and family physician Steven Hsi chronicles his "formal education as a patient" (Hsi, Belshaw, & Corbin-Hsi, 2004, p. 10). As he lived the experience of chronic, progressive, and eventually terminal heart disease, Hsi wrote in his journal, "No one can say when chronic illness begins. More often than not, the earliest signs are subtle ripples in the daily routine of our lives recognized only in retrospect to the more significant disease … this is a time of denial and recrimination as (we) confront the symptoms and try to explain the body's mysterious changes" (p. 9).

Like a stealth missile, chronic illness finds its target and disrupts and compromises the normal rhythm and landscape of life. More than 133 million Americans live with chronic illness, and one in four Americans suffers multiple, concurrent chronic conditions (Centers for Disease Control and Prevention [CDC], 2012; Parekh, Goodman, Gordon, & Koh, 2011). Managing the effects of chronic illness while maintaining quality of life is a challenging, multifaceted, complex endeavor for patients, their families, and their healthcare professionals and team.

Quality of life (QOL) and health-related quality of life (HRQOL) are terms used to describe the impact of chronic illness. These terms are often used interchangeably in the literature to describe broad concepts of life satisfaction and life concerns affected by health and illness that impact not only the person living with chronic illness, but also his or her family, the nursing profession, and the healthcare system in general. In recent years, a national healthcare dilemma and an important area of national research have evolved to address a key question related to chronic illness: How do we determine whether prolonging life is the best strategy for persons with seriously compromised quality of life? (Taylor, Gibson, & Franck, 2008).

This chapter presents an overview of how quality of life and health-related quality of life are defined, conceptualized, measured, and assessed, and offers insight and recommendations for implementing evidence-based nursing interventions to effectively care for and treat persons with chronic physical and mental illness. It is challenging to do justice to the depth and breadth of this topic.

Defining, Conceptualizing, and Measuring Quality of Life

DEFINITIONS

Quality of Life   Interest in determining the meaning and significance of quality of life began more than a half a century ago when the World

Health Organization (WHO, 1948), recognizing health's multidimensionality, defined health as a state of complete physical, mental, and social well-being and not merely the absence of disease or infirmity. Even though the WHO definition focuses on well-being, quality of life measurements in the United States have traditionally focused on health deficits and tracking morbidity, mortality, and lives saved (CDC, 2011a). As curative and treatment strategies have advanced and lifespans have been extended, the outcome measurement focus has gradually shifted from saving lives to improving quality of life. Within this context, one cannot separate the concept of health from the concept of life quality.

There is no universal definition of quality of life, and defining this concept is difficult because definitions of complex terms tend to change the longer a phenomenon is studied (Barofsky, 2012). Quality of life determinants are both subjective and objective. The uniqueness of each person's circumstances, experiences, and stages of life contribute to positive and negative *subjective* (personal perspective) determinants of life quality. Additionally, quality of life and one's overall sense of well-being are anchored to *objective* (observational perspective) factors such as good health, social and economic conditions, living arrangements, and community environment, as well as culture, personal values, happiness, life satisfaction, and spiritual well-being. A plethora of discussions in the literature have dealt with the question of defining quality of life, and the definitions vary depending on whether the terms are based on description or evaluation.

In an attempt to clarify the concept of QOL, nursing authors Mandzuk and McMillan (2005) identified three critical attributes: (1) appraisal of one's own life; (2) identification of physical, psychological, and social satisfaction in areas of one's life; and (3) objective measures to enhance personal evaluation. **Table 8-1** summarizes QOL issues specific to chronic illness identified

Table 8-1 QUALITY OF LIFE COMPONENTS IN CHRONIC ILLNESS

Source	Chronic Illness/ Patient Group	QOL Components
Garratt, Schmidt, & Fitzpatrick (2002)	Diabetes	Social, psychological, well-being
Hart, Bilo, Redekop, Stolk, Assink, & Meyboom-de-Jong (2003)		
Berra (2003)	Cardiovascular disease, patients undergoing rehabilitation	Physical, emotional, intellectual, economic, social, self-perceived health status; work-related
Shephard & Franklin (2001)	Cardiovascular disease	Personal perceptions, coping mechanisms, environmental constraints
Mackenzie & Chang (2002)	Stroke survivors	Physical and psychological aspects
Ferrans & Powers (1992)	Patients receiving dialysis	Health and functioning, socioeconomic, psychological/spiritual, and family needs satisfaction
World Health Organization (1995)	Chronic illness	Physical and psychological health, personal beliefs, social relationships, environment

by these authors. Nursing and other health disciplines have conceptualized and defined quality of life operationally so as to design quantitative index scores that drive healthcare policy and recommendations for clinical practice and educational standards (Milton, 2013).

From an ethical perspective, most quality of life definitions describe a person's satisfaction or dissatisfaction related to his or her functional ability but exclude the individual's lived experience. Excluding the qualitative lived experience has led to a confusing array of definitions that lack consensus for application in healthcare practice (Milton, 2013).

Health-Related Quality of Life   Conflicting individual, academic discipline, and group definitions of quality of life make it difficult to accurately and adequately measure HRQOL outcomes (CDC, 2011a). Since the 1980s, the term "health-related quality of life" has evolved to focus on life quality that clearly affects mental or physical health (CDC, 2011a). Cella (1995) defines HRQOL as "the extent to which one's usual or expected physical, emotional (mental) and social well-being are affected by a medical condition or its treatment" (p. 73). HRQOL is inclusive of both the subjective nature and the multidimensionality of quality of life. On an individual level, this includes health risks and conditions, social support, functional ability, and socioeconomic status; on a community level, it includes population health resources, policies, conditions, and practices in collaboration with multidisciplinary healthcare partners (CDC, 2011a).

Advanced practice nursing has a significant leadership role in diagnosing, treating, managing, and identifying evidence-based strategies to address quality of life in persons with chronic illness. Understanding the distinctions and the interconnections of quality of life, health-related quality of life, and self-perceived health is essential to patient-centered care, effective nursing practice, and improved patient outcomes.

CONCEPTUALIZING HEALTH-RELATED QUALITY OF LIFE

Application of theoretical frameworks to the concept of quality of life is key to understanding the burden that chronic illness imposes on the patient and family during the illness trajectory. Furthermore, if improved quality of life is an essential patient outcome, qualitative and quantitative measurement strategies are needed.

Theories, frameworks, and models in chronic illness provide a systematic approach to studying and explaining the complex interrelationships among the various factors that influence quality of life over the illness trajectory. Such conceptualizations are important not only to generate new evidence for best nursing practice, but also to test and evaluate existing interventions that may improve quality of life in chronic illness. It is important to consider current theoretical perspectives that nursing and other healthcare disciplines have contributed to guide the art of nursing practice and "understand the inherent indivisibility of life and its quality" (Plummer & Molzahn, 2009, p. 140).

NURSING THEORIES AND FRAMEWORKS

Plummer and Molzahn (2009) conducted a critical appraisal of nursing theories to examine quality of life as embedded within the theorists' original frameworks. They evaluated attributes of quality of life as depicted by nurse theorists Imogene King, Madeleine Leininger, Rosemarie Parse, Hildegard Peplau, and Martha Rogers. The four quality of life attributes identified were contextual, subjective, intangible, and health related. The authors concluded that there is merit in considering the term "quality of life" to be more useful to nursing than the term "health," even going as far as to recommend replacing the nursing metaparadigm concept of "health" with "quality of life." In relation to nursing practice, Plummer and Molzahn proposed that quality of life is valuable because it considers connections between the intangible and subjective aspects of the patient's environment. They recommended that (1) further research be done to develop a better understanding of quality of life for differing client populations and (2) Parse's conceptually mature theory of humanbecoming be used as a conceptual research framework.

Parse (2007) tells us that only the individual "living the life" can judge quality of life, which the theorist defines as "the incarnation of lived experiences … the indivisible human's view on living moment to moment as the changing patterns of shifting perspectives weave the fabric of life through the human–universe interconnectedness" (p. 217). Countless subjective exemplars have been described in the literature by Parse and her scholars to broaden nurses' understanding of quality of life in diverse situations and expand nursing competence to be present to persons with chronic illness in ways that "honor their lived experience" (Plummer & Molzahn, 2009, p. 138).

In a qualitative study of men suffering from chronic depression, Parse scholar Welch (2007) explored the phenomenon of taking life day-by-day. The purpose of this study was to discover the structure of the lived experience of taking life day-by-day, realize a deeper understanding of the phenomenon, and contribute to the body of nursing knowledge using the Parse research method. Three themes were captured from the study participants' dialogues. The first theme, *enduring with the burdensome*, describes moving forward in spite of day-to-day struggles. The second theme, *envisioning the possible*, focuses on looking to the future with anticipation. The third theme, *sure–unsure*, illuminates the uncertainty of moments in life. Two participants' stories reported by Welch capture the essence of these themes and the dichotomy of living with chronic illness and holding onto quality of life.

Mark's Story

Mark is 60 years of age. Taking life day-by-day, said Mark, is living "without negatives." It is to "sit on the veranda and read every day, *sitting down, and letting go of the guilt of not playing roles and not giving guilt a place or status, even though it hovers in the background."* For Mark, taking life day-by-day is to quietly live every day as it comes, having no hopes and no desires. *"It requires discipline, waking up every morning, making your first cup of tea, and purposefully electing to have no plans for the day, and let the day unfold."* Taking life day-by-day, said Mark, is harboring *"a faint feeling of loss of hope and of what was. It is dropping all the illusions that you had about yourself or the world and getting to the point {of recognizing} that in having an uneventful life, you can cope"* (Welch, 2007, p. 268).

John's Story

John is a 46-year-old man who has worked as a psychiatric nurse for the past 25 years. Presently he is working with people who have AIDS or are HIV positive. Taking life day-by-day, said John, *"is a survival strategy."* It is to leave the past in the past, not *"worrying about or looking toward the future, but rather "dealing with issues as they come up, focusing in a clear strong way on the events that happen on that day and deal with them on that day."* Taking life day-by-day for John also involves *"managing and dealing with the illness and those feelings I had on that day, and as best I could close it and start again on the following day."* John stated, *"If I felt sad, I would say to myself, 'You are sad.' Accept that is where you are at in that moment and ask, What can I do to either live with it or overcome that?"* In taking life day-by-day, John viewed the *"beginning of each day as something new and therefore seeing what that day has for me and dealing with it as it happens"* (Welch, 2007, p. 269).

Most recently, Parse (2013) has posited that the term "quality of life" is an inert concept that does not adequately represent the ever-changing facets of lived experiences (living with chronic illness), and suggested reconceptualizing it as *living quality*. Parse proposes that the concept of "living quality" better represents the changing nature of lived experiences that cannot be measured with labels, that capture only a moment in time, and concludes that nursing and other healthcare professionals honor "living quality" by acknowledging and respecting that each person within the illness trajectory has a personal sense of direction that defies labeling or criticism. Thus, rather than discerning quality of life by asking "How is your quality of life?", healthcare professionals should assess a person's living quality by asking "What is important to you now?" (p. 114).

Finally, an interesting nursing theoretical model proposed by Susan Marden (2005) explores the relationship between a patient's technology dependence and HRQOL and the unique effect that therapeutic technology has on patients' reported quality of life outcomes. This model is composed of five concepts: attitudes toward technology dependence, illness representation (commonsense beliefs), symptom distress, HRQOL, and illness history. It serves as a guide for clinical nursing research to discover the HRQOL impact of therapeutic health technology interventions.

A GLOBAL MODEL

In addition to nursing conceptual framework contributions, national and global care models have been developed to assist practitioners in the provision of care for persons with chronic illness. The chronic care model (CCM) is a global model that has been implemented nationally and internationally, emerging more than a decade ago to improve patient care and health outcomes for persons with chronic illness through a systems approach (**Figure 8-1**).

The CCM was developed and refined in response to both the escalating worldwide mortality and disease burden attributed to chronic illness and the Institute of Medicine's

Figure 8-1 The Chronic Care Model

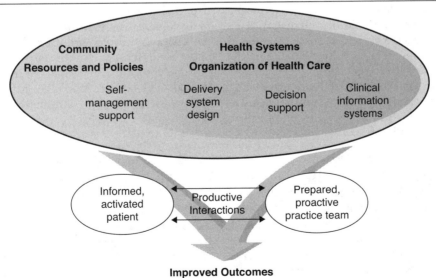

Source: Wagner, E.H. (1998). Chronic disease management: What will it take to improve care for chronic illness? *Effective Clinical Practice, 1*, 2–4.

(IOM's) challenge to healthcare organizations to improve care delivery for persons with depression, asthma, diabetes, and other chronic conditions (identified in the IOM's 2001 report, *Crossing the Quality Chasm: A New Health System for the 21st Century*). Integrating six essential elements of the healthcare system, this model directs high-quality chronic disease care and improved patient health outcomes through patient-centered, evidence-based care in ambulatory settings (Agency for Healthcare Research and Quality [AHRQ], 2008; Coleman, Austin, Brach, & Wagner, 2009). Its six essential elements include community resources, health system, self-management support, delivery system design, decision support, and clinical information. An integrated review of the CCM-based intervention literature reported that redesigning care using the CCM has improved patient care and demonstrated better health outcomes but recommended that efforts should be directed toward areas of cost-effectiveness (Coleman et al., 2009).

The CCM was an important contributor to the development of the patient-centered medical home, a new model of care being piloted across the United States (Robert Graham Center, 2007). The AHRQ (n.d.). defines a medical home not simply as a place, but rather a model of the primary care organization that delivers the core functions of primary health care using five functions and attributes: (1) comprehensive care, (2) coordinated care, (3) accessible services, (4) quality, and (5) safety.

A NATIONAL STRATEGIC FRAMEWORK

Although the CCM has demonstrated positive improvements in patient care and health outcomes, the model must be adapted specifically to each chronic disease (e.g., asthma, congestive heart failure, diabetes) and does not holistically approach persons with more than one chronic illness. For persons who suffer multiple (two or more) chronic conditions (MCC), health care and quality of life become more complicated. A staggering 80% of Americans 65 years and older live with MCC. The larger the number of chronic conditions, the higher the risk of mortality, impaired functional status, hospitalization, redundant diagnostic testing, and ambiguous medical advice (Parekh et al., 2011).

In response to these concerns, the U.S. Department of Health and Human Services (USHHS, n.d.), in collaboration with other stakeholders, developed a framework for improving health outcomes and quality of life for the MCC population (Parekh et al., 2011; Parekh & Goodman, 2013). This revised "action-oriented" *HHS Strategic Framework on Multiple Chronic Conditions* is an attempt to maximize national strategies to coordinate care and reduce health service barriers for persons with MCC. Support from the Patient Protection and Affordable Care Act (ACA) and public and private partnerships are thought to be important facilitators for this framework. The *HHS Strategic Framework on Multiple Chronic Conditions* has four interdependent major goals, each of which is associated with a set of objectives and strategies (Parekh et al., 2011). The first goal is to strengthen the healthcare and public health systems; the second goal is to empower individuals in self-care management; the third goal supplies providers with tools, interventions, and information; and the fourth goal supports research about persons with MCC and effective interventions (Parakh & Goodman, 2013). The full text of this framework is available from the Department of Health and Human Services (http://www.hhs.gov/ash/initiatives/mcc/index.html).

A poignant example of the impact of MCC on quality of life is depicted in a short animated video titled *Multiple Chronic Conditions: A Day in the Life* (http://www.ahrq.gov/professionals/prevention-chronic-care/decision/mcc/video/index.html), about a woman named Mae. Mae tries to manage just one day of her busy life, attending to the issues she faces in dealing with multiple chronic conditions in a complex healthcare maze. The complexities of a fragmented healthcare system that impact Mae are highlighted, and the video ends with a vision for individualized, coordinated, and organized provision of care, applying the principles and initiatives of the *HHS Strategic Framework on Multiple Chronic Conditions.*

MEASURING HEALTH-RELATED QUALITY OF LIFE

Theoretical frameworks provide a systematic approach to studying quality of life. Regardless of whether HRQOL is conceptualized as a complex set of relationships that influence the chronic illness trajectory, or as an outcome of the illness itself, appropriate measurement tools are crucial. Valid and reliable measures are needed to accurately capture the elements or concepts that characterize HRQOL to ensure that appropriate interventions and resources are utilized in a patient-centered, cost-effective manner. The subjective component of HRQOL is defined by each person's unique situation that reflects happiness and life satisfaction (CDC, 2011a). The general worldview of quality of life includes health as well as culture, values, beliefs, and environment. The more specific HRQOL is the relationship to health and physical function, and to emotional and mental well-being. Past measurement strategies were unable to capture the comprehensive multidimensional elements that contribute to quality to life in general or health-related quality of life more specifically.

Several popular instruments are used to assess HRQOL, measure HRQOL change over time, and evaluate quality of care in managed care plans. The Medical Outcome Study Short Forms (SF-12 and SF-36), the Sickness Impact Profile (SIP), and the Quality of Well-Being Scale have all been validated as tools for use in clinical settings for special populations (CDC, 2011a; Ware, 2004). For example, the SF-36 instrument is used in cardiac rehabilitation programs to track HRQOL in persons with chronic heart disease and the SIP is used in patients with cancer.

The CDC (2011b) is committed to tracking health-related quality of life as a health outcome to link healthcare disciplines and services. Traditional illness outcomes that measure morbidity and mortality are limiting, in that they do not consider risks, burdens, resource needs, or declines associated with illness, particularly as they relate to chronic conditions. To this end, the CDC created the HRQOL-14 Healthy Days Measure (2011c), which evaluates an individual's perception of well-being via four items: self-rated health, number of days of illness or injury, number of days of emotional distress, and number of days unable to do self-care or work. The four-item measure was later expanded to include 10 additional questions eliciting responses on individuals' days of activity limitations, pain, depression, anxiety, sleeplessness, and feeling energized. This instrument is available at http://www.cdc.gov/hrqol/hrqol14_measure.htm.

WHO (2004) has also developed a standardized tool to measure quality of life and health from the individual's perspective. In contrast to the CDC measure, the WHOQOL-BREF instrument (http://www.who.int/substance_abuse/research_tools/en/english_whoqol.pdf) has 26 items that assess an individual's feelings of satisfaction and enjoyment with life, limitations due to pain, capacity for work, ability to perform activities of daily living and to get around, access to health care, and satisfaction with relationships. Both the CDC and the WHO tools attempt to quantify and standardize quality of life. These tools are intended to measure health and well-being in healthy populations as well as to detect illness conditions that could benefit from early intervention and treatment.

The most recent and comprehensive undertaking to collect, use, and report patient-reported data on health-related quality of life is the National Institutes of Health (NIH)–funded Patient-Reported Outcome Measurement Information System (PROMIS) project (**Figure 8-2**). The PROMIS project was initiated in 2004 and re-funded in 2010 to create and test a multidimensional measurement tool using the latest advances in information technology to help patients accurately report their symptoms and health-related quality of life to their healthcare

Figure 8-2 Patient-Reported Outcomes Measurement Information System (PROMIS) Domain Framework

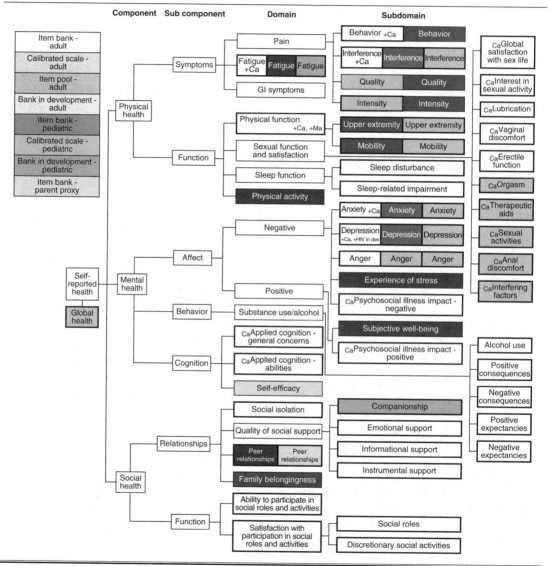

Subscripts following a + indicate bank variations for specied subgroups.
A subscript before the bank name indicates the bank was developed in this population only.
A heavy dark border indicates this instrument is currently available in Assessment Center.
Global Health includes two calibrated scales and two uncalibrated pool items.
Ca: cancer; MA: mobility; AIDS, HIV.
Reprinted with permission of the PROMIS Health Organization and the PROMIS Cooperative Group. Copyright © 2012.

providers (Cella et al., 2010; NIH, 2013, n.d.). This instrument combines generic health status, generic illness, and disease-specific instruments into a comprehensive program and is applicable across a variety of chronic illness populations, including populations with cancer (Peterman, Rothrock, & Cella, 2013). The major components and subcomponents of this computerized instrument include (1) physical health—symptoms and function; (2) mental health—affect, behavior, and cognition; and (3) social health—relationships and function. The program has adaptive testing and short-form capabilities. Although PROMIS is adult focused, pediatric instruments are also available for physical functioning, pain, fatigue, anxiety, anger, peer relationships, and asthma impact, with other item banks in development (Peterman et al., 2013).

Increasingly, the discipline of nursing is recognizing that it, too, needs to focus on measurable outcomes related to evidence-based interventions. The measurement of HRQOL has become a standard of assessment and an indicator for patient-centered nursing care and nursing practice outcomes. QOL determinations have a greater potential for holistic assessment of patients' care needs when they include consistent measures, incorporate multidimensional aspects of chronic illnesses, and use available technology support.

CONTEXT OF HEALTH-RELATED QUALITY OF LIFE IN CHRONIC ILLNESS

It is often baffling to me when I think back on this. I wonder how many people suffer from recurrent illness to which they have grown accustomed, never thinking, or worse, fearful, to seek medical advice. People who suffer from recurrent and chronic disease don't know what it is like to be normal or to feel good ... I recall having a few days last year in which I felt good. My mind was clear, my body relaxed. I felt euphoric. Today I am delighting in this good energy. I am hopeful that this is what "normal" is and that I can feel normal all the time. (Hsi et al., 2004, p. 149)

There is something to be said for the term "new normal," which is often used to describe a state of "being" when faced with long-term, life-altering changes in an individual's circumstances. Adding the dimension of quality to the term "new normal" can change the meaning, depending on whether the life circumstance change is amazing (a long-awaited positive pregnancy test) or devastating (a positive biopsy for stage 4 metastatic cancer). Many times the news of chronic illness is presented prior to a debilitated health state, and the individual wonders aloud, "How can this diagnosis be true? I feel fine!"

Perhaps for the sake of discussion, health-related quality of life in chronic illness can best be considered within the rather holistic context of the three components of the NIH-sponsored PROMIS framework: physical health (health and functioning), mental health (psychological and spiritual well-being), and social health (societal roles and economic status). The PROMIS components offer a practical way to view the tapestry of life quality for individuals living with chronic illness. However, the lived experience for each individual and the nuances of chronic illness presentation, which are further affected by age, gender, and culture, emphasize the challenge that healthcare professionals face in providing treatment and supportive interventions.

The PROMIS components are interconnected, as one cannot separate the physical, mental, and social health aspects from the whole person. The first component, physical health, includes physical symptoms and physical function, consisting of perceived health, sleep, sexual function, physical activity, energy level, pain experiences, behavior, interference, independence, capacity to meet responsibilities, access to and use of health care, and usefulness to others. Considering physical health symptoms and function together as interdependent life quality components reveals the reality that focusing on one subjective or clinical parameter may not capture an individual's true health and well-being status. Persons with chronic illness may report "good" perceived quality of life, even as the healthcare professional observes concerning, objective clinical symptoms. Knowing how symptoms affect a chronically ill individual's perception of health and function allows the healthcare professional to capture a clearer understanding of that person's life quality. Typically, the onset or worsening of symptoms prompts an individual to seek health care—for example, weakness and poor coordination in the individual with multiple sclerosis or perhaps distressing symptoms from the iatrogenic effects of a treatment. The reported symptoms may be interpreted differently by healthcare professionals and family members than by the patient, resulting in conflicting HRQOL assessment scores and treatment strategies that are not patient focused. The complexity of physical health symptoms and function in the presence of chronic illness suggests that neither good health nor optimal function is a necessary or sufficient requirement for HRQOL.

The second component, mental health, includes the subcomponents of affect, behavior, and cognition. Psychological and spiritual components of life quality include intangibles such as happiness, peace of mind, and a belief system. Psychological well-being is often considered an essential component for a quality life because of its effect on adjustment to chronic illness. More directly, spirituality has proved to be an important element in quality of life measurement across different cultures (Moreira-Almeida & Koenig, 2006). At the same time, it is important to recognize that spirituality differs from religiosity and that varying personal meanings are assigned to the concepts of life, hope, and peace. Most definitions take into consideration that spirituality affects all aspects of a person's well-being. Persons living with a chronic illness sometimes must make significant life changes to maintain their perceived quality of life and, in doing so, turn to psychological and spiritual resources or the social and emotional support offered by friends and confidantes. Spirituality that included components of life satisfaction,

reduced stress, and meaning in life was the basis for a study of women with cancer (López, McCaffrey, Quinn, Griffin, & Fitzpatrick, 2009). For these women, family activities, listening to music, and helping others were expressions of spiritual practices. López and colleagues concluded that it is beneficial to support women in their ongoing spiritual practices as they deal with a chronic illness.

Supportive care, or the lack of it, influences how individuals manage and cope with stress. Indeed, most people recognize the positive effects of having "moral support" and companionship at times of difficulty, though some may seek isolation or solitude. Family health and relationships can have positive or negative effects on quality of life. As an individual deals with the challenges of long-term illness, the persons closest to them are faced with making life adjustments as well. For example, when a family member becomes the primary caregiver for another family member with chronic illness, there are role changes, additional responsibilities, and increased stressors that have varying effects on quality of life for both the caregiver and the care receiver. Therefore, nursing interventions focused on strategies to promote quality of life must be considered in a plan of care that includes not only the patient but also his or her immediate support system. The positive effect of helping caregivers manage stress and anxiety related to caregiving duties can translate into a new sense of personal satisfaction and competent care for the patient.

The third component, social health, includes relationships and function (participation in social roles and activities). The social and cultural context of quality of life encompasses far-reaching elements. Unique cultural interpretations can influence perceptions of health and illness. Social conditions, expectations of individual behaviors, cultural regulations, and economic factors can contribute to positive or negative quality of life. Chronic illness can drain financial resources over time as the disease process affects the individual's ability to meet job responsibilities, leading to a reduction or loss of income and insurance resources. Family caregivers may also have to adjust employment responsibilities as care needs increase.

Individuals with chronic illness also suffer financially due to additional expenses incurred in the form of high medical insurance rates or out-of-pocket expenses for items not covered by insurance. Transportation to medical or treatment appointments, for example, or the extra cost of special dietary foods or supplements can add up quickly. The desperately ill person who has found little benefit from traditional therapies may expend personal funds on alternative forms of treatments that promise remission or cure. The combined effect on quality of life from the decreased income and increased expenses may not always be obvious. Continuous nursing assessment and case management may be required to meet the needs of the person with chronic illness and to address financial burdens. It is not uncommon for patients to self-manage their medications and reduce doses because they cannot afford to take the prescribed amount due to more pressing economic needs for other family members.

CASE STUDY 8-1

Kim is a 26-year-old African American woman and a single mother of 3-year-old twins. She was admitted to a long-term psychiatric facility 2 years ago after being charged with a crime and found not guilty by reason of insanity (NGIR) in a court of law. Her release date is set for 2024 based on conditions set by the court. Kim is confined to a ward but has escorted, supervised off-ward privileges twice a week to the vending machine area that offers only high-calorie, high-fat food choices. She does not qualify for a work program or the use of the fitness center. Kim has a bipolar disorder, obesity, and type 2 diabetes. Three months ago during her annual physical exam, the nurse practitioner diagnosed her with Stage 3 moderate persistent asthma. Since then, Kim has stopped her daily walking program and no longer follows her calorie-restricted diet. She tells the nurse practitioner: "What's the use, I'm falling apart! I've got sugar diabetes, now asthma, and I'll never lose all this weight. I might as well enjoy eating anything I want because there's nothing about my life right now that's any good. I thought I could get my life together but what's the use. My babies are growing up without me, I don't hear from my friends anymore, and my mom is too busy to come and visit me."

Discussion Questions

1. Explore Kim's statements for change talk that might indicate she may still be willing to work on improving the quality of her current health state.
2. Describe the mental and physical challenges Kim faces that affect her health-related quality of life in her present situation.
3. Discuss the first step the nurse practitioner could employ to create a plan of care for Kim.
4. Identify and compare what Kim's present situation is with what her lived experience might be if she were not confined in a facility. Would her quality of life be better or worse, and why?
5. Which nursing interventions or interventions by other health team members could be employed in an institutionalized setting to understand, manage, and improve quality of life in this situation?

CASE STUDY 8-2

Joe is a 95-year-old Caucasian widower and father of four adult children. His oldest daughter and one son live out of state; another daughter lives in town; and his youngest son lives at home with Joe. Joe and his son have lived in the same two-story home since 1957. He is ambulatory with a wheeled walker following bilateral hip fracture repairs and has a daytime caregiver during his son's work hours. Most of Joe's days are spent chatting with his caregiver, eating meals prepared by his daughter, talking short walks through his home, reading the newspaper, looking over his coin collection, watching TV, and "entertaining" occasional family, church, and neighborhood visitors with his jokes and opinions on current events. Joe and his daughter manage his finances. He makes the decisions, and she does the paperwork, as arthritis in his hands makes writing difficult.

During a recent hospital stay for congestive heart failure, Joe was asked what he thought about being sick and having to be in the hospital. Joe's response was "It was fun! I will miss my roommate and the nurses and therapists. They were all really nice and the food wasn't bad, either. But I couldn't wait to get home again." Joe was discharged from the hospital on continuous oxygen (a new therapy), additional cardiac medications, and a diuretic. He says the oxygen "gives me more pep!" but "I don't like that water pill and what happens after I take it." He continued, "I feel better now that the water is off me. I didn't know that I felt bad until I felt better! I think I just might make it to 100; I'll be 96 in a few months, you know."

Discussion Questions

1. Describe Joe's current health-related quality of life (give examples). How might Joe answer the question, "What is important to you now?" Identify how the two perceptions may be congruent or may conflict.
2. Identify potential barriers to quality of life in Joe's current living arrangements. Which suggestions could be made to assist Joe and his family in the short and long term?
3. Discuss nursing interventions that should be considered to promote Joe's highest level of self-care. Identify educational and service resources for Joe and his family. Might these resources be cost prohibitive?
4. Identify factors that contribute to Joe's current life quality. Would quality of life change for Joe if these factors were compromised or changed? Who would be the best judge of when and how to make changes?

QOL Guidelines, Interventions, and Outcomes in Chronic Illness

QOL Guidelines in Chronic Illness

Evidence-based practice (EBP) combines the highest-quality research evidence with clinical expertise and patient values to make clinical decisions about treatment. The building blocks for EBP decisions are four interconnected elements guided by clinical expertise (**Figure 8-3**). The first decision element is the patient's clinical state, setting, or circumstances (the severity of illness, environment, socioeconomic status, and support system). The second element incorporates the patient's preferences about healthcare options

Figure 8-3 Modified Model for Evidence-based Clinical Decisions

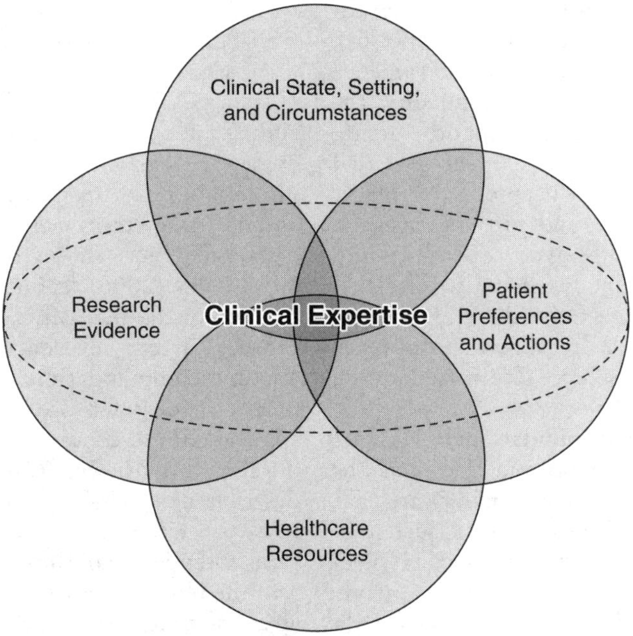

Source: DiCenso, A., Guyatt, G. & Ciliska, D. (2005). *Evidence-based nursing: A guide to clinical practice.* St. Louis, MO: Elsevier Mosby.

Evidence-Based Practice Box

Markle-Reid, Browne, and Gafni (2013) conducted a study to explore the "lessons learned" from three randomized, controlled trials designed to evaluate the effectiveness of different multicomponent health promotion and disease prevention (HPDP) interventions led by nurses to target risk factors for functional decline and frailty. Participants (*n* = 498) were community-dwelling frail, elderly (65 years or older) Canadians. The SF-36 instrument was used to measure change in HRQOL, and the Health and Social Services Utilization Inventory was used to measure cost of services from baseline to the end of intervention. The results indicated that

the nurse-led interventions improved HRQOL. It was recommended that intervention should include multiple home visits, multidimensional assessment and screening, multicomponent evidence-based (HPDP) strategies, case management, interprofessional collaboration, geriatric training, referral and coordination services, and theory use. This nurse-led, cost-effective approach optimizes HRQOL and promotes aging in place in the frail, elderly population.

Source: Markle-Reid, M., Browne, G. & Gafni, A. (2013). Nurse-led health promotion interventions improve quality of life in frail older home care clients: Lessons learned from three randomized trials in Ontario, Canada. *Journal of Evaluation in Clinical Practice, 19*, 118–131.

and his or her actions or behaviors (actions and behaviors may or may not be congruent—the patient may want to lose weight, for example, but continues to choose high-calorie food options). Identifying the best available research evidence is the third decision element. For nursing, the best research evidence should support nursing interventions that are safe and effective, based on precise nursing assessment, prognostic markers, causal relationships, and cost-effectiveness, guided by the patient's lived experience and meaning of illness. Finally, the fourth decision element weighs the benefits, risks, and management strategies needed to access appropriate, available healthcare resources (DiCenso, Guyatt, & Ciliska, 2005).

Incorporating these foundational elements into evidence-based nursing practice decisions facilitates effective, efficient nursing care that increases the potential for enhanced quality of life in persons living with chronic illness. Nurses cannot base practice decisions solely on any one element, such as tradition (how we always do things), past experience, or even outdated expert knowledge. Managing chronic illness raises the nursing practice bar, challenging nurses to apply a patient-focused, systematic, outcome-based, cost-effective, quality care model.

The National Institute of Nursing Research (NINR, 2011), as a part of the National Institutes of Health (NIH) strategic plan titled *Bringing Science to Life*, embraced this nursing challenge and pledged to invest in basic, clinical, and translational nursing research aimed at understanding symptoms and developing new strategies for symptom management to improve quality of life for persons with chronic illness. Nursing science areas of concentration include biological and genomic symptom mechanisms, disease trajectory interventions to improve assessment and symptom management, personalized interventions, strategies to improve self-management of chronic illness across the lifespan, and cost-effective, burden-reducing strategies for patients and their caregivers. According to the NINR director, Patricia Grady, "Nursing science has

positioned itself as a leader in identifying high-quality, high-value biobehavioral approaches to health promotion, disease prevention, and well-being—which are all critically linked to quality of health care and quality of life" (p. 2). Nursing's scientific research and leadership are significant contributors to national and global evidence-based clinical practice standards and guidelines that direct healthcare professionals' and healthcare team members' provision of care.

So, where is the evidence? Coopey, Nix, and Clancy (2006) report that clinical practice guidelines can be easily accessed, thereby providing current, evidence-based information about recommendations, strategies, and best practice choices for care and decision making in specific clinical conditions. A formal definition developed by the Institute of Medicine (2011) describes evidence-based clinical practice guidelines as "statements that include recommendations intended to optimize patient care that are informed by a systematic review of evidence and an assessment of the benefits and harms of alternative care options" (p. 1). The AHRQ's (2013a) National Guideline Clearinghouse (NGC) is a federally funded public Internet resource for these guidelines readily available on the AHRQ website (http://www.guideline.gov/index.aspx). Guideline categories include assessment of therapeutic effectiveness, counseling, diagnosis, evaluation, prevention, management, rehabilitation, risk assessment, screening, technology assessment, and treatment. This guideline repository provides access to major interventional strategies and outcomes, including quality of life in chronic illness, and identifies healthcare-related intended users, including nurses and advanced practice nurses. Every level of nursing practice can use this resource to evaluate quality of life management options influenced by clinical decision making and multidisciplinary research-based interventions in chronic illness.

Diagnosis, management, and treatment guidelines for chronic obstructive pulmonary disease (COPD), diabetes, and schizophrenia are presented in **Table 8-2** as examples of

Table 8-2 Comparison of Guidelines That Measure Quality of Life Outcomes

Guideline Title	Diagnosis and management of chronic obstructive pulmonary disease (COPD). December 2001 (revised March 2013) (AHRQ, 2013b)	Standards of medical care in diabetes. V. Diabetes care. 1998 (revised January 2013) (AHRQ, 2013c)	Management of schizophrenia. A national clinical guideline. (March 2013) (AHRQ, 2013d)
Guideline Developers	Institute for Clinical Systems Improvement (non-profit organization)	American Diabetes Association (professional association)	Scottish Intercollegiate Guidelines Network (national government agency [non-U.S.])
Disease/Condition	Stable COPD Acute exacerbations of COPD	Type 1 diabetes (DM) Type 2 DM Gestational DM	Schizophrenia
Clinical Specialty	Family practice, internal medicine, pulmonary medicine, thoracic surgery	Cardiology, endocrinology family practice, geriatrics, internal medicine, nephrology, neurology, nursing, nutrition, obstetrics and gynecology, ophthalmology, pediatrics, preventive medicine, psychology	Family practice, internal medicine, psychiatry, psychology

(continues)

Table 8-2 COMPARISON OF GUIDELINES THAT MEASURE QUALITY OF LIFE OUTCOMES (*Continued*)

Intended Users	Advanced practice **nurses**, allied health personnel, healthcare providers, health plans, hospitals, managed care organizations **nurses**, patients physicians, physician assistants, respiratory care practitioners	Advanced **practice nurses**, allied health personnel, dietitians, healthcare providers, health plans, hospitals, managed care organizations, **nurses**, patients, pharmacists, physicians, physician assistants, psychologists/non-physician behavioral health clinicians, public health departments	Advanced **practice nurses**, allied health personnel, occupational therapists, pharmacists, Physician Assistants Physicians Psychologists/ Non-physician behavioral health clinicians
Guideline Objectives	To improve population health through education, awareness, prevention, and evidence-based treatment To improve the patient care experience and quality of care To improve affordability through appropriate diagnosis and treatment that leads to decreasing COPD per-capita costs To increase the quality and use of spirometry testing in the diagnosis of patients with COPD To increase the number of patients with COPD who receive information on the options for tobacco cessation and information on the risks of continued smoking To increase the percentage of patients with COPD who have appropriate therapy prescribed To decrease COPD exacerbations requiring emergency department evaluation or hospital admission To increase the percentage of patients who have education and management skills with COPD	To provide evidence-based principles and recommendations for DM management To provide clinicians, patients, researchers, payers, and other interested individuals with the components of diabetes care, treatment goals, and tools to evaluate the quality of care	To provide evidence-based recommendations for the care and treatment of adults with schizophrenia

Target Population	Patients with symptoms of stable COPD as well as acute exacerbations of COPD in the outpatient setting	Adults and children with type 1 DM Adults and children with type 2 DM Pregnant women with DM Older adults with DM	Adults with schizophrenia
Major Outcomes Considered	Symptom relief; exercise tolerance; frequency of exacerbations; forced expiratory volume in 1 second (FEV$_1$) measures; quality of life; survival; adverse effects of treatment; cost-effectiveness	Changes in preprandial and postprandial blood glucose levels and HgbA$_{1c}$ levels; duration of glycemic control; hypoglycemia and hyperglycemia incidences; changes in blood pressure levels; rates of microvascular events, major adverse macrovascular events, and neuropathic complications; quality of life; mortality rate; cost	Symptom control; adherence to treatment regimen; incidence of relapse; frequency and length of hospitalizations; quality of life; global functioning; engagement in educational and/or vocational tasks
Methods Used to Assess the Quality and Strength of Evidence	Weighting according to a rating scheme	Weighting according to a rating scheme	Weighting according to a rating scheme
Methods Used to Formulate the Recommendations	Expert consensus	Expert consensus	Expert consensus

Source: Data from National Guideline Clearinghouse. (2013). Retrieved from http://www.guideline.gov

chronic illness guidelines that use quality of life as a major outcome and expert consensus as the primary means of formulating the recommendations for each guideline. Nurses can review and assess the methods and rating schemes used in guideline development as preparation for application of those guidelines in clinical practice. A determination can be made whether a recommendation is "strong"—that is, whether the intervention is always indicated and acceptable, such that it is more likely to have a positive influence on the quality of life of a patient. Conversely, nurses should consider additional information in their decision-making process when recommendations have lower ratings such as "useful," "should be considered," or "not useful." NGC guidelines are recommendations, strategies, and information based on systematic literature reviews and scientific evidence, yet they are not a substitute for clinical expertise and judgment based on patient preferences, healthcare resources, and a patient's clinical state. In the end, "evidence alone does not make decisions ... people do" (Hayes, Devereaux, & Guyatt, 2002, p. 1350).

Guidelines may not always be appropriate to all populations, however. Consider elderly persons with multiple chronic conditions (MCC) as an example. An expert panel of the American Geriatrics Society (AGS, 2012) presented an executive summary reflecting the limited evidence, the disease and treatment interactions (clinical state), and the importance of patient preferences concerning elderly persons with MCC or *multimorbidity*. The experts raised two major concerns about applying current clinical practice guidelines to this elderly population: (1) most clinical practice guidelines focus on a single disease and are impractical in the presence of MCC, and (2) older persons with MCC are most often excluded or underrepresented in clinical trials and observational studies, so there is less focus on this population in meta-analysis and systematic reviews, which ultimately skews interpretation of results used to create clinical practice guidelines. Guiding principles were

suggested as an approach to clinical management of older persons with MCC, while emphasizing that the principles were neither guidelines nor recommendations. The five guiding principles identified by the AGS include patient preferences, interpreting the evidence, considering prognosis, clinical feasibility, and optimizing therapies and care plans. Although there is some similarity to the previously discussed elements of the evidence-based clinical decision model (see Figure 8-3)—namely, clinical state, research evidence, patient preferences, and healthcare resources (DiCenso et al., 2005)—the focus and management strategies differ. Evidence for clinical MCC management in the elderly is scarce, and treatment for one condition can interfere with the treatment of another condition; furthermore, complex treatment regimens are not feasible for either the patient or the provider. Patient-centered medical homes, workforce training, reimbursement structure changes, and foundational MCC population research-focused strategies could facilitate implementation of these guiding principles into clinical practice, impacting healthcare and outcomes (AGS, 2012).

Evidence-Based QOL Interventions

I am grateful to be alive and home sitting in a chair by the fireplace ... Healing especially after a life-threatening crisis is more than simply dealing with the physical aspect of trying to get something fixed and getting on with it. It deals with the whole meaning of life. Being physically impaired requires a very different attitude. There is often a feeling of weakness and, yes, shame in not being able to do the things that once came so easily ... we are mistaken if we think we can send someone out to deal with the difficult job of healing and expect the sick person to do well when there is no community to support them. (Hsi et al., 2004, p. 149)

A review of nursing and health-related literature supports the growing interest in addressing the multidimensionality of chronic illness while attending to and preserving patients' quality of life. Most individuals with chronic illness are seen by a variety of healthcare professionals at many different points of care. Nursing is present at every level of these points of care—managing symptoms, designing and testing self-management strategies, and applying research in clinical and community health settings (NINR & NIH, 2011). Findings from many studies suggest that quality of life is a significant nurse-sensitive quality indicator and a measure of intervention effectiveness in chronic conditions. Doran and colleagues (2006) note that linking outcomes to nursing and nursing practice interventions is necessary to determine and identify those interventions that improve health outcomes and provide the evidence base to improve nursing care for the person with chronic illness. Additionally, "nurse scientists are ideally positioned to design and drive scientific discoveries that can be implemented directly and immediately into clinical practice at the point of care" (NINR & NIH, 2011, p. 6). Thus, not only does nursing involvement improve the daily lives of their patients, but it ultimately makes significant contributions to the whole of the science of nursing.

INTERVENTIONS IN CHRONIC PHYSICAL ILLNESS

Nursing researchers Axelsson, Brink, and Lövall (2014) sought to clarify the roles of gender and personality in persons with asthma in relation to adherence behavior and HRQOL. Participants (76 male, 104 female) with clinically diagnosed asthma or allergic rhinitis were randomly selected for a survey using the Neuroticism, Extraversion and Openness to Experience Five Factor Inventory (NEO-FFI), the Medication Adherence Report Scale (MARS), and the Short Form-8 Health Survey (SF-8) instruments. The study results indicated that women tended to have higher reported medication adherence rates than men; men with higher neuroticism were

less likely to follow medication treatment recommendations, whereas men with high agreeableness or conscientiousness were more likely to adhere to medication treatment. Men rated mental and physical HRQOL higher than women, with smoking having a negative influence on women's HRQOL. Because the quality of the patient–provider relationship is pivotal, the authors of this report remind nurses of their responsibility to sustain caring through human-to-human relationships with their patients. This relationship and matching of gender and personality traits is thought to support active participation and collaboration for best possible health outcomes and improved HRQOL.

Lorenzo (2013) reviewed the current literature to identify best practices for clinical management of diabetes mellitus (DM) and engage nurse practitioner (NP) clinicians into incorporating new strategies to improve management, clinical outcomes, and ultimately quality of life for persons with DM. This author identified three critical care models: (1) the chronic care model, (2) the clinical microsystem, and (3) the patient-focused medical home model. Several provider interventions were also reported. The first was DM self-management skill building and the *Healthy Interactions Conversation Map Program*, a resource used to engage persons in dialogue about their health. The second strategy included shared medical appointments and group visits, during which several patients were seen by an interprofessional team in 1- to 2-hour appointments. Diabetes teams consisting of a group of clinical staff working together with a common goal of improved patient health served as the third strategy. The fourth intervention was motivational interviewing (MI), a counseling strategy that empowers and motivates patients to move toward positive behavior changes. The final intervention was creating a behavior action plan as a planning guide (contract) to meet specific, measurable, timed goals. These primary care strategies empower patients to develop self-management skills through therapeutic partnerships with healthcare professionals and team members.

In a systematic review of 30 studies, Galway et al. (2012) assessed the effectiveness of psychosocial interventions on QOL and general psychological distress in persons ($n = 1,249$) during the first year following a cancer diagnosis. The interventions included "trained helper" therapeutic dialogue (talking therapy) with the aim of improving QOL and well-being. The results failed to show any improvement in general QOL, anxiety, or depression, but did demonstrate some improvement in illness-related QOL and mood. Telephone and face-to-face nurse-led interventions indicated promise as effective interventional methods. Further study was recommended to identify patients who could best benefit from psychosocial interventions (persons at risk for emotional problems), identify appropriate professional "trained helpers," and evaluate cost-effectiveness of the proposed interventions.

In a qualitative study to better understand interventions to support older women living at home with chronic illness, nursing researchers Lowe and McBride-Henry (2012) recruited women ($n = 3$) ages 70, 82, and 88 years to respond to unstructured interview questions posed by the researchers. Three themes were identified as ways to make meaning in these women's lives:

- *Coping with changing health* by using supportive equipment and becoming dependent on others ("I have to use my shower stool")
- *The impact of family*, which translated into family support that was essential to coping with chronic illness ("In the long run, it's your family that your world closes [down] to")
- *Attitude*—that is, accepting life circumstances with optimism ("If I have any trouble, I think, well how do I get over this?")

The authors concluded that nursing is in a position to promote successful aging. This research

allows nurses to identify ways to support healthy behaviors and assist older persons to continue to live safely in their homes. Understanding how older persons maintain quality of life can drive the development of tailored health provisions to meet their unique needs. Lowe and McBride-Henry suggest "taking time with people to listen and really hear their stories is important both for nurses and the older person" (p. 25).

A comparative correlational study by Kristofferzon, Lindqvist, and Nilsson (2011) determined differences between persons with end-stage renal disease (ESRD; $n = 41$) and those with congestive heart failure (CHF; $n = 59$) in terms of coping, sense of coherence, self-efficacy, and quality of life. Women were found to use more evasive, fatalistic, and emotional coping than men, and persons with high educational levels were more confrontational, evasive, emotional, and palliative and used more supportive coping. Older persons rated their QOL higher than younger persons. A higher sense of coherence and self-efficacy resulted in higher perceived QOL. The researchers concluded that the manner in which persons addressed their present situation was more important than the particular chronic illness they were dealing with. Women were found to experience more stress related to physical and psychological symptoms and lower QOL.

Cancer-related fatigue is frequently measured as a quality of life component, and various interventions have been proposed to reduce fatigue. A systematic review of the literature conducted by Mitchell, Beck, Hood, Moore, and Tanner (2007) applied a rating scheme to support the efficacy of different interventions to reduce cancer-related fatigue. Effectiveness was not well established for many interventions due to insufficient or poor-quality data. The interventions included alternative therapies such as yoga, acupuncture, and nutritional supplements; drugs that might help alleviate fatigue; and psychotherapy. Strategies that teach clients to manage and balance activity, rest, and sleep were rated as "likely to be effective," because the evidence was based on small, descriptive studies or expert consensus. Exercise was the one intervention that was recommended for practice because of the strength of the evidence and because the benefits outweighed the harm.

Other studies have also shown that exercise is a safe and effective intervention for reducing fatigue and promoting quality of life in persons with cancer. Exercise combined with structured group sessions appears to be effective, owing in part to the group cohesion and atmosphere and the direct effects that exercise has on reducing fatigue (Losito, Murphy, & Thomas, 2006). A growing body of evidence indicates that cancer patients may reap many benefits from exercise and provides a substantial rationale for nurses to promote and use physical activity as a means of improving health and quality of life for many persons with cancer (Hacker, 2009).

In a recent randomized, controlled trial, Brovold, Skelton, and Bergland (2013) compared the effects of high-intensity aerobic interval exercise with home-based exercise in older adults ($n =$ 115) aged 70–92 years with chronic conditions following hospital discharge. HRQOL was measured using the SF-36, physical fitness was measured using the Senior Fitness Test, and physical activity was assessed using the Physical Activity Scale for the Elderly. The high-intensity exercise group significantly improved their physical fitness, and both groups showed improvement in HRQOL and physical activity. Therefore, physical activity programs are recommended as a treatment strategy for the chronically ill elderly who are at risk for functional and life quality decline.

INTERVENTIONS IN CHRONIC MENTAL ILLNESS

Dickerson et al. (2011) conducted a research study to compare predictors of HRQOL in persons with schizophrenia ($n = 100$), major mood disorder ($n = 101$), and no mental illness ($n = 99$), all of whom had type 2 diabetes. The researcher reported that diabetes is more prevalent in persons with serious mental illness (SMI) than in the general population, and that much of the care and management

of this condition is the patient's responsibility. Persons dealing with diabetes and SMI may be more vulnerable to decreased HRQOL. The Medical Outcomes Survey, Short Form-12 (MOS SF-12) was used to measure physical and medical composite scores. For all participants, additional medical conditions exerted a strong effect on physical well-being. The HRQOL may have a stronger impact on persons without SMI than those with SMI. For persons with SMI, obesity and taking insulin also had less of an effect than on persons without SMI. The uniqueness of the SMI population should be considered when treatment strategies are planned, as their perception of QOL may be unique.

Patients with chronic mental illness benefit from interventions that augment prescribed medication and counseling therapies. Crone (2007) reported that physical activity programs enabled persons with mental illness to have positive emotional experiences, increased social interaction, and enhanced well-being. Nurses are instrumental in facilitating the development and referral programs that increase physical activity and promote quality of life for persons with mental illnesses.

Walton-Moss, Gerson, and Rose (2005) studied the effects of mental illness on families and offered insights into strategies that nurses can use to promote better quality of life for the caregivers. An important finding of their research is that nurses need to recognize the variability in response to mental illness among families. All family members, regardless of where the relative with mental illness is within the illness trajectory, need to be heard as they tell their stories and seek assistance in developing appropriate communication techniques with their loved one. This type of nursing support is critical in helping families maintain quality of life, whether their family member is coping reasonably well or is overwhelmed by numerous challenges. A family's social and emotional support and financial resources impact their quality of life. Knowledge about resources, services, and organizations for chronic illness conditions facilitate appropriate, timely referrals that better maintain quality of life and well-being in this caregiver population.

Hee (2004) reported a nursing interventional project to identify the meaning of "quality of life" for a group of eight men with mental illness who attended a community center. The goal of the project was to be truly present with these men as they explored and described the realities of their living based on Parse's practice methodology. The discussions focused on nine questions:

1. What is life like for you?
2. What contributes to your quality of life?
3. What diminishes your quality of life?
4. What are your priorities?
5. Who is most important to you?
6. Which changes in your routines or relationships might change your quality of life?
7. How would you like to change your quality of life and what can you do to make this happen?
8. What are your concerns?
9. What are your hopes and dreams?

Three quality of life themes were identified:

- Dwelling with regret while surfacing new possibilities
- Staying with and moving on with fear and confidence
- Changing while staying the same

The project offered an opportunity for the men to learn about themselves and express new insights about what they valued most and what made them happy. This project reflects themes of other research that support the value of allowing persons to tell their story—of the powerful intervention of nursing presence and the importance of listening.

Technology Interventions and Quality of Life

An entire chapter could be written discussing the possibilities and probabilities that technology can offer to improve quality of life for persons with chronic illness. In the interest of space and time, only a few examples will be presented here.

Hart and Roe (2013) developed a program to connect elderly patients in a 270-bed special-care home with the outside world through computer adaptive technology. "Adaptive technology" refers to items that are specifically designed for persons with disabilities and implemented to assist elders to eventually work independently. Computers were set up to accommodate all elders regardless of their physical or cognitive challenges. Some of the adaptive devices included large screens and keyboards; cameras; head-controlled mouse; and equipment to improve cognition and memory, physical stamina, communication skills, visual impairment, and dexterity. The technology proved to be especially stimulating and comforting for persons with Alzheimer's disease. The program authors reported, "The ability to hear and be heard, to celebrate and to explore the world beyond to ask questions, or connect with other humans has become essential for a meaningful life … adaptive technology can take elders anywhere they want to go" (p. 30).

Hirose, Beverly, and Weinger (2012) reported that QOL for children with diabetes includes the ability to enjoy meals, feel a sense of safety in school, and have positive relationships with family and friends. Diabetes imposes barriers to these QOL indicators. The authors noted that technologies that improve glycemic control for children with type 1 diabetes give them greater flexibility and better QOL. Notably, an insulin pump gives children with diabetes the flexibility to adjust insulin doses precisely, provide multiple bolus infusion patterns, and adjust hourly basal insulin doses. Continuous glucose monitoring (CGM) utilizes a wireless device system to measure glucose levels at 5-minute intervals; data can subsequently be downloaded to a computer. Web-based programs for adolescents support self-care, and mobile phones offer convenient tools for data management and medical support. An intraperitoneal insulin infusion pump has shown QOL improvement, and inhaled insulin devices are associated with improvements in glycemic control and treatment satisfaction. Finally, a new treatment strategy on the horizon—and perhaps the insulin treatment device of the future—is the closed-loop system. Understanding and appreciation of children's and parents' QOL and provision of self-management skills and support are important factors in medical and psychological treatment in this young population.

O'Dell and colleagues (2013) enrolled post-stroke survivors (*n* = 32) to test the robotic InMotion shoulder and wrist units from Interactive Motion Technologies Company over a 12-week period. The robot provides active assistance in completing movements if a participant is unable to complete a movement on his or her own. The participants engaged in 1,000 repetitions of motions during a session on the proximal and distal muscle groups of their impaired arm. The possibilities of using robot therapy for physical therapy and assistive support are exciting and without boundaries. Nursing can be involved in not only their research and development, but also the implementation and follow-up for patients utilizing these technological wonders. The only potential barrier may be the cost and availability for persons with limited financial resources.

Outcomes and Conclusions

Outcome evaluation examines the impact of an intervention, to determine if the changes that result from an intervention have the desired effect and whether the benefits of the intervention are worth the cost (DiCenso et al., 2005). In the previous discussion of interventions, many successful outcomes were identified for improving the quality of life of persons with chronic illness. Quality of life is an outcome of care, increasingly addressed by all healthcare entities, including providers, payers, and consumers. The global attention to chronic illness care makes it imperative for nursing to continue to address quality of life as a nurse-sensitive quality indicator. As an outcome of nursing practice, quality of life can be influenced by appropriate, evidence-based, well-designed care interventions.

Inability to work, unemployment, smoking, lack of exercise, asthma, obesity, and disability have been identified as strong predictors for overall poor HRQOL in some demographic areas. Not surprisingly, persons diagnosed with diabetes, asthma, obesity, and disability are significantly more likely to have poorer HRQOL than persons without these behaviors and conditions. Relationships have been identified between overall HRQOL and demographics, behavioral risk factors, and health conditions (Jiang & Hesser, 2009). Targeting healthcare interventions for at-risk populations can have a significant impact not only on individuals suffering from chronic illness, but also on communities where certain chronic illnesses are more prevalent. Efforts directed toward planning and implementing interventional treatments and therapies should include data collection and analysis of data related not only to disease management but also to improved quality of life.

Because of the growing numbers of Americans living with multiple chronic conditions and escalating healthcare costs, previous methods of evaluating interventional strategies to improve quality of life have been found to be inadequate. Managing chronic conditions creates a healthcare challenge at many levels. Identifying the patient's perspective on illness and well-being enables healthcare professionals to target the outcomes that patients value most (Chen, Baumgardner, & Rice, 2011). In other words, patients are more motivated to follow individualized treatment plans tailored to the question, "What is important to you now?" (Parse, 2013, p. 114). Self-assessments of HRQOL are being widely used to track health status, and the PROMIS initiative holds great potential to revolutionize the way HRQOL data are collected, analyzed, and utilized, all from the perspective of the person with chronic illness or illnesses.

Interventions that (1) allow patients to make choices that reflect their personal needs and goals, (2) apply motivational interviewing to help them discover health promotion activities to address health problems, and (3) customize medication and treatment regimens to empower patients to manage their chronic conditions are essential components to ensure positive quality of life outcomes (Chen et al., 2011). Successful outcome measures are also supported by new healthcare team models that use assisted care coordination such as health coaches, community health teams, guided care nurses, care navigators, and care coordinators (Schram, 2012).

Perhaps Milton (2013) sums up this discussion on quality of life and health-related quality of life in chronic illness the best. She challenges healthcare professionals by stating, "Members of the discipline of nursing have a duty and obligation to society to promote and ensure that the human experience of quality of life is at the table and adequately honored and represented in the realms of public policy and published healthcare standards ... members of professional healthcare disciplines bear responsibility for the possibilities of betrayal and violation of human trust as the current emphasis shifts from human experiences to mechanical, monetary views of quality of human life" (p. 123). Certainly, her comments are something for nursing to consider.

STUDY QUESTIONS

1. Which elements are part of quality of life evaluations in chronic illness? Discuss how the perceptions of individual patients and healthcare professionals contribute to quality of life evaluations.
2. Identify a theoretical or conceptual framework that addresses quality of life as an outcome for patients with a chronic illness. Describe an intervention using that framework that demonstrates how the discipline of nursing can impact quality of life.
3. Discuss Parse's concept of *living quality* as it pertains to chronic illness.
4. As an outcome of care, how is quality of life viewed by healthcare professionals, consumers, agencies, and third-party payers?
5. Describe how nurses use evidence-based practice guidelines to promote quality of life care to patients with chronic illness. How are guidelines impacted by multiple chronic conditions?
6. Discuss current technology that may have a significant impact on persons with chronic illness. Identify other areas of technology not mentioned in this chapter.
7. In what ways do evidence-based practice guidelines improve care for persons with chronic illness?
8. Which potential ethical dilemmas arise when evaluating quality of life in chronic illness?
9. Identify the challenges of providing interventions to improve quality of life for persons with serious mental illness.
10. What are the elements of the PROMIS initiative?

References

Agency for Healthcare Research and Quality (AHRQ). (2008). Multiple chronic conditions: A day in the life. http://www.ahrq.gov/professionals/prevention-chronic-care/decision/mcc/video/index.html

Agency for Healthcare Research and Quality (AHRQ). (2013a). National Guideline Clearinghouse. http://www.guideline.gov/index.aspx

Agency for Healthcare Research and Quality (AHRQ). (2013b). Diagnosis and management of chronic obstructive pulmonary disease (COPD). http://www.guideline.gov/content.aspx?id=44345

Agency for Healthcare Research and Quality (AHRQ). (2013c). Standards of medical care in diabetes. V. Diabetes care. http://www.guideline.gov/content.aspx?id=45153

Agency for Healthcare Research and Quality (AHRQ). (2013d). Management of schizophrenia: A national clinical guideline. http://www.guideline.gov/content.aspx?id=43956

Agency for Healthcare Research and Quality (AHRQ). (n.d.). Patient center medical home resource center. http://pcmh.ahrq.gov/page/defining-pcmh

American Geriatric Society (AGS) Expert Panel. (2012). Patient-centered care for older adults with multiple chronic conditions: A stepwise approach from the American Geriatrics Society. *Journal of the American Geriatrics Society* (Special Articles), 1–12.

Axelsson, M., Brink, E., & Lövall, J. (2014). A personality and gender perspective on adherence and health-related quality of life in people with asthma and /or allergic rhinitis. *Journal of the American Association of Nurse Practitioners*, 26(1), 32–39.

Barofsky, I. (2012). Can quality or quality-of-life be defined? *Quality of Life Research*, 21, 625–631.

Berra, K. (2003). The effect of lifestyle interventions on quality of life and patient satisfaction with health and health care. *Journal of Cardiovascular Nursing* 18(4), 319–325.

Brovold, T., Skelton, D. A., & Bergland, A. (2013). Older adults recently discharged from the hospital: Effect of aerobic interval exercise on health-related quality of life, physical fitness, and physical activity. *Journal of the American Geriatrics Society*, 61, 1580–1585.

Cella, D. F. (1995). Measuring quality of life in palliative care. *Seminars in Oncology*, 22, 73–81.

Cella, D., Riley, W., Stone, A., Rothrock, N., Reeve, B., Yount, S. ..... PROMIS Cooperative Group. (2010). The Patient-Reported Outcomes Measurement Information System (PROMIS) developed and tested its first wave of adult self-reported health outcome item banks: 2005–2008. *Journal of Clinical Epidemiology*, 63, 1179.

Centers for Disease Control and Prevention (CDC). (2011a). HRQOL concepts. http://www.cdc.gov/hrqol/concept.htm

Centers for Disease Control and Prevention (CDC). (2011b). Health-related quality of life: Methods and measures. http://www.cdc.gov/hrqol/methods.htm

Centers for Disease Control and Prevention (CDC). (2011c). Health-related quality of life: CDC HRQOL–14 "Healthy Days Measure." http://www.cdc.gov/hrqol/hrqol14_measure.htm#1

Centers for Disease Control and Prevention (CDC). (2012). Chronic diseases and health promotion. http://www.cdc.gov/chronicdisease/overview/index.htm

Chen, H.-Y., Baumgardner, D. J., & Rice, J. P. (2011). Health-related quality of life among adults with multiple chronic conditions in the United States, behavioral risk factor surveillance system, 2007. *Preventing Chronic Disease*, 8(1), A09, 1–9. http://www.cdc.gov/ped/issues/2011/jan/09_0234.htm

Coleman, K., Austin, B. T., Brach, C., & Wagner, E. H. (2009). Evidence on the chronic care model in the new millennium. *Health Affairs*, 28(1), 75–85.

Coopey, M., Nix, M. P., & Clancy, C. M. (2006). Translating research into evidence-based nursing practice and evaluating effectiveness. *Journal of Nursing Care Quality*, 21(3), 195–202.

Crone, D. (2007). Walking back to health: A qualitative investigation into service users' experiences of a walking project. *Issues in Mental Health Nursing*, 28, 167–183.

DiCenso, A., Guyatt, G. & Ciliska, D. (2005). *Evidence-based nursing: A guide to clinical practice*. St. Louis, MO: Elsevier Mosby.

Dickerson, F., Wohlheiter, K., Medhoff, D., Fang, L., Kreyenbuhl, J., Goldberg, R., ... Dixon, L. (2011). Predictors of quality of life in type 2 diabetes patients with schizophrenia, manor mood disorder, and without mental illness. *Journal Quality of Life Research*, 20, 1419–1425.

Doran, D. M., Harrison, M. B., Laschinger, H. S., Hirdes, J. P., Rukholm, E., Sidani, S., ... Tourangeau, A.E. (2006). Nursing-sensitive outcomes data collection in acute care and long-term-care settings. *Nursing Research*, 55(2S), S75–S81.

Ferrans, C., & Powers, M. (1992). Psychometric assessment of the quality of life index. *Research in Nursing & Health*, 15, 29–38.

Galway, K., Black, A., Cantwell, M., Cardwell, C. R., Mills, M., & Donnelly, M. (2012). Psychosocial interventions to improve quality of life and emotional wellbeing for recently diagnosed cancer patients (Review). *Cochrane Database of Systematic Reviews, 11,* CD007064. doi: 10.1002/14651858.CD007064. pub2

Garratt, A., Schmidt, L., & Fitzpatrick, R. (2002). Patient-assessed health outcome measure for diabetes: A structured review. *Diabetic Medicine, 19,* 1–11.

Hacker, E. (2009). Exercise and quality of life: Strengthening the connections. *Clinical Journal of Oncology Nursing, 13*(1), 31–39.

Hart, C., & Roe, P. (2013). Using adaptive technology to "make a difference" in residents' quality of life. *Canadian Nursing Home, 24*(2), 27–30.

Hart, H., Bilo, H., Redekop, W., Stolk, R., Assink, J., & Meyboom-de-Jong, B. (2003). Quality of life of patients with type 1 diabetes. *Quality of Life Research, 12,* 1089–1097.

Hayes, R. B., Devereaux, P. J., & Guyatt, G. H. (2002). Physicians' and patients' choices in evidence based practice. *British Journal of Medicine, 324,* 1350.

Hee, N. C. (2004). Meaning of the quality of life for persons living with serious mental illness: Human becoming practice with groups. *Nursing Science Quarterly, 17,* 220–225.

Hirose, M., Beverly, E. A., & Weinger, K. (2012). Quality of life and technology: Impact on children and families with diabetes. *Current Diabetes Reports, 12*(6), 711–720.

Hsi, S. D., Belshaw, J., & Corbin-Hsi, B. (2004). *Closing the chart: A dying physician examines family, faith, and medicine.* Albuquerque, NM: University of New Mexico Press.

Institute of Medicine (IOM). (2011). Graham, R., Mancher, M., Wolman, D. M., Greenfield, S., Steinberg, E. (Eds.). *Clinical practice guidelines we can trust.* Washington, DC: National Academies Press. http://www.iom.edu/Reports/2011/Clinical-Practice-Guidelines-We-Can-Trust/Standards.aspx

Jiang, Y., & Hesser, H. E. (2009). Using item response theory to analyze the relationship between health-related quality of life and health risk factors. *Preventing Chronic Disease, 6*(1), A30, 1–10. http://www.ckc.gov/pcd/issues/2009/jan07_0272.htm

Kristofferzon, M.-L., Lindqvist, R., & Nilsson, A. (2011). Relationships between coping, coping resources and quality of life in patients with chronic illness: A pilot study. *Scandinavian Journal of Caring Sciences, 25,* 476–483.

López, A., McCaffrey, R., Griffin, M., & Fitzpatrick, J. (2009). Spiritual well-being and practices among women with gynecologic cancer. *Oncology Nursing Forum, 36*(3), 300–305.

Lorenzo, L. (2013). Partnering with patients to promote holistic diabetes management: Changing paradigms. *Journal of the American Association of Nurse Practitioners, 25*(7), 351–361.

Losito, J. M., Murphy, S. O., & Thomas, M. L. (2006). The effects of group exercise on fatigue and quality of life during cancer treatment. *Oncology Nursing Forum, 33*(4), 821–825.

Lowe, P., & McBride-Henry, K. (2012). What factors impact upon the quality of life of elderly women with chronic illnesses: Three women's perspectives. *Contemporary Nurse, 41*(1), 18–27.

MacColl Institute. (1998). The chronic care model. http://www.ahrq.gov/populations/businessstrategies/busstratintro.htm

Mackenzie, A., & Chang, A. (2002). Predictors of quality of life following stroke. *Disability and Rehabilitation, 24*(5), 259–265.

Mandzuk, L. L., & McMillan, D. E. (2005). A concept analysis of quality of life. *Journal of Orthopaedic Nursing, 9,* 12–18.

Marden, S. (2005). Technology dependence and health-related quality of life: A model. *Journal of Advanced Nursing, 50*(2), 187–195.

Markle-Reid, M., Browne, G., & Gafni, A. (2013). Nurse-led health promotion interventions improve quality of life in frail older home care clients: Lessons learned from three randomized trials in Ontario, Canada. *Journal of Evaluation in Clinical Practice, 19,* 118–131.

Milton, C. L. (2013). The ethics of defining quality of life. *Nursing Science Quarterly, 26*(2), 121–123.

Mitchell, S. A., Beck, S. L., Hood, L. E., Moore, K., & Tanner, E. R. (2007). Putting evidence into practice: Evidence-based interventions for fatigue during and following cancer and its treatment. *Clinical Journal of Oncology Nursing, 11*(1), 99–113.

Moreira-Almeida, A., & Koenig, H. G. (2006). Retaining the meaning of the words religiousness and spirituality: A commentary on the WHOQOL-SRPB group's "A cross-cultural study of spirituality, religion, and personal beliefs as components of quality of life." *Social Science & Medicine, 63,* 843–845.

National Institute of Nursing Research (NINR) & National Institutes of Health (NIH). (2011). *Bringing science to life: NINR strategic plan.* NIH Publication #11-7783. Bethesda, MD: Authors.

National Institutes of Health (NIH), Office of Strategic Coordination, The Common Fund. (2013). Patient-Reported Outcomes Measurement Information System (PROMIS): Overview. http://commonfund.nih.gov/promis/overview

National Institutes of Health (NIH), Office of Strategic Coordination, The Common Fund. (n.d.). Patient-Reported Outcomes Measurement Information System (PROMIS). http://www.nihpromis.org/about/history

O'Dell, M. W., Kim, G., Rivera, L., Fieo, R., Christos, P., Polistena, C., … Gorga, D. (2013). A psychometric evaluation of the arm motor ability test. *Journal of Rehabilitation Medicine, 45*, 519–527.

Parekh, A. K., & Goodman, R. A. (2013). The HHS Strategic Framework on multiple chronic conditions: Genesis and focus on research. *Journal of Comorbidity, 3*(22), 22–29.

Parekh, A. K., Goodman, R. A., Gordon, C., & Koh, H. K. (2011). Managing multiple chronic conditions: A strategic framework for improving health outcomes and quality of life. *Public Health Reports, 126*, 460–471.

Parse, R. R. (2007). A human becoming perspective on quality of life. *Nursing Science Quarterly, 20*(3), 217–217.

Parse, R. R. (2013). Living quality: A humanbecoming phenomenon. *Nursing Science Quarterly, 26*(2), 111–115.

Peterman, A. H., Rothrock, N., & Cella, D. F. (2013). Evaluation of health-related quality of life. http://www.uptodate.com

Plummer, M., & Molzahn, A. (2009). Quality of life in contemporary nursing theory: A concept analysis. *Nursing Science Quarterly, 22*(2), 134–140.

Robert Graham Center. (2007). *The patient centered medical home history: Seven core features, evidence and transformational change.* Washington, DC: Author.

Schram, A. P. (2012). The patient-centered medical home: Transforming primary care. *Nurse Practitioner, 37*(4), 33–39.

Shephard, R., & Franklin, B. (2001). Changes in the quality of life: A major goal of cardiac rehabilitation. *Journal of Cardiopulmonary Rehabilitation, 21*(4), 189–200.

Taylor, R. M., Gibson, F., & Franck, L. S. (2008). A concept analysis of health-related quality of life in young people with chronic illness. *Journal of Clinical Nursing, 17*(14), 1823–1833.

U.S. Department of Health and Human Services (USDHHS). (n.d.). HHS initiative on multiple chronic conditions. http://www.hhs.gov/ash/initiatives/mcc/index.html

Walton-Moss, B., Gerson, L., & Rose, L. (2005). Effects of mental illness on family quality of life. *Issues in Mental Health Nursing, 26*, 627–642.

Ware, J. E. (2004). *SF-36 health survey update.* Boston, MA: Tufts University Medical School, Quality Metric Incorporated. http://www.sf-36.org/tools/sf36.shtml

Welch, A. J. (2007). The phenomenon of taking life day-by-day: Using Parse's research method. *Nursing Science Quarterly, 20*(3), 265–272.

World Health Organization (WHO). (1948). WHO definition of health. https://apps.who.int/aboutwho/en/definition.html.

World Health Organization (WHO). (1995). The World Health Organization quality of life assessment: Position paper from the World Health Organization. *Society Science & Medicine 41*(10), 1403–1409.

World Health Organization (WHO). (2004). The World Health Organization quality of life—BREF. http://www.who.int/substance_abuse/research_tools/whoqolbref/en/

Chapter 9

Adherence

Jill Berg, Robynn Zender, Lorraine S. Evangelista, and Jacqueline M. Dunbar-Jacob

Introduction

Nonadherence to prescribed treatment by healthcare professionals is now known to be a primary cause of avoidable morbidity and mortality, especially in this era of chronic and comorbid illness. Adherence, according to the World Health Organization (WHO, 2003), is defined as "the extent to which a person's behavior—taking medication, following a diet, and/or executing lifestyle changes—corresponds with agreed recommendations from a healthcare provider." Preventable diseases are estimated to consume 70% of all medical care spending in the United States (Curry & Fitzgibbon, 2009), yet adherence to medical recommendations remains poor across all chronic disease regimens, further increasing healthcare expenditures and preventing patients from achieving the full benefit of any intervention. In addition, most chronic disorders are treated with a plan of care that encompasses a variety of components, which may include medication, diet, and exercise. Therefore, patients are often asked to manage a complex treatment regimen. Medication, lifestyle, and dietary nonadherence rates are estimated to range between 50% and 80% (WHO, 2003).

The subject of adherence is multifaceted and complex, with patient, provider, and system dynamics contributing to poor adherence rates and suboptimal health. Nevertheless, it has been posited that greater health benefits worldwide would be realized with improved adherence to existing treatments than with the development of new medical treatments (Bosworth, 2010). To facilitate understanding of these complex issues, this chapter addresses factors that have an impact on adherence behavior. A discussion of the theories and a description of techniques are also presented to provide a context for the behavioral changes that are required in treatment regimens. Evidence-based guidelines adopted by national and international organizations are included, along with interventions to improve adherence behaviors, and case studies to illustrate key strategies.

Goals for Healthy People 2020

Overall goals for *Healthy People* (U.S. Department of Health and Human Services, 2010; www.healthypeople.gov) are to help Americans lead healthy and long lives and to reduce health disparities. There are nearly 600 objectives within 42 topic areas to be met by 2020, including 1,200 measures. A refined selection of "Leading Health Indicators" lists 26 high-priority indicators of *Healthy People 2020* within 12 topic areas. While the shift away from a greater focus on individual behavior to improved healthcare infrastructure is reflected in the 2020 goals, many of the objectives in these documents relate to behavior-change goals for individuals. For example, for diabetes, many of the goals in *Healthy People 2020* refer to lifestyle changes and education to better manage the disease and avoid complications such as cardiovascular disease and death. Goals for *Healthy People 2020* include health behavior change, such as adherence to chronic illness regimens, and preventive behaviors such as screenings to detect risk factors for disease.

Adherence and Chronic Illness

The predominant pattern of illness has changed from acute to chronic as science and technology have advanced. With that technology, treatment regimens have become more complex. However, because of changes in managed health care, these complex regimens are often implemented with limited or no supervision, as the patient and/or family caregivers carry out these prescribed regimens at home. Therefore, practitioners must be concerned with the extent to which patients can implement the treatment plans they design as well as the evaluation of the patient's responses.

Patient responsibility for managing chronic conditions has increased, but there is concern about adherence as it relates to medical outcomes and economic costs. For example, an individual who has insulin-dependent diabetes mellitus (IDDM) may have a computerized insulin pump and a blood-testing device. This individual may, at some point, become a candidate for hemodialysis or renal transplantation because of complications. All of these treatment modalities require adherence behaviors to ensure maximal benefit and minimal harm to the patient.

The managed care environment has also had an impact on patient burden in chronic illness. Managed care's influence on health care has been demonstrated by earlier hospital discharges, shortened office visits, and decreasing home health referrals. In addition, recent literature indicates that as many as 46% of healthcare professionals do not prescribe adequate therapy for their patients (McGlynn, Asch, Adams, Keesey, Hicks, & DeCristofaro, 2003; Roth, Ivey, Esserman, Crisp, Kurz, & Weinberger, 2013). Therefore, patients and family members have had to shoulder more of the responsibility for the treatment regimen, often in isolation. Many healthcare professionals have little time to address the management of chronic illness and adherence to the recommended regimen (Golin, Smith, & Reif, 2004; McWilliam, 2009). Even so, care providers and agencies can make a difference in health outcomes by integrating interprofessional interventions specifically aimed at assisting patients with management of their chronic disease through education, self-management instruction, prevention, outreach strategies, and technology use (Barnestine-Fonseca, Leiva-Fernández, Vidal-España, García-Ruiz, Prados-Torres, & Leiva-Fernández, 2011; Feachem, Sekhri, & White, 2002; McWilliam, 2009). The Patient Protection and Affordable Care Act (ACA, 2010) encourages monitoring of adherence behavior in an effort to improve patient outcomes.

Hundreds of studies have examined adherence behavior, but unfortunately that research has not led to significant changes in behavior (Dunbar-Jacob & Schlenk, 2001; McDonald, Garg, & Haynes, 2002). Chronic illness regimens can be exceedingly complex, and resources to assist individuals with chronic illness are often limited. Therefore, it is important that the healthcare professional understands the variables that affect the ability of the person to adhere to a regimen.

CASE STUDY 9-1

Stephanie Vu is a 17-year-old youth with asthma. Her asthma has been an issue since she was a child, and her parents have been vigilant about placing dust covers on her mattress as well as vacuuming her room frequently to cut down on triggers related to dust mites. Lately, Stephanie has been insisting that she can manage her asthma independently. Her parents have tried to help her remember to take her steroid inhaler dose in the mornings before she goes to school, but sometimes Stephanie forgets. Tonight, when she comes home from a study session at a friend's house, she has trouble breathing. After Stephanie uses her rescue inhaler and the episode passes, she confesses that she got a ride home from one of her friends and they started smoking cigarettes in the car. The next day, she and her mother visit her primary care provider, a nurse practitioner. Stephanie's mother asks you to intervene.

Discussion Questions

1. How can you help Stephanie?
2. Which strategies can you use to ensure a good relationship with Stephanie and her mother?

History and Prevalence

In 2004, Greene described the use of the terms related to a patient's suboptimal following of recommended treatment regimens. He discussed how, in the early years of scientific inquiry of adherence, a variety of patients were labeled as "uncooperative, noncompliant, poorly controlled, resistant, devious, incorrigible, and careless" (p. 330). The currently accepted term "adherence," however, recognizes the patient's active participation in and ultimate responsibility for his or her own health, implying patient empowerment to choose whether to follow health advice (Cohen, 2009). Healthcare professionals often make decisions about the effectiveness of treatments without knowing whether the patient will be able to follow the treatment or is in agreement with his or her healthcare professional (McWilliam, 2009; Rand, 2004). It is important to be aware of a tendency among care providers to see adherence behavior as positive, admirable, and wise (being the "good patient") and nonadherence behavior as being negative,

deplorable, and unwise (being the "problem patient"). It seems probable that healthcare professionals who hold this view would be less likely to make concerted efforts to search out barriers to nonadherence.

To provide efficacious treatment of chronic disease, healthcare professionals face two challenges. First, we must ascertain whether patients are following the regimen. Second, we must find effective ways of helping patients to overcome barriers in carrying out complex regimens.

Individuals with chronic medical conditions face a variety of stressful life circumstances involving a range of adaptation demands. They must deal with a loss of independence, the threat of disease progression, and the challenge of modifying their behavior to meet the demands of a prescribed regimen. Lifestyle modifications may become necessary and include, but are not limited to, dietary changes, use of medications, and change in physical activity. Adherence to these modifications has substantial implications for treatment success and decreased disease progression.

For the patient with chronic illness, failure to adhere can result in increased disease complications, increased hospitalizations, and greater treatment costs, as well as disruptions in lifestyle, family dynamics, and coping skills (WHO, 2003). Although ascertaining the true picture of nonadherence in chronic illness is difficult, several studies indicate that adherence rates in chronic illness are approximately 50% (Dunbar-Jacob, Erlen, Schlenk, Ryan, Sereika, & Doswell, 2000; Haynes, McDonald, Garg, & Montague, 2002; WHO, 2003), with ranges of nonadherence rates estimated to be 20–40% for acute illness, 20–60% for chronic illness, and an incredible 50–80% for preventive regimens (Bosworth, 2010). Of nearly 200,000 written e-prescriptions, only 78% were refilled, and only 72% of prescriptions for new medications were filled (Fischer, Stedman, Lii, Vogeli, & Shrank, 2010). Adherence rates were higher for prescriptions written by primary care specialists, especially pediatricians (84%), and for patients aged 18 and younger (87%) (Fischer et al., 2010). Self-reported adherence to cardiovascular medications in patients who have coronary artery disease is approximately 40%. Nearly 25% of patients are partially or completely nonadherent in filling prescriptions after hospital discharge for a cardiac event and, of the patients who are initially adherent, as many as 50% will discontinue antihypertensive medications within 6 to 12 months (Baroletti & Dell'Orfano, 2010). Adherence studies are typically disease-specific; that is, the study population is defined by the presence of a specific disease. However, more recent reviews of adherence behaviors in persons with chronic illness indicate that the nature and extent of adherence problems are similar across diseases, across regimens, and across age groups (Vermeire, Hearnshaw, Van Royen, & Denekens, 2001). A review of studies examining medication adherence reported rates as low as 50%, with differences in rates seen between settings and measurement methods (Dunbar-Jacob et al., 2000).

In individuals with ankylosing spondylitis, for example, adherence to exercise recommendations was about 74%, with nearly 100% adherence to anti–tumor necrosis factor (TNF) medication, and a 2-year drug continuation rate of 74% (Arturi et al., 2013; Kristensen, Karlsson, Englund, Petersson, Saxne, & Geborek, 2010). Adherence rates to exercise regimens among those with rheumatoid arthritis are slightly more than 92%, with medication adherence rates ranging between 30% and 80% (Arturi et al., 2013; Elliott, 2008; van den Bemt, Zwikker, & van den Ende, 2012). Other disease-specific adherence rates are as follows:

- Epilepsy: 34% (Paschal, Rush, & Sadler, 2013).
- Major depression in adults: 51.9% (via electronic monitoring: MEMS), 71.4% (pill count), 79.2% (clinician rating scale of compliance), and 75.3% (self-report) (Lee et al., 2010), and 42% continuation adherence (Akincigil, Bowblis, Levin, Walkup, Jan, & Crystal, 2007).
- Major depression in children and adolescents: 87.5% medication adherence (Nakonezny et al., 2010).
- Schizophrenia: Less than 55% (McCann & Lu, 2009).
- Diabetes mellitus: 67% to 85% for oral hypoglycemic medications when measured through electronic monitoring (Cramer, 2004).
- Hypertension: 62% when measured through electronic monitoring (Dunbar-Jacob, Sereika, Houze, Luyster, & Callan, 2012).
- Tuberculosis (TB): Treatment success rates can reach more than 95% in patients who are treated under optimal conditions, but actual treatment success rates are around 80% in countries with the highest TB burden (van den Boogaard, Boeree, Kibiki, & Aarnoutse, 2011; WHO, 2010). One study reported a medication adherence rate

for TB of 39% (Ailinger, Martyn, Lasus, & Garcia, 2010).

- HIV medication in adults: 62% of adults reported 90% or better adherence to highly active antiretroviral therapy (HAART) medications (Ortego et al., 2011)
- HIV medication in children: 44% to 81% via electronic monitoring (Farley, Hines, Musk, Ferrus, & Tepper, 2003; Steele et al., 2001).
- Asthma: In one study, 63 of 182 patients (35%) had filled fewer than 50% of prescriptions for inhaled combination therapy, and 57 (88%) admitted low adherence after initial denial (Gamble, Stevenson, McClean, & Heaney, 2009).
- Glaucoma: 71% (electronic monitoring), 77% (physician estimate), and 95% (patient self-report) (Okeke et al., 2009).

Components of Adherence

The most recent conceptualizations of adherence include three components: initiation, execution, and persistence (Blaschke, Osterberg, Vrijens, & Urquhart, 2012). Initiation refers to being aware that a prescription was written, filling the prescription, and taking the first dose of medication (Blaschke et al., 2012; Gadkari, 2010). Discontinuation is when a patient stops taking a medication. The time between initiation and discontinuation encompasses execution (defined as the regularity of dosing and the correspondence of behavior with prescribed regimen) and persistence (the time lapse between initiation and discontinuation) (Blaschke et al., 2012). For the purposes of clarifying the concept of adherence, and for quantification in research, these stages of adherence can be categorized as continuous actions (which include implementation and persistence) and discontinuous actions (which include initiation and discontinuation) (Lehmann et al., 2014). Continuous actions include both regularity and continuity simultaneously,

whereas discontinuous behaviors bookend continuous action. Approximately 16% of patients with a new prescription do not commence treatment (Gadkari & McHorney, 2010), and half of patients stop treatment within the first year (Haynes, McDonald, & Garg, 2002).

Another component of nonadherence that is important to determine is whether nonadherence is intentional or unintentional. Patients can purposely decide not to fill or take medication, not follow diet and exercise recommendations, or refrain from or engage in other behaviors that directly affect their health, but unintentional nonadherence should also be considered with any patient. Patients can unintentionally nonadhere to medications due to forgetfulness, carelessness, poor health literacy, socioeconomic factors, and cognitive impairment. Another factor in treatment nonadherence is the disruption of routines and schedules. Medication intakes during evening, weekend, and holiday times have been shown to contribute to incorrect timing of doses as well as missing doses entirely. Most medication intake occurs in the mornings, Monday through Thursday (96%), with the least intake occurring on Saturday evening (82%). Correctly timed intake occurs most often on Monday and Tuesday mornings (61%), in contrast to Sunday evenings (33%) (Vervloet, Spreeuwenberg, Bouvy, Heerdink, de Bakker, & van Dijk, 2013).

A more recently emerging concept important to medication adherence is that of prospective memory—that is, the neurocognitive capacity to remember to do something at a later time. Prospective memory, a subcategory within the construct of episodic memory, declines with age and neurocognitive impairment. Research has demonstrated the importance of prospective memory for medication adherence with HIV, rheumatoid arthritis, and diabetes self-management, and it may be an important avenue for interventions to increase medication adherence behaviors across disease states (Zogg, Woods, Sauceda, Wiebe, & Simoni, 2012).

The relevance of adherence to the total wellness–illness continuum was first described by Marston, a nurse, in 1970. Marston considered adherence to comprise self-care behaviors that individuals undertake to promote health, to prevent illness, or to follow recommendations for treatment and rehabilitation in diagnosed illnesses. She is notable in the history of treatment adherence as the first reviewer of literature in the field (Greene, 2004).

It may be helpful, however, to consider adherence as encompassing more than self-care behaviors; rather, it is behavior that is often shared, because patients cannot always implement their medical regimens without the participation of others, even though the delineation of responsibilities is not always clear. For example, Greenley, Josie, and Drotar (2006) note that there are misunderstandings about the responsibility for asthma treatment regimens in inner-city children, and that this misunderstanding often leads to nonadherence. This is especially true when the dependence/independence status of the patient changes, as with the teenager who assumes greater responsibility for management of his or her healthcare regimen or the older adult who now requires more supervision and assistance by family members.

Stephens, Rook, Franks, Khan, and Lida (2010) investigated both the negative and positive strategies spouses used to urge patients with type 2 diabetes to improve dietary adherence. Findings showed that cautioning the patient about the consequences of eating an inadequate diet was associated with poorer adherence, whereas encouragement to select healthier food choices was associated with better adherence. An early study of how couples managed chronic disease revealed that coordination and collaboration between the couple were necessary to carry out the work of the medical regimen (Corbin & Strauss, 1985). A 2006 study in the field of HIV describes the role that family caregivers provide in complex regimens, and explicates how various types of stigma affect caring for an HIV-infected family member (Beals, Wight, Aneshensel, Murphy, & Miller-Martinez, 2006). Likewise, family support in adolescents suffering from asthma was positively associated with asthma control and improved quality of life (Rhee, Belyea, & Brasch, 2010). A review by Knafl and Gilliss (2002) concludes that nurses need to be more involved in helping with family interventions for chronic illness management. Given that shared responsibility exists, it seems reasonable to conclude that adherence-increasing strategies should be directed toward all persons involved in the regimen, and that there may be a need for explicitly discussing the division of responsibility among family members.

Factors Contributing to Adherence Behavior

Studies have demonstrated that large numbers of individuals do not follow healthcare recommendations completely. Although nonadherence is increasingly recognized as a problem, there is no consensus about appropriate or effective methods to increase adherence. Some of the difficulty lies in the inadequacies of research on adherence, some lies in differing role expectations of patients and providers, and some relates to conflict in values. As healthcare professionals prescribe, teach, and counsel patients about medical regimens, they must be cautious in making assumptions about adherence behaviors in a given situation before imposing any specific strategy on the patient.

INDIVIDUAL CHARACTERISTICS

Several patient characteristics that influence adherence have been examined, including demographic factors, psychological factors, social support, past health behavior, somatic factors, and health beliefs (Dunbar-Jacob, Schlenk, & Caruthers, 2002). More recent literature has examined ethnicity as an influence in adherence with diagnostic testing (Cook, Kobetz, Reis, Fleming, Loer-Martin, & Amofah, 2010;

Strzelczyk & Dignan, 2002). Strzelczyk and Dignan (2002) reported that African American women were more likely to be nonadherent with mammography screening than Caucasian women. Conversely, Cook and colleagues (2010) reported that Latina and African American women were 2 and 1.45 times more likely to receive Pap smear screening, respectively, when compared to Caucasians. With respect to retention in clinical trials, African American subjects were more likely to drop out of participation in a rheumatoid arthritis treatment adherence study than were Caucasians (Dunbar-Jacob et al., 2004). An interesting study by Taira and colleagues (2007) examined predictors of medication adherence among Asian American subgroups in Hawaii and found that Filipino, Korean, and Hawaiian patients were less likely to adhere to these regimens than were Japanese patients. More research is needed to identify strategies among various ethnic groups that might increase adherence behavior.

Because of the many inconsistencies in studies that examine age and adherence behavior, no overall statement about individual factors can be made. According to Barnestein-Fonseca and colleagues (2011), a variety of factors may potentially interfere with the ability of the older adult to adhere to medical instruction. It is important to rule out cognitive changes, which may occur with aging, versus the busy lifestyle barriers that pertain to the middle-aged adult. In a study by Hinkin and colleagues (2004), patients with HIV infection who were middle aged were less adherent than older patients. For children, there are specific issues of adherence related to age that are associated with developmental stages rather than chronologic age. However, in general, such developmental issues have not been well addressed in the adherence literature (Dunbar-Jacob et al., 2000).

Psychological Factors Intuitively, healthcare professionals believe that psychological factors may affect adherence behavior. Many studies support the premise that depression is related to poor adherence. DiMatteo, Lepper, and Croghan (2000) completed a meta-analysis examining the relationship between depression and adherence and found that depressed patients were at a threefold greater risk for nonadherence. Depression has also been linked to mortality in patients not following medical recommendations in acute coronary syndromes (Kronish et al., 2006) and HIV infection (Lima et al., 2007). It may be helpful to treat depression in patients at risk for nonadherence (Berg, Nyamathi, Christiani, Morisky, & Leake, 2005). Other psychological factors, such as ambiguity, hostility, and general emotional distress, as single factors, are not predictive of adherence behavior but may, in fact, be components of motivation (Dunbar-Jacob, Schlenk, & McCall, 2012).

Social Support Social support is a variable that has frequently been explored in adherence studies. Nevertheless, it has not been demonstrated to consistently have an impact on adherence behavior. In some cases, social support increases adherence behavior, such as in pediatric patients with asthma who receive social support from family and friends (Sin, Kang, & Weaver, 2005) and in patients with HIV infection (Gonzalez et al., 2004). In contrast, other studies have found that social support has no impact on adherence (Sunil & McGehee, 2007).

Prior Health Behavior It has been suggested that adherence to a particular healthcare regimen at a single point in time may predict subsequent adherence (Dunbar-Jacob, Schlenk, Burke, & Mathews, 1997). In the 10-year study associated with the Lipid Research Clinics Coronary Primary Prevention Trial, initial medication adherence accurately predicted adherence throughout the study; however, this did not extend to other health behaviors. In general, it was found that the more similar the initial behaviors were to the behaviors that need to be developed, the greater the likelihood of accuracy (Dunbar-Jacob, Gemmell, & Schlenk, 2009). In a study examining HIV treatment adherence, attending clinic appointments was associated with medication treatment adherence (Wagner, 2003).

Somatic Factors It has been postulated that the presence of symptoms may promote greater adherence with medical recommendations. For example, hypertensive individuals who are asymptomatic indicated that they could tell when their blood pressure was high and adhered with treatment at these times because of their belief that adherence relieved the symptoms (Chen, Tsai, & Chou, 2011). In another study involving individuals with lung disease, increased dyspnea predicted greater adherence with nebulizer therapy (Laforest, Licaj, Devouassoux, Hartwig, Marvalin, & Van Ganse, 2013); in contrast, a lack of symptoms was found to be a barrier to adherence with inhaled corticosteroid therapy (Ulrik, Backer, Soes-Petersen, Lange, Harving, & Plaschke, 2006). Increased HIV symptom experience, however, was associated with decreased medication adherence, as patients' belief in the efficacy of the medication waned in the face of continued symptomatology (Cooper, 2009).

Patients who are severely ill with serious illnesses have also presented with poorer treatment adherence, as relationships with care providers decline in the face of worsening health. These patients may become depressed, pessimistic, socially withdrawn, and hopeless or ambivalent about surviving, making adherence seem futile (DiMatteo, Haskard, & Williams, 2007). Illness-related symptoms may, therefore,

be an important cue to following treatment recommendations.

Regimen Characteristics Regimen type and regimen complexity have been linked to adherence behavior, with complexity being a more important factor (Dunbar-Jacob et al., 2009). Complexity includes multiple medications, frequent treatments, a variety of treatments (e.g., diet, exercise, and medications), duration of the regimen, a complicated treatment delivery system, and irritating side effects (Chesney, 2003). Complicated regimens lead to low adherence rates (Choudhry et al., 2011). This effect has also been well documented in the HIV literature, as patients with HIV/AIDS have extremely complex medication regimens (Chesney, 2003; Hinkin et al., 2002; Waldrop-Valverde, Jones, Gould, Kumar, & Ownby, 2010).

Economic Factors Poverty, poor English-language proficiency, and limited access to health care are predictors of nonadherence (Peeters, Van Tongelen, Rousseryl, Mehuys, Remon, & Willems, 2011). The burden of financial costs alone may serve as a barrier to obtaining healthcare services, supplies, or medications needed to manage chronic illness. Another major barrier to adherence is a lack of resources, including inadequate or difficult transportation, inadequate availability of childcare, loss of time from low-paying jobs, and little job security. Socioeconomic status has recently been associated with poor adherence in individuals using hormone-replacement therapy. This needs to be examined further with other studies of adherence (Finley, Gregg, Solomon, & Gay, 2001), especially in light of the Affordable Care Act. Health literacy may also contribute to problems in managing chronic illness regimens. In some studies, limited health literacy has been associated with poor adherence to antiretroviral medications (Waldrop-Valverde et al., 2010; Wolf, Williams, Parker, Parikh, Nowlan, & Baker, 2007) and with better adherence to other HIV medications (Paasche-Orlow, Cheng, Palepu, Meli, Faber, & Samet, 2006).

Some barriers to adherence are clearly related to an ineffective healthcare system for chronic disease management. For example, some individuals with chronic disease who come to emergency departments for nonurgent care have limited access to primary care services that are more appropriate for chronic disease management (Mansour, Lanphear, & DeWitt, 2000). There is decreased availability of primary care services, particularly in inner cities and rural areas, to groups such as migrant workers, new immigrants, the homeless, and those with AIDS. In addition, the maze of governmental and third-party payers' policies and regulations often deny provider reimbursement for preventive or educational services, making these services less available to patients. How this will change in the future, as we shift to better insurance coverage and better chronic disease management, remains to be seen.

Cultural Factors   More attention is being given to the ways in which culture influences health behaviors and the interactions of patients with healthcare providers. Cultural influences affect the way adults and children experience, interpret, and respond to illness and its treatment.

Because of the changing demographics and the influx of immigrants into the United States, studies examining the behaviors of different cultural groups appear quite often in the literature. Some of these studies explore the dimension of being a member of a minority group who has a health problem. For example, minority status has been associated with lower asthma medication adherence. Minorities were found to have lower adherence and a higher prevalence of negative asthma medication beliefs compared to Caucasians. Tests of mediation have suggested that such negative medication beliefs partially mediate the relationship between minority status and adherence (Le et al., 2008). Language issues affect the utilization of health care and the ability to form relationships with healthcare professionals. Different cultural norms may also interfere with adherence behaviors. For example, in Latino families, the stigma of having tuberculosis may be a factor in poor adherence to taking medication (Cabrera, Morisky, & Chin, 2002; Hovell et al., 2003). Latinos have also been described as seeking health care late, if at all, and then using folk healers and medications for illness (Ransford, Carrillo, & Rivera, 2010). Some of the delay in healthcare utilization relates to insurance issues, language barriers, and immigration status.

Asian immigrants may have difficulty accepting and actively engaging in regimen demands. Chinese immigrants were found to have ineffective self-care and coping strategies with diabetes in a study by Jaynes and Rankin (2001). Similarly, in a study by Tanaka and colleagues (2014), Asian women ignored the symptoms of menopause until those symptoms became intolerable.

It will become increasingly important for healthcare professionals to interpret the effect of culture and ethnicity on adherence behavior. One issue that confounds the link between health behavior and culture is socioeconomic status. There is a need to distinguish whether poor adherence is related to ethnicity, cultural, or socioeconomic factors, as opposed to the interaction of these factors.

PATIENT–PROVIDER INTERACTIONS

Of all of the variables associated with nonadherence, patient–provider interactions have been highlighted as being extremely important since the year 2000. More recent studies have focused on the relationship between provider and patient as a way of encouraging health behavior change (Beach, Keruly, & Moore, 2006; O'Malley,

Sheppard, Schwartz, & Mandelblatt, 2004). Importantly, the topic of self-management is discussed in primary care consultations infrequently, as maintaining the self–other relationship remains a prime objective for both patients and professionals (Blakeman, Bower, Reeves, & Chew-Graham, 2010). Enabling the patient to self-manage his or her condition, therefore, threatens the hierarchy and is an important tension that is the foundation for care.

Perspectives of Patients and Healthcare Professionals Patients and providers are likely to have different perspectives about chronic illness, its treatment, and the relative merits of adherence behavior. The patient lives with the disease, and treatment is only one aspect of that individual's life. Living with treatment consequences is vastly different from offering advice, counsel, education, or exhortation about healthcare recommendations. Patients, on the one hand, ask for help from healthcare professionals because they feel ill, they are worried, they are responding to others' recommendations, they need evidence to validate claims for entitlement benefits, and so forth. Providers, on the other hand, are concerned about adherence, which may be seen as the desired outcome of the patient–provider interaction (Rivers, 2007).

Rivers (2007) identifies two ways in which patients' perspectives on chronic illness—in this case, diabetes mellitus—differ from those of healthcare professionals. First, there is a relative difference in understanding of the treatment regimen, not just on the level of specificity, rationale, and consequences, but also with respect to the sources of problems. Patients may see treatment as part of the problem of having diabetes, whereas providers see treatment as a solution. Second, patients are more concerned about the "here and now" experience, in contrast to providers' concern about a problem that places future health at risk. For example, patients express more concerns about

preventing hypoglycemic reactions than about managing higher than normal blood glucose levels. Providers, for their part, express more concern about the importance of achieving close to normal blood glucose levels because of their perceptions of serious long-term consequences if control of blood glucose levels is not achieved.

ETHICS AND ADHERENCE BEHAVIOR

Adherence to recommendations for health behavior is an increasingly important ethical issue in healthcare cost containment, because conflicts arise when healthcare resources are limited and decisions about the best use of time, money, and the energy of providers must be made. However, economic and ethical issues in adherence differ. Whereas economic issues are concerned with the most efficient distribution of resources, ethical issues are concerned with the most equitable distribution (Guindo et al., 2012). Bosworth (2010) believes that strategies that promote and improve a patient's active and effective self-care are both ethically and economically significant.

There is also concern about providing resources to help those persons with chronic disorders in developing countries, where treatment nonadherence is very high (WHO, 2003). Ethical issues center on reciprocal rights and responsibilities of caregivers and patients, use of paternalism and coercion by caregivers, autonomy of the patient, relative risks and benefits of proposed regimens, and the costs to society of nonadherence. Again, the focus on the patients' active participation with their healthcare professionals appears to raise ethical concerns (Bernardini, 2004; Rand & Sevick, 2000). This brings up the questions of whether health care directed solely by the practitioner without input by the patient is ethical and whether nonadherence should rest upon the shoulders of only the patient.

Theoretical Underpinnings of Adherence Behavior

Theoretical frameworks and conceptual models provide direction for healthcare professionals by guiding the assessment and providing structure for the interaction between patient and provider. At this point in time, the emphasis is on translation of theories and models into effective practice interventions. Although an extensive library devoted to adherence behavior exists, few studies support strategies to improve adherence (DiMatteo & Haskard, 2006). Models for understanding individual health behavior can be useful only if they are based on empirical research and can be used to create effective interventions. This linkage relates to the current mandate for translational research and evidence-based practice. Brief reviews of behavioral models that are currently used are presented here.

HEALTH BELIEF MODEL

The health belief model (HBM), developed by Hochman and colleagues (as cited in Rosenstock, 1974), was devised to explain health-related behaviors, especially preventive health behaviors, and contains a cluster of pertinent beliefs and attitudes (Becker & Maiman, 1975). The original model was subsequently modified to include general health motivation (Becker, 1976), and then modified again to include sick-role behaviors. The HBM's major proposition is that the likelihood of an individual taking recommended health actions is based on (1) the perceived severity of the illness, (2) the individual's estimate of the likelihood that a specific action will reduce the threat, and (3) perceived barriers to following recommendations. The HBM continues to be used to explain the relationships of attitudes and behaviors to adherence behavior, specifically in regard to perceived susceptibility, perceived severity, and perceived barriers (Jerant, Fiscella, Tancredi, & Franks, 2013; McCall & Ginis, 2004; Rodríguez-Reimann, Nicassio, Reimann, Gallegos, & Olmedo, 2004; Wutoh, Brown, Dutta, Kumoji, Clarke-Tasker, & Xue, 2005). A recent review of the efficacy of the HBM found studies utilizing this model as a theoretical foundation to inform interventions yielded significant (mostly moderate to large) improvements in adherence behaviors (Jones,

Smith, & Llewellyn, 2013). The authors concluded, however, that intervention success did not appear to be related to specific HBM constructs, as the HBM was not used in its entirety, nor were health belief outcomes measured in most studies.

HEALTH PROMOTION MODEL

A nursing model that evolved from the HBM is the health promotion model (HPM) (Pender, 1996; Pender, Murdaugh, & Parsons, 2001). Pender conceptualized health as a goal and believed that only the desire to be healthy leads to engagement in health promotion activities. Pender organized the concepts under the framework of individual characteristics and experiences, behavior-specific cognitions and affect, and behavioral outcomes. The Health-Promoting Lifestyle Profile is an instrument that assesses health promotion behaviors; it has been translated and validated in Spanish as well as English (Walker, Sechrist, & Pender, 1987), and continues to be used and adapted (D'hooghe, Nagels, De Keyser, & Haentjens, 2013; Padden, Connors, Posey, Ricciardi, & Agazio, 2013; Tucker et al., 2013). Recent studies using the HPM have found that low income and low education negatively impact involvement in health promotion activities (Chilton, Hu, & Wallace, 2006; Harley et al., 2013; Lee, Santacroce, & Sadler, 2007; Smylie et al., 2014).

COMMON SENSE MODEL OF SELF-REGULATION

The common sense model of self-regulation (CSM) was developed from two prior models. One of its antecedents, the common sense model, was developed by Leventhal, Meyer, and Nerenz in 1980 to explain how individuals process illness-related events and how this shapes coping and adherence. Early studies using this model were conducted primarily on individuals with asymptomatic illnesses (Baumann, Cameron, Zimmerman, & Leventhal, 1989; Meyer, Leventhal, & Gutmann, 1985). In brief, an individual's processing of illness-related events depends on four dimensions: cause (what was responsible for the illness), consequences (how things will change because of the illness), identity (being able to identify the illness), and timeline (the course of the illness).

In 1987, Leventhal and colleagues identified a feedback mechanism to a behavioral model and called it the self-regulation theory. The dimension of control–cure was examined as part of the illness representation.

These two models are now combined into one model known as the common sense model of self-regulation (Leventhal, Brisette, & Leventhal, 2003). Recent studies using this model have shown that beliefs about illness affect coping (Gould, 2011; Kelly, Sereika, Battista, & Brown, 2007; Ohm & Aaronson, 2006; Quinn, 2005; Searle, Norman, Thompson, & Vedhara, 2007; Snell, Hay-Smith, Surgenor, & Siegert, 2013). The CSM does not appear to be an appropriate model for predicting adherence; however, effect sizes for various mental representations and specific adherence behaviors are low across many studies, indicating weak relationships between these measures (Brandes & Mullan, 2013; Breland, McAndrew, Burns, Leventhal, & Leventhal, 2013).

THE THEORY OF REASONED ACTION AND THE THEORY OF PLANNED BEHAVIOR

The theory of reasoned action (Fishbein & Ajzen, 1975) and the theory of planned behavior (Ajzen, 1985) have intention as a main component. According to these theories, individuals engage in health behaviors intentionally, based on attitudes toward a behavior and social influence. The theory of planned behavior adds a component to the model called "perceived behavioral control," which captures the extent to which a person has control over any given behavior. Both of these theories have been useful in the examination of preventive behaviors, such as engaging in exercise programs (Martin, Oliver, & McCaughtry, 2007; Norman & Connor, 2005), condom use (Gredig, Niderost, & Parpan-Blaser, 2006), and avoiding binge drinking (Norman, Armitage, & Quigley, 2007), where intention has been found to be an important component of engaging in the desired behavior. These theories have also proved valuable in assessment of physical activity in chronic illness regimens (Eng & Martin Ginis, 2007) as well as in assessment of HAART adherence in patients with HIV infection (Vissman, Young, Wilkin, & Rhodes, 2013).

CASE STUDY 9-2

Lucille Weintraub is an 80-year-old woman who lives with her husband in an assisted-living facility. She has been depressed for years and has recently begun drinking again. When you discuss her situation with her, she admits that she took an antidepressant in the past, but ran out of the samples and is not able to get the medication now. She tells you that she does not feel as if the medication is worth the expense. She admits that she likes drinking her wine all day and it helps her feel less sad about her life. You are concerned that she is having difficulty with her balance and, with her alcohol use, she is at greater risk for falls.

Discussion Questions

1. Which suggestions can you make to ensure her safety?
2. Are there actions that you can take to solve the medication issue?

Cognitive Social Learning Theory

Cognitive social learning theory attempts to predict behavior that is dictated by outcome and efficacy expectancies. This theory combines environment, cognition, and emotion in the understanding of health behavior change (Bandura, 2004). Three necessary prerequisites to altering health behavior are the recognition that a lifestyle component can be harmful, the recognition that a change in behavior would be beneficial, and the recognition that one has the ability to adopt a new behavior (self-efficacy) (Schwarzer, 1992). To effect any change, then, each individual must be able to self-monitor and self-regulate health behavior. This aspect of self-regulation has led to a variety of self-management strategies with which to cope with illness. The additional component of self-efficacy, defined as the patient's expectations or confidence in his or her ability to perform a recommended action, has also promoted research to test efficacy-enhancing strategies important in health behavior change. Self-efficacy has been found to be an important predictor of self-management behaviors useful in the treatment of AIDS (Johnson et al., 2006), cancer (Eiser, Hill, & Blacklay, 2000), cardiac disease (Hiltunen, Winder, Rait, Buselli, Carroll, & Rankin, 2005), depression (Harrington et al., 2000), and diabetes (Ott, Greening, Palardy, Holderby, & DeBell, 2000; Stupiansky, Hanna, Slaven, Weaver, & Fortenberry, 2013).

Transtheoretical Model of Change (Stages of Change)

The stages of change (transtheoretical) model, developed by Prochaska and DiClemente (1983), is an eclectic model that aims to examine and predict the process of change. This model contains three constructs: the stages of change, the processes of change, and the levels of change. Its underlying premise proposes that people are at different stages in their intentional desire to adopt certain health behaviors with or without assistance. The model also proposes that interventions should be matched to each categorical stage of change. Although presented hierarchically, the process of change is considered to be a spiral, with relapse from a healthy behavior placing an individual in a position to move backward toward contemplation of the healthy behavior. The model also incorporates self-efficacy and decision making as key factors in the process of change, but these factors have an impact at different stages of change. The stages include the following:

- Pre-contemplation: no intention of changing behavior
- Contemplation: considering future action
- Pre-action: has a timetable for action
- Action: involved in behavior change
- Maintenance: after change is adopted; relapse is a possibility

The stages of change model of health behavior was initially applied to the treatment of addictive behaviors. Currently, other research on behavioral change for chronic illness has embraced this model. Clinical interventions have been proposed at each stage. The use of motivational interviewing has been examined as a means to move patients to an action phase of readiness (Jackson, Asimakopoulou, & Scammell, 2007; Johnson et al., 2007), although critics warn that there is no theoretical link between motivational interviewing and the transtheoretical model.

Three-Factor Model

With decades of research on behavior change and adherence behaviors to review, consistent findings across meta-analyses and large-scale studies have led to the identification of a three-factor model for clinical action to promote patient adherence. The three factors are information, motivation, and strategy (DiMatteo, Haskard-Zolnierek, & Martin, 2012).

- Providing *information* to patients and ensuring their understanding is essential to treatment adherence, but insufficient to ensure adherence. Essential elements in providing useful information to patients include clinician–patient communication, accurate patient recall of information, adapting information to compensate for any extant cognitive deficits, and shared decision making.

- Patient *motivation* for adherence is ignited by the patient's belief in the efficacy, appropriateness, and feasibility of any treatment, and is strengthened by "informed collaborative choice" (p. 81). Motivation requires ongoing reinforcement to be maintained.
- *Strategy* refers to a patient's ability to adhere to the treatment, where identification and overcoming of obstacles improves his or her capacity for adherence. Commonly encountered barriers include medication cost and side effects, cognitive deficits, inability to perform ongoing difficult lifestyle changes, mental health, and highly complex treatment regimens.

ECOLOGICAL PERSPECTIVE

Broadening adherence beyond individual and/or patient–provider (dyad-level) considerations to include system-level factors can expand intervention options to improve modifiable aspects of adherence. Such factors include clinicians' patient load, available consultation time, provider training, and policies and regulations (Berben, Dobbels, Engberg, Hill, & De Geest, 2012). Such multilevel attention, including individual-, micro-, and macro-level implementation, can support individuals' success in caring for themselves and their families.

In summary, many models have been used to study adherence behavior in chronic illness. It is important to have a theoretical basis for proposed interventions; however, more work needs to be accomplished to evaluate the effectiveness of theory-based strategies.

Measuring Adherence Behaviors

When a treatment is prescribed, the efficacy of that recommendation hinges on the follow-through by the patient. If a prescribed treatment does not appear to be working, clinicians often change medication dose, question the diagnosis, or take a more (sometimes harmful) aggressive approach. What is sometimes missed in the face of an apparently ineffective treatment response is an assessment of the degree to which the patient adhered to the prescribed action.

Measuring patient behavior can be complex, and different methodologies exist for different contexts and diseases. Important aspects of choosing appropriate measurement methods include the need for accuracy, comprehensiveness, ease, and cost of administration (Riekert, 2009).

There is no gold standard to measure medication, lifestyle, or dietary adherence, and current evidence suggests several strategies besides disease outcomes may be used to capture treatment adherence to medication (Desroches, Lapointe, Ratté, Gravel, Légaré, & Turcotte, 2013; Krapek et al., 2004; Lehmann et al., 2014; Wagner & Rabkin, 2000; Wendel, Mohler, Kroesen, Ampel, Gifford, & Coons, 2001). Electronic monitoring is often used as the reference method for determining medication adherence in most studies (Erdine & Arslan, 2013). Polypharmacy in chronic disorders adds another variable when observing and measuring medication adherence (Vik, Maxwell, & Hogan, 2004). Each measurement is prone to some error, usually consisting of a bias toward an overestimation of adherence (Dunbar-Jacob et al., 2002; Lehmann et al., 2014). However, using a combination of methods to measure a specific adherence behavior is recommended to increase accuracy and reliability of the results, compared with a single method of measurement (WHO, 2003).

An assessment of the patient's overall well-being and psychological structure is also essential to attain a better understanding of his or her adherence behaviors. A systematic assessment of the patient includes the patient's family, sociocultural and economic factors, knowledge level, beliefs, attitudes, and current understanding of the proposed regimen. Likewise, attention should be given to the patient's perceptions of the illness threat, the efficacy of recommendations, and the patient's ability to carry these out. There should be a determination of the "rightness" of the prescriptions for the particular patient, including an estimation of the relative harm or benefit that is expected. This assessment allows the nurse to determine which aspects of the regimen management are most *unlikely* to achieve adherent behavior, are most important in attaining therapeutic goals, and require the most learning to attain the desired behavioral change.

The following questions should be asked in an adherence-oriented history (Hingson, Scotch, Sorenson, & Swazey, 1981):

- Have you been taking anything for this problem already?
- Does anything worry you about the illness?
- What can happen if the recommended regimen is not followed?
- How likely is it that you will not follow the recommended regimen?
- How effective do you feel the regimen will be in treating the disorder?
- Can you think of any problems you might have in following the regimen?
- Do you have any questions about the regimen or how to follow it?

Several widely used methodological approaches focus on adherence, and it has been suggested that adherence assessment should always focus squarely on adherence as a behavior—not on its predictors or its consequences (Morisky & DiMatteo, 2011, p. 255). Primary methods include self-report, practitioner report, observation, physiologic measures, medication monitoring, and electronic monitors.

INDIRECT MEASURES

Self-Report   Patient self-reports of adherence behaviors are the simplest and least expensive method of gathering nonadherence information and are feasible in virtually all care settings. Self-reports also allow the collection of more detailed information on the circumstances surrounding poor adherence than any other type of measure (Dunbar-Jacob et al., 2009). They may be elicited through simple questions; through a more complex, structured interview schedule; or through a validated questionnaire. Common self-report measures include medication and symptom diaries, structured questionnaires, and interviews.

Self-reported adherence behavior has come under scrutiny because this methodology is widely believed to be invalid and unreliable (Berg & Arnstein, 2006; Liu, Miller, Hays, Wagner, Golin, & Hu, 2006; Smith, Wahed, Kelley, Conjeevaram, Robuck, & Fried, 2007). There are many reasons why a patient's self-reported adherence may be inaccurate. While patients who report nonadherence tend to report their behavior accurately (Bosworth, 2010), some may honestly not remember whether they took their medications, may be unaware that they are not following recommendations, or may have misconceptions about their dosing schedule (Barfod, Hecht, Rubow, & Gerstoft, 2006; Bosworth, 2010; Sankar, Nevedal, Neufeld, & Luborsky, 2007). Other reasons for nonadherence may include economic factors, lack of resources, or the patient's discomfort with being honest with healthcare providers. In any event, it is incumbent on the provider to be able to assess whether a patient can and is willing to follow a recommendation. Toward this end, researchers recommend asking questions in a nonjudgmental way to elicit valid responses about regimen adherence (Berg & Arnstein, 2006).

Several studies have attempted to evaluate and define the accuracy of self-reported adherence. Many of these have compared patient reports with pill counts, electronic monitoring, drug levels, or biological markers in body fluids. Most have found that individuals overestimate their adherence (Garfield, Clifford, Eliasson, Barber, & Willson, 2011; Liu et al., 2006; Shi, Liu, Koleva, Fonseca, Kalsekar, & Pawaskar, 2010).

Despite its inherent problems, self-reports are still the measure most commonly used in adherence behavior assessment, and they have the potential to provide the most accurate record of what a given patient has done, as long as the patient can remember taking the medication and is motivated to be absolutely truthful about what is remembered (Morisky & DiMatteo, 2011, p. 255–257). Thus, establishing trust within the patient–provider relationship and developing strategies to enhance recall are essential to obtaining accurate information.

Observation and Clinical Judgment   Direct observation of the patient is rarely possible, making it an impractical method of assessing adherence. Theoretically, this method would be an ideal way to provide evidence of adherence behavior; however, individuals often "play to an audience," and the knowledge that someone is watching affects behavior. Direct observation is thought of as a passive method of medication distribution; it limits patients' active participation in treatment and is inflexible to adaptation in real-life contexts (Erdine & Arslan, 2013).

An example of this behavior for the individual with asthma is the demonstration/return demonstration of the correct method of using metered-dose inhalers (MDIs). Patients with asthma are assessed on their ability to carry out the instructed regimen and adherence with teaching. Although nurses assess a patient's behavior in carrying out tasks related to healthcare management, the assumption cannot be made that this activity will continue at home.

Clinical judgment of patients' adherence to medication regimens has also been shown to be poor, with rates of adherence to cystic fibrosis medication ranging from 50% to 60%, compared to 36% when measured via electronic monitoring (Daniels, Goodacre, Sutton, Pollard, Conway, & Peckham, 2011). Clinician assessment of medication adherence is often incorrect, with overestimation being more common than underestimation (Burrows, Bunting, Masel, & Bell, 2002).

Monitoring   Other methods for measuring medication adherence (drug-dosing recall, pill counts, self-report surveys, and pharmacy refills) have been used and have indicated similar rates of adherence (DiMatteo, 2004; Dunbar-Jacob et al., 2002). In a study that enrolled patients with chronic pain, paper diaries and electronic diaries were compared. The electronic diaries offered a time-stamped variation on the paper diary and outperformed the latter with regard to adherence of use by the patient (Stone, Shiffman, Schwartz, Broderick, & Hufford, 2003).

Pill counts, pharmacy-refill monitoring, and MDI canister weighing can all be used to measure medication adherence. In studies that use pill counts, the subject is given a vial each month that contains a certain number of tablets, and this vial is exchanged for a new one each month. The medication left in the vial can be compared with the number that was supposed to be left if the medication were taken. Similarly, when a patient requests a refill from the pharmacy, the time of the request is compared with the expected date of refill if the medication were taken as prescribed. Such methods do not take into account whether patients are sharing medications with others or "dumping" pills prior to refill. MDI canister weighing is used with patients who have respiratory illnesses. The canister is weighed before it is given to the patient and then reweighed at specific times during treatment.

Although medication-monitoring methods appear highly accurate, they may overestimate adherence behavior (Jentzsch, Camargos, Colosimo, & Bousquet, 2009; Rapoff, 2010). Berg and Arnstein (2006) further suggest that asking a patient to bring in the medications for a check of pill count may, in fact, be offensive and counterproductive to building rapport between patient and provider.

Electronic monitors are the newest technology for the assessment of adherence behaviors. The most commonly used of these devices is the electronic medication monitor. Electronic monitors may also be used to capture heart rate and muscle movement with exercise adherence (Sylvia, Bernstein, Hubbard, Keating, & Anderson, 2013) or to monitor nasal continuous positive airway pressure adherence for patients with sleep apnea (Fox et al., 2012).

Electronic monitors that assess medication adherence are used with tablets, eye drops, and MDIs (Berg & Arnstein, 2006). With this technology, microprocessors are placed in special bottle caps or blister packs and can monitor the date and time of day for each manipulation of the drug container and provide information on drug-taking behavior for days or weeks. Knowing the pattern of pill taking (or not taking) can be useful in evaluating clinical responses (or lack thereof) or side effects, and can provide guidance for interventions specifically tailored for each patient (Quittner, Modi, Lemanek, Ievers-Landis, & Rapoff, 2007).

Electronic monitors have been used to assess medication adherence in many studies. Studies of treatment adherence in HIV-infected populations, for example, have used self-reports, diaries, and medication event monitors (MEMs). This technology is not specific to HIV-infected populations, however.

Electronic monitoring typically provides lower estimates of adherence than self-report data (Wagner & Rabkin, 2000). The following adherence rates are provided for the sake of comparison:

- Rheumatoid arthritis: consistently below 50% (Elliott, 2008)
- Epilepsy: 34% (Cramer, Vachon, Desforges, & Sussman, 1995)
- Ankylosing spondylitis: 22% (de Klerk & van der Linden, 1996)
- Major depression: 51% upon initiation, 42% upon continuation/follow-up (Akincigil et al., 2007; Carney, Freedland, Eisen, Rich, & Jaffe, 1995; Demyttenaere, Van Ganse, Gregoire, Gaens, & Mesters, 1998)
- Schizophrenia: less than 55% (Duncan & Rogers, 1998; McCann & Lu, 2009)
- Diabetes mellitus: 47% (Mason, Matsayuma, & Jue, 1995)
- Hypertension: 30–47% (Le et al., 1996; Mounier-Vehier, Bernaud, Carre, Lequeuche, Hotton, & Charpentier, 1998)
- Tuberculosis: 39% (Ailinger et al., 2010)
- Ischemic heart disease: 38–45% (Carney, Freedland, Eisen, Rich, Skala, & Jaffe, 1998; Straka, Fish, Benson, & Suh, 1997)
- Use of inhaled corticosteroids in asthma: 44–72%, with only 13% continuing to fill prescriptions after 1 year (Borrelli, Reikert, Weinstein, & Rathier, 2007)

An innovative use of technology was reported in a pilot trial to monitor lung transplant recipients' adherence to self-care behaviors—namely, a Pocket Personal Assistant for Tracking Health device (Pocket PATH) (De Vito Dabbs et al., 2009). This mobile, hand-held device significantly improved self-care behaviors of monitoring vital signs, medical regimens, health habits, and communicating important changes to the transplant team between scheduled visits, as compared to standard pencil-and-paper methods.

DIRECT MEASURES

Physiologic Measures   Physiologic measures of adherence include serum drug levels, heart rate monitoring, muscle strength, urine sample analysis, cholesterol levels, and glycosylated hemoglobin levels. The advantage of physiologic methods is that these measures are not dependent on the patient's memory or veracity.

Of all of the physiologic measures, measurement of drug levels is most commonly used. Although drug-level measurements offer a greater degree of accuracy than self-reports and practitioner reports, there are some difficulties with this type of assessment. First, these measures do not reflect the level of adherence (Dunbar-Jacob, Burke, & Puczynski, 1995), but merely classify a person as having followed or not followed some of the regimen (Burke & Dunbar-Jacob, 1995). Second, although biochemical assays offer a direct and objective approach to the measurement of nonadherence, this method is neither affordable nor available for every drug, is applicable only to medications with a long half-life, and may vary from individual to individual (de Geest, Abraham, & Dunbar-Jacob, 1996). Third, physiologic technologies are often unable to detect dosage levels. For example, many asthma medications are so rapidly absorbed systemically that it is not possible to detect them by biochemical assay (Rand & Wise, 1994). Finally, accurate detection of nonadherence through drug-level testing offers no explanation or insight into the reasons for nonadherence (Besch, 1995).

In the end, no single measure of adherence can compete with the accuracy of a multi-method approach that combines feasible self-reporting and reasonable objective measures amidst an effective patient–provider relationship (Bosworth, 2010). Assessment should also lead to a determination of the proper focus of adherence-increasing strategies. It was mentioned earlier that the notion of adherence as self-care may be too restrictive in situations where adherence with medical regimens cannot be achieved without the assistance of others. For instance, the combination of marked disability and chronic illness makes the conceptualization of adherence as self-care ability inappropriate. In such instances, a social support network may be the most important influence on adherence and, therefore, should become the focus

of adherence-increasing strategies. However, the nurse should carefully assess the impact of social support on adherence. Although social support—by significant others or through support networks—may help patients cope with chronic illness and reinforce adherence behavior in some populations (McWilliam, 2009), this relationship may not hold true for all individuals, because patients do not always want or cannot always receive tangible help from others.

Interventions to Enhance Behavior

The complexity of the variables associated with nonadherence should not deter the healthcare professional from working with the patient to achieve maximum possible integration of optimal health recommendations. To accomplish maximum adherence, those who use adherence-increasing strategies have a responsibility to ensure the patient's safety and comprehension. For the nurse, who frequently serves as liaison between patient and physician, communicating with either or both is often necessary before matters are sufficiently clear to select and begin specific adherence-increasing strategies. Enhancing adherence behaviors is not as simple as telling patients what to do and then telling them again when the desired effect is not achieved. It is necessary to understand that it is not the length of their life that is of concern to many people with chronic illness, but rather their perception that the recommended behavior change will be worth the effort (Rapley, 1997). Understanding and respecting the social, cultural, and psychological factors that influence adherence behaviors may enhance efforts to manage the problem of nonadherence. Furthermore, the patient or caregiver simply may not understand, or remember, instructions. If patients lack the knowledge or skills to undertake a recommended behavior or treatment, it is unlikely that they will do so. Instructions related to treatment regimens need to be reinforced continually over time to enhance adherence behaviors.

It is generally believed that adherence increases when patients actively participate in learning and deciding how to implement prescribed regimens. However, insistence by the healthcare professional on a preconceived or stereotyped notion of the most desirable level of participation may be inappropriate. A mismatch between an authoritarian provider and an assertive, active learner may influence adherence adversely. Conversely, the provider who expects an active involvement process can overwhelm a passive and nonactive learner.

The power differential between patients and providers constitutes an important aspect of adherence behaviors. It has been posited that providers inadvertently transmit their expectations to their patients, and that this subtle projection may be even more determinative for health effects than the expectations of the patient (McWilliam, 2009; Van Dulmen & Bensing, 2002). A clinician's belief in his or her own ability to enhance adherence significantly predicts actual efforts to enhance adherence and raises expectations about adherence outcomes (Byrne, Deane, & Caputi, 2008). Interestingly, empathy for the patient on the part of the provider has been shown to lower adherence expectations, possibly indicating that understanding the difficulty in adhering to medications reduces the provider's belief in his or her ability to effect change (Byrne et al., 2008).

Enhancing a patient's motivation requires careful assessment of his or her readiness to make and maintain behavioral changes. Building skills requires that the patient be ready to learn tasks such as reading food labels, selecting appropriate foods in restaurants, and incorporating the taking of medications into his or her daily routine. In other words, patients must learn new strategies to help them adopt and maintain new behaviors, especially when their daily routines are interrupted (Bandura, 1997; Barnestein-Fonseca et al., 2011; Miller, Hill, Kottke, & Ockene, 1997).

There is universal agreement that it is important for patients with chronic illness to follow evidence-based provider recommendations

(WHO, 2003). To enhance adherence to treatment, healthcare professionals can employ a variety of strategies. Some of these strategies are educational, some are behavioral, and some are organizational. WHO (2003) has suggested adopting the use of the five "As" to assist patients with self-management of their chronic disease: assess, advise, agree, assist, and arrange (Locke & Latham, 2002). Advising the patient of the importance of treatment adherence, establishing agreement with a treatment plan, and arranging adequate follow-up are necessary steps for healthcare professionals who are interested in providing treatment adherence interventions to their patients. Additionally, four phases of treatment adherence have been identified—contemplating, initiating, maintaining, and sustaining long-term behavior—with each phase having different barriers and facilitators (Bosworth, 2010). Discrepancies between a patient's stage of treatment adherence and a provider's intervention may yield nonadherence due to a patient's lack of readiness for the intervention. The interventions suggested in this chapter are adaptable within these frameworks.

Education and Coaching

Educational interventions should be developed based on an assessment of the patient's level of knowledge, cultural background, and particular goals. Educational information should be presented in manageable segments, with additional information and reinforcement being provided at subsequent meetings. The nurse should focus on key issues in the management of the regimen and should select the most important aspects necessary for health maintenance. Difficult skills should be demonstrated, and then the patient is allowed to practice and perform a return demonstration. Difficult skills should also be reviewed each time the patient visits.

Written material should be geared to the patient's reading level and language. Glazer, Kirk, and Bosler (1996) evaluated printed materials to teach breast self-examination and found that, although the materials provided were written at a ninth-grade reading level, the average reading level of the target population was the sixth grade. Health information has not improved over the past decade (Ngoh, 2009). Another study on health literacy found that 24% of patients could not understand even the most basic written medication instructions and that an additional 12% had very limited literacy (Gazmararian, Williams, Peel, & Baker, 2003). These findings underscore the need to prepare materials that can be used by the maximum number of patients. Other educational materials can be provided, such as videotapes, audiotapes, and computer-assisted instruction.

Health numeracy is the capacity of an individual to assess, process, interpret, communicate, and act on numerical quantitative, graphical, biostatistical, and probabilistic health information so as to make effective health decisions (Golbeck, Ahlers-Schmidt, Paschal, & Dismuke, 2005). Examples of numeracy include being able to understand food labels; manage weights, portions, and size estimations; and interpret blood sugar or blood pressure readings (Cavanaugh et al., 2008; Huizinga, Beech, Cavanaugh, Elasy, & Rothman, 2008).

While health numeracy is discussed less than literacy, it is a skill of equal importance when self-management, family involvement in management of a loved one's health, and adherence behaviors are at stake (Gaglio, Glasgow, & Bull, 2012).

Often patients rely on family members to interpret regimen details at home and may feel embarrassed about their issues with health literacy (Williams et al., 2007). Therefore, when educating those with chronic illnesses, family members or significant others should be involved in the teaching session. Emphasis in teaching needs to be directed toward not only knowledge of the disease, but also the skills needed for the regimen (Burke & Dunbar-Jacob, 1995; Morello, Chynoweth, Kim, Singh, & Hirsch, 2011). In addition, the regimen should be simplified as much as possible.

Given the recognition of the prevalence and complexity of managing chronic illness, nurses are increasingly being trained in coaching techniques. Health coaching, whether carried out by nurses or by other healthcare professionals, utilizes multiple consultations between the participant and coach to improve disease management (Melko, Terry, Camp, Xi, & Healey, 2010). Coaching has been effective in improving patients' adherence to diabetes regimens, obesity treatment, and adoption of healthier lifestyle habits, including diet, physical activity, weight management, medication adherence, tobacco cessation, avoidance of excess alcohol consumption, and preventive healthcare practices (DiLillo, Siegfried, & West, 2003; Olsen & Nesbitt, 2010; Palmer, Tubbs, & Whybrow, 2003; Schafer, Koltes, Anderson, Rickheim, & Kendall, 2005; Vincent & Birkhead, 2013; Whittemore, Melkus, Sullivan, & Grey, 2004). Numerous coaching techniques and theoretical frameworks inform various coaching practices, but generally have their foundation in the chronic care model. Health coaching utilizes motivational interviewing and cognitive-behavioral therapeutic techniques to improve self-efficacy. Wong-Rieger and Rieger (2013) have identified the following health coaching principles as being most often utilized:

- The patient is the best source of information for personal behavior change strategies.
- Education is provided when the patient is ready.
- Goals are aligned with the patient's vision of health and personal values.
- Emphasis is placed on how to change behavior, not why current behaviors exist.
- Plans are established for how to deal with setbacks.
- The coach reinforces accountability using the patient's own values and stories.
- Only the patient is able to choose goals that are the most motivating.
- Priorities are established by balancing long-term vision and what is most salient in the patient's present life.
- Patience and belief in the patient are critical to establish trust in the coaching relationship.
- Coaches guide patients in linking behavior change to their life purpose.

Strategies such as motivational interviewing have also been used successfully by healthcare professionals who are advocating health behavior change (Carels et al., 2007; Cook, Emiliozzi, & McCabe, 2007). Motivational interviewing is a "client-centered, directive style for enhancing intrinsic motivation to change by exploring and resolving ambivalence" (Miller & Rollnick, 2002, as cited in Lane & Rollnick, 2009, p. 154). Through the utilization of four core principles, practitioners can harness the spirit of motivational interviewing and guide patients toward greater self-motivated change: expressed empathy, rolling with resistance, supporting self-efficacy, and developing discrepancy (the last means discovering how one's personal values are at odds with current behavior through careful listening). Through the use of open-ended questions, summarizing, reflective listening directed toward empathy, and eliciting "change talk," practitioners can gain an understanding of the importance of change to a patient and determine how much confidence the patient has in his or her ability to effect such change (Rollnick, Butler, Kinnersley, Gregory, & Mash, 2010). Motivational interviewing was originally developed for the treatment of addictions (Levensky, Forcehimes, O'Donohue, & Beitz, 2007), but has since been modified for use in different contexts, including adaptation to the healthcare setting, sometimes termed "behavior change counseling" (Lane & Rollnick, 2009). This technique—whether termed motivational interviewing or behavior change counseling—has been used effectively to realize better treatment adherence through improving body mass index, cholesterol, and systolic blood pressure (Lane & Rollnick, 2009); hypertension, diet and exercise regimens, and smoking cessation (Anshel & Kang, 2008; Levensky et al., 2007); asthma medication adherence (Borelli et al., 2007); and weight loss in diabetic women (West, DiLillo, Bursac, Gore, & Greene, 2007).

Abilities beyond knowledge and comprehension are required as well. Therefore, educational goals must be broader than solely the acquisition of knowledge if adherence is to result from the intervention. The outcome of adherence depends on participation of the learner beyond simply listening, reading, or assimilating information. That is, clinicians should encourage patients' participation in their own care. Flexible self-care regimens enable people to exercise a larger degree of autonomy than is incorporated in standard regimens, even when these regimens are adapted to some extent for individuals. The flexibility of instructions, such as "If you have this sign or this symptom, then try this activity," allows people some freedom to make informed choices, and having choices fosters independence and a better quality of life (McWilliam, 2009; Rapley, 1997).

Behavioral Strategies to Enhance Adherence

Behavioral strategies attempt to influence specific adherence behaviors directly through the use of various techniques. These strategies may be used either as single interventions or in combination to achieve the desired results. Cognitive-behavioral techniques such as goal setting and self-monitoring, and behavioral techniques such as cueing, chaining (associating new behaviors with established ones), positive reinforcement, and patient contracting are a few examples of strategies that have demonstrated a positive impact on adherence behaviors (Rains, Penzien, & Lipchik, 2006). Interventions employing education with behavioral support with continued contact over several weeks or months via phone, mail, and/or video have shown the greatest success in increasing medication compliance across several diseases, including hypertension, hyperlipidemia, heart failure, and myocardial infarction (Viswanathan et al., 2012).

Tailoring

At a minimum, the outcome of patient participation with the nurse in developing an adherence strategy should be tailoring of the treatment to the patient's needs, preferences, daily behaviors, and cultural values. Patient-centered tailored interventions are probably necessary for improved treatment adherence, as no single intervention strategy has been shown to be effective across all patients, conditions, and settings (Bosworth, 2010). Effectively tailored treatment regimens incorporate strategies that address unique barriers such as intermittent illness, the burden of caregiving, and changing schedules. Integrating treatment activities so that they coincide with routine activities is an important way of individualizing and enhancing the treatment plan. The daily schedule of eating, arising and retiring, hygiene, favorite television program, and so on, identifies rituals that may be used to incorporate health behaviors into daily life.

Ongoing contact with the healthcare professional also improves adherence within a tailored intervention. Such continuity allows the patient and healthcare professional to assess changes in the patient's stage of readiness for adopting the recommended behavioral activities. Tailoring adherence-oriented interventions toward an individual can be accomplished through written materials, phone contact, text and email messaging, and the Internet (Hugtenburg, Timmers, Elders, Vervloet, & van Dijk, 2013). Interventions also need to be targeted to barriers that inhibit adherence, such as cognitive deficits, stigma, social barriers, lack of autonomy, medication side effects, and absence of symptoms.

Simplifying the Regimen

As a result of discussions between patient and nurse, it may become apparent that the patient is unable to manage the complexity of the prescribed regimen. Negotiation with the prescribing source may result in better adherence if this barrier is cleared away and the regimen is simplified. As a general rule, the number of times medications are taken and the number of doses should be kept to a minimum (Schernthaner, 2010).

Providing Reminders

Reminders or memory aids are useful when the problem is a failure of the behavior to occur because patients have forgotten to perform one or more aspects of the desired behavior. Calendars, clocks, and individually prepared posters with medication and food reminders can be very helpful in this regard. Separating a day's supply of medications can also help the person who has difficulty remembering if a particular dose was taken.

The healthcare professional can reinforce the importance of adherence at episodic visits. Such reinforcement may involve pill counting, attention to patient diaries or to other reports of behavior, and self-monitoring. All of these methods are intended to remind the patient of the value of adherence and elicit participation.

Reminder interventions that include all manner of methods (telephone, text, email, pagers, interactive voice response systems, videotelephone calls, and programmed electronic audiovisual reminder devices) can effectively improve treatment adherence, although not all methods are practical or economical (Fenerty, West, Davis, Kaplan, & Feldman, 2012). Progressive telephone calls have been shown to be superior to one-time brief educational sessions in increasing self-care behaviors among patients with heart failure (Baker et al., 2011); in encouraging adherence with medications in the elderly (Doggrell, 2010); and in promoting adherence among low-income, minority populations with diabetes (Walker, Shmukler, Ullman, Blanco, Scollan-Koliopoulus, & Cohen, 2011). Bosworth and colleagues (2008) used a telephone intervention for patients with hypertension and found a significant change in medication-taking behavior. The use of text messaging to adolescents with diabetes increased disease self-efficacy and adherence to the medical regimen (Franklin, Waller, Pagliari, & Greene, 2006). SMS intervention (text messaging) in sub-Saharan Africa also improved patients' adherence to antiretroviral therapy, perhaps through an improved patient–provider relationship (Chi & Stringer, 2010; Lester et al., 2010).

Ethnocultural Interventions

Recognition that the patient's and family's patterns of communication may differ from the provider's own pattern is important to ensure effective interactions. In addition, cultural components need to be integrated into any strategies that are proposed. Attention to some basics in delivering culturally competent care can enhance treatment adherence. Most of these strategies have been addressed in other documents—for example, *Healthy People 2020*. One goal for providers is to eliminate the disparities that currently exist in providing care, thereby improving health for all. Flaskerud (2007) acknowledges that the provision of culturally competent care rests on the shoulders of the healthcare provider. Therefore, it is up to healthcare professionals, on an individual basis, to include these key ingredients in their practices:

- Ask about health practices that may interfere with a treatment regimen.
- Seek understanding when a patient says something that you do not understand.
- Acknowledge to patients that there may be additions to recommendations that stem from culture and tradition, and inquire about these.
- Listen carefully to verbal communication and pay close attention to nonverbal communication.

For effective interaction with persons of a different culture, "cultural translation" may be needed. One requisite for a cultural translator is learning about the historical rituals and norms that relate to health of the particular group. Another requisite is evaluating health behaviors in the patient's cultural context to determine competing priorities, environmental obstacles, or degree of knowledge and skills (George, 2001). One cultural intervention study successfully improved tuberculosis (TB) medication adherence among Latino immigrants by building relationships and implementing Latino values of personal attention (seeing the same nurse during the 9-month treatment period), asking about family members, incorporating a common Latino proverb into each session (translating to "It is better to prevent than to lament"), adapting written materials to be easily understood (in Spanish at a sixth-grade level) with photos of Latino families, and use of culturally appropriate, nonverbal language of touching the arm of the woman or shoulder of the man at the end of each visit (Ailinger et al., 2010).

Healthcare professionals need to recognize that *their* belief system, values, and attitudes toward healthcare management are also culturally determined and may be responsible for ideologic or philosophic differences (McWilliam, 2009). The emphasis on self-care in Western medical systems is ideologically consistent with the value of individual enterprise in Western cultures (Anderson, Tang, & Blue, 2007). Persons of other cultures, however, may find this value of self-care to be foreign.

Outcomes

There has been a blossoming interest in documenting the evidence of particular strategies to improve health outcomes. Evidence-based practice guidelines for a variety of physiologic and behavioral interventions are now readily available to all healthcare practitioners (through the Agency for Healthcare Research and Quality, National Guideline Clearinghouse). This means that what we recommend to patients is based on evidence of efficacy. Nevertheless, we continue to face the challenge of helping patients follow recommendations. No matter the quality of our interventions, they will be beneficial only if patients actually use them. It is up to healthcare professionals to more effectively assess whether patients can do what we suggest, and then to evaluate the outcomes.

Evidence-Based Practice Box

Purpose: The purpose of this study was to assess the effect of a community health worker (CHW) intervention on blood pressure and HgbA$_{1c}$ levels on Mexican American adults with diabetes.

Method: The participants were randomized to either an attention control group or an intervention group. The attention control group received a bilingual newspaper about diabetes care. Subjects assigned to the treatment group received the intervention described as follows.

Sample: The study enrolled 144 adults with type 2 diabetes who were taking at least one oral hypoglycemic medication. Study participants were followed for 2 years.

Intervention: Members of the intervention group received 36 home visits from a CHW over the 2 years of the study. The intervention consisted of a behavioral self-management program derived from the American Academy of Diabetes Educators. CHWs were bilingual Mexican Americans working for a nonprofit agency who received extensive training before the intervention was initiated.

Results and Implications for Nursing Practice: Participants visited by CHW had lower HgbA$_{1c}$ levels in years 1 and 2 compared to the control group subjects. There was no effect on blood pressure between the two groups. The use of CHWs is an important and effective mechanism for chronic disease management and should be implemented by those caring for patients with diabetes.

Source: Rothschild, S. K., Martin, M. A., Swider, S. M., Tumialán Lynas, C. M., Janssen, I., Avery, E. F., & Powell, L. H. (2013). Mexican American trial of community health workers: A randomized controlled trial of a community health worker intervention for Mexican Americans with Type 2 diabetes mellitus. *American Journal of Public Health.* doi: 10.2105/AJPH2013.301439.

STUDY QUESTIONS

1. Why is trying to increase adherence behaviors important for patients with chronic illness?
2. Which factors are involved in adhering to medical regimens? Discuss them.
3. How prevalent is nonadherence? Can you think of examples from your own practice?
4. How does adherence behavior affect evidence-based practice?
5. Which ethical issues arise when a healthcare professional tries to increase a patient's adherence behavior? Discuss an ethical approach.
6. Using your own or a patient's culture, identify how norms, rituals, and practices affect adherence with healthcare recommendations.
7. What are the strengths and weaknesses of education as a means of increasing adherence?
8. How does health literacy influence adherence behavior?
9. How can you encourage patient participation to increase adherence? Discuss tailoring, simplifying the regimen, and reminders.
10. How can you enhance coping to increase adherence?
11. What are the advantages and disadvantages of support groups to aid adherence behavior?

References

Ailinger, R. L., Martyn, D., Lasus, H., & Lima Garcia, N. (2010). Populations at risk across the lifespan: Population studies: The effect of a cultural intervention on adherence to latent tuberculosis infection therapy in Latino immigrants. *Public Health Nursing, 27*(2), 115–120.

Ajzen, I. (1985). From intention to action: A theory of planned behavior. In J. Kuhl & J. Beckman (Eds.), *Action control: From cognition to behavior* (pp. 11–39). Heidelberg, Germany: Springer.

Akincigil, A., Bowblis, J. R., Levin, C., Walkup, J. T., Jan, S., & Crystal, S. (2007). Adherence to antidepressant treatment among privately insured patients diagnosed with depression. *Medical Care, 45*(4), 363–369.

Anderson, J. M., Tang, S., & Blue, C. (2007). Health care reform and the paradox of efficiency: "Writing in" culture. *International Journal of Health Services, 37*(2), 291–320.

Anshel, M., & Kang, M. (2008). Effectiveness of motivational interviewing on changes in fitness, blood lipids, and exercise adherence of police officers: An outcome-based action study. *Journal of Correctional Health Care, 14*(1), 48–62.

Arturi, P., Schneeberger, E. E., Sommerfleck, F., Buschiazzo, E., Ledesma, C., Cocco, J. A. M., & Citera, G. (2013). Adherence to treatment in patients with ankylosing spondylitis. *Clinical Rheumatology, 32*(7), 1007–1015.

Baker, D. W., DeWalt, D. A., Schillinger, D., Hawk, V., Ruo, B., Bibbins-Domingo, K., … Pignone, M. (2011). The effect of progressive, reinforcing telephone education and counseling versus brief educational intervention on knowledge, self-care behaviors and heart failure symptoms. *Journal of Cardiac Failure, 17*(10), 789–796.

Bandura, A. (1997). *Self-efficacy: The exercise of control.* New York, NY: W. H. Freeman.

Bandura, A. (2004). Swimming against the mainstream: The early years from chilly tributary to transformative mainstream. *Behavior Research and Therapy, 42*(6), 613–630.

Barfod, T. S., Hecht, F. M., Rubow, C., & Gerstoft, J. (2006). Physicians' communication with patients about adherence to HIV medication in San Francisco and Copenhagen: A qualitative study using grounded theory. *BMC Health Services Research, 6*, 154.

Barnestein-Fonseca, P., Leiva-Fernández, J., Vidal-España, F., García-Ruiz, A., Prados-Torres, D., & Leiva-Fernández, F. (2011). Efficacy and safety of a multifactor intervention to improve therapeutic adherence in patients with chronic obstructive pulmonary disease (COPD): Protocol for the ICEPOC study. *Trials, 14*(12), 40.

Baroletti, S., & Dell'Orfano, H. (2010). Medication adherence in cardiovascular disease. *Circulation, 121*(12), 1455–1458.

Baumann, L. J., Cameron, L. D., Zimmerman, R. S., & Leventhal, H. (1989). Illness representations and matching labels with symptoms. *Health Psychology, 8*(4), 449–469.

Beach, M. C., Keruly, J., & Moore, R. D. (2006). Is the quality of the patient–provider relationship associated with better adherence and health outcomes for patients with HIV? *Journal of General Internal Medicine, 21*(6), 661–665.

Beals, K. P., Wight, R. G., Aneshensel, C. S., Murphy, D. A., & Miller-Martinez, D. (2006). The role of family caregivers in HIV medication adherence, *AIDS Care, 18*(6), 589–596.

Becker, M. H. (1976). Socio-behavioral determinants of compliance. In D. L. Sackett & R. Haynes (Eds.), *Compliance with therapeutic regimens* (pp. 40–50). Baltimore, MD: Johns Hopkins University Press.

Becker, M. H., & Maiman, L. A. (1975). Sociobehavioral determinants of compliance with health and medical care recommendations. *Medical Care, 13*, 10–24.

Berben, L., Dobbels, F., Engberg, S., Hill, M. N., & De Geest, S. (2012). An ecological perspective on medication adherence. *Western Journal of Nursing Research, 34*(5), 635–653.

Berg, J., Nyamathi, A., Christiani, A., Morisky, D., & Leake, B. (2005). Predictors of screening results for depressive symptoms among homeless adults in Los Angeles with latent tuberculosis. *Research in Nursing & Health, 28*(3), 220–229.

Berg, K. M., & Arnstein, J. H. (2006). Practical and conceptual challenges in measuring antiretroviral adherence. *Journal of Acquired Immune Deficiency Syndromes, 43*(suppl 1), 79–87.

Bernardini, J. (2004). Ethical issues of compliance/adherence in the treatment of hypertension. *Advances in Chronic Kidney Disease, 11*(2), 222–227.

Besch, C. L. (1995). Compliance in clinical trials. *AIDS, 9*(1), 1–10.

Blakeman, T., Bower, P., Reeves, D., & Chew-Graham, C. (2010). Bringing self-management into clinical view: A qualitative study of long-term condition management in primary care consultations. *Chronic Illness, 6*(2), 136–150.

Blaschke, T. F., Osterberg, L., Vrijens, B., & Urquhart, J. (2012). Adherence to medications: Insights arising from studies on the unreliable link between prescribed and actual drug dosing histories. *Annual Review of Pharmacology and Toxicology, 52*, 275–301.

Borrelli, B., Riekert, K. A., Weinstein, A., & Rathier, L. (2007). Brief motivational interviewing as a clinical strategy to promote asthma medication adherence. *Journal of Allergy and Clinical Immunology, 120*(5), 1023–1030.

Bosworth, H. B. (2010). *Improving patient treatment adherence: A clinician's guide.* New York, NY: Springer.

Bosworth, H. B., Olsen, M. K., Neary, A., Orr, M., Grubber, J., Svetkey, L., ... Oddone, E.Z.. (2008). Take Control of Your Blood Pressure (TCYB) study: A multifactorial tailored behavioral and educational intervention for achieving blood pressure control. *Patient Education and Counseling, 70*(3), 338–347.

Brandes, K., & Mullan, B. (2013). Can the common-sense model predict adherence in chronically ill patients? A meta-analysis. *Health Psychology Review*, 1–25. Epub ahead of print.

Breland, J. Y., McAndrew, L. M., Burns, E., Leventhal, E. A., & Leventhal, H. (2013). Using the common sense model of self-regulation to review the effects of self-monitoring of blood glucose on glycemic control for non–insulin-treated adults with type 2 diabetes. *Diabetes Educator, 39*(4), 541–559.

Burke, L. E., & Dunbar-Jacob, J. (1995). Adherence to medication, diet and activity recommendations: From assessment to maintenance. *Journal of Cardiovascular Nursing, 9*(2), 62–79.

Burrows, J. A., Bunting, J. P., Masel, P. J., & Bell, S. C. (2002). Nebulised dornase alpha: Adherence in adults with cystic fibrosis. *Journal of Cystic Fibrosis, 1*(4), 255–259.

Byrne, M., Deane, F., & Caputi, P. (2008). Mental health clinicians' beliefs about medicines, attitudes, and expectations of improved medication adherence in patients. *Evaluation & the Health Professions, 31*(4), 390–403.

Cabrera, D. M., Morisky, D. E., & Chin, S. (2002). Development of a tuberculosis education booklet for Latino immigrant patients. *Patient Education and Counseling, 46*(2), 117–124.

Carels, R. A., Darby, L., Cacciapaglia, H. M., Konrad, K., Coit, C., Harper, J., . . Versland, A.. (2007). Using motivational interviewing as a supplement to obesity treatment: A stepped-care approach. *Health Psychology, 26*(3), 369–374.

Carney, R. M., Freedland, K. E., Eisen, S. A., Rich, M. W., & Jaffe, A. S. (1995). Major depression and medication adherence in elderly patients with coronary artery disease. *Health Psychology, 14*(1), 88–90.

Carney, R. M., Freedland, K. E., Eisen, S. A., Rich, M. W., Skala, J. A., & Jaffe, A. S. (1998). Adherence to

a prophylactic medication regimen in patients with symptomatic versus asymptomatic ischemic heart disease. *Behavioral Medicine, 24*(1), 35–39.

Cavanaugh, K., Huizinga, M. M., Wallston, K. A., Gebretsadik, T., Shintani, A., Davis, D., ... Rothman, R. L. (2008). Association of numeracy and diabetes control. *Annals of Internal Medicine, 148*, 737–746.

Chen, S. L., Tsai, J. C., & Chou, K. R. (2011). Illness perceptions and adherence to therapeutic regimens among patients with hypertension: A structural modeling approach. *International Journal of Nursing Studies, 48*(2), 235–245.

Chesney, M. (2003). Adherence to HAART regimens. *AIDS Patient Care and STDs, 17*(4), 169–177.

Chi, B. H., & Stringer, J. S. (2010). Mobile phones to improve HIV treatment adherence. *Lancet, 376*(9755), 1807–1808.

Chilton, L., Hu, J., & Wallace, D. C. (2006). Health-promoting lifestyle and diabetes knowledge in Hispanic American adults. *Home Health Care Management Practice, 18*, 378–385.

Choudhry, N. K., Fischer, M. A., Avorn, J., Liberman, J. N., Schneeweiss, S., Pakes, J., ... Shrank, W. H. (2011). The implications of therapeutic complexity on adherence to cardiovascular medications. *Archives of Internal Medicine, 171*(9), 814–822.

Cohen, S. M. (2009). Concept analysis of adherence in the context of cardiovascular risk reduction. *Nursing Forum, 44*(1), 15–36.

Cook, N., Kobetz, E., Reis, I., Fleming, L., Loer-Martin, D., & Amofah, S. A. (2010). Role of patient race/ethnicity, insurance and age on Pap smear compliance across ten community health centers in Florida. *Ethnic Disease, 20*(4), 321–326.

Cook, P. F., Emiliozzi, S., & McCabe, M. M. (2007). Telephone counseling to improve osteoporosis treatment adherence: An effectiveness study in community practice settings. *American Journal of Medical Quality, 22*(6), 445–456.

Cooper, L. (2009). A 41-year-old African American man with poorly controlled hypertension: Review of patient and physician factors related to hypertension treatment adherence. *Journal of the American Medical Association, 301*(12), 1260–1284.

Corbin, J. A., & Strauss, A. L. (1985). Managing chronic illness at home: Three lines of work. *Qualitative Sociology, 8*(3), 224–247.

Cramer, J. A. (2004). A systematic review of adherence with medications for diabetes. *Diabetes Care, 27*(5), 1218–1224.

Cramer, J., Vachon, L., Desforges, C., & Sussman, N. (1995). Dose frequency and dose interval compliance with multiple antiepileptic medications during a controlled clinical trial? *Epilepsia, 36,* 1111–1117.

Curry, S., & Fitzgibbon, M. (2009). Theories of prevention. In S. A. Schumaker, J. K. Ockene, & K. A. Riekert (Eds.), *The handbook of health behavior change* (3rd ed., pp. 3–17). New York, NY: Springer.

Daniels, T., Goodacre, L., Sutton, C., Pollard, K., Conway, S., & Peckham, D. (2011). Accurate assessment of adherence to nebulizer treatments. Self-report and clinical report vs electronic monitoring of nebulizers. *Chest Journal, 140*(2), 425–432.

de Geest, S., Abraham, I., & Dunbar-Jacob, J. (1996). Measuring transplant patients' compliance with immunosuppressive therapy. *Western Journal of Nursing Research, 18*(5), 595–605.

de Klerk, E., & van der Linden, S. (1996). Compliance monitoring of NSAID drug therapy in ankylosing spondylitis, experiences with an electronic monitoring device. *British Journal of Rheumatology, 35,* 60–65.

Demyttenaere, K., Van Ganse, E., Gregoire, J., Gaens, E., & Mesters, P. (1998). Compliance with depressed patients treated with fluoxetine or amitriptyline. *International Clinical Psychopharmacology, 13*(1), 11–17.

Desroches, S., Lapointe, A., Ratté, S., Gravel, K., Légaré, F., & Turcotte, S. (2013). Interventions to enhance adherence to dietary advice for preventing and managing chronic diseases in adults. *Cochrane Database of Systematic Reviews, 2,* CD008722. doi: 10.1002/14651858.CD008722. pub2

De Vito Dabbs, A., Dew, M. A., Myers, B., Begey, A., Hawkins, R., Ren, D., ... McCurry, K.R. (2009). Evaluation of a hand-held, computer-based intervention to promote early self-care behaviors after lung transplant. *Clinical Transplantation, 23*(4), 537–545.

D'hooghe, M. B., Nagels, G., De Keyser, J., & Haentjens, P. (2013). Self-reported health promotion and disability progression in multiple sclerosis. *Journal of the Neurological Sciences, 325*(1–2), 120–126.

DiLillo V., Siegfried N. J., & West, D. S. (2003) Incorporating motivational interviewing into behavioral obesity treatment. *Cognitive Behavioral Practice, 10,* 120–130.

DiMatteo, M. R. (2004). Variations in patients' adherence to medical recommendations: A quantitative review of 50 years of research. *Medical Care, 42*(3), 200–209.

DiMatteo, M. R., & Haskard, K. B. (2006). Further challenges in adherence research: Measurements, methodologies, and mental health care. *Medical Care, 44*(4), 300–303.

DiMatteo, M. R., Haskard, K. B., & Williams, S. L. (2007). Health beliefs, disease severity, and patient adherence: A meta-analysis. *Medical Care, 45*(6), 521–528.

DiMatteo, M. R., Haskard-Zolnierek, K. B., & Martin, L. R. (2012). Improving patient adherence: A three-factor model to guide practice. *Health Psychology Review, 6*(1), 74–91.

DiMatteo, M. R., Lepper, H. S., & Croghan, T. W. (2000). Depression is a risk factor for noncompliance with medical treatment. *Archives of Internal Medicine, 160,* 2101–2107.

Doggrell, S. A. (2010). Adherence to medicines in the older-aged with chronic conditions. *Drugs & Aging, 27*(3), 239–254.

Dunbar-Jacob, J., Burke, L. E., & Puczynski, S. (1995). Clinical assessment and management of adherence to medical regimens. In P. M. Nicassio & T. W. Smith (Eds.), *Managing chronic illness: A biopsychosocial perspective* (pp. 313–349). Washington, DC: American Psychological Association.

Dunbar-Jacob, J., Erlen, J. A., Schlenk, E. A., Ryan, C. M., Sereika, S. M., & Doswell, W. M. (2000). Adherence in chronic disease. *Annual Review of Nursing Research, 18,* 48–90.

Dunbar-Jacob, J., Gemmell, L. A., & Schlenk, E. A. (2009). Predictors of patient adherence: Patient characteristics. In S. A. Shumaker, J. K. Ockene, & K. A. Riekert (Eds.), *The handbook of health behavior change* (pp. 397–410). New York, NY: Springer.

Dunbar-Jacob, J., Holmes, J. L., Sereika, S., Kwoh, C. K., Burke, L. E., Starz, T. W., . . Foley, S.M. (2004). Factors associated with attrition of African Americans during the recruitment phase of a clinical trial examining adherence among individuals with rheumatoid arthritis. *Arthritis & Rheumatology, 51*(3), 422–428.

Dunbar-Jacob, J., & Schlenk, E. (2001). Patient adherence to treatment regimen. In A. Baum & T. Revenson (Eds.), *Handbook of health psychology* (pp. 321–657). Mahwah, NJ: Lawrence Erlbaum Associates.

Dunbar-Jacob, J., Schlenk, E., & Caruthers, D. (2002). Adherence in the management of chronic disorders. In A. Christensen & M. Antoni (Eds.), *Chronic physical disorders: Behavioral medicine's perspective* (pp. 69–82). Malden, MA: Blackwell.

Dunbar-Jacob, J., Schlenk, E., & McCall, M. (2012). Patient adherence to treatment regimen. In A. Baum, T. A. Revenson, & J. Singer (Eds.), *The handbook of health psychology* (pp. 271–292). New York, NY: Psychology Press.

Dunbar-Jacob, J., Sereika, S. M., Houze, M., Luyster, F. S., & Callan, J. A. (2012). Accuracy of measures of medication adherence in a cholesterol-lowering regimen. *Western Journal of Nursing Research, 34*(5), 578–597.

Duncan, J., & Rogers, R. (1998). Medication compliance in patients with chronic schizophrenia: Implications for the community management of mentally disordered offenders. *Journal of Forensic Sciences, 43,* 1133–1137.

Eiser, C., Hill, J. J., & Blacklay, A. (2000). Surviving cancer: What does it mean for you? An evaluation of a clinic based intervention for survivors of childhood cancer. *Psycho-Oncology, 9,* 214–220.

Elliott, R. (2008). Poor adherence to medication in adults with rheumatoid arthritis: Reasons and solutions. *Disease Management & Health Outcomes, 16*(1), 13–29.

Eng, J. J., & Martin Ginis, K. (2007). Using the theory of planned behavior to predict leisure time physical activity among people with chronic kidney disease. *Rehabilitation Psychology, 52*(4), 435–442.

Erdine, S., & Arslan, E. (2013). Monitoring treatment adherence in hypertension. *Current Hypertension Reports, 15*(4), 269–272.

Farley, J., Hines, S., Musk, A., Ferrus, S., & Tepper V. (2003). Assessment of adherence to antiviral therapy in HIV-infected children using the Medication Event Monitoring System, pharmacy refill, provider assessment, caregiver self-report, and appointment keeping. *Journal of Acquired Immune Deficiency Syndrome, 33,* 211–218.

Feachem, R. G., Sekhri, N. K., & White, K. L. (2002). Getting more for their dollar: A comparison of the NHS with California's Kaiser Permanente. *British Medical Journal, 324*(7330), 135–141.

Fenerty, S. D., West, C., Davis, S. A., Kaplan, S. G., & Feldman, S. R. (2012). The effect of reminder systems on patients' adherence to treatment. *Patient Prefer Adherence, 6,* 127–135.

Finley, C., Gregg, E. W., Solomon, L. J., & Gay, E. (2001). Disparities in hormone replacement therapy use by socioeconomic status in a primary care population. *Journal of Community Health, 26*(1), 39–50.

Fischer, M. A., Stedman, M.R., Lii, J., Vogeli, C., & & Shrank, W. H. (2010). Primary medication non-adherence: Analysis of 195,930 electronic prescriptions. *Journal of General Internal Medicine, 25*(4), 284–290.

Fishbein, M., & Ajzen, I. (1975). *Belief, attitude and intention: An introduction to theory and research.* Reading, MA: Addison-Wesley.

Flaskerud, J. H. (2007) Can we achieve it? *Issues in Mental Health Nursing, 28*(3), 309–311.

Fox, N., Hirsch-Allen, A. J., Goodfellow, E., Wenner, J., Fleetham, J., Ryan, C. F., ... Ayas, N. T. (2012). The impact of a telemedicine monitoring system on positive airway pressure adherence in patients with obstructive sleep apnea: A randomized controlled trial. *Sleep, 35*(4), 477.

Franklin, V. L., Waller, A., Pagliari, C., & Greene, S. A. (2006). A randomized controlled trial of Sweet Talk, a text-messaging system to support young people with diabetes. *Diabetic Medicine, 23*(12), 1332–1338.

Gadkari, A. S., & McHorney, C. A. (2010). Medication nonfulfillment rates and reasons: Narrative systematic review. *Current Medical Research & Opinion, 26*(3), 683–705.

Gaglio, B., Glasgow R. E., & Bull, S. S. (2012). Do patient preferences for health information vary by health literacy or numeracy? A qualitative assessment. *Journal of Health Communication, 17*(suppl 3), 109–121.

Gamble, J., Stevenson, M., McClean, E., & Heaney, L.G. (2009). The prevalence of non-adherence in difficult asthma. *American Journal of Respiratory and Critical Care Medicine, 180*(9), 817–822.

Garfield, S., Clifford, S., Eliasson, L., Barber, N., & Willson, A. (2011). Suitability of measures of self-reported medication adherence for routine clinical use: a systematic review. *BMC Medical Research Methodology, 11*(1), 149.

Gazmararian, J. A., Williams, M. V., Peel, J., & Baker, D. W. (2003). Health literacy and knowledge of chronic disease. *Patient Education and Counseling, 51*(3), 267–275.

George, M. (2001). The challenge of culturally competent health care: Applications for asthma. *Heart and Lung, 30*(5), 392–400.

Glazer, H., Kirk, L., & Bosler, F. (1996). Patient education pamphlets about prevention, detection, and treatment of breast cancer in low literacy women. *Patient Education and Counseling, 27,* 185–189.

Golbeck, A. L., Ahlers-Schmidt, C. R., Paschal, A. M., & Dismuke, S. E. (2005). A definition and operational framework for health numeracy. *American Journal of Preventive Medicine, 29,* 375–376.

Golin, C. E., Smith, S. R., & Reif, S. (2004). Adherence counseling practices of generalist and specialist physicians caring for people living with HIV/AIDS in North Carolina. *Journal of General Internal Medicine, 19*(1), 16–27.

Gonzalez, J. S., Penedo, F. J., Antoni, M. H., Durán, R. E., McPherson-Baker, S., Ironson, G., ... Schneiderman, N. (2004). Social support, positive states of mind, and HIV treatment adherence in men and women living with HIV/AIDS. *Health Psychology, 23*(4), 413–418.

Gould, K. A. (2011). A randomized controlled trial of a discharge nursing intervention to promote self-regulation of care for early discharge of interventional cardiology patients. *Dimensions of Critical Care Nursing. 30*(2), 117–125.

Gredig, D., Niderost, S., & Parpan-Blaser, A. (2006). HIV-protection through condom use: Testing the theory of planned behaviour in a community sample of heterosexual men in a high-income country. *Psychology & Health*, 21(5), 541–555.

Greene, J. A. (2004). "Noncompliance" enters the medical literature, 1955–1975. 2002 Roy Porter Memorial Prize Essay, Therapeutic Infidelities. *Social History of Medicine*, 17(3), 327–343.

Greenley, R. N., Josie, K. L., & Drotar, D. (2006). Perceived involvement in condition management among inner-city youth with asthma and their primary caregivers. *Journal of Asthma*, 43(9), 687–693.

Guindo, L. A., Wagner, M., Baltussen, R., Rindress, D., Van Til, J., Kind, P., & Goetghebeur, M. M. (2012). From efficacy to equity: Literature review of decision criteria for resource allocation and healthcare decision making. *Cost Effective Resource Allocation*, 10(1), 1–13.

Harley, A. E., Yang, M., Stoddard, A. M., Adamkiewicz, G., Walker, R., Tucker-Seeley, R. D., ... Sorensen, G. (2013). Patterns and predictors of health behaviors among racially/ethnically diverse residents of low-income housing developments. *American Journal of Health Promotion*. http://dx.doi.org/10.4278/ajhp.121009-QUAN-492

Harrington, R., Kerfoot, M., Dyer, E., McNiven, F., Gill, J., Harrington, V., ... Woodham, A.. (2000). Deliberate self-poisoning in adolescence: Why does a brief family intervention work in some cases and not others? *Journal of Adolescence*, 23, 13–20.

Haynes, R. B., McDonald, H. P., & Garg, A. X. (2002). Helping patients follow prescribed treatment. *Journal of the American Medical Association*, 288(22), 2880–2883.

Haynes, R. B., McDonald, H., Garg, A. X., & Montague, P. (2002). Interventions for helping patients to follow prescriptions for medications. *Cochrane Database of Systematic Reviews*, 2, CD000011. doi: 10.1002/14651858.CD000011

Healthy people 2020. (n.d.). http://www.healthypeople.gov/2020/default.aspx

Hiltunen, E. F., Winder, P. A., Rait, M. A., Buselli, E. F., Carroll, D. L., & Rankin, S. H. (2005). Implementation of efficacy enhancement nursing interventions with cardiac elders. *Rehabilitation Nursing*, 30(6), 221–229.

Hingson, R., Scotch, N., Sorenson, J., & Swazey, J. (1981). *In sickness and in health*. St. Louis, MO: Mosby.

Hinkin, C. H., Castellon, S. A., Durvasula, R. S., Hardy, D. J., Lam, M. N., Mason, K. I., ... Stefaniak, M.. (2002). Medication adherence among HIV positive adults: Effects of cognitive dysfunction and regimen complexity. *Neurology*, 59(12), 1944–1950.

Hinkin, C. H., Hardy, D. J., Mason, K. I., Castellon, S. A., Durvasula, R. S., Lam, M. N., ... Stefaniak, M..

(2004). Medication adherence in HIV-infected adults: Effect of patient age, cognitive status, and substance abuse. *AIDS*, 18(1), 19–25.

Hovell, M. F., Sipan, C. L., Blumberg, E. J., Hofstetter, C. R., Slymen, D., Friedman, L., ... Vera, A.Y. (2003). Increasing Latino adolescents' adherence to treatment for latent tuberculosis infection: A controlled trial. *American Journal of Public Health*, 93(11), 1871–1877.

Hugtenburg, J. G., Timmers, L., Elders, P. J., Vervloet, M., & van Dijk, L. (2013). Definitions, variants, and causes of nonadherence with medication: A challenge for tailored interventions. *Patient Preference and Adherence*, 7, 675.

Huizinga, M. M., Beech, B. M., Cavanaugh, K. L., Elasy, T. A., & Rothman, R. L. (2008). Low numeracy skills are associated with higher BMI. *Obesity*, 16, 1966–1968.

Jackson, R., Asimakopoulou, K., & Scammell, A. (2007). Assessment of the transtheoretical model as used by dietitians in promoting physical activity in people with type 2 diabetes. *Journal of Human Nutrition & Dietetics*, 20(1), 27–36.

Jaynes, R., & Rankin, S. (2001). Application of Leventhal's self-regulation model to Chinese immigrants with type 2 diabetes. *Journal of Nursing Scholarship*, 31, 333–338.

Jentzsch, N. S., Camargos, P. A. M., Colosimo, E. A., & Bousquet, J. (2009). Monitoring adherence to beclomethasone in asthmatic children and adolescents through four different methods. *Allergy*, 64(10), 1458–1462.

Jerant, A., Fiscella, K., Tancredi, D. J., & Franks, P. (2013). Health insurance is associated with preventive care but not personal health behaviors. *Journal of the American Board of Family Medicine*, 26(6), 759–767.

Johnson, M. O., Chesney, M. A., Goldstein, R. B., Remien, R. H., Catz, S., Gore-Felton, C., ... NIMH Healthy Living Project Team. (2006). Positive provider interactions, adherence self-efficacy, and adherence to antiretroviral medications among HIV-infected adults: A mediation model. *AIDS Patient Care and STDs*, 20(4), 258–268.

Johnson, S. S., Paiva, A. L., Cummins, C. O., Johnson, J. L., Dyment, S. J., Wright, J. A., .. Sherman, K. (2007). Transtheoretical model-based multiple behavior intervention for weight management: Effectiveness on a population basis. *Preventive Medicine*, 46(3), 238–246.

Jones, C. J., Smith, H., & Llewellyn, C. (2013). Evaluating the effectiveness of health belief model interventions in improving adherence: A systematic review. *Health Psychology Review*, 1–17. Epub ahead of print.

Kelly, M. A., Sereika, S. M., Battista, D. R., & Brown, C. (2007). The relationship between beliefs about depression and coping strategies: Gender differences. *British Journal of Clinical Psychology*, 46(3), 315–332.

Knafl, K. A., & Gilliss, C. L. (2002). Families and chronic illness: A synthesis of current research. *Journal of Family Nursing*, 8(3), 178–198.

Krapek, K., King, K., Warren, S. S., George, K. G., Caputo, D. A., Mihelich, K., ... Lubowski, T.J. (2004). Medication adherence and associated hemoglobin A_{1c} in type 2 diabetes. *Annals of Pharmacotherapy*, 38(9), 1357–1362.

Kristensen, L. E., Karlsson, J. A., Englund, M., Petersson, I. F., Saxne, T., & Geborek, P. (2010). Presence of peripheral arthritis and male sex predicting continuation of anti–tumor necrosis factor therapy in ankylosing spondylitis: An observational prospective cohort study from the South Swedish Arthritis Treatment Group Register. *Arthritis Care & Research*, 62(10), 1362–1369.

Kronish, I. M., Rieckmann, N., Halm, E. A., Shimbo, D., Vorchheimer, D., Haas, D. C., ... Davidson, K.W. (2006). Persistent depression affects adherence to secondary prevention behaviors after acute coronary syndromes. *Journal of General Internal Medicine*, 21(11), 1178–1183.

Laforest, L., Licaj, I., Devouassoux, G., Hartwig, S., Marvalin, S., & Van Ganse, E. (2013). Factors associated with early adherence to tiotropium in chronic obstructive pulmonary disease. *Chronic Respiratory Disease*, 10(1), 11–18.

Lane, C., & Rollnick, S. (2009). Motivational interviewing. In S. A. Shumaker, J. K. Ockene, & K. A. Riekert (Eds.), *The handbook of health behavior change* (3rd ed., pp. 151–167). New York, NY: Springer.

Lee, J. Y., Kusek, J. W., Greene, P. G., Bernhard, C., Norris, K., Smith, D., ... Wright, J.T.. (1996). Assessing medication adherence by pill count and electronic monitor in the African American study of kidney disease and hypertension (AASK) pilot study. *American Journal of Hypertension*, 9(8), 719–725.

Le, T. T., Bilderback, A., Bender, B., Wamboldt, F. S., Turner, C. F., Turner, C. F., Rand, C. S. ... Bartlett, S.J. (2008). Do asthma medication beliefs mediate the relationship between minority status and adherence to therapy? *Journal of Asthma*, 45(1), 33–37.

Lee, M. S., Lee, H. Y., Kang, S. G., Yang, J., Ahn, H., Rhee, M., ... Kim, S. H. (2010). Variables influencing antidepressant medication adherence for treating outpatients with depressive disorders. *Journal of Affective Disorders*, 123(1), 216–221.

Lee, Y. L., Santacroce, S. J., & Sadler, V. (2007). Predictors of healthy behavior in long-term survivors of childhood cancer. *Journal of Clinical Nursing*, 16(11a), 285–295.

Lehmann, A., Aslani, P., Ahmed, R., Celio, J., Gauchet, A., Bedouch, P., ... Schneider, M. P. (2014). Assessing medication adherence: Options to consider. *International Journal of Clinical Pharmacy*, 36(1), 55-69.

Lester, R. T., Ritvo, P., Mills, E. J., Kariri, A., Karanja, S., Chung, M. H., ... Plummer, F.A.. (2010). Effects of a mobile phone Short Message Service on antiretroviral treatment adherence in Kenya (WelTel Kenya1): A randomised trial. *Lancet*, 376(9755), 1838–1845.

Levensky, E. R., Forcehimes, A., O'Donohue, W. T., & Beitz, K. (2007). Motivational interviewing: An evidence-based approach to counseling helps patients follow treatment recommendations. *American Journal of Nursing*, 107(10), 50–58.

Leventhal, H., Brisette, I., & Leventhal, E. (2003). The common-sense model of self-regulation of health and illness. In L. Cameron (Ed.), *The self-regulation of health and illness behaviour* (pp. 42–65). New York, NY: Routledge.

Leventhal, H., Glynn, K., & Fleming, R. (1987). Is the smoking decision an "informed choice"? Effect of smoking risk factors on smoking beliefs. *Journal of the American Medical Association*, 257, 3373–3377.

Leventhal, H., Meyer, D., & Nerenz, D. (1980). The common sense representations of illness danger. In S. Rachman (Ed.), *Contributions to medical psychology* (pp. 27–30). Oxford, UK: Pergamon Press.

Lima, V. D., Geller, J., Bangsberg, D. R., Patterson, T. L., Daniel, M., Kerr, T., ... Hogg, R.S.. (2007). The effect of adherence on the association between depressive symptoms and mortality among HIV-infected individuals first initiating HAART. *AIDS*, 21(9), 1175–1183.

Liu, H., Miller, L. G., Hays, R. D., Wagner, G., Golin, C., & Hu, W. (2006). A practical method to calibrate self-reported adherence to antiretroviral therapy. *Journal of Acquired Immune Deficiency Syndromes*, 43(suppl 1), 104–112.

Locke, E. A., & Latham, G. P. (2002). Building a practically useful theory of goal setting and task motivation: A 35-year odyssey. *American Psychologist*, 57(9), 705–717.

Mansour, M. E., Lanphear, B. P., & DeWitt, T. G. (2000). Barriers to asthma care in urban children: Parent perspectives. *Pediatrics*, 106, 512–519.

Marston, M. (1970). Compliance with medical regimens: A review of the literature. *Nursing Research*, 19, 312–323.

Martin, J., Oliver, K., & McCaughtry, N. (2007). The theory of planned behavior: Predicting physical activity in Mexican American children. *Journal of Sport & Exercise Psychology, 29*(2), 225–232.

Mason, B., Matsayuma, J., & Jue, S. (1995). Assessment of sulfonylurea adherence and metabolic control. *Diabetes Educator, 21*, 52–57.

McCall, L. A., & Ginis, K. A. (2004). The effects of message framing on exercise adherence and health beliefs among patients in a cardiac rehabilitation program. *Journal of Applied Biobehavioral Research, 9*(2), 122–135.

McCann, T. V., & Lu, S. (2009). Medication adherence and significant others' support of consumers with schizophrenia in Australia. *Nursing and Health Sciences, 11*(3), 228–234.

McDonald, H. P., Garg, A. X., & Haynes, R. B. (2002). Interventions to enhance patient adherence to medication prescriptions: Scientific review. *Journal of the American Medical Association, 288*(22), 2868–2879.

McGlynn, E., Asch, S., Adams, J., Keesey, J., Hicks, J., & DeCristofaro, A. (2003). The quality of health care delivered to adults in the United States. *New England Journal of Medicine, 348*(26), 2635–2645.

McWilliam, C. L. (2009). Patients, persons or partners? Involving those with chronic disease in their care. *Chronic Illness, 5*(4), 277–292.

Melko, C. N., Terry, P. E., Camp, K., Xi, M., & Healey, M. L. (2010). Diabetes health coaching improves medication adherence: A pilot study. *American Journal of Lifestyle Medicine, 4*(2), 187–194.

Meyer, D., Leventhal, H., & Gutmann, M. (1985). Common-sense models of illness: The example of hypertension. *Health Psychology, 4*(2), 115–135.

Miller, N. H., Hill, M., Kottke, T., & Ockene, I. (1997). The multilevel compliance challenge: Recommendations for a call to action: A statement for healthcare professionals. *Circulation, 95*, 1085–1090.

Miller, W. R., & Rollnick, S. (2002). *Motivational interviewing: Preparing people for change.* New York, NY: Guilford Press.

Morello, C. M., Chynoweth, M., Kim, H., Singh, R. F., & Hirsch, J. D. (2011). Strategies to improve medication adherence reported by diabetes patients and caregivers: Results of a Taking Control of Your Diabetes survey. *Annals of Pharmacotherapy, 45*(2), 145–153.

Morisky, D., & DiMatteo, M. (2011). Improving the measurement of self-reported medication nonadherence: Response to authors. *Journal of Clinical Epidemiology, 64*(3), 255–257.

Mounier-Vehier, C., Bernaud, C., Carre, A., Lequeuche, B., Hotton, J. M., & Charpentier, J. C. (1998). Compliance and antihypertensive efficacy of amlodipine compared with nifedipine slow-release. *American Journal of Hypertension, 11*, 478–486.

Nakonezny, P. A., Hughes, C. W., Mayes, T. L., Sternweis-Yang, K. H., Kennard, B. D., Byerly, M. J., & Emslie, G. J. (2010). A comparison of various methods of measuring antidepressant medication adherence among children and adolescents with major depressive disorder in a 12-week open trial of fluoxetine. *Journal of Child and Adolescent Psychopharmacology, 20*(5), 431–439.

Ngoh, L. N. (2009). Health literacy: A barrier to pharmacist–patient communication and medication adherence. *Journal of the American Pharmacists Association, 49*(5), e132–e149.

Norman, P., Armitage, C. J., & Quigley, C. (2007). The theory of planned behavior and binge drinking: Assessing the impact of binge drinker prototypes. *Addictive Behaviors, 32*(9), 1753–1768.

Norman, P., & Conner, M. (2005). The theory of planned behavior and exercise: Evidence for the mediating and moderating roles of planning on intention–behavior relations. *Journal of Sport and Exercise Psychology, 27*, 488–504.

Ohm, R., & Aaronson, L. S. (2006). Symptom perception and adherence to asthma controller medications. *Journal of Nursing Scholarship, 38*(3), 292–297.

Okeke, C. O., Quigley, H. A., Jampel, H. D., Ying, G. S., Plyler, R. J., Jiang, Y., & Friedman, D. S. (2009). Adherence with topical glaucoma medication monitored electronically: The Travatan Dosing Aid study. *Ophthalmology, 116*,191–199.

Olsen, J. M., & Nesbitt, B. J. (2010). Health coaching to improve healthy lifestyle behaviors: An integrative review. *American Journal of Health Promotion, 25*(1), e1–e12.

O'Malley, A. S., Sheppard, V. B., Schwartz, M., & Mandelblatt, J. (2004). The role of trust in use of preventive services among low-income African-American women. *Preventive Medicine, 38*(6), 777–785.

Ortego, C., Huedo-Medina, T. B., Llorca, J., Sevilla, L., Santos, P., Rodríguez, E., ... Vejo, J. (2011). Adherence to highly active antiretroviral therapy (HAART): A meta-analysis. *AIDS and Behavior, 15*(7), 1381–1396.

Ott, J., Greening, L., Palardy, N., Holderby, A., & DeBell, W. K. (2000). Self efficacy as a mediator variable for adolescents' adherence to treatment for insulin dependent diabetes mellitus. *Children's Health Care, 29*, 47–63.

Paasche-Orlow, M. K., Cheng, D. M., Palepu, A., Meli, S., Faber, V., & Samet, J. H. (2006). Health literacy, antiretroviral adherence, and HIV-RNA suppression: A longitudinal perspective. *Journal of General Internal Medicine, 21*(8), 835–840.

Padden, D. L., Connors, R. A., Posey, S. M., Ricciardi, R., & Agazio, J. G. (2013). Factors influencing a health promoting lifestyle in spouses of active duty military. *Health Care for Women International, 34*(8), 674–693.

Palmer, S., Tubbs, I., & Whybrow, A. (2003). Health coaching to facilitate the promotion of healthy behaviors and achievement of health-related goals. *International Journal of Health Promotion Education, 41*, 91–93.

Paschal, A. M., Rush, S. E., & Sadler, T. (2013). Factors associated with medication adherence in patients with epilepsy and recommendations for improvement. *Epilepsy & Behavior, 31*, 346–350.

Patient Protection and Affordable Care Act, Section 3503, Public Law 111-148, 111th Cong., Stat. 119 (March 2010).

Pender, N. J. (1996). *Health promotion in nursing practice* (2nd ed.). Norwalk, CT: Appleton-Century-Crofts.

Pender, N. J., Murdaugh, C. L., & Parsons, M. A. (2001). *Health promotion in nursing practice.* Upper Saddle River, NJ: Prentice Hall.

Peeters, B., Van Tongelen, I., Roussery, K., Mehuys, E., Remon, J. P., & Willems, S. (2011). Factors associated with medication adherence to oral hypoglycemic agents in different ethnic groups suffering type 2 diabetes: A systematic literature review and suggestions for future research. *Diabetic Medicine, 28*(3), 262–275. doi: 10.1111/j.1464-5491.2010.03133.x

Prochaska, J., & DiClemente, C. (1983). Stages and processes of self-change of smoking: Toward an integrative model of change. *Journal of Consulting & Clinical Psychology, 51*, 390–395.

Quinn, J. R. (2005). Delay in seeking care for symptoms of acute myocardial infarction: Applying a theoretical model. *Research in Nursing & Health, 28*(4), 283–294.

Quittner, A. L., Modi, A. C., Lemanek, K. L., Ievers-Landis, C. E., & Rapoff, M. A. (2007). Evidence-based assessment of adherence to medical treatments in pediatric psychology. *Journal of Pediatric Psychology. 33*(9), 916–936.

Rains, J. C., Penzien, D. B., & Lipchik, G. L. (2006). Behavioral facilitation of medical treatment for headache. Part II: Theoretical models and behavioral strategies for improving adherence. *Headache, 46*(9), 1395–1403.

Rand, C. (2004). Non-adherence with asthma therapy: More than just forgetting. *Journal of Pediatrics, 146,* 157–159.

Rand, C. S., & Sevick, M. A. (2000). Ethics in adherence promotion and monitoring. *Controlled Clinical Trials, 21*(suppl 5), 241–247.

Rand, C. S., & Wise, R. A. (1994). Measuring adherence to asthma medication regimens. *American Review of Respiratory and Critical Care Medicine, 149,* 289–290.

Ransford, H. E., Carrillo, F. R., & Rivera, Y. (2010). Health care-seeking among Latino immigrants: Blocked access, use of traditional medicine, and the role of religion. *Journal of Health Care for the Poor and Underserved, 21*(3), 862–878.

Rapley, P. (1997). Self-care: Re-thinking the role of compliance. *Australian Journal of Advanced Nursing, 15,* 20–25.

Rapoff, M. A. (2010). *Adherence to pediatric medical regimens.* New York: Springer.

Rhee, H., Belyea, M. J., & Brasch, J. (2010) Family support and asthma outcomes in adolescents: Barriers to adherence as a mediator. *Journal of Adolescent Health, 47*(5), 472–478.

Riekert, K. A. (2009). Measurement. In S. A. Shumaker, J. K. Ockene, & K. A. Riekert (Eds.), *The handbook of health behavior change* (3rd ed., p. 307). New York, NY: Springer.

Rivers, D. A. (2007). *An examination of the relationship among patient factors, patient–physician interaction, and utilization of health services in adults with diabetes.* Doctoral dissertation, Texas A&M University, College Station, TX.

Rodríguez-Reimann, D. I., Nicassio, P., Reimann, J. O., Gallegos, P. I., & Olmedo, E. L. (2004). Acculturation and health beliefs of Mexican Americans regarding tuberculosis prevention. *Journal of Immigrant Health, 6*(2), 51–62.

Rollnick, S., Butler, C. C., Kinnersley, P., Gregory, J., & Mash, B. (2010). Motivational interviewing. *British Medical Journal, 340,* 1900.

Rosenstock, I. M. (1974). Historical origins of the health belief model. *Health Education Monographs, 2,* 354–386.

Roth, M. T., Ivey, J. L., Esserman, D. A., Crisp, G., Kurz, J., & Weinberger, M. (2013). Individualized medication assessment and planning: Optimizing medication use in older adults in the primary care setting. *Pharmacotherapy: The Journal of Human Pharmacology and Drug Therapy, 33*(8), 787–797.

Rothschild, S. K., Martin, M. A., Swider, S. M., Tumialan Lynas, C. M., Janssen, I., Avery, E. F., & Powell, L. H. (2013). Mexican American trial of community health workers: A randomized controlled trial of community health worker intervention for Mexican Americans with type 2 diabetes mellitus. *American Journal of Public Health,* (0), e1–e9. doi: 10.2105/AJPH.2013.301439

Sankar, A. P., Nevedal, D. C., Neufeld, S., & Luborsky, M. R. (2007). What is a missed dose? Implications for construct validity and patient adherence. *AIDS Care, 19*(6), 775–780.

Schafer, L. C., Koltes, L. D., Anderson, R. L., Rickheim, P. L., & Kendall, D. M. (2005). *Behavioral coaching improves diabetes management and A₁c in worksite settings.* Abstract 78-OR. Abstract presented at American Diabetes Association, San Diego, CA.

Schernthaner, G. (2010). Review Article: Fixed-dose combination therapies in the management of hyperglycaemia in type 2 diabetes: An opportunity to improve adherence and patient care. *Diabetic Medicine, 27*(7), 739–743.

Schwarzer, R. (1992). Self-efficacy in the adoption and maintenance of health behaviors: Theoretical approaches and a new model. In R. Schwarzer (Ed.), *Self-efficacy: Thought control of action* (pp. 217–243). Washington, DC: Hemisphere.

Searle, A., Norman, P., Thompson, R., & Vedhara, K. (2007). A prospective examination of illness beliefs and coping in patients with type 2 diabetes. *British Journal of Health Psychology, 12*(4), 621–638.

Shi, L., Liu, J., Koleva, Y., Fonseca, V., Kalsekar, A., & Pawaskar, M. (2010). Concordance of adherence measurement using self-reported adherence questionnaires and medication monitoring devices. *Pharmacoeconomics, 28*(12), 1097–1107.

Sin, M. K., Kang, D. H., & Weaver, M. (2005). Relationships of asthma knowledge, self-management, and social support in African American adolescents with asthma. *International Journal of Nursing Studies, 42*(3), 307–313.

Smith, S. R., Wahed, A. S., Kelley, S. S., Conjeevaram, H. S., Robuck, P. R., & Fried, M. W. (2007). Assessing the validity of self-reported medication adherence in hepatitis C treatment. *Annals of Pharmacotherapy, 41*(7), 1116–1123.

Smylie, J., Fell, D. B., Chalmers, B., Sauve, R., Royle, C., Allan, B., & O'Campo, P. (2014). Socioeconomic position and factors associated with use of a nonsupine infant sleep position: Findings from the Canadian Maternity Experiences Survey. *American Journal of Public Health, 104*(3), 539–547.

Snell, D. L., Hay-Smith, E. J. C., Surgenor, L. J., & Siegert, R. J. (2013). Examination of outcome after mild traumatic brain injury: The contribution of injury beliefs and Leventhal's common sense model. *Neuropsychological Rehabilitation, 23*(3), 333–362.

Steele, R. G., Anderson, B., Rindel, B., Dreyer, M. L., Perrin, K., Christensen, R. … Flynn, P. M.. (2001). Adherence to antiretroviral therapy among HIV-positive children: Examination of the role of caregiver health beliefs. *AIDS Care, 13*, 617–629.

Stephens, M. A., Rook, K. S., Franks, M. M., Khan, C., & Lida, M. (2010). Spouses' use of social control to improve diabetic patients' dietary adherence. *Family System Health, 28*(3), 199–208.

Stone, A., Shiffman, S., Schwartz, J., Broderick, J., & Hufford, M.R. (2003). Patient compliance with paper and electronic diaries. *Controlled Clinical Trials, 24*(2), 182–199.

Straka, R., Fish, J., Benson, S., & Suh, J. (1997). Patient self-reporting of compliance does not correspond with electronic monitoring: An evaluation using isosorbide dinitrate as a model drug. *Pharmacotherapy, 17*, 126–132.

Strzelczyk, J. J., & Dignan, M. B. (2002). Disparities in adherence to recommended follow-up on screening mammography: Interaction of sociodemographic factors. *Ethnic Disparities, 12*(1), 77–86.

Stupiansky, N. W., Hanna, K. M., Slaven, J. E., Weaver, M. T., & Fortenberry, J. D. (2013). Impulse control, diabetes-specific self-efficacy, and diabetes management among emerging adults with type 1 diabetes. *Journal of Pediatric Psychology, 38*(3), 247–254.

Sunil, T. S., & McGehee, M. A. (2007). Social and religious support on treatment adherence among HIV/AIDS patients by race/ethnicity. *Journal of HIV/AIDS & Social Services, 6*(1–2), 83–99.

Sylvia, L. G., Bernstein, E. E., Hubbard, J. L., Keating, L., & Anderson, E. J. (2013). Practical guide to measuring physical activity. *Journal of the Academy of Nutrition and Dietetics, 114*(2), 199–208.

Taira, D. A., Gelber, R. P., Davis, J., Gronley, K., Chung, R. S., & Seto, T. B. (2007). Antihypertensive adherence and drug class among Asian Pacific Americans. *Ethnicity & Health, 12*(3), 265–281.

Tanaka, E., Momoeda, M., Osuga, Y., Rossi, B., Nomoto, K., Hayakawa, M., … Wang, E. C. (2014). Burden of menstrual symptoms in Japanese women: An analysis of medical care-seeking behavior from a survey-based study. *International Journal of Women's Health, 6*, 11.

Tucker, C. M., Butler, A., Kaye, L. B., Nolan, S. E., Flenar, D. J., Marsiske, M., … Daly, K. (2013). Impact of a culturally sensitive health self-empowerment workshop series on health lifestyles, body mass index, and blood pressure of culturally diverse overweight/obese adults. *American Journal of Lifestyle Medicine.* doi: 10.1177/1559827613503117

Ulrik, C. S., Backer, V., Soes-Petersen, U., Lange, P., Harving, H., & Plaschke, P. (2006). The patient's perspective: Adherence or non-adherence to asthma controller therapy. *Journal of Asthma, 43*(9), 701–704.

van den Bemt, B. J., Zwikker, H. E., & van den Ende, C. H. (2012). Medication adherence in patients with rheumatoid arthritis: A critical appraisal of the existing literature. *Expert Review of Clinical Immunology*, 8(4), 337–351.

van den Boogaard, J., Boeree, M. J., Kibiki, G. S., & Aarnoutse, R. E. (2011). The complexity of the adherence–response relationship in tuberculosis treatment: Why are we still in the dark and how can we get out? *Tropical Medicine & International Health*, 16(6), 693–698.

Van Dulmen, A. M., & Bensing, J. M. (2002). Health promoting effects of the physician–patient encounter. *Psychology, Health and Medicine*, 7(3), 289–300.

Vermeire, E., Hearnshaw, H., Van Royen, P., & Denekens, J. (2001). Patient adherence to treatment: Three decades of research: A comprehensive review. *Journal of Clinical Pharmacological Therapy*, 26(5), 331–342.

Vervloet, M., Spreeuwenberg, P., Bouvy, M. L., Heerdink, E. R., de Bakker, D. H., & van Dijk, L. (2013). Lazy Sunday afternoons: The negative impact of interruptions in patients' daily routine on adherence to oral antidiabetic medication: A multilevel analysis of electronic monitoring data. *European Journal of Clinical Pharmacology*, 69(8), 1599–1606.

Vik, S. A., Maxwell, C. J., & Hogan, D. B. (2004). Measurement, correlates, and health outcomes of medication adherence among seniors. *Annals of Pharmacotherapy*, 38(2), 303–312.

Vincent, A. E., & Birkhead, A. C. S. (2013). Evaluation of the effectiveness of nurse coaching in improving health outcomes in chronic conditions. *Holistic Nursing Practice*, 27(3), 148–161.

Vissman, A. T., Young, A. M., Wilkin, A. M., & Rhodes, S. D. (2013). Correlates of HAART adherence among immigrant Latinos in the southeastern United States. *AIDS Care*, 25(3), 356–363.

Viswanathan, M., Golin, C. E., Jones, C. D., Ashok, M., Blalock, S. J., Wines, R. C., ... Lohr, K. N. (2012). Interventions to improve adherence to self-administered medications for chronic diseases in the United States: A systematic review. *Annals of Internal Medicine*, 157(11), 785–795.

Wagner, G. (2003). Placebo practice trials: The best predictor of adherence readiness for HAART among drug users? *HIV Clinical Trials*, 4(4), 269–281.

Wagner, G., & Rabkin, J. G. (2000). Measuring medication adherence: Are missed doses reported more accurately than perfect adherence? *AIDS Care*, 12(4), 405–408.

Waldrop-Valverde, D., Jones, D. L., Gould, F., Kumar, M., & Ownby, R. L. (2010). Neurocognition, health-related reading literacy, and numeracy in medication

management for HIV infection. *AIDS Patient Care STDS*, 24(8), 477–484.

Walker, E. A., Shmukler, C., Ullman, R., Blanco, E., Scollan-Koliopoulus, M., & Cohen, H. W. (2011). Results of a successful telephonic intervention to improve diabetes control in urban adults: A randomized trial. *Diabetes Care*, 34(1), 2–7.

Walker, S. N., Sechrist, K. R., & Pender, N. J. (1987). The health-promoting lifestyle profile: Development and psychometric characteristics. *Nursing Research*, 36, 76–80.

Wendel, C. S., Mohler, M. J., Kroesen, K., Ampel, N. M., Gifford, A. L., & Coons, S. J. (2001). Barriers to use of electronic adherence monitoring in an HIV clinic. *Annals of Pharmacotherapy*, 35(9), 1010–1015.

West, D. S., DiLillo, V., Bursac, Z., Gore, S. A., & Greene, P. G. (2007). Motivational interviewing improves weight loss in women with type 2 diabetes. *Diabetes Care*, 30(5), 1081–1087.

Whittemore, R., Melkus, G. D., Sullivan, A., & Grey, M. (2004). A nurse-coaching intervention for women with type 2 diabetes. *Diabetes Educator*, 30, 795–804.

Williams, L. K., Joseph, C. L., Peterson, E. L., Wells, K., Wang, M., Chowdhry, V. K., ... Pladevall, M. (2007). Patients with asthma who do not fill their inhaled corticosteroids: A study of primary nonadherence. *Journal of Allergy & Clinical Immunology*, 120(5), 1153–1159.

Wolf, M. S., Williams, M. V., Parker, R. M., Parikh, N. S., Nowlan, A. W., & Baker, D. W. (2007). Patients' shame and attitudes toward discussing the results of literacy screening. *Journal of Health Communication*, 12(8), 721–732.

Wong-Rieger, D., & Rieger, F. P. (2013). Health coaching in diabetes: Empowering patients to self-manage. *Canadian Journal of Diabetes*, 37(1), 41–44.

World Health Organization (WHO). (2003). *Adherence to long-term therapies: Evidence for action*. Geneva, Switzerland: Author.

World Health Organization (WHO). (2010). Global tuberculosis control 2010. Geneva, Switzerland: WHO /HTM/TB/2010.7.

Wutoh, A. K., Brown, C. M., Dutta, A. P., Kumoji, E. K., Clarke-Tasker, V., & Xue, Z. (2005). Treatment perceptions and attitudes of older human immunodeficiency virus–infected adults. *Research in Social and Administrative Pharmacy*, 1(1), 60–76.

Zogg, J. B., Woods, S. P., Sauceda, J. A., Wiebe, J. S., & Simoni, J. M. (2012). The role of prospective memory in medication adherence: A review of an emerging literature. *Journal of Behavioral Medicine*, 35(1), 47–62.

Chapter 10

Family Caregiving

Linda L. Pierce and Barbara J. Lutz

Introduction

Mr. J. is the caregiver for his 55-year-old wife, who has heart disease that has caused her increasing fatigue, shortness of breath, and chest pain over the past 12 months. The couple has no children or close family. Mr. J. has refused help from friends, saying this is his "job." Mrs. J. is unable to climb stairs in their two-story home due to her shortness of breath and fatigue. The living room has been converted into her bedroom; she uses a wheelchair for mobility. Mr. J. placed a toilet commode near her wheelchair and bed, but he has difficulty transferring her from bed to chair to toilet. He is feeling hopeless and helpless, as his back pain makes it hard for him to move. Mr. J. shares that he is short-tempered and is tired all the time. He becomes upset as he begins to think that he can no longer care for his wife at home because of her increasing weakness and his health issues. However, Mr. J. promised her that he would never place her in a nursing home, stating that "only family can take care of family."

This story demonstrates family caregiving. Few adults receive paid homecare services. Outside support is not always welcome, and caregivers often refuse any type of help and resources. Caregivers frequently feel guilty about using outside help, and they may feel that professionals are prying into their private lives (Bursack, 2011; Pierce, 2001).

It has been estimated that 65.7 million family caregivers provide care to adults who are disabled, ill, or aged (Johnson & Wiener, 2006; National Alliance for Caregiving [NAC], 2013). The value of this care in the United States was estimated at $405 billion in 2009 and is expected to grow (NAC & AARP, 2012). The term *unpaid caregiver* refers to a range of kin and non-kin individuals who provide both functional (task-oriented) and affective (emotional) assistance to a dependent person with whom a long-term or lifelong commitment usually exists (Shirey & Summer, 2000). Family members, friends, and neighbors who provide unpaid care may also be referred to as *informal caregivers*. These individuals care for spouses, other relatives, friends, and disabled children (Pierce, Steiner, Govoni, Thompson, & Friedemann, 2007; Reinhard, Given, Petlick, & Bemis, 2008). The most common informal caregiving relationship is between an adult child, usually a woman, and an aging parent (Office on Women's Health, 2008). However, a study financed by the U.S. Department of Health and Human Services' Administration on Aging (AOA) found that more than 906,000 households include a child caregiver between the ages of 8 and 18 years who cares for an ill or disabled family member (American Psychological Association [APA], 2013; NAC, 2005). Moreover, the number of male caregivers is increasing. It is estimated that

47% of the caregivers for younger adult care recipients (between the ages of 18 and 49 years) are male (NAC & American Association of Retired Persons [AARP], 2009).

Decisions about caring for a person with chronic illness are complex and multifaceted for caregivers. Each choice an individual makes has both advantages and disadvantages for the person with chronic illness, the caregiver, and the family. Healthcare professionals generally find that no two situations are alike. Each and every situation needs to be individualized to best meet the needs of everyone involved. This chapter focuses on the multiple aspects of caregiving for someone with a chronic illness and the issues and concerns that caregivers face, often on a daily basis.

Current Family Caregiving

With advances in health care, the number of adults and children living with debilitating and/or chronic conditions is expected to grow. More than 133 million adults in the United States live with chronic conditions such as diabetes, heart disease, and cancer (Bodenheimer, Chen, & Bennett, 2009), and approximately 25% of these individuals report significant limitations in performing at least one activity of daily living (Centers for Disease Control and Prevention [CDC], 2009). Approximately 25% of adults aged 18 to 64 years suffer from two or more chronic conditions (Ward & Schiller, 2013). Most importantly, the number of adults older than 65 years (39.6 million people in 2009) will rise by more than 19 million by 2020; by 2030, there will be approximately 72.1 million adults 65 years and older in the United States (AOA, 2010; Moore, 2006). Recent estimates suggest that 90% of all Medicare beneficiaries have at least one chronic condition (Machlin, Cohen, & Beauregard, 2008). Furthermore, in 2010 more than two-thirds of the Medicare beneficiaries had multiple chronic conditions, and more than half of them had four or more chronic conditions (Center for Medicare and Medicaid

Services [CMS], 2012). Individuals with more than one chronic condition accounted for 93% of total Medicare spending and 98% of hospital readmissions in 2010 (CMS, 2012).

At the other end of the age spectrum is the growing number of children with chronic illness, disabilities, or both. Advances in neonatal care can now save increasing numbers of preterm and low-birth-weight infants. According to the World Health Organization (WHO, 2012a), 15 million babies are born preterm (fewer than 37 completed weeks of gestation), and this number is rising. In 2010, the United States ranked sixth in the world with the greatest number of preterm births (Blencowe et al., 2012). A fact long recognized is that low birth weight and prematurity can lead to an increased incidence of chronic health problems in the pediatric population. Approximately 15% to 18% of children have a chronic disease that continues into adulthood (University of Michigan Health System, 2006).

A 2009 study by the National Alliance for Caregiving and the American Association of Retired Persons (now known simply as AARP) estimated that 28.5% of the American population serves as unpaid family caregivers to an adult or child with special needs. This translates into 65.7 million caregivers in the United States (NAC & AARP, 2009). The duration of caregiving can last from a few months to decades. Caregivers, on average, report approximately 21 hours per week in caring for a person with a chronic condition (NAC & AARP, 2009). Nearly half of these caregivers spent 8 hours or less per week providing assistance. However, 13% of the sample spent more than 40 hours per week in caregiving activities. Primary caregivers spent almost 27 hours per week while secondary caregivers, who assist in providing that care, spent an average of 12 hours per week. Caregivers who lived with the care recipient provided three times as many hours of care per week as those who did not. Additionally, caregivers caring for a child or older adult with a chronic illness spent more time in caregiving activities. More than half of the caregivers provided help with at least one activity of daily living, such as bathing, dressing, or toileting (NAC & AARP, 2009).

PREFERENCES FOR FAMILY CARE

It is important to clarify that some dependent individuals will always need the level of care provided in institutional settings and that not all families are willing or able to provide care over the long term. However, for all but the most severely impaired individuals, most chronically ill, dependent persons have their long-term care needs met in the home or with community-based care arrangements. Approximately two-thirds of dependent persons in the community rely solely on informal caregivers (Colello, 2009; Mittelman, 2003). For these arrangements to work, family members, friends, or neighbors must play central roles in long-term plans of care.

The decision about where and how to provide care for family members with chronic conditions is emotionally charged and multifaceted. Home-based care can be financially cost-effective for the healthcare system. However, the reliance on family members as care providers creates multiple stressors for the family due to their own life circumstances, which may include competing demands of work, childcare responsibilities, and chronic diseases and decline in the caregivers' own personal health (Colello, 2009). When formal assistance is required, married persons prefer help in the home regardless of the level of disability of the care recipient; however, financial difficulty and the strain of extended caregiving, especially on the caregiver's health, often lead family caregivers to decisions that favor institutionalized care (Family Caregiver Alliance [FCA], 2006).

CHARACTERISTICS OF FAMILY CAREGIVERS

Today, the term *family caregiver* extends beyond the traditional family boundaries. *Caregiver* is defined as anyone who provides assistance to another in need. An *informal caregiver* is anyone who provides care without pay and who may have personal ties to the care recipient. *Family caregiver* is a term used interchangeably with informal caregiver and can include family, friends, or neighbors. *Caregiver coalition* is a term used to describe the addition of a support person or persons in traditional relationships when the caregiver–recipient arrangement is no longer sufficient (Haigler, Bauer, & Travis, 2004; Reinhard et al., 2008).

Motivations for caregiving, such as love, duty, or obligation (often based on ethnicity and culture), strongly influence a caregiver's willingness to accept primary caregiving status (Geister, 2005; WHO, 2012b). Additional reasons given by family caregivers for accepting their role are their expectations of themselves and others, religious training and spiritual experiences, and role modeling (Piercy & Chapman, 2001; WHO, 2012b).

CAREGIVER DYADS AND CAREGIVER SYSTEMS

Early caregiving research identified a care recipient and a caregiver as separate entities; the caregiver had primary responsibility for the care and well-being of the care recipient. These studies often did not recognize that caregiving usually occurs within the context of larger, more complex family systems (Palmer & Glass, 2003) or other social networks (Weitzner, Haley, & Chen, 2000). Furthermore, the helping networks used by widowed and never-married individuals may be larger than those of married people (Barrett & Lynch, 1999).

In recent years, caregiving research has placed more emphasis on the dynamics of the family relationships (Palmer & Glass, 2003) and the dyadic relationship (Badr & Actielli, 2005; Sebern & Whitlatch, 2007). As would be expected, these studies indicate that the dynamics of the family or other close personal relationships that existed before the illness experience can influence caregiving relationships post-illness. The increasing number of stepfamilies also adds to the complexity of caregiving.

Today, people of both genders and all ages, ethnicities, and economic classes occupy positions as caregivers with varying levels and types of responsibilities, especially in long-term care arrangements (Desilver, 2013). Because caregivers have varying degrees of responsibility for providing or arranging for care, the terms *care provider* and *care manager* may be used to differentiate two types of caregivers (Stoller & Cutler, 1993). This designation helps clarify the previously invisible contributions of all family caregivers. If a son is close to his dependent parents, especially if he is not married, he is likely to be accountable for seeing that things get done, even if he does not provide all of the direct care that is required (Allen, Goldscheider, & Ciambrone, 1999; Keith, 1995; Thompson, Tudiver, & Manson, 2000). Similarly, an adult grandchild may help a grandparent in the absence of a nearby adult child, or children-in-law may find their relationships to relatives with chronic illness make them better suited to caregiving roles than the biological children (Bursack, 2013; Travis & Bethea, 2001).

Changes in the modern family social structure have resulted in more families in which both adults work outside the home. The adults in this so-called sandwich generation are often not available to provide care for aging family members, which creates a new level of caregivers—children and adolescents. These young caregivers may assist with or even assume the care of adults with chronic illness (Austin, 2013; Hunt, Levine, & Naiditch, 2005).

RACIAL AND ETHNIC DIVERSITY

The family caregiving experience is also shaped by race and ethnicity. In chronic illness, preferences for certain types of assistance often vary along racial and ethnic lines. The percentage of racial and ethnic minority older adults (65 years and older) has increased from 16.3% of the elderly population in 2000 to 21% in 2011. From 2012 to 2030, the white (non-Hispanic) elderly population in the United States is expected to

increase by 54%, while older ethnic minorities are expected to increase by 125% in the same time period (AOA, 2012).

The percentage of individuals engaging in caregiving activities also varies across ethnic groups, with the number of minority caregivers increasing. In an analysis of caregiver characteristics from the 2009 Behavioral Risk Factor Surveillance System (BRFSS) data, 21.4% of Hispanics, 24.8% of whites, 28.6% of blacks, and 24% of members of other ethnic groups indicated that they provided health-related care or assistance to a family member or friend (Anderson, Edward, Pearson, Talley, McGuire, & Andresen, 2013).

In another survey conducted by the NAC and AARP (2009), estimates of the percentage of people who served as caregivers were somewhat higher: white, 30.5%; African American, 33.6%, Hispanic, 36.1%; and Asian American, 20%. This same survey found that white respondents were more likely to be older than nonwhite respondents. Thirty-eight percent of African American caregivers were single/never married, compared to 16% of all caregiver respondents. More than 50% of the African American caregivers reported that they provide care for both an older person and a younger person at the same time. The study also found that more Hispanic caregivers (27%) rated their health as fair or poor when compared with white or Asian caregivers (15%) (NAC & AARP, 2009).

Minority caregivers are more likely to be employed (Seifert, Williams, Dowd, Chappel-Aiken, & McCorkle, 2008) and report having more unmet needs (Scharlach, Giunta, Chow, & Lehning, 2008) than their white counterparts. Results from the study by Scharlach and colleagues (2008), which included more than 1,500 ethnically diverse caregivers in California, found that being a minority does not significantly affect service use after controlling for other variables such as "age, education, emotional support, family contribution, care recipient service use, and care recipient impairment"

(p. 326). Another study of 595 caregivers in Florida found that once other social determinants, such as age, education, income, caregiver health, and care recipient impairment, were controlled, patterns of caregiving were not significantly different among different ethnic groups (Friedemann, Buckwalter, Newman, & Mauro, 2013). Based on these and other studies, the influence of race and ethnicity on caregiving may be in part a proxy for other demographic and social determinants that influence health, such as age, education, income, and social support. All of these factors must be carefully evaluated when assessing the needs of family caregivers.

GENDER DIFFERENCES

The choice of who becomes the primary caregiver and what the family caregiving system looks like depends on many factors. In a spousal relationship, the unaffected spouse usually assumes the caregiving role. Often, both spouses are forced to cope with role renegotiation in addition to their new roles as the giver and the receiver of care.

Among married adult children, daughters or daughters-in-law are most often the primary caregivers for aging parents (NAC & AARP, 2012; Office on Women's Health, 2008; Shirey & Summer, 2000). Daughters are more likely to offer assistance to their father when he is serving in a caregiving role than to their mother when she is filling this role. This may be because daughters are more comfortable with their mother in that role and feel that their father needs additional assistance performing the tasks required of a caregiver (Mittelman, 2003). Sarkisian and Gerstel (2004) found that much of the relationship between gender and helping parents is explained by gender differences in employment patterns. They suggest that gender differences in adult care may be fading as women's and men's work lives become more similar (Sarkisian & Gerstel, 2004). Although some men are just as likely as women to be involved in caring for and

helping seniors, women, wives, mothers, and adult daughters spend more time as the designated primary caregiver (FCA, 2012). The most recent statistics from 2009 indicate approximately two-thirds of family caregivers for older adults are female, while caregivers for adults ages 19 to 49 are more equally split, with males accounting for approximately 47% of the caregiver population (FCA, 2012; NAC & AARP, 2009). However, men are less likely to be involved in personal care such as toileting and bathing and are more likely to supplement their caregiving tasks with paid caregivers (NAC & AARP, 2009).

The gendered nature of caregiving is one important characteristic of long-term caregiving that is likely to continue in the future. All things being equal, the person who is closest to and the most involved in the daily life of the dependent person is usually the person most accountable for either doing or seeing that care is done.

TYPES OF CARE PROVIDED BY FAMILY CAREGIVERS

Over the long term, a dependent person requires two types of care: social care and health-related care. Social care includes both functional and affective assistance in daily living, while health-related care refers to specialized care by professionals and daily treatments performed by family caregivers, such as medication administration.

Functional assistance is determined by the care recipient's ability to perform various tasks of daily living, which are categorized as either instrumental or basic activities of daily living. Instrumental activities of daily living (IADLs) are the functions an adult would be expected to perform in the process of everyday life, including cooking, cleaning, buying groceries, doing yard work, and paying bills. Basic activities of daily living (ADLs) are personal care and basic survival tasks, such as eating, bathing, dressing, going to the bathroom, maintaining personal hygiene, and getting around (mobility).

Affective assistance, also called emotional support, includes behaviors that convey caring and concern to the care recipient. The relationship between the caregiver and the care recipient is a shared one involving emotions, experiences, and memories, which can place a caregiver at higher risk for psychological and physical illness (FCA, 2012). For the caregiver, affective assistance can lead to anxiety, depression, and other mental health consequences. However, affective assistance can be rewarding and is often linked with enhanced feelings of autonomy, personal growth, self-esteem, contentment, life satisfaction, hope of recovery, dignity, and general well-being (FCA, 2012).

In the past, there was a somewhat clearer division between formal and informal care networks. The informal network—family caregivers or significant others—provided both emotional and functional aspects of care and monitored the care provided by formal providers. The formal network provided specialized care that was highly task oriented and goal directed. Today, however, the roles of the formal and informal network have merged to create a blended approach to caregiving. Family caregivers may perform highly skilled tasks formerly reserved for the professional. Professional caregivers function as a team with the family in making care decisions for the client (Day, 2013; Haigler et al., 2004).

Caregiving Histories and Maturation over Time

Longitudinal studies of family caregiving have documented the many changes that occur in the role of family caregiver and note that family caregiving is not a static event. Some time ago, Pearlin (1992) equated caregiving to career development. Two factors contribute to this notion of a caregiving career or caregiving history: maturation of the caregiver over time, and ongoing role development associated with the inevitable transitions in care over the long term.

The expectations of the family caregiver are many. Family caregivers often begin their roles with little or no training or support. In addition to the psychological aspects of caregiving, they are expected to provide competent, skilled health care for their loved ones, such as medication management, skin care, and tube feedings (Elliot & Shewchuk, 2003; HealthNetCafé, 2013). Most caregivers begin their experiences as novices with little or no experience or knowledge of how to navigate the healthcare system (FCA, 2009). Over time, mature caregivers master a new language system of entitlements (Medicare, Medicaid) and treatments (medication administration, illness symptomatology), and learn how to incorporate the needs of a dependent person into their daily lives (Leavitt et al., 1999). Some caregivers mature quickly and with ease, whereas other caregivers are never able to achieve adequate skill or confidence in the caregiver role. Thus, tremendous variability can be found in the levels and types of care provided by family caregivers, which are at least partially attributed to successful mastery of their roles (Reinhard et al., 2008; Seltzer & Wailing, 2000).

Transitions in care occur at three points: entry into a caregiving relationship (e.g., help with cooking, cleaning, and money management, moving to help with bathing, dressing, grooming, toileting, and so on), institutionalization (or transitions into other formal care arrangements), and bereavement (Hill, 2009; Seltzer & Wailing, 2000). Unlike acute or episodic care that has an end point, the only natural end to long-term caregiving is the death of the care recipient. Even families that ultimately opt for institutional placement of their dependent family members do not abandon their relatives over the long term. Most caregivers stay engaged as care managers following the institutional placement decision (Hill, 2009; Seltzer & Wailing, 2000).

One of the reasons that family caregiving precipitated by acute hospitalization is so stressful for new caregivers is that they have not had a period of maturation and development before facing the intense caregiving demands and the decision-making requirements that follow (Feinberg, Reinhard, Houser, & Coula, 2011; Lutz, Young, Cox, Martz, & Creasy, 2011). In addition, the transitions in care occur rapidly and over a highly compressed period. In a matter of days, the caregiver may transition from having no care responsibilities to being fully engaged in rehabilitation after hospitalization, or home or institutional long-term care (Feinberg et al., 2011; Lutz et al., 2011). Many caregivers have said, "All of a sudden you're labeled as the caregiver and you really have no clue what that is. You know that you just take care of them."

POSITIVE ASPECTS OF CAREGIVING

In the past, research on stress, strain, burden, and burnout overshadowed the positive aspects of providing care to a dependent family member. As a result, little was understood about how and why caregivers provide care even under difficult circumstances. Of late, more has become known about the positive aspects of caregiving. For example, Mackenzie and Greenwood (2012) report that when care recipients show progress, this results in a positive experience for the caregivers, strengthening the pair's relationships with each other. Caregivers may report more satisfaction in caring if the care recipient is only mildly disabled and if relatives, friends, or both are able to help provide the needed assistance (Pierce, 2001). Strengthened relationships with care recipients, especially when caring for spouses, are seen as positive aspects of being caregivers (Mackenzie & Greenwood, 2012). These experiences are connected to caregivers feeling appreciated and an increase in perceived self-esteem and self-efficacy (Mackenzie & Greenwood, 2012; Semiatin & O'Connor, 2012). Caregivers view their role as an opportunity to

give back and to discover personal strengths (Peacock et al., 2010). Coherence—that is, a sense of togetherness in caring for others—is important for maintaining stability within the family. Through coherence, family caregivers feel connected, which helps them survive the stressful times related to caring situations and, therefore, leads to positive aspects of caregiving (Peacock et al., 2010; Pierce, 2001). Longitudinal research and research with caregivers in diverse arrangements are needed to provide a more comprehensive view of what contributes to a positive caregiving experience.

THE FUTURE OF CAREGIVING

Looking to the future, the caregiving landscape will be very different from past decades and will further confound the current reliance on family caregivers. Parents of the baby boomer generation had several children from whom to seek assistance, while aging baby boomers typically have smaller families and, therefore, less available assistance. The aging of the population, sometimes referred to as the "silver tsunami," and the decrease in the number of family members available to provide care is expected to significantly affect the long-term care of older adults with chronic illnesses.

In 2013, an AARP policy paper reported on the potential decline of available family caregivers during the first half of the 21st century. From 1990 to 2010, as individuals in the baby boomer generation became the primary caregivers of their older parents, the ratio of potential caregivers to care recipients actually increased to 7 to 1. However, from 2010 to 2030, as baby boomers become the group who needs care, the ratio of potential caregivers to care recipients will decline. The projected ratio will decrease to 4 to 1 in 2030 and 3 to 1 in 2050 (Redfoot, Feinberg, & Houser, 2013).

Declining family sizes, increasing childlessness, more households with two working adults, and rising divorce rates further limit the number of family caregivers (Johnson, Toohey, &

Wiener, 2007). One adult daughter who was caring for her father with Parkinson's disease sums it up:

> I think with my dad's generation, they didn't put their parents in different types of homes. We always had my grandparents at home. They never went anywhere because the family always took care of everything, but back then, not everybody was working either, the way that we are today in our society.

Additionally, the mobility of families often separates individuals by thousands of miles, making family assistance impossible. It remains to be seen what this societal trend will mean to this cohort. Most researchers agree, however, that any predictions about family caregiving in the future are tenuous because public policy is difficult to predict from one generation to the next. The need for policy to change to accommodate the caregiving needs of the aging population both in the United States and globally is the only certainty.

Problems and Issues

Family caregivers face multiple problems, issues, and concerns throughout their caregiving experiences. The case study of Z and her family that appears at the end of the chapter is typical of the effort that most family caregivers put into fulfilling their responsibilities, attending to the wants and needs of the care recipient, and continuously adjusting their lives to the physical and emotional requirements of the caregiving situation.

Family caregiving experiences incorporate societal values and are shaped by governmental policy. These values and policies presume that families are responsible for caring for their disabled members and will provide the majority of the care that is needed—a view shared by 68% of Americans age 40 and older (Thompson, Benz, Agiesta, Junius, Nguyen, & Lowell, 2013). However, with changing demographics and fewer potential caregivers, the resources available to meet the long-term care needs of an aging population will be significantly affected in the future (Redfoot et al., 2013).

Increased technology, greater acuity of those in need of assistance, and competing demands on available caregivers create an imbalance between the demand for family care and the ability of family caregivers to provide care. Family caregivers are being asked to provide highly technical treatments; administer complex medication regimens; provide labor-intensive, hands-on care; and monitor the medical conditions of very ill family members.

A checklist was developed to identify the needs and concerns of caregivers after a patient's discharge from the hospital or rehabilitation facility following a stroke. It includes the following categories: getting information about stroke, dealing with the care recipient's emotions and behaviors, providing physical and instrumental care, and caring for self and managing other roles and responsibilities (Bakas, Austin, Oknokwo, Lewis, & Chadwick, 2002, p. 245). This checklist has been adapted for use with caregivers of individuals receiving home dialysis (Welch et al., 2013).

The one responsibility that has remained constant over time, whether the family caregiver is a direct care provider or arranges care as a care manager, is the extensive decision-making demands placed on family caregivers. When the dependent family member cannot make decisions or has difficulty communicating choices, the responsibility for countless decisions associated with managing daily life falls to the caregiver. These decisions include the initiation, timing, and provision of assistance from informal and formal sources; integration of caregiving demands into work and family life; planning for future long-term care needs (Travis & Bethea, 2001); and consideration of advanced and end-of-life care preferences of the care recipient (Michael, O'Callaghan, Baird, Hiscock, & Clayton, in press).

The Influence of Public Policy on Family Caregiving

Containing the rising costs of healthcare services has become a national policy imperative. This goal is demonstrated through policies that promote prevention of premature or unwanted institutionalization of disabled elders in nursing homes, limit publicly funded homecare services to individuals with the lowest incomes, and curtail the Medicare home health benefit. Such policies limit the amount and scope of services that can be provided to families because of financial concerns. Cost-containment measures are occurring precisely when the demand for help in providing long-term care at home is increasing (Redfoot et al., 2013). These changes in government-sponsored services mean that many families—particularly low- and middle-income families—face difficult decisions about providing assistance while receiving minimal help from healthcare professionals.

In the past two decades, several government initiatives have attempted to address the needs of family caregivers. In 1993, the Family and Medical Leave Act (FMLA) became law. This act gives qualified caregivers the option of taking up to 12 weeks of unpaid leave from their jobs to care for a family member (U.S. Department of Labor, 1993). The FMLA was updated in 2008 to increase this leave to 26 weeks for qualifying military families and in 2013 for family members of qualifying veterans (U.S. Department of Labor, 2013). In 2011, approximately 16% of eligible employees used family and medical leave. Six percent of the qualified employees who needed FMLA did not take it. The top barriers were not being able to afford unpaid leave (46%) or being worried about losing their job (17%). These barriers disproportionately affect lower-income workers. Moreover, nearly one-third of eligible employees are unaware of the FMLA benefit and approximately 40% of the U.S. workforce is not covered by FMLA (Klerman, Daley, & Pozniak, 2012).

In addition to barriers associated with FMLA, many caregiving situations require that the caregiver be available for a longer period of time than the 12 to 26 weeks afforded by the FMLA. These barriers present difficult choices for family members of individuals in need of caregiving assistance—many are faced with the prospect of leaving or reducing gainful employment to provide the necessary care because they have no other options.

The Older Americans Act Amendments of 2000 established the National Family Caregiver Support Program (NFCSP) (AOA, 2011a). Federal funds are given to states based on their proportionate share of the population aged 70 years or older. States, working in partnership with local agencies on aging and faith and community service providers and tribes, offer five direct services to best meet the range of caregiver needs. The services include provision of the following:

- Information to caregivers about available services
- Assistance to caregivers in gaining access to supportive services
- Individual counseling, organization of support groups, and caregiver training to assist caregivers in making decisions and solving problems related to their roles
- Respite care to enable caregivers to be temporarily relieved from their caregiving responsibilities
- Supplemental services, on a limited basis, to complement the care provided by caregivers

Family caregivers eligible for the NFCSP are those who care for adults aged 60 years or older and grandparents and relatives of children not more than 18 years of age, including grandparents who are sole caregivers of grandchildren and those individuals who have developmental disabilities. Priority is given to caregivers with social and economic needs, particularly low-income and minority individuals, or older individuals providing care and support to persons with mental retardation and related developmental disabilities. While the NFCSP has been lauded as an important step in recognizing the needs of family caregivers, the appropriate funding for its implementation has not been allocated to support the needs of caregivers at any meaningful level. Furthermore, each state decides how the funds are used, resulting in inconsistencies of services across states.

Currently, public financing of long-term care in the home setting is minimal. Medicare offers a hospice benefit for a time-limited period at the end of life, and some states have limited home- and community-based waiver programs that provide some home-based services for low-income residents. Often the waiting lists for these services are long, with residents never receiving the services for which they are eligible. Many private insurers offer long-term care policies through employers, fraternal organizations, retirement communities, and health management organizations. Unfortunately, in the past, most of these policies did not cover many aspects of the personal care provided by family caregivers, leaving in-home care to be paid as an out-of-pocket expense. Current long-term care policies on the market are more comprehensive, but are expensive to purchase.

In 2010, Congress passed the Patient Protection and Affordable Care Act (ACA). The ACA provides additional assistance for caregivers of persons with chronic illness in the United States. Medicaid-funded home- and community-based care includes programs that provide attendant care services for individuals with disabilities and protection against spousal impoverishment. Care coordination provides incentives to physicians and healthcare organizations to improve postdischarge patient outcomes and reduce hospital readmission for Medicare beneficiaries. The law also includes stipulations for caregiver and care recipient involvement in decision making about care options and promotes family-centered models of care. However, the ACA has been hotly contested and the extent to which these reforms will remain in effect is a highly debated issue (Feinberg & Reamy, 2011).

Emotional Effects of Being a Caregiver

Although not all persons experience stress when providing care, many do. A number of factors influence caregiving and the stress it may cause—for example, the intensity of the care provided, the types of care tasks performed, gender, personal characteristics of the caregiver, the relationship between the caregiver and the person receiving care, support from other family members, and competing obligations of the caregiver. Financial hardship also contributes to caregiver stress (Evercare & NAC, 2007). Researchers have labeled caregiver stress as either strain or burden.

STRAIN AND BURDEN

Caregiver strain and burden are multidimensional constructs that include both subjective perceptions of caregivers, such as role overload, and objective factors, such as physical care needs of the care recipient. One caregiver shared that she "wakes up with dread of caregiving for another day." Another caregiver said, "Sometimes, you just feel like you want a truck to hit you but you don't want to leave someone else with the mess" (Pierce, Thompson, Govoni, & Steiner, 2012, p. 263). The most common theory that underpins research on caregiver strain and burden is Lazurus and Folkman's (1984) *theory of stress and coping* (Bakas, Champion, Perkins, Farran, & Williams, 2006; Oberst, Thomas, Gass, & Ward, 1989; Zarit, Reever, & Bach-Peterson, 1980).

According to Hunt (2003), caregiver burden is defined as "the oppressive or worrisome load borne by people providing direct care for the chronically ill" (p. 28). By comparison, strain is related to the stress, hardship, or conflicting feelings one has when performing the caregiving role (Hunt, 2003). However, for practical purposes, these two terms are often used interchangeably in the literature. Furthermore, caregivers have indicated that they prefer the term "strain" over "burden" because they do not view caring for a family member as a burden (Abendroth, Lutz, & Young, 2012; Greenwood, Mackenzie, Cloud, & Wilson, 2009).

Several validated tools are used to measure strain or burden (Deeken, Taylor, Mangran, Yarbroff, & Ingham, 2003). Some of the more commonly used tools include the Caregiver Strain Index (Robinson, 1983), Bakas Caregiving Outcomes Scale (Bakas et al., 2006), Zarit Burden Inventory (Zarit et al., 1980), Caregiver Burden Inventory (Novak & Guest, 1989), Caregiving Stress Inventory (Pearlin, Mullan, Semple, & Skaff, 1990), and Appraisal of Caregiving Scale (Oberst et al., 1989). In a 2009 study, 32% of the 1,480 caregivers surveyed indicated they had high levels of burden and another 19% had medium levels of burden (NAC & AARP, 2009). Furthermore, caregivers who indicated that they did not have a choice in assuming the caregiving role experienced more strain than those who took on the role willingly. One study reported that as many as 44% of the caregivers did not feel they were given a choice in assuming the caregiving role (Schulz, Beach, Cook, Martire, Tomlinson, & Monin, 2012).

One area of caregiver research that has focused heavily on caregiver strain is dementia care. In particular, caregiving is more stressful and produces more emotional and physical strain when the caregiver is caring for a person who has disruptive or problematic behaviors, such as someone with cognitive impairments as is common with dementia or Alzheimer's disease. For example, in one study, caregivers of persons with dementia were more likely than caregivers of persons without dementia to say that they suffered from depressive symptoms as

a result of caregiving. However, this difference was mediated by problematic behaviors of the care recipient (Givens, Mezzacappa, Heeren, Yaffe, & Fredman, 2013). Therefore, interventions designed to minimize problematic or disruptive behaviors in care recipients may help reduce caregiver strain.

Caregivers with higher levels of strain are also at higher risk for poorer health, such as depression and depressive symptoms, than non-caregivers (FCA, 2006; NAC & AARP, 2009). The Family Caregiver Alliance (2006) estimates that between 40% and 70% of caregivers have "clinically significant" depressive symptoms.

Research focusing on the impact of strain on caregiver mortality has yielded mixed results. In a longitudinal study of 3,710 caregivers of care recipients with disability or chronic illness, the mortality rates for caregivers who reported high strain were more than one and half times those for caregivers who reported no or minimal strain (Perkins et al., 2013). In another study of 3,503 stroke caregivers, there were no differences in mortality when compared to non-caregivers even within subgroup analysis, where subgroups were defined on characteristics including race, gender, strain, and relationship (Roth, Haley, Hovater, Perkins, Wadley, & Judd, 2013).

Caregivers for spouses report a higher incidence of depression and stress than those caring for a disabled parent. The caregiving roles and responsibilities may have a major impact on the relationship itself. Healthcare professionals must realize that the relationship between the caregiver and the spouse receiving the care needs to be supported and nurtured in terms of love, affection, and intimacy (Gordon & Perrone, 2004).

Few studies have addressed the effects of caregiving on children and adolescents (younger than age 18). In addition to assuming more roles and responsibilities within their families, these caregivers report increased stress and anxiety, interrupted sleep, back pain from lifting, bullying from peers, and pronounced effects on their school, social, and recreational activities (Action Canada, 2013). They also report difficulty watching their loved one progress with a chronic problem and feeling helpless because of their lack of knowledge and fear that they will not be able to deal with a crisis (Lackey & Gates, 2001). A Canadian task force investigating the effects of caregiving on children and adolescents recommends raising awareness, increasing research, and developing a "multisector approach" to address the needs of these young, often invisible, caregivers (Action Canada, 2013).

There also appears to be a gender component associated with caregiver strain. Female caregivers experience more strain than do male caregivers (Kim, Chang, Rose, & Kim, 2012) and are much more likely than men to report being depressed or anxious and to experience lower levels of life satisfaction. The irony is that, while they report more caregiver strain and role conflict, women are more likely than male caregivers to continue caregiving responsibilities over the long term (NAC & AARP, 2009).

Research has found that caregivers who have a higher sense of self-efficacy and control over their life situations (e.g., personal mastery) have less strain and fewer depressive symptoms (Chumbler, Rittman, Van Puymbroeck, Voegl, & Qin, 2004; Chumbler Rittman, & Wu, 2007; Mausbach et al., 2007). These studies suggest that interventions that enhance self-efficacy or personal mastery might decrease health risks and improve health-related outcomes for caregivers (Chumbler et al., 2007; Halm & Bakas, 2007; Rabinowitz, Mausbach, Thompson, & Gallagher-Thompson, 2007).

COMPASSION FATIGUE

Compassion fatigue is a term coined by Figley (1995) to describe the impact of caregiving on professional caregivers (e.g., nurses and social workers). The concept of compassion fatigue has implications for family caregivers. In Figley's model, compassion fatigue begins with a caregiver's stress response, which is "the stress connected with exposure to a sufferer" (Figley, 1998, p. 21). In this case, the sufferer is the care recipient. When compassion stress is accompanied by prolonged exposure to the suffering or unresolved trauma, compassion fatigue sets in. Compassion fatigue can also be exacerbated by a substantial degree of life disruption. These factors lead to caregiver burnout, which may be dealt with by placing the care recipient in an institution, by having another family member assume primary caregiver duties, or, in some cases, by neglecting or abusing the care recipient. Parents caring for children with severe developmental disabilities or others caring for individuals with Alzheimer's disease are especially at risk for compassion fatigue due to prolonged exposure and high levels of life disruption (Day & Anderson, 2011). However, to date, little research has addressed the incidence of compassion fatigue in informal caregivers (Lynch & Lobo, 2012).

GRIEF, LOSS, AND BEREAVEMENT

One area of caregiving in chronic illness that has received attention is the grief and loss that caregivers and care recipients experience at the onset of a debilitating chronic illness and, as that illness progresses, often at the eventual death of the care recipient. Caregivers grieve the loss of the previous relationship, the loss of future and hoped-for plans, and the losses their loved one is facing. Caregivers and care recipients need support and assistance to help them work through the grief they are experiencing. Caregivers should be provided with opportunities to talk about their experiences, concerns, and fears. Referrals to family therapists who can help them learn to manage the challenges they are facing, reframe their relationships and their lives in light of the effects of chronic illness, and help them to adjust to the changes they are experiencing should be considered (Boerner & Schulz, 2010; Lutz & Young, 2010).

FAMILY RELATIONSHIPS AND SHIFTING ROLES

Providing care to others, especially spouses and parents, often requires changes in the ways that family members interact with each other. For the care provider, this decision may be a lifelong commitment to another family member (Elliot & Shewchuk, 2003). These changes in family interactions represent a complex phenomenon that often involves *role renegotiation* or *role reconstruction*. Although most family caregivers and care recipients handle these role changes over time, some struggle with changes in their family relationships (Lutz, Chumbler, & Roland, 2007).

Previously, these changes in roles have been defined as *role reversal*, but this term may be inadequate for describing family relationships in late life and also can reinforce negative stereotypes of dependency in general and old age in particular. If being a parent, child, or spouse is a social position in a family, then these positions do not change during the lifetime of the family. A parent is always a parent; a spouse is always a spouse. Although the family members' behaviors toward each other may change as health or functioning decline, the roles remain stable. Therefore, the terms *role renegotiation* and *role reconstruction* may more accurately describe changes in familial relationships due to caregiving.

Studies have found that adult child caregivers respect traditional parental autonomy for as long as possible. The caregivers in one study described sensitivity to the parents' wishes, even when they disagreed with the parent, and well beyond the point at which the parent experienced significant cognitive or physical decline (Piercy, 1998). This is particularly evident in studies of nonwhite cultures in which familial roles are revered and respected (Evans, Coon, & Crogan, 2007). However, Lackey and

Gates (2001) found that in some cases children younger than 18 years of age who provide care to their parents at times perceived a reversal of roles. When caring for a parent, children reported serving as the personal confidant of the parent.

ELDER ABUSE AND NEGLECT

According to the Centers for Disease Control and Prevention (CDC, 2013), more than 500,000 adults older than the age of 60 years are abused or neglected annually in the United States. Much abuse and neglect goes unreported, however, and the American Psychological Association (APA, 2012) estimates that the actual number of abused and neglected elders may be as high as 4 million. Most elder abuse and neglect occurs in the older person's home (APA, 2012), and most often the perpetrators of abuse and neglect are family members (spouse, parents, children, grandchildren, siblings, and other family members), with spouses or partners being the most frequent perpetrators.

The Administration on Aging (2009) defines the following types of abuse and neglect: physical abuse, sexual abuse, neglect, financial abuse and exploitation, emotional abuse, abandonment, and self-neglect.

- Physical abuse is defined as the willful infliction of physical pain or injury. Examples include slapping, bruising, and restraining.
- Sexual abuse is the infliction of nonconsensual sexual contact of any kind.
- Neglect is failing to provide shelter, health care, or protection.
- Financial abuse and exploitation is the illegal taking, misuse, or concealment of funds, property, or assets.
- Emotional abuse includes inflicting pain, anguish, or distress through verbal and nonverbal acts.
- Abandonment is desertion of the elder by anyone who is responsible for care.

- Self-neglect is failure of a person to perform essential self-care tasks, such that this failure creates an unsafe environment for the elder.

It is important for healthcare professionals to recognize the precipitating factors for caregiver abuse of an elder. There appears to be a strong link between the likelihood of abuse and the caregiver's perception of his or her situation. Caregivers who have had a positive relationship with care recipients in the past are less likely to become abusive. In certain situations, the risk of abuse increases in direct relationship to the amount of care required. The personality characteristics and behaviors of the care recipient have also been identified as factors in relation to the caregiver's stress level. Finally, an abusive incident may be triggered by the use of alcohol, substance abuse, or psychiatric illness (APA, 2012; Nerenberg, 2002).

Although it is more common to think about the potential abuse of a dependent person by a family caregiver, it is also possible that a caregiver may be the victim of an abusive care recipient. Patterns of dysfunctional behavior in families can extend over decades. If a wife was abused by her husband before he became ill or dependent on her for assistance, there is no reason to believe that the husband would suddenly discontinue all forms of abusive behavior because of illness.

Family caregivers, especially women, who have not managed the family finances and must always ask the care recipient or other family members for money, or who rely solely on the care recipients' families for other types of assistance, may be very vulnerable to neglect. In addition, self-neglect—a behavior that threatens a person's own health or safety—can be an adverse consequence of profound caregiving stress and associated depression.

Financial Impact of Caregiving

Caregiving has different degrees of financial impact on families, depending on their particular caregiving situations and financial resources. The impact may range from minimal to considerable, depending on the extent to which other family help is available, how formal services are used, and how they are financed.

The current public financing system for in-home and community-based services targets persons with the lowest incomes. Affluent family caregivers can afford to pay for home or community-based care out of pocket, regardless of the financial eligibility of the care recipient. However, families in the middle and low-middle ranges of income (less than 250% of the poverty level) may be unable to purchase in-home services or receive public financing for needed care. In other words, these care recipients are not financially eligible for assistance, nor are their family caregivers able to purchase services for them.

The cost of caregiving is associated with the level of need for the affected individual. According to the Administration on Aging (2011b), caregivers spend an average of 11% of their annual income on out-of-pocket expenditures for services not covered by Medicare. In a survey of 1,000 caregivers, Evercare and the National Alliance for Caregiving (2007) found that the average annual cost of caregiving was $5,531, which represented approximately 13% of the median annual income ($43,026) of the caregivers surveyed. However, in a smaller subsample of caregivers ($n = 41$) who maintained a 1-month diary of expenses, the annualized expenses were $12,348. The most common expenses were in the areas of "household goods, food, and meals" (42%), travel and transportation costs (40%), and medical care copayments and pharmaceuticals (31%)" (p. 7). These caregivers found they had to cut back on expenditures on their own needs to meet the expenses of the care recipient. For example, 34% of caregivers used their savings, 32% deferred home maintenance, and 23% cut back on their own healthcare expenditures.

Those in the lowest income categories provided the most number of hours of care per week. Caregivers whose income was less than $25,000 per year provided an average of 41 hours of care each week. The estimated cost of care for these caregivers was more than $5,000 annually (or approximately 20% of their income). Of the total sample, 43% reported that their financial worries had increased since taking on the role of caregiver. Those reporting higher expenses also reported poorer physical and emotional health (Evercare & NAC, 2007).

EMPLOYMENT

In a 2009 survey of 1,480 caregivers, approximately 57% reported being employed in the past 12 months while also serving in a caregiving role for a family member. Of these, almost 80% were employed full-time while 19% had part-time employment. As would be expected, older caregivers were more likely to be retired (72% of those age 65 years and older). Furthermore, caregivers were more likely to be employed if they were male, were college graduates, had lower caregiver burden, provided less than 20 hours of care per week, were not the primary caregiver, or had been providing care for more than a year (NAC & AARP, 2009). Seventy percent of the caregivers responded that they had to reduce their working hours, change jobs, take a leave of absence, or quit their jobs because of their caregiving responsibilities, representing a 7% increase from the share of caregivers who reported doing so in 2004 (NAC & AARP, 2009).

The employees most in need of support are those who function as primary caregivers and those whose care recipients have higher care needs (Evercare & NAC, 2007; NAC & AARP, 2009). Being female, Caucasian, and in fair to poor health increases the caregiver's likelihood of needing some assistance to accommodate work and caregiving demands. There is also evidence to suggest that caregivers who have less education and those less likely to view their work as a career are more likely than others to decide to leave paid employment altogether. Research reveals that the daughter living closest to the parent needing care is most likely to be called upon for caregiving duties (Pillemer & Suitor, 2013).

Clearly, there are hidden costs, both economic and noneconomic, of informal care for caregivers, care recipients, and other family members (Evercare & NAC, 2007; NAC & AARP, 2009). Unfortunately, these costs are frequently ignored by policy makers who are focused primarily on containing costs of services. The most dramatic economic costs to caregivers include giving up paid employment, lost income from unpaid leave or time off work, relinquishment of career advancement opportunities, and the prospect of out-of-pocket expenses to support home care. Those in the lowest income categories experience the highest economic burden. Employers need to consider flexible options to help the caregiver/employee meet the demands of his or her multiple roles.

Caregiver Assessment

Several studies have indicated the need for a systematic assessment of caregivers' needs and the impact of caregiving (Messecar, 2012). There are many tools designed to assess effects of caregiving after the caregiver has been providing care for some period of time (Deeken et al., 2003; van Exel, Scholte op Reimer, Brouwer, van den Berg, Koopmanschap, & van den Bos, 2004; Visser-Meily, Post, Riphagen, & Lindeman, 2004). For example, the *Caregiver Strain Index* was designed to assess strain in caregivers of postdischarge heart failure and hip surgery patients (Robinson, 1983). The *Mutuality and Preparedness Scales of the Family Care Inventory* were developed for use with caregivers 6 months postdischarge to evaluate the quality of the caregiver–care recipient relationship and to screen for the level of caregiver preparedness and recommend further assessment, respectively (Archbold, Stewart, Greenlick, & Harvath, 1990, 1992). Bakas developed two scales focusing on stroke caregivers post discharge: The *Bakas Caregiving Outcomes Scale* assesses caregiver life changes (Bakas et al., 2006) and the *Needs and Concerns Checklist* assesses postdischarge caregiver needs (Bakas et al., 2002).

These tools can be used to assess the impact of caregiving on the caregiver's health and well-being and to help target interventions specifically to the caregiver's needs. However, they do not assess a family member's commitment, capacity, and preparedness for assuming the caregiving role. Studies indicate that a systematic assessment of family members who are planning to assume the caregiving role should be conducted to identify areas of need (Lutz, Young, Creasy, & Cox, in press). This is especially important for first-time caregivers of care recipients who are hospitalized with a condition that results in functional limitations, such as stroke, cancer, brain injury, and spinal cord injury (Lutz, 2004; Lutz & Young, 2010; van Heugten, Visser-Meily, Post, & Lindeman, 2006).

Several authors have identified specific assessment domains that should be considered when evaluating caregivers. In 2003, Feinberg identified 12 caregiver assessment domains. These are included in the "Nursing Standard of Practice Protocol: Family Caregiving" by the Hartford Institute for Geriatric Nursing, in which the following areas of caregiver assessment are recommended: (1) caregiving context—including relationship to patient, roles and responsibilities, physical environment, resources, and cultural background; (2) caregiver's understanding of the patient's health and functional limitations; (3) level of preparation for and knowledge about the caregiving role; (4) quality of family relationships; (5) preexisting issues, such as marital discord or poor management of finances; and (6) the caregiver's physical, mental, and emotional health (Messecar, 2012).

Feinberg (2003) identified five often-neglected areas of caregiving assessment: "(1) actual tasks performed by family caregivers

beyond personal care functions; (2) skills necessary to provide the care; (3) quality of care provided; (4) values and preferences of the care recipient and the caregiver; and (5) positive aspects of caregiving" (p. 28). Clinical practice guidelines indicate that there is "level A" evidence that "caregivers should have their individual psychosocial and support needs reviewed on a regular basis" (Lindsay et al., 2010, p. 148). Level A evidence is the strongest recommendation and includes evidence from randomized controlled trials (RCTs) or meta-analyses where "desirable effects [of the interventions] clearly outweigh undesirable effects" (p. 232).

Feinberg and Houser (2012) identified "fundamental principles for caregiver assessment." These include the importance of (1) recognizing, respecting, assessing, and addressing the needs of caregivers; (2) including the preferences of both the caregiver and the care recipient; (3) developing a plan of care with measurable outcomes and regular updates; (4) using a multidimensional approach; and (5) reflecting cultural respect and competence. The assessment should be completed by practitioners with specialized knowledge about caregiving and should be covered by insurance as part of providing care for older persons with chronic illnesses. Unfortunately, these types of caregiver assessments are often overlooked.

Interventions

The Interface of Informal and Formal Caregiving Networks

The interface of a formal caregiving network with the family caregiver is important for the long-term emotional and physical health of the individual with chronic illness and his or her family caregiver(s). Recognizing the importance of family caregivers as integral to the care team and implementing models of care that view the family—not just the patient—as the unit of care is important to improve outcomes for patients and caregivers over the long term. Family caregivers rely on nurses and other healthcare professionals to assist them in navigating the caregiving role, especially when they are inexperienced. They also want to be included in treatment and care decisions and want providers to understand the care recipients' preferences for care (Creasy, Lutz, Young, Ford, & Martz, 2013).

Most interventions related to caregiving comprise a blend of both formal and informal networks of care and include providing information, skill building and problem solving, and support services. These interventions need to be individualized to address the caregiving needs and preferences, which are unique for each person with chronic illness and cannot be generalized to others (Lutz & Young, 2010).

Family-Centered Care

Knowledge of family systems theories provides a basis for understanding family-centered care. A family-centered model of care acknowledges the importance of considering the family system when caring for children or adults with chronic illnesses. In the 1970s, parents of children with chronic illness advocated for a family-centered approach to care; decades later, this practice is slowly being integrated into adult health care. The family-centered model of care evolved from earlier patient-centered models to a focus on the family as the unit of care. According to the Institute for Patient- and Family-Centered Care (IPFCC):

> *Patient- and family-centered care is an approach to the planning, delivery, and evaluation of health care that is grounded in mutually beneficial partnerships among health care providers, patients, and families. It redefines the relationships in health care. Patient- and family-centered practitioners recognize the vital role that families play in ensuring the health and well-being of infants, children, adolescents, and family members of all ages. They acknowledge that emotional, social, and developmental support are integral components of health care. They promote the health and well-being of individuals and families and restore dignity and control to them. Patient- and family-centered care is an approach to health care that shapes policies, programs, facility design, and staff day-to-day interactions. It leads to better health outcomes and wiser allocation of resources, and greater patient and family satisfaction. (IPFCC, 2010, para 1-3)*

Family members are defined by the patient and family unit and can be related biologically, emotionally, or legally. There are four core concepts of a family-centered model of care:

- Members of the interprofessional team demonstrate respect and dignity for patients and their family members by incorporating the knowledge, values, beliefs, and cultural practices that families bring to the healthcare interaction.
- The healthcare team provides unbiased, accurate, and complete information to patients and families that is useful and understandable so that family members and patients can effectively participate in team meetings and decisions about their care.
- Patients and their families are encouraged and supported to actively participate in care in ways that are meaningful to them through collaboration with the interprofessional team.
- Patients and family members are encouraged to collaborate in program and policy development to help advance the practice of family-centered care within the organization and healthcare policy (IPFCC, 2010).

By incorporating a family-centered approach to health care, the needs of caregivers and care recipients are considered in tandem and plans of care that take into account the needs and preferences of the family unit are developed.

Lifespan Development and Developmentally Appropriate Care

Knowledge of growth and development helps caregivers separate normal changes from disease-related changes in the dependent family member, regardless of the client's age. This knowledge helps caregivers deal more effectively with decision-making issues, obtain appropriate available community resources, and secure emotional support for themselves. Specialty organizations, such as the March of Dimes, provide this type of educational material for families of children and adolescents.

The Need for Culturally Sensitive Interventions

The United States and Canada have experienced massive waves of immigration as well as growing populations of native-born minorities. Given the diversity of racial, ethnic, and religious groups in North America, there is a need for healthcare professionals to learn more about the cultural groups with which they work so that they can provide culturally sensitive interventions. To that end, there has been a rapid rise of multicultural consciousness in the United States. Unfortunately, cultural awareness among healthcare professionals remains largely inadequate.

Awareness that the definition of family differs from one cultural group to another is important. For example, African American families may focus on a wider network of kin and community, and they often include non-biological family members in their family networks. The Chinese culture includes a person's ancestors and descendants in the definition of family, and the needs of the family are valued more highly than the needs of the individual. However, these values may be changing

because of globalization and the influence of Western values (Lee, 2007). Who the client considers to be family and who is providing care influences who should be included in interventions.

Cultural groups vary greatly in how they respond to problems and their attitudes toward seeking help. For example, Hispanic families may want to keep problems confidential and view caregiving as a responsibility of the female family members (Evans et al., 2007). To assist a Hispanic family, a healthcare professional will have to work on *personalismo*, knowing the older adult and her caregiver as total persons, before focusing on personal matters; *dignidad*, developing a working relationship that reflects dignity and self-worth; *respeto*, respect between the helping professional and Hispanic elder; and *confianza*, trust between the two parties (Evans et al., 2007; Gallagher-Thompson, Solano, Coon, & Areán, 2003).

Ethnic differences exist in attitudes toward caregiving and caregiving responsibilities. For example, Cuban Americans often have a hierarchical relational orientation and adhere to traditional family roles. Because of this factor, female caregivers may have difficulty in adopting the leadership role of caregiving (Mitrani & Czaja, 2000). Other cultural characteristics of Cubans are collectivism, giving precedence to the needs of the family over the individual, and the high degree of emotional and psychological closeness or enmeshment between caregiver and care recipient. Enmeshment, observed more frequently in Cuban families than in white American families, can produce a lack of objectivity and an unwillingness to delegate care tasks, making it difficult for the caregiver to be an effective care manager (Mitrani & Czaja, 2000). To work effectively with families from varied ethnic and cultural heritages, the nurse must tailor family interventions to be culturally congruent.

Providing assistance to family caregivers of minority elders for any number of issues is most effective when the members of the targeted minority group are represented in the provider or intervention group. For this reason, neighborhood-centered services, in which minority caregivers can interact with bilingual professionals, tend to be highly effective. These programs are well suited to respecting the values and customs of families in need of help and to offering culturally relevant solutions to the caregivers (Spector, 2000).

Providing Support and Building Skills

Part of the maturation of individual family caregivers and caregiving systems involves the development of realistic expectations of the individual member's abilities and limitations, as well as an understanding of the anticipated trajectory of dependent care that lies ahead. To provide adequate care for a dependent relative and at the same time secure their own well-being, family caregivers need support, aid, and understanding from their families and friends and from the healthcare system. To get that support, it is crucial that family caregivers learn to recognize when they need help, which kind of help to ask for, how to ask for the help they need, and who to ask (Mittelman, 2003). In doing so, caregivers may need assistance in developing skills and acquiring the information, support, and services to meet those needs (Bakas et al., 2002, Elliott & Shewshuk, 2003; Piercy & Chapman, 2001). Individual family caregivers and their caregiving systems may need assistance in learning how to cope with the positive and negative feelings and the emotional and social impacts of caregiving. Healthcare professionals need to promote family caregivers' well-being, which is a complex, multidimensional concept that includes personal meanings.

Family caregivers need formal providers who have time and the training necessary to help them develop effective skills for managing their day-to-day caregiving responsibilities. Because nurses with clinical training also understand behavioral and counseling techniques, they are often considered the most appropriate member of the team to work with family caregivers and to oversee educational programs.

In general, programs that build family caregiver confidence and skill and provide a feeling of support are more effective than those that simply impart knowledge (Piercy & Chapman, 2001; Smith, Forster, & Young, 2009). Problem-solving and skill-building interventions that target the specific concerns of family caregivers are especially effective and can reduce caregiver depression and distress (Elliott & Shewshuk, 2003). Kaye and colleagues (2003) found that early intervention screening of family caregivers of older relatives resulted in caregivers accessing sources of community support before a crisis and impending compassion fatigue. In all cases, intervention programs must be developmentally appropriate and tailored to be culturally relevant and learner specific.

The time constraints of most contemporary family caregivers are now being addressed by such strategies as telephone conferencing, Internet chat rooms, and email. Link2Care (http://www.link2care.net) and Caring~Web (http://caringweb.utoledo.edu/) are examples of successful, innovative Internet-based programs that combine high technology with traditional service to increase caregiver well-being and coping skills (Kelly, 2003–2004; Pierce & Steiner, 2013; Pierce, Steiner, Govoni, Hicks, Thompson, & Friedemann, 2004; Steiner & Pierce, 2002). Caregivers using both of these sites found features of updated news and research, information articles and fact sheets, online discussion groups, and "ask an expert" to be of value.

The Veterans Administration (VA) is using home-telehealth and web-based technologies to link caregivers and veterans with chronic conditions to primary care providers at the VA (Lutz, Chumbler, Lyles, Hoffman, & Kobb, 2008; Lutz et al., 2007). It is no longer the case that an intervention program can be effective only when it includes direct, face-to-face contact. The key is to make the interventions relevant, multicomponent, tailored to caregivers' needs, and accessible when the caregiver needs support (Chambers & Connor, 2002; Elliott & Shewchuk, 2003; Gitlin et al., 2003; Mittelman, 2003). Many of the caregiving Internet site resources identified at the end of the chapter contain specific support interventions.

Caregivers also need the opportunity for activities other than providing care to avoid a sense of entrapment and feelings of loss of self and burnout. Attention to self-help activities sustains one's sense of well-being and revitalizes energy that can later be used in providing care to the client, but many caregivers feel guilty about engaging in activities that focus on themselves (Abdendroth et al., 2011).

Spirituality and Caregiving

Spiritual beliefs and faith-based behaviors play multiple roles in caregivers' lives. This point was evidenced by caregivers feeling the presence of a greater power described by a caregiver as "watching over them, giving them strength, providing meaning to life, and working in mysterious ways" (Pierce, Steiner, Havens, & Tormoehlen, 2008, p. 7). Spirituality involves connectedness not only with a sacred other, but also with other people, perspectives, and sources of value and meaning beyond oneself (Faver, 2004). Such connectedness can produce happiness and energy to sustain a caregiver's ability to care for a family member with chronic illness (Faver, 2004; Haley & Harrigan, 2004; Pierce et al., 2008). Whether caregivers hold religious beliefs or not, they have needs for love, meaning, purpose, and, sometimes, transcendence in their lives (Murray, Kendall, Boyd, Worth, Boyd, & Benton, 2004). Caregivers draw strength from maintaining relationships with their families and value opportunities to give and receive love, to feel connected to their social world, and to feel useful (Abendroth et al., 2012; Murray et al., 2004).

Religious beliefs and formal religious practices can be essential aspects of caregiving.

Heavy reliance on prayer to cope with adversity has been reported by many caregivers (Paun, 2004; Stuckey, 2001). African American women caregivers describe their prayer as an ongoing dialogue that keeps them connected with their God rather than as a formal religious ritual (Paun, 2004). Religiosity is also demonstrated by the belief that God has a plan, belief in a loving God, hope in an afterlife, and a sense of the evidence of God all around (Hamilton, Moore, Johnson, & Koenig, 2013; Stuckey, 2001). Reading the Bible and other religious materials and listening to music are also aspects of formal religion used by caregivers (Hamilton et al., 2013; Theis, Biordi, Coeling, Nalepka, & Miller, 2003). Churches provide an important source of encouragement and social support for caregivers (Faver, 2004; Murray et al., 2004; Theis et al., 2003). A strong connection with a caring community is what caregivers value in their church relationships. Caregivers find that the consistent presence of fellow parishioners is a powerful sustaining force (Faver, 2004). Efforts to maintain chronically ill spouses' engagement in religious practices, such as church attendance, are important for caregivers. When church attendance is no longer possible, caregivers substitute televised or recorded services and arrange for other formal religious practices like communion to be given at their home (Paun, 2004).

Churches and Communities in Care Solutions

In addition to government-sponsored programs to help caregivers, churches have a potentially important role to play in caregivers' lives. Although to date little research has been conducted on the role of churches in elder care, Stuckey (2001) found that churches supported caregivers by encouraging continued church participation whenever possible and by taking services to the care recipient and caregiver when needed.

An example of a church collaboration is the Interfaith CarePartners (www.interfaith-carepartners.org). This innovative church collaboration began in 1985 in the Greater Houston, Texas, area. The focus of the program is a care team concept of caregiving that provides in-home support to individuals with chronic health conditions and offers respite support to their caregivers. Individuals with AIDS/HIV were the first to benefit from the care team approach. Caring for those persons with Alzheimer's disease and dementia began in 1992, followed by caring for the elderly or those with disabling conditions in 1994, and lastly caring for families with impaired children in 2000 (Interfaith CarePartners, 2011).

Communities also have a role in providing assistance to those in need of care. An excellent example of a community partnership is the Gatekeeper Model developed in Spokane, Washington (Substance Abuse & Mental Health Services Administration, 2004). Employees of community businesses and corporations who work with the public (the "gatekeepers") are trained to identify and refer community-dwelling older adults who may be in need of aid. Upon referral by these gatekeepers, home-based assessments are conducted by interprofessional teams provided by the local mental health services, with referrals made for additional services as needed.

Programs, Services, and Resources for Family Caregivers

A multitude of information and referral links, products and services, educational sites, and caregiver support groups are available online. There is no shortage of programs, services, and resources for family caregivers. However, one problem is finding affordable programs that are accessible and convenient for overwhelmed family caregivers. In addition, narrowing an Internet search from a broad term like "family caregiving" to a search for agencies and organizations to assist family caregivers or books for

caregivers and professionals still yields an enormous number of results. An easy-to-use, comprehensive list of agencies and organizations with resources for family caregivers, plus a list of books for caregivers and professionals, can be found on the Family Caregiver Alliance website (www.caregiver.org).

Utilization of community services by family caregivers provides a range of benefits for caregivers. Unfortunately, barriers to services persist. Benefits reported by caregivers include renewal, sense of community, and knowledge and belief that their family member also benefited from the service. Barriers include care recipient resistance, reluctance of the caregiver, hassles for the caregiver, concerns about quality, and concerns about finances (Reinhard et al., 2008; Winslow, 2003). Nurses and other healthcare professionals involved in community services need to work to decrease or eliminate these barriers faced by family caregivers.

Respite Programs and Services

Respite is temporary relief from caregiving responsibilities that provides intervals of rest and relief for the caregiver. Family members may provide respite for the primary caregiver by taking over some tasks; for example, children may assist their caregiving parents shopping, cleaning, and so forth. There ar formal sources of respite, such as adult programs, in-home companions, an weekend respite programs.

It is important for caregiver the warning signs that indic skills are deteriorating and outside help. For many est step is acknowledgi the next most difficu effort to seek this guilty about see formal respite and debilita lenges nor particularly for spousal caregivers who feel it is their role to provide assistance that is needed in the home.

> *In retrospect, I see that I was hanging on by a thread as Randy's health continued to decline. I was too close to the situation and trying to be the perfect family caregiver for my husband. When you are so close to the situation, you're often numb and unable to even figure out that you need help. During the last 2 weeks of his life, some nights Randy and I were up 20 times. Now, I wonder why our hospice nurse and social worker couldn't see that I was losing it. Yes, I've been an RN for 40-plus years, so maybe they thought I could handle the situation. But this was my husband of 43 years who was dying, and when that happens, you lose prospective.*

—Jenny

Caregivers need to see respite services as a reasonable and appropriate action, not as a sign of personal failure, if they plan to continue caregiving without being overwhelmed by the physical and social demands; as this caregiver describes: "Respite would help because I know I've tried ⌐d my attitude changed during that ⌐e rested and felt like I ⌐ get away

comparable to what is provided at home and that the relative is not negatively affected by the hospital stay (Gilmour, 2002; Phillipson & Jones, 2011).

Both Medicare and many long-term care insurance policies provide a short-term nursing home placement for a dependent family member. Longer or more frequent temporary stays are also possible, if the family has the financial resources to do so.

Adult Day Services

Adult day services (formerly known as adult daycare) are congregate programs that provide opportunities for impaired adults to socialize and participate in organized activities, and for their families to receive respite time. Use of adult day services results in decreased caregiver worry and stress and improved psychological well-being (Ritchie, 2003; Zarit, Kim, Femia, Almeida, Savla, & Molenaar, 2011). Caregivers appreciate the client socializing and improved health (behavior and sleep patterns) as well as the respite for themselves on the day(s) this service is used (Warren, Kerr, Smith, Godkin, & Schalm, 2003; Zarit et al., 2011).

Great variation exists in the type and amount of services that these centers provide. In general, the centers are broadly classified as ⌐ or social models of care. Social models ⌐asize socialization and cognitive stimula- ⌐. Health models of care are often supported ⌐ a state's Medicaid program and include ⌐lthcare monitoring in the day program. In ⌐eral, the major difference between the two ⌐pes of programs is the presence or absence ⌐ a registered nurse on site. Some health pro- ⌐rams with advanced rehabilitation or restor- ⌐tive programs are certified by Medicare as day treatment hospitals and include rehabilitation specialists on staff.

Social day programs have a variety of funding options, but most reimbursement sources are limited to low-income families or those with long-term care insurance (AOA, 2011b).

Day health programs are primarily Medicaid-funded programs or those skilled rehabilitation programs that are eligible for Medicare reimbursement. The out-of-pocket cost of day care to the family caregivers varies widely, depending on the region of the country and the type of program offered.

FAMILY COUNSELING INTERVENTIONS

Individual, couple, group, or family counseling may be needed to help families respond to the changes associated with chronic illness and the demands of caregiving. Individual counseling is directed toward enhancing the caregiver's capacity to deal with the day-to-day rigors of caregiving. Family counseling can be complex because of the multiple issues involved, such as changes in relationships and roles, dependency, grief over the losses, uncertainty, and fear. When peer interaction and feedback seem appropriate, group therapy can be effective in assisting family caregivers in decision making and problem solving associated with the caregiving role.

Using a family-centered approach, New York University has been conducting a longitudinal study of a family and spousal caregiver counseling intervention for caregivers with dementia since 1987. The intervention includes two individual caregiver counseling sessions, four family sessions, a support group, and additional telephone counseling as needed for crisis management. Over the more than 25 years that the program has been providing this support to caregivers, researchers have found that individual, family, and group counseling can have positive effects on caregivers. These include a reduction in depression, delays in institutionalization, improved family relationships, and improved caregiver health and well-being (Mittelman, 2002).

SUPPORT GROUPS

Also called self-help groups, support groups are forums that focus on specific client populations and related caregivers' needs. Self-help groups for caregivers have been established in many communities throughout the United States. Some are self-directed or run by volunteers; others are led by healthcare professionals who act as group facilitators. These groups provide information, emotional support, advocacy, or a combination of these services. Telephone support networks and Internet chat rooms are simply contemporary versions of the traditional face-to-face support group.

> *Each month I put on my calendar when the support group was meeting at the oncology office. Randy would never go. It just wasn't his thing. But initially the idea of a support group appealed to me. But as the day of the support group meeting approached, I would get cold feet and not go. What was I afraid of? That I would hear worse stories than Randy's? That I would cry the whole time? I might have learned something from the people there. But I never gave it a chance.*
>
> —Jenny

Evidence-Based Practice

Evidence-based practice is based on the demonstrated effectiveness of interventions tested in multiple clinical trials. Systematic reviews of research are considered to be the highest level of evidence. As described in the previous sections, numerous studies have tested a variety of interventions intended to help improve the health and well-being of caregivers. However, there are limited systematic reviews of the literature that focus on these widely varying interventions. Furthermore, the reviews available cite the lack of high-quality evidence and poor consistency in the clinical trials testing these interventions (Boots, de Vugt, van Knippenberg, Kempen, & Verhey, 2013; Glasdam, Timm, & Vitrrup, 2010; Smith et al., 2009). Therefore, it is imperative that more intervention research is conducted with a focus on replicating previous clinical trials. Researchers also suggest the inclusion of qualitative findings in the systematic reviews to better determine the specific effects of the interventions from caregivers' perspectives (Thompson et al., 2007). **Table 10-1** includes examples of systematic reviews of the literature on caregiver interventions.

Outcomes

Care Recipient, Caregiver, and Caregiving System Outcomes

Providing care to another person has both positive and negative outcomes for the primary caregiver and the caregiver system. Because caregiving is a very personal journey, it is almost impossible to predict how each caregiver or care recipient will respond to the demands of dependency and caregiving support. Therefore, all of the interventions provided by an interprofessional team should ultimately be directed toward supporting family caregivers when the situation is going well and not so well.

As noted earlier, much of the caregiving literature reflects a focus on the negative aspects of caregiving. Nevertheless, a growing body of literature is available on the positive aspects of the caregiver role. The literature continues to need studies that identify the potential benefits of caregiving for the purpose of increasing our understanding of the caregiving experience (Tarlow et al., 2004) as well as preventing the likelihood of viewing caregiving only from a pathologic perspective and thus socializing caregivers to expect this role to be a burden (Gaugler, Kane, & Langlois, 2000). The study of caregiver benefits can also provide data for the development of evidence-based supportive care strategies and interventions to help families and family caregivers develop the skills needed to manage caregiving responsibilities on a long-term basis (Harding & Higginson, 2003).

Despite the paucity of information regarding the benefits derived from the caregiver role, the available studies indicate that most caregivers find some element of satisfaction in the caregiving experience (Hudson, 2004; Kate, Grover, Kulhara, & Nehra, 2013; Nolan, 2001; Scott, 2001). Kate and associates (2013) suggest that higher positive caregiving experiences are associated with better quality of life in family caregivers of persons with schizophrenia. Hudson (2004) reported that 60% of caregivers readily identified positive aspects of the caregiver role. Given what is known about long-term family caregiving, several outcomes are commonly monitored. Together, these outcomes form a gold standard by which caregiving experiences can be measured. Outcomes for both the family caregivers and their care recipients include assessment of quality and meaning in life; levels of family stress and coping, including signs of anxiety and depressive symptoms; and impact on social functioning.

QUALITY OF LIFE

Chronic illness can have profound effects on the quality of life for both care recipients and family members. It has been written that human beings "can be at their best when they are behaving with altruism and commitment to a person they love" (Lattanzi-Licht, Mahoney, & Miller, 1998, p. 31). Evidence of enhanced meaning of life can be seen in caregivers' comments about positive aspects of caregiving: "Love doing it—we've been given an opportunity we'd never thought we'd have" (Hudson, 2004, p. 62).

However, quality of life can be negatively impacted by the day-to-day responsibilities of caregiving, as well as by a care recipient whose health is declining and moving toward the end of life. To minimize these negative effects on the quality of life of the family unit, nurses and other healthcare professionals need to conduct periodic assessments of the family caregiver's needs and capacity to assume and/or continue in the caregiving role and implement interventions to help prepare the family on its journey through the chronic illness trajectory (Lutz & Young 2010; Lutz et al., in press). Enhancing caregiver preparedness and support can help

Table 10-1 EXAMPLES OF SYSTEMATIC REVIEWS OF RESEARCH ON CAREGIVING INTERVENTIONS

Authors (Date)	Focus of Review and Number of Studies Reviewed	Findings	Recommendations
Selwood, Johnston, Katona, Lyketsos, & Livingston (2007)	Effectiveness of psychological interventions for family CGs of persons with dementia (n = 62 RCTs)	Individual behavioral management therapy with 6 or more sessions is effective in decreasing CG depression. Group behavioral management therapy is not as effective. Individual or group therapy focusing on coping strategies is effective. Education on dementia and supportive therapy are not effective.	Individual behavioral management and individual and group coping strategy therapy improve CG mental health. Educational sessions should be individualized to each CG. More research is needed.
Smith, Forster, & Young (2009)	Effectiveness of information provision on improving outcomes for patients with stroke and their CGs (n = 11 RCTs)	Providing information improves knowledge of patients and CGs, but shows no effect on CG stress.	Limited evidence. More research on information provision interventions is needed, with a focus on active strategies that involve the patient and CG.
Glasdam, Timm, & Vitrrup (2010)	Describe and critically evaluate support interventions for caregivers of chronically ill persons (n = 32 studies: 29 RCTs, 3 clinical trials published from 1997 to 2007)	Incomplete description of the research design in many of the studies reviewed. An aim of all interventions was to improve CG knowledge and support. Education and counseling were provided at individual and/or group levels. Mode of delivery included in-home visits, face-to-face counseling, and telephone support.	Insufficient evidence to make a recommendation. Effect of support interventions for CG is inconclusive. Quality of the studies is questionable. Future research should include interventions that go beyond knowledge transfer and cognitive-behavioral therapy, focusing instead on interventions that support CG relationships and activities in their home or local environments.
Boots, de Vugt, van Knippenberg, Kempen, & Verhey (2013)	Review of Internet interventions for CGs of CRs with dementia (n = 12 studies)	Studies employed various types, dosage, and duration of intervention. CGs of persons with mild cognitive impairment exhibited symptoms of depression, stress, and burden.	Internet interventions may improve CG confidence, depression, and self-efficacy. However, the level of evidence is not strong and the methodological quality of the studies varied widely. More research is needed in this area.

CG = caregiver; CR = care recipient; RCT = randomized controlled trial.

Note: See individual citations for more details.

family members feel that they are able to be confident in this role. This, in turn, can help contribute to a positive caregiving experience—for example, "Taking responsibility for things I had not previously been responsible for"; "I feel like I'm a stronger person now"; and "I've been able to undertake much more than I thought I could" (Hudson, 2004, p. 62).

FAMILY STRESS AND COPING

As previously discussed, the adverse effects of caregiving include an array of affective responses by caregivers to the demands of long-term caregiving. An important goal of the care team is to evaluate the level of stress and anxiety and implement interventions to reduce it to a level that is perceived by the caregiver to be manageable. Caregivers are able to voice positive aspects in their role despite the negative aspects (Hudson, 2004; Roff et al., 2004). Perhaps caregivers use positive emotions to augment and maintain their coping strategies when faced with an ongoing stressor like caregiving (Folkman, 1997).

SOCIAL FUNCTIONING

Social functioning is an important component of quality of life. Caregivers of all ages often limit or give up leisure, work, and social activities to provide care for a family member with a chronic illness, sacrificing activities and leading to social isolation. It is critical that nurses and other healthcare professionals work with caregivers to identify strategies to help maintain social interactions. Research has demonstrated that when caregivers are satisfied with their social lives, they are less likely to experience depressive and other negative symptoms associated with caregiving (Brodaty, 2009).

Societal Outcomes

Studies have examined the cost-effectiveness of community-based home services to groups of individuals at risk for nursing home placement. In a 2012 survey of 15,300 long-term care providers, in-home services for a certified nursing assistant cost an average of $19/hour; adult day-care services, $61/day; assisted living, $3,300/month; and nursing home care, $6,000/month (Genworth, 2013). These calculations do not take into consideration the out-of-pocket expenses and subsidized programs and services that family caregivers must use to make community-based care a viable long-term care option for them and their dependent family members. Furthermore, in many states Medicaid covers the cost of nursing home care for low-income residents, and Medicare and some insurance policies include short-term nursing home benefits after hospital discharge under certain circumstances. In contrast, the costs of in-home and community-based services are not often covered by third-party payers unless the care recipient has private long-term care insurance.

Despite the fact that home- and community-based care may not be less costly than institutional care, providing such care remains a goal for many families and a priority of policy makers. This is because institutional care is perceived as more expensive by most policy makers, and as less desirable than home care by older adults and policy makers alike, who clearly prefer non-institutional solutions to long-term care.

Institutional placement is typically a very difficult decision for caregivers to make. A study of how caregivers decided on long-term care placement for persons with Parkinson's disease found that as the caregiving load increased, so did caregiver strain. This increasing load and strain led to nursing home placement, which was usually precipitated by a trigger event, such as an injurious fall, depletion of informal and formal resources, high safety risk for the caregiver and/or care recipient, or the caregiver's inability to manage the high level of care required. However, caregivers were left feeling guilty and remorseful after making this decision. Comments from one caregiver are representative: "It was, and still is, something—a decision that I agonize over every day. Every time I go [to the nursing home], I leave in tears because it breaks my heart" (Abendroth et al., 2012, p. 50).

CASE STUDY 10-1

Z. is a 90-year-old woman who lives alone in her own two-story home. During this past year, she has fallen once and been treated for a broken left hip at a local hospital and rehabilitation facility. Z. reports her health as "good," although she is often tired. Recently she placed her husband in a dementia care unit in a Veterans Administration facility 1 hour from her home. She cries when she shares that while she visits him every day, she feels "emotionally drained." Her son lives in another state, but is the primary caregiver. The son is concerned about his mother's home environment, her chance of falling again, and her emotional stability in dealing with her husband, his father. The son wants to assist his mother, but he is physically unable to provide aid and is at a loss on how to help.

Discussion Questions

1. What are the advantages and disadvantages of Z. living in her own home? For her? For her son?
2. What are some emotional responses to family caregiving?
3. How can healthcare professionals support family caregivers?
   - Which ideas might be offered to her son in helping his mother decrease her fatigue and feeling "emotionally drained"?
   - Suggest a first step for this son to prevent his mother from a fall at home.

     If you chose a home assessment targeted at preventing falls, so did the son. There are many home safety checklists available online to evaluate the home setting, as well as professional checklists. The son contacted the local rehabilitation facility and scheduled a home assessment. The assessment results were as follows:
   - Medication and alcohol use: Z. takes medicine for high blood pressure (metoprolol [Lopressor] 50 mg every morning) and diabetes (pioglitazone [Actos] 30 mg in the evening and glimepiride [Amaryl] 5 mg in the morning). She denies any side effects of the medicines or use of alcohol.
   - Vision problems: Z.'s vision with glasses is corrected to 20/20.
   - Neurological deficits (e.g., balance problems, mental confusion, and faulty judgment): There are no uncovered deficits for Z.
   - Incontinence/urgency: Z. reports no problems.
   - Fear of falling: Z. shares that she is "afraid of falling again."
   - Environmental factors: No deficits were found in Z.'s home.
4. Where can family caregivers go for assistance and information?
   - For example, are any of Z.'s medications a potential cause for falls? Search the Internet and find at least one website that describes these medications and the associated side effects that will be useful for the son in caring for his mother.
   - To combat the "fear of falling again," which strategies can be offered to her son to keep Z. connected to others in times of emergencies?

CASE STUDY 10-2

Mr. and Mrs. R. have been married for 65 years. They emigrated to the United States from Mexico as a young couple and have lived here since then. They are 85 and 87 years old, respectively. The R.s are devout Catholics and live in the same two-story home in a mid-sized community where they raised their children. Slowly, their older friends are moving out of the neighborhood, and the houses are being sold as rental properties to younger, working families. Mrs. R. walks her dog a few blocks every day. However, Mr. R. has developed severe arthritis and has difficulty walking without the assistance of a walker. The R.s have one friend, a widow in the neighborhood, whom they see a couple of times each week. The couple own a car and while Mr. R. used to be the primary driver, his vision has declined and he no longer drives. Mrs. R. is now the driver; so far, she can get to the grocery store, doctor's appointments, the pharmacy, and other places they need to go.

The R.'s have four adult children—two sons and two daughters, all of whom have moved to other states. Until recently, one of their daughters lived close by, and she saw her parents frequently. However, the daughter has moved to another state to help her own daughter, who is single, care for her children. Since moving, the daughter notes that when she talks to her parents, both seem to be getting more frail. Her mother's short-term memory is getting poorer. She repeats the same stories frequently and has trouble remembering recent events and appointments—she missed her most recent appointment with her primary care provider and had to reschedule. Her father has had two falls without injury. The daughter is worried about her parents' safety and her mother's ability to continue to care for her father, who needs help with basic and instrumental activities of daily living. The daughter believes that in the next year her mother will have to quit driving and will not be able to care for her father. She is also concerned that her father's balance is getting worse and that he is at increased risk for an injurious fall. The daughter is trying to decide how to approach her parents about relocating to a retirement community in the daughter's city. Her father has repeatedly said he will never move; Mrs. R. seems a little more amenable to the idea, but she generally lets her husband make the decisions.

The R.'s sons think their parents are doing fine and they should be able to stay in their home. Furthermore, the sons believe it is up to their sister, as the oldest, to care for their parents and do not understand why she cannot just move back to care for them. The youngest daughter is ambivalent: She wants her parents to be happy, but she understands both her brothers' and sister's concerns.

It is difficult to figure out what is best for Mr. and Mrs. R. over the long term. The oldest daughter is anxious about approaching her parents about a possible move to a retirement community. She plans to call their primary care provider, a nurse practitioner who cares for both of them, to discuss her concerns.

Discussion Questions
1. What are the "at-risk" variables of Mr. and Mrs. R.?
2. Which factors should the daughter consider when she talks with her parents about her concerns?
3. What are potential drawbacks to having Mr. and Mrs. R., as a couple, move to the retirement community?
4. What is the impact of the family's cultural background on these decisions?

Internet Resources

AARP Caregiving Resource Center: http://www.aarp.org/home-family/caregiving/

AssistGuide Information Services: http://www.agis.com

"Caregiver Resources: Because We Care," Administration on Aging and the U.S. Department of Health and Human Services: http://www.aasa.dshs.wa.gov/caregiving/documents/BecauseWeCare.pdf

Caregiving Resources from the American College of Physicians, Internal Medicine: http://www.acponline.org

Caring for someone with Alzheimer's: http://nihseniorhealth.gov/alzheimerscare/afterthediagnosis/01.html

Caring from a distance: http://www.cfad.org

Empowering caregivers: http://www.care-givers.com

Family Caregiver Alliance: http://caregiver.org/caregiver/jsp/home.jsp

Institute for Patient- and Family-Centered Care: http://www.ipfcc.org

Interfaith CarePartners: http://www.interfaithcarepartners.org

National Alliance for Caregiving: http://www.caregiving.org

National Cancer Institute, Coping with Cancer: http://www.cancer.gov/cancertopics/coping

National Family Caregivers' Association: http://www.nfcacares.org

References

Abendroth, M. A., Lutz, B. J., & Young, M. E. (2012). Family caregivers' decision process to institutionalize persons with Parkinson's disease: A grounded theory study. *International Journal of Nursing Studies, 49*(4), 445–454.

Action Canada. (2013). Who cares about young carers? http://www.scribd.com/doc/124089317/Who-Cares-About-Young-Carers-Raising-Awareness-for-an-Invisible-Population

Administration on Aging (AOA). (2009). National Center on Elder Abuse (Title II). http://aoa.gov /AoARoot/AoA_programs/elder_rights/NCEA/Index .aspx

Administration on Aging (AOA). (2010). *A profile of older Americans: 2009.* Washington, DC: U.S. Department of Health and Human Services.

Administration on Aging (AOA). (2011a). National family caregiver support program (OAA Title III E). http://www.aoa.gov/AoAroot/AoA_programs/HCLTC /Caregiver/index.aspv

Administration on Aging (AOA). (2011b). AOA programs. http://aoa.gov/AoARoot/AoA_Programs/index .aspx

Administration on Aging (AOA). (2012). *A profile of older Americans: 2012.* Washington, DC: U.S. Department of Health and Human Services. http://www.aoa.gov /AoARoot/Aging_Statistics/Profile/2012/4.aspx

Allen, S. M., Goldscheider, F., & Ciambrone, D. (1999). Gender roles, marital intimacy, and nomination of spouses as primary caregivers. *The Gerontologist, 39,* 150–158.

American Psychological Association (APA). (2012). *Elder abuse and neglect.* Washington, DC: Author. http:// www.apa.org/pi/aging/resources/guides/elder-abuse.pdf

American Psychological Association (APA). (2013). Who are family caregivers? http://www.apa.org/pi/about /publications/caregivers/faq/statistics.aspx

Anderson, L. A., Edward, V. J., Pearson, W. S., Talley, R. C., McGuire, L.C., & Andresen, E. M. (2013). Adult caregivers in the United States: Characteristics and differences in well-being, by caregiver age and caregiving status. *Preventing Chronic Disease, 10.* http://dx.doi .org/10.5888/pcd10.130090

Archbold, P. G., Stewart, B. J., Greenlick, M. R., & Harvath T. (1990). Mutuality and preparedness as predictors of caregiver role strain. *Research in Nursing and Health, 13*(6), 375–384.

Archbold, P. G., Stewart, B. J., Greenlick, M. R., & Harvath, T. A. (1992). The clinical assessment of mutuality and preparedness in family caregivers to frail older people. In S. Funk, E. Tornquist, M. Champagne, & R. Wiese (Eds.), *Key aspects of elder care: Managing falls, incontinence, and cognitive impairments* (pp. 328-339). New York, NY: Springer.

Austin, L. (2013). Children as caregivers. http://caregiver. com/articles/children/children_as_caregivers3.htm

Badr, H., & Acitelli, L. K. (2005). Dyadic adjustment in chronic illness: Does relationship talk matter? *Journal of Family Psychiatry, 19*(2), 465–469.

Bakas, T., Austin, J. K., Okonkwo, K. F., Lewis, R. R., & Chadwick, L. (2002). Needs, concerns, strategies,

and advice of stroke caregivers: The first 6 months after discharge. *Journal of Neuroscience Nursing, 34*(5), 242–251.

Bakas, T., Champion, V., Perkins, S. M., Farran, C. J., & Williams, L. S. (2006). Psychometric testing of the revised 15-item Bakas Caregiving Outcomes Scale. *Nursing Research, 55*(5), 346–355.

Barrett, A. E., & Lynch, S. M. (1999). Caregiving networks of elderly persons: Variation by marital status. *The Gerontologist, 39,* 695–704.

Blencowe, H., Cousens, S., Oestergaard, M., Chou, D., Moller, A. B., Narwal, R., … Lawn, J. E. (2012). National, regional and worldwide estimates of preterm birth. *Lancet, 9*(379), 2162–2172.

Bodenheimer, T., Chen, E., & Bennett, H. D. (2009). Confronting the growing burden of chronic disease: Can the U.S. health care workforce do the job? *Health Affairs, 28*(1), 64–74.

Boerner, K., & Schulz, R. (2010). Caregiving, bereavement and complicated grief. *Bereavement Care 28*(3), 10–13. doi: 10.1080/02682620903355382

Boots, L. M. M., de Vugt, M. E., van Knippenberg, R. J. M., Kempen, G. I. J. M., & Verhey, R. J. (2013, August). A systematic review of Internet-based supportive interventions for caregivers of patients with dementia. *International Journal of Geriatric Psychiatry.* Epub ahead of print. http://www.ncbi.nlm.nih.gov .lp.hscl.ufl.edu/pubmed/23963684

Brodaty, H. (2009). Family caregivers of people with dementia. *Dialogues in Clinical Neuroscience, 11*(2), 217–228.

Bursack, C. (2011). You are still a caregiver when you need outside help. http://www.eldercarelink.com /In-Home-Care/You-Are-Still-a-Caregiver-When-You- Get-Outside-Help.htm

Bursack, C. (2013). When adult grandchildren become the primary caregiver. http://www.agingcare.com /Articles/grandchildren-caring-for-their-grandparents-149490.htm

Centers for Disease Control and Prevention (CDC). (2009). Chronic diseases: The power to prevent, the call to control—at a glance 2009. http://www.cdc.gov /nccdphp/publications/AAG/chronic.htm

Centers for Disease Control and Prevention (CDC). (2013). Elder abuse prevention. http://www.cdc.gov /features/elderabuse/

Center for Medicare and Medicaid Services (CMS). (2012). *Chronic conditions among Medicare beneficiaries: Chartbook, 2012 edition.* Baltimore, MD: Author.

Chambers, M., & Connor, S. L. (2002). User-friendly technology to help family carers cope. *Journal of Advanced Nursing, 40*(5), 568–577.

Chumbler, N. R., Rittman, M., Van Puymbroeck, M., Vogel, W. B., & Qin, H. (2004). The sense of coherence, burden, and depressive symptoms in informal caregivers during the first month after stroke. *International Journal of Geriatric Psychiatry, 19*(10), 944–953.

Chumbler, N. R., Rittman, M. R., & Wu, S. S. (2007). Associations of sense of coherence and depression in caregivers of stroke survivors across 2 years. *Journal of Behavioral Health Services Research, 35*(2), 226–234.

Colello, K. (2009). *Family caregiving to the older population: Background, federal programs and issues for congress.* Washington, DC: Congressional Research Service.

Creasy, K. R., Lutz, B. J., Young, M. E., Ford, A., & Martz, C. (2013). The impact of interactions with providers on stroke caregivers' needs. *Rehabilitation Nursing, 38*(2), 786–797.

Day, J. R., & Anderson, R. A. (2011). Compassion fatigue: An application of the concept to informal caregivers of family members with dementia. *Nursing Research and Practice, 2011*(408024), 1–10. doi: 10.1155/2011/408024

Day, T. (2013). About caregiving. http://www.long-termcarelink.net/eldercare/caregiving.htm

Deeken, J. F., Taylor, K. L., Mangan, P., Yabroff, K. R., & Ingham, J. M. (2003). Care for the caregivers: A review of self-report instruments developed to measure the burden, needs, and quality of life of informal caregivers. *Journal of Pain and Symptom Management, 26*(4), 922–953.

Desilver, D. (2013). As population ages, more Americans becoming caregivers. Pew Research Center. http://www.pewresearch.org/fact-tank/2013/07/18/as-population-ages-more-americans-becoming-caregivers/

Elliot, T. R., & Shewchuk, R. M. (2003). Social problem-solving and distress among family members assuming a caregiving role. *British Journal of Health Psychology, 8*, 149–163.

Evans, B. C., Coon, D. W., & Crogan, N. L. (2007). *Personalismo* and breaking barriers: Accessing Hispanic populations for clinical services and research. *Geriatric Nursing 28*(5), 289–296.

Evercare & National Alliance for Caregiving (NAC). (2007). *Evercare study of family caregivers: What they spend, what they sacrifice.* Minnetonka, MN: Author. http://www.caregiving.org/data/Evercare_NAC_CaregiverCostStudyFINAL20111907.pdf

Family Caregiver Alliance (FCA). (2006). *Fact sheet: Caregiver health.* San Francisco, CA: Author. http://caregiver.org/caregiver/jsp/content_node.jsp?nodeid=1822

Family Caregiver Alliance (FCA). (2009). Caregiving. http://www.caregiver.org/caregiver/jsp/content_node.jsp?nodeid=2313

Family Caregiver Alliance (FCA). (2012). Selected caregiver statistics. http://www.caregiver.org/caregiver/jsp/content_node.jsp?nodeid=439&expandnodeid=384

Faver, C. A. (2004). Relational spirituality and social caregiving. *Social Work, 49*(2), 241–249.

Feinberg, L. (2003). The state of the art of caregiving assessment. *Generations, 27*(4), 24–32.

Feinberg, L., & Houser, A. (2012). *Assessing family caregiver needs: Policy and practice considerations.* Washington, DC: AARP Public Policy Institute. http://www.caregiving.org/wp-content/uploads/2010/11/AARP-caregiver-fact-sheet.pdf

Feinberg, L., & Reamy, A. M. (2011). *Health reform law creates new opportunities to better recognize and support family caregivers.* Washington, DC: AARP Public Policy Institute. http://assets.aarp.org/rgcenter/ppi/ltc/fs239.pdf

Feinberg, L., Reinhard, S., Houser, A., & Coula, R. (2011). *Valuing the invaluable: 2011 update the growing contributions and costs of family caregiving.* Washington, DC: AARP Public Policy Institute. http://www.aarp.org/relationships/caregiving/info-07-2011/valuing-the-invaluable.html

Figley, C. R. (1995). Compassion fatigue: Toward a new understanding of the costs of caring. In B. Hudnall Stamm (Ed.), *Secondary traumatic stress: Self-care issues for clinicians, researchers, and educators* (pp. 3–28). Baltimore, MD: Sidran Press.

Figley, C. R. (1998). Burnout as systemic traumatic stress: A model for helping traumatized family members. In C. R. Figley (Ed.), *Burnout in families: The systemic costs of caring* (pp. 15–28). Boca Raton, FL: CRC Press.

Folkman, S. (1997). Positive psychological states and coping with severe stress. *Social Science & Medicine, 45*(8), 1207–1221.

Friedemann, M. L., Buckwalter, K. C., Newman, F. L., & Mauro, A. C. (2013). Patterns of caregiving of Cuban, other Hispanic, Caribbean black, and white elders in south Florida. *Journal of Cross-Cultural Gerontology, 28*, 137–152. doi: 10.1007/s10823-013-9193-6

Gallagher-Thompson, D., Solano, N., Coon, P., & Areán, P. (2003). Recruitment and retention of Latino dementia family caregivers in intervention research: Issues to face, lessons to learn. *The Gerontologist, 43*, 45–51.

Gaugler, J., Kane, R., & Langlois, J. (2000). Assessment of family caregivers of older adults. In R. Kane & R. Kane (Eds.), *Assessing older persons: Measures, meaning and practical applications* (pp. 321–359). New York, NY: Oxford University Press.

Geister, C. (2005). The feeling of responsibility as core motivation for caregiving – Why daughters care for their mothers. *Pflege, 18*(1), 5–14.

Genworth. (2013). *Cost of care survey: Home care providers, adult day health care facilities, assisted living facilities, and nursing homes* (10th ed.). New York, NY: Genworth Financial.

Gilmour, J. A. (2002). Disintegrated care: Family caregivers and in-hospital care. *Journal of Advanced Nursing, 39*(6), 546–553.

Gitlin, L.N, Belle, S.H., Burgio, L.D., Czaja, S.J., Mahoney, D., Gallagher-Thompson, D., ... REACH Investigators (2003). Effect of multicomponent interventions on caregiver burden and depression: The REACH Multisite Initiative at 6-month follow-up. *Psychology and Aging, 18*(3), 361–374.

Givens, J. L., Mezzacappa, C., Heeren, T., Yaffe, K., & Fredman, L. (2013). Depressive symptoms among dementia caregivers: Role of mediating factors. *American Journal of Geriatric Psychiatry.* Epub ahead of print. doi: 10.1016/j.jagp.2012.08.010

Glasdam, S., Timm, H., & Vittrup, R. (2010). Support efforts for caregivers of chronically ill persons. *Clinical Nursing Research, 19*(3), 233–265.

Gordon, P. A., & Perrone, K. M. (2004). When spouses become caregivers: Counseling implications for younger couples. *Journal of Rehabilitation, 70*(2), 27–32.

Greenwood, N., Mackenzie, A., Cloud, G. C., & Wilson, N. (2009). Informal primary carers of stroke survivors living at home challenges, satisfactions and coping: A systematic review of qualitative studies. *Disability & Rehabilitation, 31*(5), 337–351.

Haigler, D. H., Bauer, L. J., & Travis, S. S. (2004). Finding the common ground of family and professional caregiving: The education agenda at the Rosalynn Carter Institute. *Educational Gerontology, 30,* 95–105.

Haley, J., & Harrigan, R. C. (2004). Voicing the strengths of Pacific Island parent caregivers of children who are medically fragile. *Journal of Transcultural Nursing, 15*(3), 184–194.

Halm, M. A., & Bakas, T. (2007). Factors associated with depressive symptoms, outcomes, and perceived physical health after coronary bypass surgery. *Journal of Cardiovascular Nursing, 22*(6), 508–515.

Hamilton, J. B., Moore, A. D., Johnson, K. A., & Koenig, H. G. (2013). Reading the Bible for guidance, comfort, and strength during stressful life events. *Nursing Research, 62*(3), 178–184. doi: 10.1097/NNR.0b013e31828fc816.PMID:23636344

Harding, R., & Higginson, I. (2003). What is the best way to help caregivers in cancer and palliative care? A systematic literature review of interventions and their effectiveness. *Palliative Medicine, 17,* 63–74.

HealthNetCafé. (2013). Your role as caregiver. http://www.healthnetcafe.com/content/the_caregiver/your_roles_as_caregiver.html

Hill, C. (2009). Caregiver transitions. http://alzheimers.about.com/od/caregiving/qt/transitions.htm

Hudson, P. (2004). Positive aspects and challenges associated with caring for a dying relative at home. *International Journal of Palliative Nursing, 10*(2), 58–64.

Hunt, C. K. (2003). Concepts in caregiver research. *Journal of Nursing Scholarship, 35*(1), 27–32.

Hunt, G., Levine, C., & Naiditch, N. (2005). *Young caregivers in the U.S.* New York, NY: National Alliance for Caregiving & United Hospital Fund.

Institute for Patient- and Family-Centered Care (IPFCC). (2010). What is patient- and family-centered care? http://www.ipfcc.org/faq.html.

Interfaith CarePartners. (2011). Home page. http://www.interfaithcarepartners.org/index/php/home/c/home

Johnson, R., Toohey, D., & Wiener, J. (2007). Meeting the long-term care needs of the baby boomers. http://www.urban.org/publications/311451.html

Johnson, R., & Wiener, J. (2006). *A profile of frail older Americans and their caregivers: The retirement project.* Washington, DC: Urban Institute. http://www.urban.org/UploadedPDF/311284_older_americans.pdf

Kate, N., Grover, S., Kulhara, P., & Nehra, R. (2013). Positive aspects of caregiving and its correlates in caregivers of schizophrenia: A study from north India. *Archives of Psychiatry, 23*(2), 45–55.

Kaye, L. W., Turner, W., Butler, S. S., Downey, R., & Cotton, A. (2003). Early intervention screening for family caregivers of older relatives in primary care practices: Establishing a community health service alliance in rural America. *Family Community Health, 26*(4), 319–328.

Keith, C. (1995). Family caregiving systems: Models, resources, and values. *Journal of Marriage and the Family, 57,* 179–190.

Kelly, K. (2003–2004, Winter). Link2Care: Internet-based information and support for caregivers. *Family Caregiving,* 87–88.

Kim, H., Chang, M., Rose, K., & Kim, S. (2012). Predictors of caregiver burden in caregivers of individuals with dementia. *Journal of Advanced Nursing, 68*(4), 846–855.

Klerman, J. A., Daley, K., & Pozniak, A. (2012). *Family and medical leave in 2012: Technical report.* Cambridge, MA: Abt Associates. http://www.dol.gov/asp/evaluation/fmla/FMLA-2012-Technical-Report.pdf

Lackey, N. R., & Gates, M. F. (2001). Adults' recollections of their experiences as young caregivers of family members with chronic physical illnesses. *Journal of Advanced Nursing, 34*(3), 320–328.

Lattanzi-Licht, M., Mahoney, J. J., & Miller, G. W. (1998). *The hospice choice: In pursuit of a peaceful death.* New York, NY: Simon & Schuster.

Lazarus, R. S., & Folkman, S. (1984). *Stress, appraisal, and coping.* New York, NY: Springer.

Leavitt, M., Martinson, I. M., Liu, C. Y., Armstrong, V., Hornberger, L., Zhang, J., & Han, X. (1999). Common themes and ethnic differences in family caregiving the first year after diagnosis of childhood cancer: Part II. *Journal of Pediatric Nursing, 14*, 110–122.

Lee, M. D. (2007). Correlates of consequences of intergenerational caregiving in Taiwan. *Journal of Advanced Nursing, 59*(1), 49–56.

Lindsay, M. P., Gubitz, G., Bayley, M., Hill, M. D., Davies-Schinkel, C., Singh, S., & Phillips, S. (2010). *Canadian best practice recommendations for stroke care.* Ottawa, ON: Canadian Stroke Network.

Lutz, B. J. (2004). Determinants of discharge destination for stroke patients. *Rehabilitation Nursing, 29*(5), 154–163.

Lutz, B. J., Chumbler, N. R., Lyles, T., Hoffman, N., & Kobb, R. (2008). Testing a home-telehealth programme for US veterans recovering from stroke and their family caregiver. *Disability and Rehabilitation, 7*, 1–8.

Lutz, B. J., Chumbler, N. R., & Roland, K. (2007). Care coordination/home-telehealth for veterans with stroke and their caregivers: Addressing an unmet need. *Topics in Stroke Rehabilitation, 14*(4), 32–42.

Lutz, B. J., & Young M. E. (2010). Rethinking intervention strategies in stroke family caregiving. *Rehabilitation Nursing, 35*(4), 296–305.

Lutz, B. J., Young, M. E., Cox, K. C., Martz, C., & Creasy, K. (2011). The crisis of stroke: Experiences of caregivers and patients. *Topics in Stroke Rehabilitation 18*(6), 786–797.

Lutz, B. J., Young, M. E., Creasy, K. R., & Cox, K. (In press). A comprehensive assessment of family caregivers of stroke survivors during inpatient rehabilitation. *Disability and Rehabilitation.*

Lynch, S. H. & Lobo, M. L. (2012, March 21). Compassion fatigue in family caregivers: A Wilsonian concept analysis. *Journal of Advanced Nursing, 68*(9), 2125–2134. doi: 10.1111/j.1365-2648.2012.05985. PMID: 22435873

Machlin, S., Cohen, J., & Beauregard, K. (2008). *Health care expenses for adults with chronic conditions, 2005.* (Statistical Brief #203). Agency for Healthcare Research and Quality. http://www.meps.ahrq.gov/mepsweb/data_files/publications/st203/stat203.pdf

Mackenzie, A., & Greenwood, N. (2012). Positive experiences of caregiving in stroke: A systematic review. *Disability and Rehabilitation, 34*(17), 1413–1422.

Mausbach, B. T., Patterson, T. L., Von Känel, R., Mills, P. J., Dimsdale, J.E., Ancoli-Israel, S., & Grant, I. (2007). The attenuating effect of personal mastery on the relations between stress and Alzheimer caregiver health: A five-year longitudinal analysis. *Aging & Mental Health, 11*(6), 637–644.

Messecar, D. C. (2012). Nursing standard of practice protocol: Family caregiving. In M. Boltz, E. Capezuti, T. T. Fulmer, & D. Zwicker, (Eds.), *Evidence-based geriatric nursing protocols for best practice* (4th ed.). New York, NY: Springer. http://consultgerirn.org/topics/family_caregiving/want_to_know_more#item_4

Michael, N., O'Callaghan, C., Baird, A., Hiscock, N., & Clayton, J. (In press). Cancer caregivers advocate a patient- and family-centered approach to advance care planning. *Journal of Pain and Symptom Management.*

Mitrani, V. B. & Czaja, S. J. (2000). Family-based therapy for dementia caregivers: Clinical observations. *Aging & Mental Health, 4*(3), 200–209.

Mittelman, J. S. (2003). Community caregiving. *Alzheimer's Care Quarterly, 4*(4), 273–285.

Mittelman, M. S. (2002). Family caregiving for people with Alzheimer's disease: Results of the NYU spouse caregiver intervention study. *Generations, 26*(1), 102–106.

Moore, J. (2006). *The impact of the aging population on the health workforce in the United States.* Rensselaer, NY: University at Albany. http://www.albany.edu/news/pdf_files/impact_of_aging_full.pdf

Murray, S. A., Kendall, M., Boyd, K., Worth, A., Boyd, K., & Benton, T. F. (2004). Exploring the spiritual needs of people dying of lung cancer or heart failure: A prospective qualitative interview study of patients and their carers. *Palliative Medicine, 18*, 39–45.

National Alliance for Caregiving (NAC). (2005). Young caregivers in the U.S. http://www.caregiving.org/data/youngcaregivers.pdf

National Alliance for Caregiving (NAC). (2013). Research. http://www.caregiving.org/research

National Alliance for Caregiving (NAC) & American Association of Retired Persons (AARP). (2009). Caregiving in the U.S. 2009. http://www.caregiving.org/data/Caregiving_in_the_US_2009_full_report.pdf

National Alliance for Caregiving (NAC) & AARP. (2012). Fact sheet: Selected caregiver statistics.

http://www.caregiver.org/caregiver/jsp/content_node
.jsp?nodeid=439

Nerenberg, L. (2002). *Preventing elder abuse by family caregivers.* Washington, DC: National Center of Elder Abuse.

Nolan, M. (2001). Positive aspects of caring. In S. Payne & C. Ellis-Hill (Eds.), *Chronic and terminal illness: New perspectives on caring and carers* (pp. 22–44). Oxford, UK: Oxford University Press.

Novak, M., & Guest, C. (1989). Application of a multidimensional caregiver burden inventory. *The Gerontologist, 29*(6), 798–803. doi: 10.1093/geront/29.6.798

Oberst, M. T., Thomas, S. E., Gass, K. A., & Ward, S. E. (1989). Caregiving demands and appraisal of stress among family caregivers. *Cancer Nursing, 12*(4), 209–215.

Office on Women's Health. (2008). Caregiver stress fact sheet. http://www.womenshealth.gov/publications /our-publications/fact-sheet/caregiver-stress.cfm

Palmer, S., & Glass, T. A. (2003). Family function and stroke recovery: A review. *Rehabilitation Psychology, 48*(4), 255–265.

Paun, O. (2004). Female Alzheimer's patient caregivers share their strength. *Holistic Nursing Practice, 18*(1), 11–17.

Peacock, S., Forbes, D., Markle-Reid, M., Hawranik, P., Morgan, D., Jansen, L., … Henderson, S. (2010). The positive aspects of the caregiving journey with dementia: Using a strengths-based perspective to reveal opportunities. *Journal of Applied Gerontology, 29*(5), 640–659.

Pearlin, L. I. (1992). The careers of caregivers. *The Gerontologist, 32*, 647.

Pearlin, L. I., Mullan, J. T., Semple, S. J., & Skaff, M. M. (1990). Caregiving and the stress process: An overview of concepts and their measures. *The Gerontologist, 30*(5), 583–594.

Perkins, M., Howard, V. J., Wadley, V.G., Crowe, M., Safford, M. M., Haley, W. E., … Roth, D. L. (2013). Caregiving strain and all-cause mortality: Evidence from the Regards study. *Journals of Gerontology Series B: Psychological Sciences and Social Sciences, 68*(4), 504–512. doi: 10.1093/geronb/gbs084

Phillipson, L., & Jones, S. (2011). "Between the devil and the deep blue sea": The beliefs of caregivers of people with dementia regarding the use of in-home respite services. *Home Health Care Services Quarterly, 30*(2), 43–62.

Pierce, L. (2001). Coherence in the urban family caregiver role with African American stroke survivors. *Topics in Stroke Rehabilitation, 8*(3), 64–72.

Pierce, L., & Steiner, V. (2013). Usage and design evaluation by family caregivers of a stroke intervention website. *Journal of Neuroscience Nursing, 45*(5), 254–261.

Pierce, L., Steiner, V., Govoni, A., Hicks, B., Thompson, T., & Friedemann, M. (2004). Caring~Web: Internet-based support for rural caregivers of persons with stroke shows promise. *Rehabilitation Nursing, 29*(3), 95–99, 103.

Pierce, L., Steiner, V., Govoni, A., Thompson, T., & Friedemann, M. (2007). Two sides to the caregiving story. *Topics in Stroke Rehabilitation, 14*(2), 13–20.

Pierce, L., Steiner, V., Havens, H., & Tormoehlen, K. (2008). Spirituality expressed by caregivers of stroke survivors. *Western Journal of Nursing Research, 30*(5), 606–619.

Pierce, L., Thompson, T., Govoni, A., & Steiner, V. (2012). Caregivers' incongruence: Emotional strain in caring for persons with stroke. *Rehabilitation Nursing, 37*(5), 368–366.

Piercy, K. W. (1998). Theorizing about family caregiving: The role of responsibility. *Journal of Marriage and the Family, 60*, 109–118.

Piercy, K. W., & Chapman, J. G. (2001). Adopting the caregiver role: A family legacy. *Family Relations, 50*, 386–393.

Pillemer, K., & Suitor, J. J. (2013). Who provides care? A prospective study of caregiving among adult siblings. *The Gerontologist.* Epub ahead of print. doi: 10.1093/geront/gnt066. http://gerontologist.oxfordjournals .org.lp.hscl.ufl.edu/content/early/2013/07/08/geront .gnt066.full.pdf+html?sid=c52c9fe0-b6af-48f7-ac4b-e4e38150cbf3

Rabinowitz, Y. G., Mausbach, B. T., Thompson, L. W., & Gallagher-Thompson, D. (2007). The relationship between self-efficacy and cumulative health risk associated with health behavior patterns in female caregivers of elderly relatives with Alzheimer's dementia. *Journal of Aging and Health, 19*(6), 946–964.

Redfoot, D., Feinberg, L., & Houser, A. (2013). *The aging of the baby boom and the growing care gap: A look at future declines in the availability of family caregivers.* Washington, DC: AARP Public Policy Institute. http://www.aarp.org/research/ppi

Reinhard, S., Given, B., Petlick, N., & Bemis, A. (2008). Supporting family caregivers in providing care. In R. Hughes (Ed.), *Patient safety and quality: An evidence-based handbook for nurses* (pp. 341-363). Rockville, MD: Agency for Healthcare Research and Quality.

Ritchie, L. (2003). Adult day care: Northern perspectives. *Public Health Nursing, 20*(2), 120–131.

Robinson, B. C. (1983). Validation of a caregiver strain index. *Journal of Gerontology, 38*(3), 344–348.

Roff, L., Burgio, L., Gitlin, L., Nichols, L., Chaplin, W., & Hardin, J.M. (2004). Positive aspects of Alzheimer's caregiving: The role of race. *Journals of Gerontology Series B: Psychological Sciences and Social Sciences*, 59B(4), 185–190.

Roth, D. L., Haley, W. E., Hovater, M., Perkins, M., Wadley, V. G., & Judd, S. (2013, October 3). Family caregiving and all-cause mortality: Findings from a population-based propensity-matched analysis. *American Journal of Epidemiology*, 178(10), 1571–1578. doi: 10.1093/aje/kwt225. PMID: 24091890

Sarkisian, N., & Gerstel, N. (2004). Explaining the gender gap in help to parents: The importance of employment. *Journal of Marriage and Family*, 66, 431–451.

Scharlach, A. E., Giunta, N., Chow, J. C., & Lehning, A. (2008). Racial and ethnic variations in caregiver service use. *Journal of Aging and Health*, 20(3), 326–346. doi: 10.1177/0898264308315426

Schulz, R., Beach, S. R., Cook, T. B., Martire, L. M., Tomlinson, J. M., & Monin, J. K. (2012, February 24). Predictors and consequences of perceived lack of choice in becoming an informal caregiver. *Aging in Mental Health*, 16(6), 712–721. doi: 10.1080/13607863.2011.651439. PMID: 22360296

Scott, G. (2001). A study of family carers of people with a life-threatening illness 2: The implications of the needs assessment. *International Journal of Palliative Nursing*, 7(7), 323–330.

Sebern, M. D., & Whitlatch, C. J. (2007). Dyadic relationship scale: A measure of the impact of the provision and receipt of family care. *The Gerontologist*, 47(6), 741–751.

Seifert, M. L., Williams, A., Dowd, M. F., Chappel-Aiken, L., McCorkle, R. (2008). The caregiver experience in a racially diverse sample of cancer family caregivers. *Cancer Nursing*, 31(5), 399–407.

Seltzer, M. M., & Wailing, L. (2000). The dynamics of caregiving: Transitions during a three-year prospective study. *The Gerontologist*, 40, 165–178.

Selwood, A., Johnston, K., Katona, C., Lyketsos, C., & Livingston, G. (2007). Systematic review of the effect of psychological interventions on family caregivers of people with dementia. *Journal of Affective Disorders*, 101, 75–89.

Semiatin, A., & O'Connor, M. (2012). The relationship between self-efficacy and positive aspects of caregiving in Alzheimer's disease caregivers. *Aging & Mental Health*, 16(6), 683–688.

Shirey, L., & Summer, L. (2000). *Caregiving: Helping the elderly with activity limitations*. Washington, DC: National Academy on Aging Society.

Smith, J., Forster, A., & Young, Y. (2009). Cochrane review: Information provision for stroke patients and their caregivers. *Clinical Rehabilitation*, 23, 196–206.

Spector, R. E. (2000). *Cultural diversity in health and illness* (5th ed.). Upper Saddle River, NJ: Prentice Hall Health.

Steiner, V., & Pierce, L. (2002). Building a web of support for caregivers of persons with stroke. *Topics in Stroke Rehabilitation*, 9(3), 102–111.

Stoller, E. P., & Cutler, S. J. (1993). Predictors of use of paid help among older people living in the community. *The Gerontologist*, 33(1), 31–40.

Stuckey, J. C. (2001). Blessed assurance: The role of religion and spirituality in Alzheimer's disease caregiving and other significant life events. *Journal of Aging Studies*, 15(1), 69–84.

Substance Abuse and Mental Health Services Administration. (2004). SAMHSA model programs. http://nrepp.samhsa.gov/

Tarlow, B., Wisniewski, S., Belle, S., Rubert, M., Ory, M.G., & Gallagher-Thompmson, D. (2004). Positive aspects of caregiving: Contributions of the REACH project to the development of new measures for Alzheimer's caregiving. *Research on Aging*, 26(4), 429–453.

Theis, S. L., Biordi, D. L., Coeling, H., Nalepka, C., & Miller, B. (2003). Spirituality in caregiving and care receiving. *Holistic Nursing Practice*, 17(1), 48–55.

Thompson, B., Tudiver, F., & Manson, J. (2000). Sons as sole caregivers for their elderly parents. How do they cope? *Canadian Family Physician*, 46, 360–365.

Thompson, C.A., Spilsbury, K., Hall, J., Birks, Y., Barnes, C., & Adamson, J. (2007). Systematic review of information and support interventions for caregivers of people with dementia. *BMC Geriatrics*, 7, 18

Thompson, T., Benz, J., Agiesta, J., Junius, D., Nguyen, K., & Lowell, K. (2013). Long-term care: Perceptions, experiences, and attitudes among Americans 40 or older. Associated Press, NORC Center for Public Affairs Research. http://www.apnorc.org/projects/Pages/long-term-care-perceptions-experiences-and-attitudes-among-americans-40-or-older.aspx

Travis, S. S., & Bethea, L. S. (2001). Medication administration by family members of elders in shared care arrangements. *Journal of Clinical Geropsychology*, 7, 231–243.

University of Michigan Health System. (2006). *Children with chronic conditions*. Ann Arbor, MI: Author. http://www.med.umich.edu/1libr/yourchild/chronic.htm

U.S. Department of Labor. (1993). *The family and medical leave act of 1993*. Washington, DC: U.S. Department of Labor, Wage and Hour Division.

U.S. Department of Labor. (2013). Family and Medical Leave Act: Protections expanded for military families and airline flight crews. http://www.dol.gov/WHD /fmla/2013rule/index.htm

van Exel, N. J., Scholte op Reimer, W. J., Brouwer, W. B., van den Berg, B., Koopmanschap, M. A., & van den Bos, G. A. (2004). Instruments for assessing the burden of informal caregiving for stroke patients in clinical practice: A comparison of CSI, CRA, SCQ and self-rated burden. *Clinical Rehabilitation, 18*(2), 203–214.

van Heugten, C., Visser-Meily, A., Post, M., & Lindeman, E. (2006). Care for carers of stroke patients: Evidence-based clinical practice guidelines. *Journal of Rehabilitation Medicine, 38*(3), 153–158.

Visser-Meily, J. M., Post, M.W., Riphagen, I. I., & Lindeman, E. (2004). Measures used to assess burden among caregivers of stroke patients: a review. *Clinical Rehabilitation, 18*(6), 601–623.

Ward, B. W., & Schiller, J. S. (2013). Prevalence of multiple chronic conditions among US adults: Estimates from the National Health Interview Survey, 2010. *Preventing Chronic Disease, 10*. http://dx.doi. org/10.5888/pcd10.120203

Warren, S., Kerr, J., Smith, D., Godkin, D., & Schalm, C. (2003). The impact of adult day programs on family caregivers of elderly relatives. *Journal of Community Health Nursing, 20*(4), 209–221.

Weitzner, M. A., Haley, W. E., & Chen, H. (2000). The family caregiver of the older cancer patient. *Hematology and Oncology Clinics of North America, 14,* 269–281.

Welch, J. L., Thomas-Hawkins, C., Bakas, T., McLennon, S. M., Byers, D. M., Monetti, C. J., & Decker, B. S. (2013). Needs, concerns, strategies, and advice of daily home dialysis caregivers. *Clinical Nursing Research*. doi: 10.1177/1054773813495407

Winslow, B. W. (2003). Family caregivers' experiences with community services: A qualitative analysis. *Public Health Nursing, 20* (5), 341–348.

World Health Organization (WHO). (2012a). Preterm birth: Fact sheet. http://www.who.int/mediacentre /factsheets/fs363/en/

World Health Organization (WHO). (2012b). *Dementia: A public health priority.* United Kingdom: Author. http://www.who.int/mental_health/publications /dementia_report_2012/en/index.html

Zarit, S., Kim, K., Femia, E., Almeida, D., Savla, J., & Molenaar, P. (2011). Effects of adult day care on daily stress of caregivers: A within-person approach. *Journals of Gerontology: Series B, Psychological Sciences and Social Sciences, 66B*(5), 538–546.

Zarit, S. H., Reever, K. E., & Bach-Peterson, J. (1980). Relatives of the impaired elderly: Correlates of feelings of burden. *The Gerontologist, 20,* 649–655.

Chapter 11

Intimacy

Pamala D. Larsen

Introduction

In previous editions, this chapter was titled "sexuality," with the "physicalness" of sexuality—and particularly sexual intercourse—being the focus. Thus, tables about erectile dysfunction, ways in which radiation and chemotherapy affected sexual intercourse, and the part that medications play in sexuality were part of the chapter. Even in the current literature, sexual intercourse appears to be the pinnacle of sexuality and sexual health. In the sexuality and cancer chapter of the prominent nursing textbook about cancer, titled *Cancer Symptom Management* (Yarbro, Wujcik, & Gobel, 2014), the focus is sexual intercourse. In the *MD Anderson Manual of Psychosocial Oncology* (Duffy & Valentine, 2011), the chapter on sexuality and cancer gives five short "bullets" on what this author would suggest is intimacy, while the rest of the chapter is devoted to sexual intercourse and sexual dysfunction in cancer.

In an excellent review of sexuality and chronic illness, Steinke (2013) examines cardiovascular conditions, chronic obstructive pulmonary disease (COPD), sleep apnea, and cancer and describes their effects on sexuality. However, the focus for each condition is sexual intercourse and the dysfunction that may occur after a diagnosis, along with interventions that include sexual counseling being tailored to the

patient's specific condition, based on exercise capacity; any risks with sexual activity; and specific concerns of the patient and partner (p. 25).

If patients and partners are candid about what they are experiencing with chronic illness, then it becomes clear that sexual intercourse makes up only a small part of sexuality for those couples. The term "intimacy" better describes the personal, private, and sexual relationships that patients and their partners experience with chronic illness. In many ways, intimacy becomes *more* important after a diagnosis, as a way of reaffirming human connection, aliveness, and continued desirability and caring (Wilmoth, 2013, p. 289).

Definitions

Sexuality is a complex construct with terminology that has yet to be defined in a manner that is accepted by everyone. The clearest and most inclusive definition comes from a World Health Organization (WHO) document published in 2006. If one takes WHO's definition literally, then activities other than sexual intercourse fit within that definition. Intimacy is generally considered part of sexuality. When the term "sexuality" is used, however, particularly with patients, the automatic response/thinking in their mind is sexual intercourse. That is the "normal" response of society as well. However, for many patients with chronic disease, sexual intercourse may not be possible. "Intimacy," therefore, better defines what patients and partners are experiencing or want to experience, and is a term that may include sexual intercourse. As Rainey (2011) states, intimacy is an umbrella term and includes feelings of love and devotion as well as sexual desire and attraction (p. 18). Not finding a definition of intimacy that is inclusive, this author has included descriptors of intimacy.

- *Sexuality*: A central aspect of being human throughout life encompasses sex, gender identities and roles, sexual orientation, eroticism, pleasure, intimacy, and reproduction. Sexuality is experienced and expressed in thoughts, fantasies, desires, beliefs, attitudes, values, behaviors, practices, roles, and relationships. While sexuality can include all of these dimensions, not all of them are always experienced or expressed. Sexuality is influenced by the interaction of biological, psychological, social, economic, political, cultural, legal, historical, religious, and spiritual factors (WHO, 2006, p. 5).
- *Intimacy*: Relationship driven; a feeling of belonging; touch demonstrated in a variety of ways; verbal and nonverbal communication; affection.

Sexual Physiology

A brief summary of sexual physiology is described here. For more information, the reader is encouraged to refer to focused literature on the topic.

Masters and Johnson (1966) described the sexual response cycle as a four-stage model of sexual response of the male and the female. The four phases of the Masters and Johnson model are excitement, plateau, orgasm, and resolution. In the male, the excitement stage causes an increase in the heart rate and vasocongestion to the penis. In the female, there is lengthening and widening of the vagina, elevation of the cervix and uterus, and initial swelling of the labia minora (Hall, 2011). These changes are caused by vasocongestion and occur secondary to a parasympathetic response mediated at S2 and S4 through the pudendal nerve and sacral plexus in both men and women (Hall, 2011).

The second stage in the Masters and Johnson model is the plateau stage, which is an increased state of arousal causing the heart rate and blood pressure to increase, with a subsequent increase in respiratory rate (Katz, 2007). The third stage is the orgasm, the phase of maximal muscular contraction (male ejaculation; female pelvic muscle contraction), with a peak of respirations and heart rate, and a subjective feeling of intense pleasure that radiates throughout the body (Katz, 2007). Orgasm is mediated by the sympathetic nervous system and is the physical release and peak of pleasurable expression, followed by relaxation. The sympathetic nerves between T12 and L2 control ejaculation (Hall, 2011). The intensity of orgasm in women depends on the duration and intensity of sexual stimulation. The final stage is resolution, when vasocongestion resolves and the body returns to its normal nonaroused state.

The neurohormonal system influences sexual hormone production. The hypothalamic–hypophysial portal system plays an important role in sexual functioning in both genders through the production of gonadotropin-releasing hormone (GnRH), which in turn triggers the pituitary gland to secrete follicle-stimulating hormone (FSH) and luteinizing hormone (LH). In men, LH influences the production of testosterone by the interstitial cells of Leydig in the testes through a negative feedback loop (Hall, 2011). Production of GnRH is reduced once a satisfactory level of testosterone has been attained. A negative feedback loop also exists in women, although it is much more complex, given the concurrent production of estrogen and progesterone by the ovaries and the production of androgens by the adrenal cortex.

Psychological factors appear to play a larger role in the sexual functioning in women than in men, particularly in relation to sexual desire. Multiple neuronal centers in the brain's limbic system transmit signals into the arcuate nuclei in the mediobasal hypothalamus. These signals modify the intensity of GnRH release and the frequency of the impulses (Hall, 2011). This may explain why desire in women is more vulnerable to emotions and distractions than it is in men.

Intimacy and Chronic Illness

Sexuality and intimacy are seen as central to psychological well-being and quality of life. However, how intimacy is shown by patients and partners varies significantly. Numerous articles focus on sexuality and specific chronic illnesses and the impact of each illness on sexuality. However, the majority of these articles describe how each chronic illness and treatment affect sexual intercourse and then propose interventions to achieve intercourse. Unfortunately, there is a dearth of information or data about intimacy in the literature.

This chapter uses cancer as the example of chronic disease, partly because it is associated with survivors who remain cancer-free, but also because of the roller coaster of health status that often occurs during the illness as well as the possibility of cancer being a terminal illness. Unlike other side effects of cancer and its treatment, sexual issues do not tend to resolve, even after several years of survivorship (Hughes, 2011, p. 125). Intimacy can be demonstrated in many ways throughout the disease course—from diagnosis, to remission, to recurrence, to palliative care and hospice.

Although this chapter focuses on intimacy, healthcare professionals need to be aware of the psychosocial effects that cancer may have on sexuality in general. Cort, Monroe, and Oliviere (2004, p. 341) summarize those effects as follows:

- Vulnerability implicit in the illness itself—how it is perceived, including the threat to the future and the fear of death and dying
- Helplessness, including loss of control of the body; invasion of the body by others and dependence on others for survival

- Altered body image, which may include distaste and feeling dirty, smelly, abnormal, or unwholesome
- Anxieties about treatment and pain
- Guilt and self-blame for the possibility of having caused or contributed to the illness
- Anger and resentment—"Why has this happened to me?"

Cost-effective care has become one of the hallmarks of the healthcare system, as healthcare payers and providers try to tie patient outcomes to costs of care. In 2004, the National Institutes of Health (NIH) began development of PROMIS (Patient Reported Outcomes Measurement System). As of 2010, this system was measuring patient-reported health status markers for physical, mental, and social well-being. The PROMIS tools can be used across a wide variety of chronic diseases and conditions and in the general population. The data collected measure effects of treatment that cannot be assessed with traditional clinical measures. These data can then be used to design treatment plans, but also used by patients and physicians to improve communication and manage chronic disease (NIH, n.d.). Pertinent to the topic of this chapter, PROMIS has been used to explore the scope and importance of sexual functioning and intimacy in cancer patients in sites across the United States and along the care continuum. The study described next was undertaken to inform the development of an improved measure of sexual function for cancer patients.

Patients were recruited into 16 diagnosis- and sex-specific focus groups from the oncology/hematology clinical and tumor registry at Duke University. Across cancers, the most commonly discussed cancer- or treatment-related effects on sexual functioning and intimacy were fatigue, treatment-related hair loss, weight gain, and organ loss or scarring (Flynn et al., 2011). Of note were some unusual findings from the focus groups about intimacy, sexual functioning, and relationships. The data revealed the complexity of relationships among functioning, intimacy, and overall satisfaction with the person's sex life. Evaluations of satisfaction with sex life did not necessarily correspond to specific aspects of functioning, as many participants described satisfaction with their sex life and intimacy *despite* decreased sexual function (p. 385). For the researchers, this finding meant it was critical to measure satisfaction with sex life as a separate concept from functioning. Another important finding was the role of the partner for those participants in a committed relationship. Due to the complexity and importance of partner issues, the PROMIS sexual domain group will address that topic at a later time (Flynn et al., 2011).

Influences on Intimacy

A general list of influences on intimacy include religious beliefs, age, education, level of comfort with one's body and physical functioning, experience of sexual abuse and trauma, one's partner's wishes, comfort level with one's own sexual orientation, and the health of each partner (Hughes, 2011, p. 126).

Numerous physical influences on intimacy exist for a patient and partner. These factors may be a direct result of treatment, such as fatigue, nausea and vomiting, or pain, or just inherent in cancer, even if the patient is not in treatment. Often the inconsistencies of the symptoms for the patient affect intimacy.

> *He usually feels bad in the afternoon. There is something about lunch that signals a downward spiral in how he feels. It's the nausea and dizziness that are the worst. But today those symptoms started by 9 in the morning. We can't seem to predict anything anymore. What triggers these miserable symptoms? Something different every day.*

> —Jenny

For many cancer patients, treatment brings a change in body image, which is often accompanied by a change in self-concept. However, a change in body image does not occur in isolation, but rather is an experience that is contextually and relationally based (Varela, Nelson, & Bober, 2011, p. 2464). Such a change may involve the removal of a breast, disfigurement due to surgery, radiation burns, or a stoma on the abdomen. It could also stem from the presence of a feeding tube into the stomach or jejunum, a nasal cannula that delivers a continuous flow of oxygen, an insulin pump, or another device that others do not have. So the questions begin for the couple: Will the stoma bag remain in place? Will the feeding tube be displaced or even come out? What if my legs start to spasm and it is too painful to continue? The thoughts that go through each partner's minds suggest, "We must be very careful"—and soon any pleasure and intimacy that the partners could have felt has been displaced by anxiety and fear.

For other patients, there may be not be a visible change in body image, but in his or her gut, the patient knows that he or she is different from other people. This type of change is very real to the patient and adds more complexity to issues of intimacy.

The Western culture context for intimacy emphasizes the self and describes the key ingredient of intimacy development as an individual being understood, validated, and cared for by his or her partner. Other cultures may not view intimacy in the same way. However, research is lacking on the effect of culture and intimacy with chronic illness.

There are differences in how men and women view intimacy. Men more often report sex or physical contact as the key feature of intimacy, while women often do not refer to sex in describing intimate situations (Graber, Laurenceau, & Belcher, 2009, p. 900).

Frameworks for Viewing Intimacy in Cancer

The Interpersonal Process Model of Intimacy

One model of intimacy is the interpersonal process model of intimacy, initially proposed by Harry Reis and Phillip Shaver (1988). In this model, intimacy is defined as a process in which one person expresses important self-relevant feelings and information to another, and as a result of the other's response, comes to feel understood, validated, and cared for. The model conceptualizes intimacy as a personal, subjective (and often momentary) sense of connectedness that is the outcome of a dynamic, interpersonal process (Graber et al., 2009; Laurenceau, Rivera, Schaffer, & Pietromonaco, 2004). The key elements that foster the development of intimacy are self-disclosure, partner responsiveness, and perceived partner responsiveness. Intimacy and self-disclosure, however, are not synonymous constructs. One study noted that self-disclosure had been found to account for slightly less than half of the variance in ratings of couples' level of intimacy (Laurenceau et al., 2004).

Research indicates that sharing of emotional information versus factual information leads to greater feelings of intimacy (Graber et al., 2009, p. 899). This model views intimacy not as a single construct and/or outcome, but rather as a *process* based on communication between partners. Often communication may be one of the few ways in which couples can express intimacy.

Manne and colleagues (2004) completed a study validating the interpersonal process model of intimacy in a sample of 98 women with breast cancer and their partners. Couples engaged in two discussions and rated self- and partner disclosure, perceived partner responsiveness, and intimacy experienced. For patients, perceived responsiveness partially mediated the association between partner disclosure and intimacy. By comparison, for partners, perceived responsiveness mediated the association between self-disclosure and perceived partner disclosure and intimacy. For these breast cancer patients, then, partner disclosure predicted patient feelings of intimacy and feelings of acceptance, understanding, and caring (Manne et al., 2004, p. 589).

Additionally, interpersonal shifts may take place over the course of the disease and subsequently affect sexuality throughout the cancer continuum (Laurenceau et al., 2004). Thus the process is dynamic and not static. At any point in this process, interpersonal silence may become "the elephant in the room" (Varela et al., 2011).

RELATIONSHIP INTIMACY MODEL

Manne and Badr (2008) view cancer from a relationship perspective. The relationship as it exists, both prediagnosis and postdiagnosis, sets the tone for intimacy. Not only does this perspective consider the marital relationship as a resource for each partner to draw upon, but it highlights the importance of focusing attention on the relationship and engaging in communication behaviors aimed at sustaining or enhancing the relationship (p. 2541).

During the last 20 years or so, researchers have begun to view cancer within a family context instead of a patient context. However, much of the focus of the literature has been on the caregiving aspect, as one partner cares for the other. Typically this literature has focused on the negative aspects of caregiving, such as caregiver strain or burden. What Manne and Badr's work brings into focus is the adoption of a couple-level perspective, whereby the cancer experience is viewed in relational terms (p. 2542), thereby leading to couple-focused interventions versus patient-focused interventions. The development of this relationship intimacy model (RIM) is key in understanding how relationship factors influence psychosocial adaptation to cancer (p. 2550).

If the relationship is poor before the diagnosis, the chances of it improving following a cancer diagnosis are small. Research suggests that the ways that patients and partners cope with the cancer-induced stressors in trying to maintain a sense of normalcy in their relationship may impact the relationship, and that the relationship may in turn impact the psychosocial adaptation of the couple (Manne, Badr, Zaider, Nelson, & Kissane, 2010).

Researchers examined couples' communication and their perceptions of relationship intimacy in a study that enrolled 139 patients who were coping with head and neck and lung cancers and their partners (Manne, Badr, & Kashy, 2012). The diagnosis of lung or head and neck cancer is a stressful event for couples. Particularly with head and neck cancer, changes in body image occur and ability to eat and/or talk may be affected. With lung cancer, the biggest stressor is the poor survival rate. The study assessed whether the way couples communicated about cancer and whether their perceptions of relationship intimacy influenced both the patient's and the partner's psychosocial adjustment. The findings demonstrated that individuals who engaged in more positive spousal communication experienced less distress, whereas the partners of individuals who engaged in more negative communication experienced greater distress (p. 342). Patients and partners who reported greater baseline distress at diagnosis also reported more negative baseline communication as well as lower levels of intimacy and greater levels of distress over time. Although these findings are not surprising, they are revealing precisely because there has been little research about relationship intimacy.

What Is Intimacy for a Patient and Partner?

For an interaction to be intimate, the individuals need to be in a state of positive involvement with each other. Involvement refers to the partner's attentional focus on the unfolding interaction; an involved partner devotes full attention to the encounter (Prager & Roberts, 2004, p. 45).

Hawkins and colleagues (2009) surveyed 156 informal carers who were partners with individuals with cancer. Analysis of these open-ended questionnaires helped inform the interview questions for the next phase of the study. Interviews were then conducted with 20 of these participants. The aim of the interviews was to examine the subjective experience of sexuality and intimacy after diagnosis and treatment of cancer from the perspective

of the partner. Two themes characterized the responses of the partners on the current status of their sexual relationship: (1) cessation or decreased frequency of sex or intimacy and (2) renegotiation of sex or intimacy. Many of the partners who reported cessation or decreased frequency of sex also reported decreased closeness and intimacy (p. 276).

We hadn't been able to have sexual intercourse since February. Neither of us really knew why nothing worked, but the sexual relationship we had had in the past wasn't possible anymore. Perhaps it was the cumulative effect of the cancer and its treatment or knowing that the cancer had metastasized. But it was another loss for both of us.

However, entering hospice care and knowing that our time together was limited (it ended up being 6 weeks), we concentrated on what we called our evening cuddles in addition to being more affectionate in general. At times Randy's nausea, fatigue, or pain would dictate what we could or could not do, so sometimes the cuddling time was during the day. We tried so hard to have a special time together each day. No, it wasn't 'sex', but a time of intimacy for both of us.

—Jenny

Communication with Healthcare Professionals

As healthcare professionals, we have little idea of what intimacy might mean to patients and their partners. Perhaps it is a hug, a massage, or quiet conversation. The definition of intimacy may change as the patient moves along the cancer continuum. It is a part of the lived experience of the person with cancer and his or her partner.

A study by Lindau, Surawska, Paice, and Baron (2011) explored the patient's, partner's, and healthcare professional's perspective on three issues: (1) the effects of lung cancer on physical and emotional intimacy; (2) the ways in which intimacy affects the experience of living with lung cancer; and (3) communication about intimacy and sexuality in the context of lung cancer. Completing qualitative in-depth interviews with 8 cancer care providers and 13 married couples, aged 43–79, provided the following results:

Healthcare Providers' Perspectives and Attitudes

- Communication about sexuality and intimacy is poor in provider–patient relationships.
- Emotional intimacy: Mixed responses were found, as some providers claimed that cancer had a negative impact on emotional intimacy, while others added there could be positive effects, such as increased closeness.
- Physical intimacy: Providers shared predominantly negative assumptions about the effects of lung cancer on physical intimacy; however, providers did not distinguish between sexual intercourse and other forms of physical intimacy.

Patients' and Partners' Perspectives and Attitudes

- A recurrent theme was that emotional intimacy increased and that sexual intimacy decreased, but was replaced by noncoital physical intimacy such as hugging and touching.
- Increased relationship solidarity was observed.
- Role changes and shifting balance of dependency were reported.
- An increase in physical contact occurred, particularly noncoital physical intimacy.
- Some couples described improved communication due to an increased awareness of time.

Caregiving

In a unique book about love, sex, and disabilities, Rainey (2011) interviewed numerous couples in which one of the partners in each couple was physically disabled. The couples talked about the ways in which caregiving and sexual intimacy frequently intersected. In fact, most of the couples felt that physical caregiving activities enhanced intimacy. Here is an example:

Richard: It enhances it, I think {laughter}.

Emma: [inaudible] When you're in the shower and he is bathing me it's … it's not sexual, but yet it is. I can't explain it the right way.

Richard: It's a … um, high-level sexual, but I mean, it is certainly not, certainly not intercourse, but it's, it's pleasurable, it's pleasurable.

Emma: It is very intimate…. it is a very loving, sensual state-of-being. (p. 145)

From a partner whose loved one is in a wheelchair:

I'm trying to think of the best way to put this. There are times when it kind of increases intimacy, and I'm talking about sexual intimacy and just the closeness. In fact, I think we get a lot more closeness out of those up-close and personal moments that we have together…. Looking at other relationships before her, I would say this is the closest, strongest relationship, and I'm sure that {physical care} has a lot to do with it. (p. 150)

Interventions

Typically, the prevailing model of "treating" sexual dysfunction has been the biomedical model. Finding the pathophysiology that is contributing to the problem is the first step, with interventions then being implemented based almost exclusively on medical or pharmacologic treatments. This approach deals with the physicalness of sexuality activity—namely, sexual intercourse. Intimacy, however, can be approached in a different manner.

Because chronic illness is seen as a dyadic stressor, any interventions must be focused on both partners of the relationship (Revenson & DeLongis, 2011). Healthcare professionals should also remember that the partner—that is, the person without cancer—is expected to provide support to the partner while coping with his or her own emotional distress (p. 103).

Both the flexible coping model and the renegotiation model are based on relationship-focused coping. This refers to efforts to attend to the other partner's needs while maintaining the integrity of the relationship, and efforts to manage one's own stress without creating upset or problems for others. In other words, there needs to be a balance between self and other (Revenson & DeLongis, 2011, p. 105).

Flexible Coping Model

Barsky and colleagues (2006) proposed a model of coping with sexual dysfunction that emphasizes the construct of flexibility. Originally proposed for a general medical population, the authors' most recent work has included cancer survivors. Their model identifies two potential domains of response that can be altered to be more flexible in sexual activity: (1) the definition of sexual function and activity and (2) the centrality (importance) of sexual function and activity (Reese, Keefe, Somers, & Abernethy, 2010, p. 789). A flexible definition of sexual activity would include non-intercourse forms of sexual intimacy as well as sexual intercourse (Barsky et al., 2006, p. 238). Underlying the model is the notion that flexibility in responding "in the moment" when faced with a sexual difficulty is critical in the face of uncontrollable biological effects of chronic illness on sexual functioning. **Table 11-1** and **Table 11-2** demonstrate inflexible and flexible coping in sexual functioning.

The authors argue that sexual functioning, as one aspect of the self, may exist on a continuum between extreme to little or no importance to the individual's self-concept. This part of the model about the centrality (importance) of sexual function within the self-concept is supported by literature that shows the beneficial effect of making shifts in psychological well-being (p. 243). Changes in centrality

Table 11-1 EXAMPLES OF STAGES OF INFLEXIBLE AND FLEXIBLE COPING IN THE DEFINITION OF SEXUAL FUNCTIONING

Stage in Coping Process	Inflexible	Flexible
Cognition	"Intercourse is the only real form of sexual activity that counts."	"Intercourse is only one way to be sexually intimate with my partner."
Behavior	Abstaining from sexual activity	Engaging in oral sex
Psychosocial outcomes	Negative mood; poor sexual functioning; impaired relationship functioning	Positive mood; enhanced sexual functioning; enhanced relationship functioning

Source: Sexual dysfunction and chronic illness: The role of flexibility in coping, Barsky, J.L., Friedman, M.A., & Rosen, R.C., *Journal of Sex & Marital Therapy 32*(3), 2006, p. 240. Reprinted by permission of the publisher, Taylor & Francis Ltd, http://www.tandf.co.uk/journals.

(importance) of sexual function and activity within a person's self-concept can be made by relinquishing a focus on sexual function (e.g., erection) as key in the self-concept when this focus is no longer possible (Reese et al., 2010, p. 789). An individual with sexual concerns may benefit from shifting efforts toward more feasible goals such as enjoying alternative activities that foster intimacy. Both behavioral and cognitive shifts characterize changes in the centrality of sexual function that are likely to lead to positive outcomes for both the patient and the partner (pp. 789–790).

Table 11-2 Examples of Stages of Inflexible and Flexible Coping in the Centrality of Sexual Functioning

Stage in Coping Process	Inflexible	Flexible
Cognition	"Nothing could replace intercourse in our relationship anyway."	"Intimacy is a better focus for us than sex."
Behavior	Neglecting intimacy in relationship	Enrolling in dancing lessons together
Psychosocial outcomes	Negative mood; poor relationship functioning	Positive mood; enhanced relationship functioning

Source: Sexual dysfunction and chronic illness: The role of flexibility in coping, Barsky, J.L., Friedman, M.A., & Rosen, R.C., *Journal of Sex & Marital Therapy 32*(3), 2006, p. 242. Reprinted by permission of the publisher, Taylor & Francis Ltd, http://www.tandf.co.uk/journals.

In Reese and colleagues' (2010) review of the literature, one of their findings in studies of cancer patients and their partners was that over the course of the disease, couples were able to shift their perspectives on intimacy and sexuality. Additionally, their review supported the contention that the context of the relationship was important in addressing sexual concerns for cancer patients (p. 793).

As flexible coping relates to individuals' own perceptions of sexuality and self-concept related to sexuality, it is conceptualized on an individual level. Because sexuality is typically occurring in the context of an interpersonal relationship, the context of that relationship should be considered. Flexible coping will be most successful if both the patient and the partner are willing to possibly challenge their cognitive perceptions of sexuality (Reese et al., 2010, pp. 795–796).

Renegotiation

Changes to sexuality in the context of cancer can also have ramifications beyond sex as an activity. It has been argued that when sexual intercourse stops, other forms of intimacy and affectionate physical contact also decrease (Gilbert, Ussher, & Perz, 2010). If this occurs, both patients and partners can feel isolated, anxious, depressed, and inadequate, and the partners may develop an emotional distance from each other (p. 998). Few studies to date have examined sexual negotiation; in those that have, couples have been found to be unable to renegotiate sexuality and intimacy. Gilbert and colleagues' study (p. 999) asked two questions: (1) How do carers who are the intimate partner of a person with cancer renegotiate their sexual relationship following the onset of cancer and the caring role? and (2) Which factors are associated with successful or unsuccessful renegotiation? Participants in the sample (*n* = 20) were informal carers and intimate partners of patients with cancer. Semi-structured interviews were used, and data were analyzed using a grounded theory approach.

For 11 of the participants in this study, after sexual intercourse could no longer be performed, all sexual intimacy ceased. However, for the other 9 participants, when sexual intercourse was no longer possible, there was renegotiation of sexual intimacy behaviors. For these individuals, alternative practices could include masturbation (both self and mutual), the use of vibrators, and oral sex. Hugging, kissing, and giving and receiving affection were mentioned by all 9 of the renegotiators and were considered sexually satisfying and rewarding (p. 1002). These individuals also described their positive communication with their partners and having a good relationship.

The other study participants, who had not renegotiated sexuality, gave personal accounts that were in accordance with the coital imperative. Participants talked about "full" sex and "real" sex, meaning sexual intercourse. The assumption of these individuals was that "real sex" consisted of penetrative vaginal intercourse, and there were no other viable options. Women carers of husbands with cancer who were unable to have sexual intercourse reported that considering their own sexual needs would not be appropriate: "Their own sexual needs were positioned as secondary to the risk of their partners' feeling inadequate about their masculinity" (p. 1002).

The biomedical model of sex positions sex as a physiologically driven act, and heterosexual penis–vagina intercourse as "natural" or "real" sex. Described as the "coital imperative," this model of sex is enshrined in the definitions of sexual dysfunction in the *Diagnostic and Statistical Manual of Mental Disorders* published by the American Psychiatric Association (Ussher, Perz, Gilbert, Wong, & Hobbs, 2013, pp. 455–456). The coital imperative is not confined to the biomedical domain, but is also reflected as "normal" or "real" in popular culture.

In a follow-up study to Gilbert et al.'s investigation, Ussher and colleagues (2013) interviewed 44 persons with a variety of reproductive and nonreproductive cancers and 35 partners. An analysis of the results revealed that renegotiation of sex or intimacy was reported by 70% of the participants and categorized into three themes:

- Resisting the coital imperative: Redefining sex
- Resisting the coital imperative: Embracing intimacy
- Adopting the coital imperative: Refiguring the body through techno-medicine (Ussher et al., 2013, p. 457)

Another theme that researchers identified from the study was "the intersubjective nature of sexual renegotiation: relationship context and communication." Sexual negotiation is primarily an intersubjective experience, which takes place between persons with cancer and their partners. In this study, the context of a couple's relationship and effective communication was identified as the major factor that facilitated renegotiation of sex. Participants talked about being honest and allowing their partner to ask anything, communicating their needs and desires, being open about which sexual or intimate act they could try, and saying what they did not want to do (p. 458).

Communication with Healthcare Professionals

Healthcare professionals have often underrated the side effects of chronic disease as related to sexuality as part of their assessment, believing that "others" should discuss the topic (Krebs, 2014). In fact, the literature notes that neither patients, nor partners, nor healthcare professionals bring up the subject on their own, preferring to avoid it (Hawkins et al., 2009; Lindau et al., 2011; Perz, Ussher, & Gilbert, 2013; Ussher et al., 2013). On the one hand, many healthcare professionals fear privacy issues if the topic of sexuality and intimacy is brought up. On the other hand, patients and partners feel embarrassed about bringing up the intimate subject, and wonder what their healthcare professional could do about it.

Studies have shown that patients, both male and female, are often disappointed by the lack of information, support, and practical strategies provided by their clinicians to help manage sexual changes secondary to cancer and treatment (Varela et al., 2011). Moreover, some healthcare professionals may have little sensitivity when discussing the subject or its consequences.

Randy had been in the surgical intensive care unit (SICU) for slightly over a week, and was still on the ventilator when I developed a urinary tract infection. Perhaps stress played

Table 11-3 PLISSIT MODEL

Permission (P)	(Assessment) Actions taken by the nurse to let the patient/partner know that sexual issues are a legitimate aspect in providing nursing care. This could include questions about sexuality that are incorporated into the general admission assessment or questions specifically related to their disease process or treatment.
Limited Information (LI)	(Education) Sharing of information regarding the effects of disease, treatments, and medications. Examples of limited information include discussing when sexual intercourse may be resumed after surgery, the possibility of menopause occurring in conjunction with chemotherapy, or medications leading to erectile dysfunction.
Specific Suggestions (SS)	(Counseling) This level of care requires specialized knowledge about specific conditions and their relationship to sexual functioning. Various techniques and positions that can be useful in achieving sexual satisfaction are examples of counseling concerns.
Intensive Therapy (IT)	(Referral) Treatment of sexual dysfunction requires specialized training in psychotherapy, sex therapy techniques, crisis intervention, and behavior modification.

Source: Data from Annon, J. S. (1976). *The behavioral treatment of sexual problems: Volume I: Brief therapy.* New York, NY: Harper & Row.

into the infection, or me not drinking water as I should have, as I had Randy on my mind, not me. I don't know why, but it was clear to me that I had an infection. There was only one physician available in the clinic to see me that day. I had not seen him before (my physician was booked that day, as well as others whom I knew). In the past some members of my family had expressed some concern with this particular physician's "bedside manner," but I had no choice. I was miserable, and I needed to be on top of my game for Randy.

A urine sample quickly found bacteria in my urine. Then the physician started asking me questions. Had I had intercourse lately? I replied no, not recently, as my husband had cancer, and in fact was currently in the SICU on a ventilator. "That's funny," he said. "I thought that sex was the last thing a man gave up, even if he had cancer." I was stunned and said nothing. I quickly took my prescription

and left the office in tears, determined that I would never schedule an appointment with him again. If need be, I'd go to the ER if no one else was available in the practice.

—Jenny

Sexuality is a part of a person's quality of life, so assessing sexuality and intimacy and responding to problematic issues are essential in caring for the whole patient. Many healthcare professionals use the PLISSIT model (Annon, 1976) to assist them in their sexual assessments. In this model, P stands for permission; LI, for limited information; SS, for specific suggestions; and IT, for intensive therapy (**Table 11-3**). Nurses should be able to intervene at the first two levels.

The BLISSS Communication model is another model for an individual intervention (de Vocht, Notter, & van de Weil, 2010):

- B: Bring up the topic in an appropriate way
- LI: Listen to the individual experience

- S: Support the individual and partner
- S: Stimulate communication between the partners
- S: Supply personalized advice and information; where necessary, refer in an appropriate way

Outcomes

Desired client and partner outcomes may include the following:

- The ability to identify potential/actual changes in sexuality, sexual functioning, or intimacy related to disease and treatment
- The ability to express feelings about alopecia, body image changes, and altered sexual functioning
- The ability to engage in open communication with a partner regarding changes in sexual functioning or desire within a relationship framework

Evidence-Based Practice Box

The aim of this study was to explore renegotiation of sex in individuals with cancer and in partners across a broad range of cancer types and relational contexts. Semi-structured interviews were conducted with 44 persons with cancer. Renegotiation of sex or intimacy was reported by 70% of the participants and reflected three themes: (1) resisting the coital imperative: redefining sex; (2) resisting the coital imperative: embracing intimacy; and (3) adopting the coital imperative: refiguring the body through techno-medicine. Resistance of the coital imperative should be a fundamental aspect of information and support that healthcare providers should share with patients to reduce the distress associated with sexual changes after cancer.

Source: Ussher, J. M., Perz, J., Gilbert, E., Wong, W. K. T., & Hobbs, K. (2013). Renegotiating sex and intimacy after cancer: Resisting the coital imperative. *Cancer Nursing, 36*(6), 454–462.

CASE STUDY 11-1

Rebecca is newly diagnosed with Stage II breast cancer. She is having a lumpectomy followed by radiation therapy. The surgical procedure reveals that all nodes are clear. Rebecca's husband comes with her to the appointment. He asks the oncologist, "Is my wife's breast ever going to look normal again?" Her husband had to return to work as soon as the oncologist left the office. It seems as if Rebecca wants to ask you some questions, but you are not sure.

Discussion Questions

1. How would you draw out Rebecca's questions and concerns?
2. Rebecca mentions to you that her husband is "kind of a man's man" and does not really understand what the lumpectomy and radiation therapy are all about. How do you respond to Rebecca?

CASE STUDY 11-2

Bob has been diagnosed with prostate cancer that appears to be localized at this point in time. He and his wife have some "personal" questions for the oncologist, and it is apparent that they are not willing to talk with you about the issue. You sense it has something to do with possible sexual changes to Bob's body.

Discussion Questions

1. How do you create an environment where personal questions are welcomed?
2. How do you, as a female oncology nurse, work with your male patients with reproductive cancers?

STUDY QUESTIONS

1. How would you attempt to talk with a patient and partner about intimacy? Which cues from the couple might give you the opportunity to bring up the subject?
2. Describe how physical caregiving could be an intimate experience.
3. How would you apply both the renegotiation and flexible coping models to a partner with breast cancer, a patient with multiple sclerosis, and a patient with an ileostomy?
4. Describe your role in working with patients and partners with intimacy issues.

References

Annon, J. S. (1976). A proposed conceptual schema for the behavioural treatment of sexual problems. *Journal of Sex Education and Therapy, 2*(1), 1–15.

Barsky, J. L., Friedman, M. A., & Rosen, R. C. (2006). Sexual dysfunction and chronic illness: The role of flexibility in coping. *Journal of Sex & Marital Therapy, 32,* 235–253. doi: 10.1080/00926230600575322

Cort, E., Monroe, B., & Oliviere, D. (2004). Couples in palliative care. *Sexual and Relationship Therapy 19*(3), 337–354. doi: 10.1080.14681990410001715454

de Vocht, J. M., Notter, J., & van de Weil, H. B. M. (2010, June). *Sexuality and intimacy: Impact of cancer and discussion with health care professionals from a client's perspective.* Paper presented at the 2nd Rotterdam Symposium on Cancer and Sexuality, Rotterdam, Netherlands. http://www.issc.nu /uploads/07-hildedevocht.pdf

Duffy, J. D., & Valentine, A. D. (2011). *MD Anderson manual of psychosocial oncology.* New York, NY: McGraw-Hill.

Flynn, K. E., Jeffery, D. D., Keefe, F. J., Porter, L. S., Shelby, R. A., Fawzy, M. R., ... Weinfurt, K. P. (2011). Sexual functioning along the cancer continuum: Focus group results from the Patient-reported Outcomes Measurement Information System (PROMIS®). *Psycho-Oncology, 20,* 378–386. doi: 10.1002/pon.1738

Gilbert, E., Ussher, J. M., & Perz, J. (2010). Renegotiating sexuality and intimacy in the context of cancer: The experience of carers. *Archives of Sexual Behavior, 39*(4), 998–1009. doi: 10.1007/s/0508-008-9416-z

Graber, E., Laurenceau, J., & Belcher, A. (2009). Interpersonal process model of intimacy. In H. Reis

& S. Sprecher (Eds.), *Encyclopedia of human relationships* (pp. 899–901). Thousand Oaks, CA: Sage. doi: http://dx.doi.org/10.4135/9781412958479.n289

Hall, J. E. (2011). *Guyton and Hall textbook of medical physiology* (12th ed.) Philadelphia, PA: Elsevier Saunders.

Hawkins, Y., Ussher, J., Gilbert, E., Perz, J., Sandoval, M., & Sundquist, K. (2009). Changes in sexuality and intimacy after the diagnosis and treatment of cancer: The experience of partners in a sexual relationship with a person with cancer. *Cancer Nursing, 32*(4), 271–280.

Hughes, M. K. (2011). Sexuality and cancer. In J. D. Duffy & A.D. Valentine (Eds.), *MD Anderson manual of psychosocial oncology* (pp. 125–137). New York, NY: McGraw–Hill.

Katz, A. (2007). *Breaking the silence on cancer and sexuality: A handbook for healthcare providers.* Pittsburgh, PA: Oncology Nursing Society.

Krebs, L. U. (2014). Altered body image and sexual health. In C. H. Yarbro, D. Wujcik, D., & B. H. Gobel (Eds.), *Cancer symptom management* (4th ed., pp. 507–528). Burlington, MA: Jones & Bartlett Learning.

Laurenceau, J. P., Rivera, L. M., Schaffer, A. R., & Pietromonaco, P. R. (2004). Intimacy as an interpersonal process: Current status and future directions. In D. J. Mashek & A. Aron (Eds.), *Handbook of closeness and intimacy* (pp. 61–78). Mahwah, N.J.: Lawrence Erlbaum Associates.

Lindau, S. T., Surawska, H., Paice, J., & Baron, S. R. (2011). Communication about sexuality and intimacy in couples affected by lung cancer and their clinical care providers. *Psychooncology, 29*(2), 179–185. doi: 10.1002/pon.1787

Manne, S., & Badr, H. (2008). Intimacy and relationship processes in couples' psychosocial adaptation to cancer. *Cancer, 112*(11 suppl), 2541–2555.

Manne, S., Badr, H., & Kashy, D. (2012). A longitudinal analysis of intimacy processes and psychological distress among couples coping with head and neck or lung cancers. *Journal of Behavioral Medicine, 35*, 334–346.

Manne, S., Badr, H., Zaider, T., Nelson, C., & Kissane, D. (2010). Cancer-related communication, relationship intimacy and psychological distress among couples coping with localized prostate cancer. *Journal of Cancer Survivorship, 4*, 74–85. doi: 10.1007/s11764-009-0109-y

Manne, S., Ostroff, J., Rini, C., Fox, K., Goldstein, L., & Grana, G. (2004). The interpersonal process model of intimacy: The role of self-disclosure, partner disclosure, and partner responsiveness in interactions between breast cancer patients and their partners. *Journal of Health Psychology, 18*(4), 589–599. doi: 10.1037/0893-3200.18.4.589

Masters, W. H, & Johnson, V. E. (1966). *Human sexual response.* Philadelphia: Lippincott-Raven.

National Institutes of Health (NIH). (n.d.). PROMIS. http://www.nihpromis.org/about/overview

Perz, J., Ussher, J. M., & Gilbert, E. (2013). Constructions of sex and intimacy after cancer: Q methodology study of people with cancer, their partners and health professionals. *BMC Cancer, 13,* 270.

Prager, K. J., & Roberts, L. J. (2004). Deep intimate connection: Self and intimacy in couple relationships. In D. J. Mashek & A. Aron (Eds.), *Handbook of closeness and intimacy* (pp. 43–60). Mahwah, NJ: Lawrence Erlbaum Associates.

Rainey, S. S. (2011). *Love, sex and disability: The pleasures of care.* Boulder, CO: Lynne Rienner.

Reese, J. B., Keefe, F. J., Somers, T. J., & Abernethy, A. P. (2010). Coping with sexual concerns after cancer: The use of flexible coping. *Supportive Care in Cancer, 18,* 785–800. doi: 10.1007/s00520-010-0819-8

Reis, H. T., & Shaver, P. (1988). Intimacy as an interpersonal process. In S. Duck (Ed.), *Handbook of personal relationships* (pp. 367–389). Chichester, UK: Wiley.

Revenson, T. A., & DeLongis, A. (2011). Couples coping with chronic illness. In S. Folkman (Ed.), *The Oxford handbook of stress, health and coping* (pp. 101–123). Oxford, UK: Oxford University Press.

Steinke, E. E. (2013). Sexuality and chronic illness. *Journal of Gerontological Nursing, 39*(11), 18–27.

Ussher, J. M., Perz, J., Gilbert, E., Wong, W. K. T., & Hobbs, K. (2013). Renegotiating sex and intimacy after cancer: Resisting the coital imperative. *Cancer Nursing, 36*(6), 454–462. doi: 10.1097/NCC.0b013e3182759e21

Varela, V. S., Nelson, C. J., & Bober, S. L. (2011). Sexual problems. In V. T. Devita, T. S. Lawrence, & S. A. Rosenberg (Eds.), *Devita, Hellman and Rosenberg's cancer: Principles and practice of oncology* (9th ed., pp. 2456–2466). Philadelphia, PA: Lippincott Williams and Wilkins.

Wilmoth, M. C. (2013). Sexuality. In P. Larsen & I. Lubkin, *Chronic illness: Impact and intervention* (8th ed., pp. 289–313). Burlington, MA: Jones & Bartlett Learning.

World Health Organization (WHO). (2006). Defining sexual health: Report of a technical consultation in sexual health, 28–31 January, 2002. http://www.who.int/reproductivehealth/publications/sexual_health/defining_sexual_health.pdf?ua=1

Yarbro, C. H., Wujcik, D., & Gobel B. H. (Eds.). (2014). *Cancer symptom management* (4th ed.) Burlington, MA: Jones & Bartlett Learning.

Chapter 12

Powerlessness

Faye I. Hummel

It was only yesterday I was at the top of my game ... it felt good to be settled, content, and confident about most everything. Honestly, I never dreamed I would be where I am today ... I can't believe it even now ... oh my, ... my strength, my spirit, my control are fading. My professional career and personal life are crumbling at my feet ... it's like a landslide ... no stopping it. It was just today with great regret and sorrow, I resigned as the president of Faculty Senate of my university. The control, the power, the autonomy I once had over my life and my body are slipping away ... no stopping it.

—Margaret, 55-year-old university professor with multiple sclerosis

Introduction

Powerlessness diminishes health and quality of life for persons with chronic illness. Chronic illness changes one's sense of self and one's sense of time. Living with chronic illness requires one to adapt to a continuous changing of outlooks in which the existence of dualities, such as hope and despair, self-control and loss of power, dependence and independence, can elicit feelings of ambiguity, anxiety, and frustration (Delmar et al., 2006). Chronic illness creates threats to well-being and produces multidimensional changes and challenges for the individual and family. Whether these changes occur suddenly or over a long period, chronic illness requires that individuals and families deal with and adapt to an unrelenting altered reality. Managing real and perceived powerlessness is significant. Lack of control and the incapacity to act and change may dominate everyday life for persons with chronic illnesses. Accepting and acknowledging one's limitations as a result of chronic illness

may result in a sense of helplessness and loss, as evidenced in the case of Margaret:

Last week I watched Emma, my 8-year-old granddaughter, playing in my backyard. She called to me to play tag with her, a game we've enjoyed so many times. I can't run anymore; I can barely keep my balance, I have difficulty walking and I've been falling more often lately. I'm heartbroken to see the disappointment in her eyes when I tell her "I'm sorry, I can't." The weakness throughout my body is getting so much worse and so fast ... my fatigue is crushing and I'm having more difficulty managing my pain. I am worried I won't be able to continue my work as a professor at the local university. I've been elected to numerous leadership positions but I've had to give them up ... one by one. I miss my interactions with my colleagues, the challenges of problem solving, debating issues, the intellectual discourse. This MS is a confusing and emotional experience for me ... in my mind, I'm willing and able ... I'm capable of anything and everything just like always. Yet at the same time, I feel distant and separate from my body.... . I don't recognize those flaccid legs, those limp arms. I have no energy ... what happened? I'm losing control of my body, of my daily routines, of my relationships with my family and work colleagues ... not to mention those life pleasures and joys, those bike rides in the evenings and those mountain hikes on the weekends with my husband.

—Margaret, 55-year-old university professor
with multiple sclerosis

The Phenomenon of Powerlessness in Chronic Illness

At some point in the course of chronic illness, individuals experience powerlessness. Ill health is powerlessness created by a self-image of worthlessness, a sense of imprisonment in one's life situation, and emotional suffering (Strandmark, 2004). Powerlessness may consist of a real loss of power or a perceived loss of power. For some persons, the feelings of powerlessness may be short lived; for others, they are persistent.

What and who determine powerlessness and which factors facilitate powerlessness? The natural history of chronic illness is highly variable and does not conform to a predictable course of events. The uncertainty of chronic illness, exacerbation of symptoms, failure of therapy, physical deterioration despite adherence to treatment regimens, side effects of drugs, iatrogenic influences, depletion of social support systems, and disintegration of the client's psychological stamina can all contribute to powerlessness (Miller, 2000). Chronic illness results in a pronounced loss of functioning over time, disrupts and depletes social roles and activities, and limits fulfillment of role expectations (Beal, 2007). Fatigue and inability to participate and engage in social activities contribute to social withdrawal (Beal, 2007) and loss of relationships. Loss of employment, social contacts, and physical and mental function can contribute to

disempowerment of individuals with chronic illness

Powerlessness occurs when an individual is controlled by external forces rather than the individual controlling the environment. Therefore, powerlessness is a situational attribute (Miller, 2000). For Margaret, powerlessness arises in part because of the degenerative nature of her disease. Despite her previous life successes, she now feels powerless over her own circumstances. Although Margaret experienced physical limitations associated with her chronic disease for a number of years, she was able to successfully adapt and respond to the slow progressive deterioration of her physical condition. Margaret maintained power and control over her daily life. When she began to experience the crushing effects of her illness symptoms and physical limitations, Margaret felt a loss of control, a sense of powerlessness. No longer was she able to maintain her veneer of normalcy, nor was she able to sustain her work and social obligations. Margaret ultimately withdrew from leadership positions at her university. When she began to consider herself without worth in terms of social norms and expectations, feelings of powerlessness emerged. Her autonomy and existence were threatened. Over time, Margaret became exhausted from fatigue and grief and felt powerless over her life situation (Strandmark, 2004).

Dorothy Johnson was one of the first individuals to explore the concept of powerlessness in nursing. Johnson (1967) defined powerlessness as a "perceived lack of personal or internal control of certain events or in certain situations" (p. 40) and urged nurses to take into account the concept of powerlessness inasmuch as nursing interventions—particularly health education—would not be effective if the client felt powerless.

The work of Miller (1983, 1992, 2000) has also been instrumental in the development of the concept of powerlessness in chronic illness. Miller (1983, 1992, 2000) differentiates powerlessness from similar constructs, including helplessness, learned helplessness, and locus of control. Helplessness and locus of control are based on a reinforcement paradigm, whereas powerlessness is an existential construct (Miller, 2000). Miller (2000) categorizes locus of control as a personality trait; in contrast, powerlessness is situationally determined. Locus of control refers to the degree to which people attribute accountability to themselves (internal control), such as owing to their personal behavior or characteristics, versus to uncontrollable forces (external control), such as fate, chance, or luck (Rotter, 1966). The physical and psychosocial outcomes of seeking and gaining control over chronic illness have been the focus of research by social scientists for decades. Locus of control and the beliefs of individuals about who and what controls their lives are linked to physical and psychological health (Bandura, 1989).

Chronic illness erodes individual control, and this loss of personal control results in powerlessness. Progressive physiologic changes resulting from chronic illness may limit mobility or diminish cognitive abilities. The progressive nature of chronic illness limits possibilities and opportunities to exert control over daily life events as well as plans for the future. Chronic illness sharply delineates the nature and quality of control, often resulting in a sense of powerlessness in individuals and their families.

Chronic illness disrupts personal control and changes life activities and expectations. Maintaining personal control is important for persons with chronic illness; lack of self-management and inability to predict the course of their disease can be distressing. Decision making to manage and control everyday life with a chronic illness is complex and bound to individually constructed lives (Thorne, Paterson, & Russell, 2003). Perceptions of control are associated with greater levels of psychosocial well-being, whereas perceptions of powerlessness are associated with poorer health and psychosocial outcomes (Hay, 2010). Persons with

inflammatory bowel disease reported personal control required maintaining a balance between what one could control versus what one needed to control for everyday life (Cooper, Collier, James, & Hawkey, 2010). Using grounded theory methodology, Pihl-Lesnovska, Hjortswang, Ek, and Frisman (2010) interviewed 11 persons with Crohn's disease. Dominant themes that emerged from analysis of the interview data included quality of life, self-image, confirmatory relations, powerlessness, attitude toward life, and a sense of well-being.

Rånhein and Holand (2006) conducted a hermeneutic–phenomenologic study of women's lived experience with chronic pain and fibromyalgia. Themes of powerlessness, ambivalence, and coping emerged from interviews with 12 women with fibromyalgia. The stories of these women revealed their struggles to manage and control the severe symptoms of their disease and their efforts to reduce their feelings of powerlessness that surfaced with pain, fatigue, and immobility. Individuals with chronic illness who develop effective systems for controlling their most severe symptoms have a more positive outlook and a lessened sense of powerlessness. The main challenge facing women with chronic pain was to maintain a sense of control of self and pain so as to avoid becoming discouraged. In a theory synthesis, Skuladöttir and Halldorsdöttir (2008) postulated that women with chronic pain face multiple challenges and the threat of demoralization. Notably, interactions with healthcare professionals may be either positive or negative. Positive interactions can result in empowerment, as a sense of control is maintained; conversely, negative interactions can disempower clients and diminish a sense of control over self and the situation.

Persons whose health fails experience increasing powerlessness (Falk, Wahn, & Lidell, 2007). A systematic review of 14 qualitative research studies conducted with older adults found that living with chronic heart failure was characterized by physical limitations and stressful symptoms, feelings of powerlessness and hopelessness, and social and role interruptions (Yu, Lee, Kwong, Thompson, & Woo, 2008). Aujoulat, Luminet, and Deccache (2007) conducted interviews with 40 individuals with various chronic conditions and asked them to discuss their experiences of powerlessness. The researchers found that powerlessness extends beyond medical and treatment issues to feelings of insecurity and threats to individuals' social and personal identities. Desperation and powerlessness were expressed by women with long-term urinary incontinence. Women who lacked control over their urinary incontinence reported their autonomy was threatened, which promoted a sense of powerlessness to control their own bodies (Hägglund & Ahlström, 2007).

The phenomenon of powerlessness in chronic illness is a dynamic and complex issue. It can be triggered by individual attributes and perceptions or stimulated by the evolving nature of the chronic disease. Powerlessness is inherent and impending in chronic illness. Nevertheless, feelings of powerlessness may ebb and flow, receding and advancing throughout the course of the chronic illness as individuals negotiate between control and loss and navigate the changing landscape of their daily realities. Variables such as the degree of physical limitation and ability to manage symptoms of chronic illness can also influence an individual's experience with powerlessness.

The Paradox of Powerlessness in Chronic Illness

The paradox of powerlessness in chronic illness is that power and powerlessness coexist simultaneously within a social context. A dichotomy, power and powerlessness are two mutually exclusive, interactive experiences: In the absence of power, powerlessness emerges, and vice versa. Power and powerlessness are a process as well as a condition. On the one hand, power is defined as the "ability to act or produce an effect" and "possession of control, authority, or influence over others" (*Merriam-Webster*, 2014a). On the

other hand, powerlessness is "devoid of strength or resources" and "lacking the authority or capacity to act" (*Merriam-Webster*, 2014b). Power is essential to enable and enhance one's autonomous ability and capacity. Despite the limiting effects of chronic illness and feelings of powerlessness, individuals strive to exert power and control in areas of their lives through adaptation and accommodation to their evolving abilities and selves. Power is a personal resource inherent in all individuals. Seeking, getting, and preserving power is a dynamic process that reflects a human being's ability to achieve a desired goal in the face of personal, social, cultural, and environmental facilitators and barriers (Efraimsson, Rasmussen, Gilje, & Sandman, 2003).

In the individual-oriented society of the United States, power is associated with independence and self-determination. Although we may think of power as an individual quality, in reality power is a relational attribute. Power has no meaning in the absence of relationships with others and the context of the interaction. It is developed and maintained in relationships. Power can restrict self-determination with forcefulness or authority by restricting the autonomy of another in personal relationships as well as hierarchical organizations (Moden, 2004). It is a "social, political, economic, and cultural phenomenon, since all these dimensions of human societies determine who has power and what kind" (McCubbin, 2001, p. 76).

Theoretical Perspectives of Powerlessness and Power

Persons with chronic illness live in a dual world, that of wellness and illness, of control and powerlessness, and of hope and despair. The shifting perspectives model of chronic illness (Paterson, 2001, 2003) describes chronic illness as a complex dialectic between the individual and his or her world. This model posits that persons with chronic illness shift between the perspective of wellness in the foreground and illness in the background, and vice versa. Further, this model suggests that the experience of living with a chronic illness is a dynamic process reflecting the elements of both wellness and illness. A perspective shift is a cognitive and affective strategy to negotiate the effects of chronic illness and to make sense of the experience. The perspectives of wellness and illness are not mutually exclusive; rather, the degree to which illness or wellness is in the foreground or background fluctuates over time (Paterson, 2001).

Rather than a static outlook, a continual shifting of perspectives occurs (Paterson, 2003). Persons living with chronic illness have a preferred perspective that is assumed most frequently. Therefore, persons with an illness perspective in the foreground focus on their illness, their symptoms, and the negative impact their chronic condition has on them and others. Conversely, from a perspective of wellness in the foreground, the individual views the chronic illness at a distance and focuses on his or her abilities to navigate daily life and to perform roles and responsibilities; the negative aspects of the chronic illness recede into the background. In addition to illness and wellness, this shifting perspectives model acknowledges parallel and simultaneous contradictions in the chronic illness experience such as loss and gain, control, and powerlessness (Paterson, 2003). Hence, persons with a wellness perspective will likely exert greater power and control over their daily routines and social interactions.

The illness and wellness perspective is dynamic, so it can be interrupted and changed at a moment's notice. Such a shift in perspective can be precipitated by physiologic changes, events, fears, and other individuals (Paterson, 2003). Social support, competent care professionals, hope, and humor are factors that influence a shift from illness in the foreground to wellness in the foreground (Freeman, O'Dell, & Meola, 2003). Exacerbations of symptoms and other forms of illness intrusiveness such as

pain, diminished physical strength, depression, and feelings of loss of a planned future may shift an individual's perspective and put the disease state in the foreground, with an accompanying sense of loss of control and powerlessness. The "relative importance of the illness, physical experiences with the illness, and biomedical uncertainties" (Sutton & Treloar, 2007, p. 338) can also trigger a shift in perspective. Clinical indicators of chronic disease progression may not be congruent with individual perceptions of health and illness inasmuch as health and illness views are constructed within the individual's physical, emotional, and social spheres and may not be compatible with healthcare priorities (Sutton & Treloar, 2007). Although the focus of illness in the foreground can be self-absorbing, this perspective may provide the individual with an opportunity to learn more about his or her illness and effective strategies to treat and manage symptoms. **Figure** 12-1 illustrates the shift of perspectives in chronic illness.

Figure 12-1 Shifting Perspectives in Chronic Illness

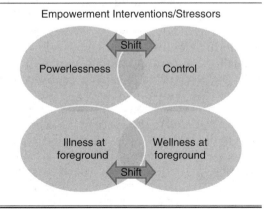

Source: Adapted from Paterson, B.L. (2001). The shifting perspectives model of chronic illness. *Journal of Nursing Scholarship, 33,* 21–26A; Paterson, B.L. (2003). The koala has claws: Applications of the shifting perspectives model in research of chronic illness. *Qualitative Health Research, 13*(7), 987–994.

SELF-DETERMINATION THEORY

Self-determination theory (SDT) highlights the psychological processes that promote optimal functioning and health. This theory posits three basic, innate psychological needs that are the basis for optimal functioning and personal well-being: competence, relatedness, and autonomy. These psychological needs are universal and must be satisfied for all people to achieve optimal health. They provide a framework that specifies the conditions in which people can maximize their human potential.

The need for competence reflects an individual's ability to adapt to new challenges in a changing context. It stimulates unique talents of individuals and produces adaptive competencies and flexible functioning in the context of changing demands.

The need for relatedness focuses on the integration of the individual into the social world in which the individual seeks attachments, security, and a sense of belonging and intimacy with others. The tendencies of relatedness are to cohere to one's group and to feel connection with and care of others. However, the need for relatedness can compete or conflict with autonomy.

Autonomy, according to SDT, refers to self-organization and self-regulation, and conveys adaptive advantage. Autonomous individuals function and respond effectively within changing contexts and circumstances. When behavior is regulated by outside pressures and expectations, holistic functioning is precluded. Therefore, autonomous individuals are better able to regulate their actions in accordance with their perceived needs and available capacities as well as coordinate and prioritize courses of action that will maximize self-maintenance (Deci & Ryan, 2000; Ryan & Deci, 2000).

Self-determination theory distinguishes between autonomous and controlled behavior regulation. Behaviors are autonomous when persons experience a sense of choice to act because of the personal importance of the behavior. Controlled behaviors, in contrast, are performed when persons feel pressured to act by external forces (Deci & Ryan, 1985, 1991). Autonomous regulation—that is, the choice to do what is important and relevant to the individual—is associated with subjective experiences of vitality and energized behavior and differentiated controlled and autonomous choice (Moller, Deci, & Ryan, 2006).

Clients whose needs for autonomy, competence, and connectedness are met during healthcare delivery are more likely to engage in health behaviors that enhance health outcomes (Ryan, Patrick, Deci, & Williams, 2008) and demonstrate enhanced adjustment and adaptation to chronic illness. Thus, patient-centered care is fundamental in self-determination theory. In *Crossing the Quality Chasm,* the Institute of Medicine (IOM, 2001) recognized the patient as the source of control. Patient-centered care focuses on the patient rather than the disease and gives the responsibility for disease management to the patient, along with the resources and support needed to assume that responsibility, reinforcing client power and control. Conversely, provider-centered care that focuses on the goals of the healthcare system inhibits client self-control, which in turn promotes dependency, leads to powerlessness, and erodes client autonomy (McCann & Clark, 2004).

DETERMINANTS OF HEALTH AND SOCIAL DETERMINANTS OF HEALTH

Determinants of health are factors that contribute to the health and illness of individuals and communities. They include biology and genetics, health services, and individual behavior, both physical and social.

Biology and genetic factors such as age, gender, and family history increase the risk for chronic illness. Many chronic illnesses such as cystic fibrosis and sickle cell disease have a genetic basis.

The health services determinant includes access to and quality of healthcare services. Lack of or limited access to healthcare services impacts the health status of individuals. Persons with chronic illness may experience barriers to health care due to lack of availability, affordability, accessibility, and acceptability of services. These barriers can result in unmet healthcare needs, delay the receipt of appropriate health care, and lead to otherwise avoidable hospitalizations. Where someone lives may determine the type of services available to that person. For example, Joan, a woman with HIV disease who lives in a rural community, may not have access to adequate healthcare services to manage her chronic illness due to her geographic location. For Jose, an undocumented farm worker with diabetes, healthcare services to manage his chronic illness may not be available; may not be affordable due to his lack of health insurance; or may not be acceptable due to language differences between him and the healthcare professional. For both Joan and Jose, their unmet healthcare needs may result in the progression of their chronic illness and/or avoidable hospitalizations.

The individual behavior determinant plays a significant role in health outcomes and the development of chronic illness. Individual determinants include diet, physical activity, sleep, use of substances such as tobacco or alcohol, levels of stress, and other individual factors that influence a person's health (*Healthy People 2020*, n.d.).

A growing body of evidence supports the sensitivity of health to the social environment (Wilkinson & Marmot, 2003), prompting researchers to focus more intently on the social determinants of health. Social determinants of health (SDH) are social factors that influence the overall health of an individual and determine levels of vulnerability to disease or poor health status (Shi & Singh, 2011); they must be considered in the context of powerlessness and chronic illness. Social determinants of health encompass a range of personal, social, economic, and environmental factors that interact to influence the health of individuals and populations. These major determinants act as vertical hierarchies wherein one's position on the hierarchy relates to susceptibility to a disease and illness (Shi & Singh, 2011). In other words, persons with

fewer social resources are more likely to experience poor health. Poverty, minority status, and lower educational levels are related to higher rates of chronic illness, including cancer, heart disease, stroke, and diabetes (National Center for Health Statistics [NCHS], 2010).

SDH are those factors and conditions in the environment in which people live, learn, work, play, and age. These determinants, which impact health, functioning, and quality of life, include education and employment, socioeconomic conditions such as income and wealth, social support and social interactions, public safety, social norms, and attitudes such as bias and stigma. Physical determinants include the natural environment, housing, work and school settings, exposure to toxins, other physical hazards or physical barriers, and aesthetic elements. Social and physical determinants are fundamental causes of a range of health outcomes (*Healthy People 2020*, n.d.).

Chronic illnesses may be exacerbated by the interaction between individuals and their social and physical environment. For example, children with asthma who live in neighborhoods with poor air quality tend to experience worse asthma symptoms and more difficulty in managing their asthma. Those who are poor and powerless have higher rates of disease and are less able than those with money, power, and prestige to minimize the consequences of a disease once it occurs (Phelan, Link, & Tehranifar, 2010). Socioeconomic determinants of health, powerlessness, poor health, risk factors, and health outcomes are all interconnected and reinforce one another. In the absence of appropriate and adequate resources, vulnerability and powerlessness increase.

SDH provide a framework for healthcare professionals to engage in holistic health services with clients with chronic illness. That is, interventions that address multiple determinants of health enhance health outcomes. Healthcare professionals must incorporate determinants of health into their interventions and plans of care to improve the health status of their clients with chronic illness. Assessing where clients engage in their daily activities of living—whether at work, school, or home—is essential for chronic illness management.

Problems and Issues Associated with Powerlessness

There are a number of issues associated with powerlessness. The issues discussed here are examples of what individuals and their families may experience, but are presented with the caveat that all individual intricacies and experiences with powerlessness in chronic illness will not be presented.

Loss

From a medical viewpoint, chronic illness is composed of physical symptoms and limitations. From a broader perspective, chronic illness brings multiple losses for individuals and their families on the physical side, but perhaps even more so on the psychosocial level, such as the loss of future hopes and dreams, a diminished quality of life, and the erosion of independence. The diagnosis of a chronic illness may, in and of itself, represent a loss to the individual; for some persons, the diagnosis may be as significant as a death. The loss of mobility and agility as a result of chronic illness affects one's ability to participate in social activities and to maintain social ties (Beal, 2007). Loss of paid employment due to chronic illness has a significant impact on one's life. Leaving work not only results in the loss of income and daily routines, but also triggers a loss of positive social identity (Walker, 2010).

Persons with chronic illness have restrictions in their daily lives, experience social isolation, feel they are discounted, and fear becoming a burden to others (Charmaz, 1983). Loss of self is felt by many persons with chronic illness (Charmaz, 1983), as the serious debilitating effects of chronic illness erode the former self-image of the individual. Over time, accumulated loss of self-image can result in diminished self-concept. Loss of self is a result of chronic illness that diminishes control over one's life

and future (Charmaz, 1983). Consequently, lack of self-confidence and disrupted identity are two major factors of powerlessness. In-depth interviews with clients with various chronic conditions have revealed numerous losses experienced by these individuals, including loss of self-control and confidence as their environment and possibilities become diminished (Aujoulat, Luminet, & Deccache, 2007).

Uncertainty

Chronic illness generates a wide array of emotions and reactions and engenders anxiety and uncertainty. The uncertainty of chronic illness promotes feelings of loss of control and a sense of powerlessness in individuals and families (Mishel, 2014). Content analysis from interviews with fathers of adult children with various forms of long-term mental illness revealed uncertainty about how to act and feelings of powerlessness, despair, and a sense of insufficiency (Johansson, Anderzen-Carlsson, Åhlin, Andershed, & Sköndal, 2012). Narratives of persons diagnosed with multiple sclerosis revealed concerns about the unpredictable progression of the disease and fear and anxiety relative to the unknown (Barker-Collo, Cartwright, & Read, 2006). Severity of the illness, the erratic nature of symptomatology, and the ambiguity of symptoms promote uncertainty in persons with chronic illness (Mishel, 2014). Anticipating and planning for the future become complicated. The unpredictability of physical symptoms and capabilities interferes with the individual's ability to schedule activities and events in the future and may result in an unwillingness to plan in advance.

Individuals with fibromyalgia participated in email interviews exploring their experiences with their diagnosis. Respondents expressed relational uncertainty that undermined the security of their connections to family, friends, colleagues, and the workplace (Dennis, Larkin, & Derbyshire, 2013). The uncertainty associated with their chronic illness raises salient concerns for persons about their future, their ability to control their illness and symptoms, and their capacity to garner the necessary personal and financial resources to manage their illness.

Chronic Illness Management

Chronic illness management often entails a multifaceted self-management regimen. The complexity of chronic illness has the potential to strip away a client's sense of self-worth and confidence. Clients who lack confidence often are unable to assess their needs accurately; consequently, they are at risk of being manipulated or coerced by others and may capitulate to the wishes of family members or healthcare professionals. Self-management of complex chronic disease is often difficult to achieve and is reflected in low rates of adherence to treatment guidelines (Newman, Steed, & Mulligan, 2004). Although some healthcare professionals believe they can motivate persons with chronic illness to follow a treatment regimen, the impetus to follow a plan of care is internal. Healthcare professionals may possess scientific expertise about a chronic condition, but they lack knowledge of the details of a person's daily life or the barriers that individual may face in managing a chronic illness.

Additionally, persons with a chronic illness may not be willing or capable of carrying out the complex tasks and activities required to manage their chronic illness; thus, words of admonition from the healthcare professional are inadequate to promote adherence and may be inappropriate. Clients' realization that their days are built around their healthcare regimen—that is, specific treatments they must perform every day, doctor visits, lab tests, body scans, consults with other healthcare professionals, physical therapy, and *not the other aspects of their lives*—can become unbearable. In many cases, the ability to "control" their day is gone.

For example, Sara, a 61-year-old woman with multiple myeloma, must spend three days a week at an infusion center two hours from her rural home. Even though she has accepted the time involved to adhere to her treatment regimen and has changed her lifestyle accordingly, Sara schedules a three-week visit to her childhood home in Germany to rekindle fond memories with family and friends. Her decision to forego the prescribed chemotherapy was triggered by her personal desire to exert power and control over her life.

In another example, John, a 50-year-old man with type 2 diabetes, experiences difficulties adhering to a complex pharmacologic regimen because of financial constraints. John finds himself consumed with the ongoing process of seeking resources to maintain his prescribed treatment, which takes away his ability to participate in other areas of his life.

The lives of Sara and John are centered on their chronic illness and treatment regimens. Both have experienced a loss of control over time management, personal choice, and quality of life. Their chronic illness and treatment regimens consume their daily lives to the detriment of other activities, causing feelings of powerlessness to arise. Other persons dealing with chronic illness may have similar experiences to Sara and John, in which the lack of self-control inherent in their disease and treatment fosters feelings of dependence and powerlessness, and undermines client autonomy (McCann & Clark, 2004).

Can we just have one day when we do not see a healthcare provider? It's either a doctor's appointment, rechecking lab results, radiation therapy, outpatient IV antibiotics, a port that is clogged, etc. This is a life? Where is our relationship of old when we used to talk about things other than "lab results," how much you've vomited, when the next appointment is? Why is every day of the weekend filled with an ER visit or an outpatient procedure of some type?

—Jenny

Adherence to treatment regimens requires active and meaningful collaboration of those with chronic conditions in the healthcare decisions that affect them. Choice of treatment regimen and control of that regimen are central to self-determination in persons with chronic conditions. To provide appropriate information, the nurse must listen to the needs, wants, and desires of the client. When clients feel unheard and have no voice, they feel invalidated and dismissed, and they feel powerless (Courts, Buchanan, & Werstlein, 2004). As a result of this powerlessness, the opportunity for the nurse to enhance client outcomes diminishes greatly.

Lack of Knowledge and Health Literacy

Knowledge about chronic illness is essential for effective disease management and control. Conversely, lack of knowledge or skills related to the disease may affect the dynamics of the disease. Often, information and education about the chronic illness occur during the acute phase of the illness or during hospitalization—overwhelming periods when the client and family may not be able to fully grasp the concepts. Unfamiliar surroundings coupled with the insecurities of a new or recurrent chronic illness diagnosis may also negatively influence learning. Although the client may have listened intently to the instructions and education, he or she may not have been able to internalize and actualize the content. As a result, after discharge from the acute care setting, the client may lack sufficient knowledge to effectively manage issues and problems that arise from the chronic condition. Lack of information to successfully meet the challenges of daily living further reinforces feelings of powerlessness.

Feelings of powerlessness have been noted to be rooted in the experience of living with limited health literacy in adults with chronic illness (King & Taylor, 2010). Nearly half of all American adults have difficulty in understanding and using health information. Health literacy impacts health outcomes and adherence to treatment regimens in chronic illness. Health literacy is the ability to understand verbal and written healthcare language and directions, including those on prescription bottles, procedure consent forms, and patient education materials. Having a specific educational level and reading ability does not ensure the individual will have the capacity to understand graphs and visual data, interpret test results, analyze risks and benefits, or calculate medication dosage. Low health literacy has been associated with poorer health, higher medical expenses, medication errors and nonadherence, increased hospitalizations, and poor disease outcomes (IOM, 2004). For all these reasons, healthcare professionals must ensure that clients have a clear understanding of health information related to management of their chronic illness.

Dignity

Human dignity is the value that belongs to every human by virtue of being human, whereas social dignity is shaped from the interactions among individuals, groups, and societies. Dignity is the subjective valuing of one's self (internal) and the valuing of one's self by others (external) (Eanes, 2003; Franklin, Ternestedt, & Nordenfelt, 2006). Dignity is affected by the inevitable decline and loss of function associated with chronic illness. An investigation of the concept of dignity of persons living at home with a variety of illnesses found that illness impacts an individual's dignity by one or more of three identified components shaping self-perception: (1) the individual self—that is, the subjective experiences; (2) the relational self—that is, the self in interactions with others; and (3) the societal self—that is, the self as perceived by others. Dignity was associated with social value and a feeling of being a burden or sensing stigmatization by others (van Gennip, Pasman, Oosterveld-Vlug, Willems, & Onwuteaka-Philipsen, 2013). These social forces have important implications for healthcare professionals as they seek to preserve dignity for those with chronic illnesses.

Dignity in healthcare interactions is an essential component of quality care and influences outcomes. Clients treated with dignity in their healthcare exchanges are more likely to adhere to treatment recommendations and regimens (Beach, Sugarman, Johnson, Arbelaez, Duggan, & Cooper, 2005). Preservation of dignity is a significant predictor of satisfaction in nursing home residents (Burack, Weiner, Reinhardt, & Annunziato, 2012), whereas a diminished sense of dignity is associated with depression, hopelessness. and a desire for death (Oosterveld-Vlug et al., 2014).

Dignity can be threatened in asymmetric relationships in which one person has more power, authority, knowledge, or wealth than the other. Jacobson (2009) conducted a grounded theory analysis to understand dignity violation in health care. Informants reported their dignity was harmed and violated by healthcare professionals through numerous processes of interaction and communication. Oosterveld-Vlug and colleagues (2014) interviewed nursing home residents and found many felt discarded and discounted simply due to their age and illness. Their personal dignity was diminished by having to wait for assistance, their lack of input into decisions, and their isolation. Further, these informants believed threats to their personal dignity could be diminished by good professional care that included active listening and attention as well as respect and honoring their point of view and perspectives. Strengthening a client's coping abilities, developing a caring and helpful social network, and ensuring appropriate and compassionate professional care can diminish threats to personal dignity associated with chronic illness.

Vulnerability

Vulnerability implies susceptibility. Vulnerability is a condition and process. It is a level of well-being—the degree of exposure to risk and the capacity to manage risk effectively. Some groups of people are more likely than others to suffer harm from exposure to health risks. Those identified as vulnerable lack the physical abilities, educational achievements, communication skills, or economic resources to protect their health. Vulnerable individuals and populations have increased levels of illness, experience poorer access to health care and receive poorer quality of healthcare services (Shi & Stevens, 2010), and are at greater risk of poor physical, psychological, and social health, with higher rates of morbidity

and mortality (Aday, 2001). Vulnerable individuals experience higher rates of chronic illnesses, including asthma and diabetes; are more likely to die from cardiovascular disease; and report more depression and exclusion from social groups. Even though vulnerable individuals have greater health needs, they experience greater barriers to timely and needed care. When they do receive care, they experience poorer health outcomes than others. Vulnerability to poor health is not a personal deficiency, but rather arises from the effects of the interaction among individual, community, social, and political forces over which individuals have little or no control (Shi & Stevens, 2010).

The social determinants of health are central to the concept of vulnerability and must be considered in the context of chronic illness management. Persons who experience a marginalized sociocultural status and have limited access to economic resources have a greater than average risk of developing health problems and have higher rates of morbidity and mortality associated with chronic illness (Aday, 2001). Vulnerability implies powerlessness (Strandmark, 2004). Vulnerable clients are the most powerless and the least able to identify and express their needs and desires beyond the completely obvious (Niven & Scott, 2003). Chronic conditions are a significant healthcare challenge, and one's vulnerability is often brought into sharp focus by a chronic disease.

Stigma

Stigma diminishes power. Persons with chronic illnesses are at risk for stigma based on the negative perceptions held by society. Stigma is a response to any physical or social attribute or characteristic that devalues a person's social identity and disqualifies him or her from full social acceptance (Goffman, 1963). Thus stigma and the associated stereotypes and misconceptions about chronic illness lead to exclusion and feelings of powerlessness. Confusion and misinformation about chronic illness can lead to discrimination and stigma, and result in unintended, harmful effects for persons with a chronic condition.

For example, family and friends of persons with hepatitis C may be fearful and lack knowledge about the virus. For the individual with hepatitis C, the ignorance of others may stimulate feelings of helplessness and infectiousness (Zickmund, Ho, Masuda, Ippolito, & LaBrecque, 2003) or fear of judgment and stigma from those around the individual (Sutton & Treloar, 2007). In this way, external societal pressures can create and perpetuate feelings of powerlessness in individuals with chronic illness.

Some clients are viewed as having less social value than others (Glaser & Strauss, 1968). Social value is subjective and influenced by such factors as age, marital status, income, living conditions, hygiene, and behavior. Some clients with chronic illnesses may be perceived as having low moral worth. The nurse may believe the client's illness or condition is the result of poor or risky behaviors chosen by the client. Clients who do not behave within the prescribed norms and expectations of the institution or agency may be labeled as undesirable or noncompliant and may not have the opportunity to engage in decision making and control over their healthcare regimen.

Culture

The concepts of powerlessness and power are grounded in the context of cultural values, beliefs, and practices of persons with chronic illness and their families. The traditional power and control culture in the healthcare setting may conflict with the cultural customs and beliefs of an individual with a chronic illness. Many cultural groups view the individual as embedded in a web of social relationships; thus, the role of the individual in decision making is not recognized. For group-oriented persons or families, power and control may reside within the family rather than with the individual. For example, in some Native American families, healthcare decisions are made by the matriarch of the family rather than the individual with chronic illness. Failure to include the family matriarch in the decision-making process is, therefore, likely to diminish adherence to the prescribed treatment

regimen by the Native American client. In some cultures, the oldest male holds the power and control to make decisions. Cultural conflicts may arise when families are not consulted before an intervention or staff interfere with rituals deemed necessary by the client's family to promote healing.

Conversely, when a client chooses to go against his or her cultural norm or custom, the client must have the power to do so. In situations where families are in disagreement with the client about compliance with cultural customs, the nurse must support the client and give him or her the resources necessary for self-determination. The desires and wishes of the individual client supersede the values, beliefs, and practices of the culture regarding which the individual and family are in disagreement (Tang & Lee, 2004).

Culture is the context in which individuals, families, and groups make healthcare decisions. In Western society, power and control tend to be based on the concept of individualism—that is, the notion that a society consists of autonomous individuals. While Western societies typically promote the actualization of the individual self as the goal, other cultures do not. The Western principle of autonomy is self-determination. In other cultures, the principle of autonomy is family determination—that is, the family is the autonomous social unit in which the entire family, not the individual, has real authority in decision making. For example, for Chinese cancer patients living in Hong Kong, emphasizing the Chinese cultural beliefs of loyalty to family, letting go, harmony with the universe, and the cycles of life and nature have been found to be essential to the development of feelings of empowerment (Mok, Martinson, & Wong, 2004).

Values, beliefs, practices, and responses to chronic illness vary by culture and within a given culture. Culture influences and dictates one's responses to normal events of everyday life and is a driving force in the decisions and choices that individuals and families make about health and care. Some individuals experiencing chronic illness may remain silent about their experiences with chronic illness. This is not an indicator of indifference or incompetence, but rather a reflection of cultural differences in the use of silence. Culturally appropriate care can occur only when cultural care values, expressions, or patterns are known and used appropriately (Leininger, 1995). Life experiences and situations of the past influence the present. For many African Americans, for example, religion and spiritual values provide a method for coping with chronic conditions. Their faith and belief in God give them power to endure pain and suffering associated with their chronic conditions (Anthony, 2007).

The centrality of cultural values to healthcare decisions is highlighted by the findings of a survey of 1,253 African Americans in Alabama churches. In this study, 59% of the respondents reported they believed in fate or destiny in relation to healthcare decisions and health-seeking behaviors. Women who believed in fate or destiny were less likely than those who did not to have breast examinations (Green, Lewis, Wang, Person, & Rivers, 2004).

Knowledge of cultural values, beliefs, and practices provides an invaluable blueprint for healthcare providers in caring for diverse clients with chronic illness. Furthermore, the promotion of cultural values can help clients with chronic illness mitigate their experiences of powerlessness.

Healthcare System

Power and powerlessness are inherent in the healthcare system. Education and professional status are sources of power for healthcare professionals. The procedures and language used by healthcare professionals are foreign and strange to the client and leave many persons with chronic conditions unable or unwilling to be an active participant in their health care (Anthony, 2007). The healthcare system perpetuates client vulnerability upon entry into the healthcare system. Clients relinquish control and surrender their independence to this system, where the healthcare professional is omniscient and clients begin the process of learned helplessness and inability

to speak for themselves. The client loses self-identity and initiative, and becomes distant from supportive networks. The client's voice may be ignored by healthcare professionals or quieted by dwindling energy levels that come from the disease process itself or the side effects of treatment. The healthcare system provides fragmented care for persons with chronic illness and leaves individuals feeling isolated and left to care for themselves with inadequate knowledge and resources. Frustration and inability to overcome obstacles in accessing, receiving, and paying for services may further add to feelings of powerlessness.

The healthcare system is designed for acute, episodic treatment and strives for efficient and cost-effective care. While this type of complex process is essential for those with acute illness who lack expertise to make appropriate decisions, such a system is counterproductive for those with chronic illness who develop competency and expertise regarding management of their illness (Thorne, 2006). The fast-paced and impersonal care system leaves little time and individual focus for a chronic illness management approach. Thus, clients with chronic conditions are vulnerable and powerless within the acute care structure.

Interventions

Persons with chronic illness feel overwhelmed, exhausted, and discouraged at times. Therefore, one of the most important challenges for nurses working with these clients is to help them overcome feelings of powerlessness. Factors that affect powerlessness in persons with chronic illness are complex and multidimensional. Nursing interventions to address powerlessness in chronic illness, in turn, should be equally multifaceted and require attention to the complex nature of the healthcare situation.

Appropriate and relevant nursing interventions are based on ongoing assessments and observations of the client with chronic illness in his or her environment, the context in which the person manages and copes with chronic illness. This includes not only the physical surroundings, but also the psychosocial dimensions of the client's life. Because of the dynamic nature of chronic illness, continuing evaluation of interventions with subsequent modifications to meet the current needs of the client are required. The goals of nursing interventions are to assist the client to manage the realities of his or her limitations, illuminate strengths to reduce the sense of powerlessness and loss and create new boundaries for the client's changed life. Persons with chronic illness seek a sense of normalcy and a sense of dignity by focusing on personal strengths and remaining engaged in family and social activities to diminish isolation and loneliness (Skuladóttir & Halldorsdóttir, 2011).

Nursing interventions to restore client control and increase power resources in clients with chronic illness are discussed in this section. Strategies and tools to strengthen the client's power base are highlighted as part of this coverage.

Empowerment

Empowerment is a health-enhancing process. The outcome of client empowerment is self-efficacy, mastery and control, and a renewed and valued sense of self. Key issues for empowerment are self-awareness and self-determination. Self-determination is the ability to make choices and accept responsibility for one's choices (Aujoulat, d'Hoore, & Deccache, 2007). Client empowerment in chronic illness entails a personal transformation through a dialectic process of (1) "holding on" to former self-representations and roles and learning to manage the disease and treatment so as to differentiate oneself from the illness, and (2) "letting go" or relinquishing control to integrate the chronic illness into a reconciled self. "Holding on" is linked to efforts to gain control and maintain a sense of mastery, whereas "letting go" is connected to a search for meaning and an acceptance that chronic illness is not always controllable (Aujoulat, Marcolongo, Bonadiman, & Deccache, 2008).

The nurse–client relationship emphasizes the primacy of the client's own ideas, emotions,

and beliefs about the chronic illness. Within this relationship, the nurse must provide information and opportunities for choice and negotiation regarding treatment-related issues. The nurse must be attentive to individual beliefs and desires with regard to choice and control. Some persons with chronic illness may choose to rely on others, such as family members or healthcare professionals, to make healthcare decisions for them. These individual desires and wishes must be honored and respected by healthcare professionals.

Empowerment strategies and efforts increase power and strengthen individual life circumstances. Two dimensions of empowerment emerge from the literature. One dimension is psychological, which includes self-esteem and self-efficacy. The other dimension of empowerment is social and action oriented, comprising power, involvement, and control over individual life circumstances (Hansson & Bjorkman, 2005). Key features of empowering provider–client relationships include continuity of care, patient-centeredness, and mutual acknowledgment and relatedness (Aujoulat, d'Hoore, & Deccache, 2007).

Empowerment is important for clients with chronic illness because it increases perceived quality of life and promotes self-esteem. For empowerment, clients need access to information, resources, support, and opportunity (Laschinger, Gilbert, Smith, & Leslie, 2010). Healthcare professionals can promote client empowerment by providing access to relevant, timely, and appropriate information about an illness or treatment. Ongoing information can be provided through the use of information technology, including email and vetted Internet sites. Client access to necessary support and resources further enhances empowerment. Nurses can assist clients with identifying sources of social support and introduce them to alternative resources within the family or community systems (Laschinger et al., 2010). For example, one such resource—peer support—enhanced the sense of empowerment and agency in a group of persons with kidney disease (Hughes, Wood, & Smith, 2009).

HEALTH COACHING

A variety of patient-centered strategies can be developed, such as incorporating lifestyle changes, engaging in prevention strategies, and making decisions to promote self-management of chronic illness. Although not a new idea in the practice of nursing, the reemergence of the idea of client-centered care is central in health coaching. In health coaching, clients become actively involved in determining what is important and what they want to accomplish relative to the management of their chronic illness. Health coaching motivates behavior change in clients through collaboration, open-ended inquiry, and questions and reflection (Huffman, 2007).

CARE TRANSITION

Effective care transition across the healthcare continuum is essential to facilitate empowerment. Care transition planning strengthens the client's position and role in social and healthcare systems. A client-tailored, well-orchestrated plan of care enhances coping when the client must deal with relocation from one healthcare setting to another. Open and clear communication among all participants in this process—the client, the family, and healthcare professionals—is essential for mutual understanding and successful transition. Nurses may think of care transition simply in terms of discharge from the acute healthcare setting to another care setting. The concept of transitions of care, however, emphasizes the collaboration and communication among and between healthcare professionals and the family and client necessary to facilitate restoration of client power and autonomy for effective chronic illness management.

COLLABORATION

Successful management of chronic illness and optimal wellness is based on collaboration and partnership with clients to establish mutually negotiated and established healthcare and treatment goals. Collaboration is promoted when the client is encouraged and expected to participate in his or her own care and make decisions that are based on the client's self-determined needs (Laschinger et al., 2010). Standardized approaches to empowering clients and improving the quality of life in persons with chronic illness are not appropriate. The lack of a match between a person's readiness and the healthcare professional's interventions may result in lack of adherence to the prescribed treatment regimen; as such, tailoring of the approach is essential. Adherence is a dynamic process that may be compromised by barriers related to different aspects of the chronic illness. Such barriers include determinants of health such as social and economic factors, the healthcare team and system, characteristics of the disease, therapies, and client-related factors. Solving problems related to each of these factors is necessary to promote client adherence (World Health Organization [WHO], 2003).

The client with a chronic illness must be a full partner with the healthcare professional in decision making. Indeed, imparting knowledge and information to clients is an exchange process that requires active client participation. Sometimes, however, the client may not desire information because of fear of the information, information overload, or lack of ability to understand the information. The nurse needs to assess client readiness for receiving information by acknowledging clients' concerns, listening to their perspectives, and respecting their desire for new information.

SELF-MANAGEMENT

Persons with chronic illness must be empowered to be managers of their own care within their capabilities and settings. The opportunities to manage self-control are dependent on the context in which the clients live their everyday lives (Delmar et al., 2006). Psychological, behavioral, environmental, social, and socioeconomic factors determine one's ability to self-manage one's chronic illness and adhere to a complex treatment regimen (Granger, Moser, Germino, Harrell, & Ekman, 2006). In an institutional setting (acute or long-term care), clients with a chronic illness may be highly motivated to manage their own care. However, the clients' environment dictates the parameters of activities of daily living and may severely limit the opportunity to fully operationalize self-management despite ability and desire to do so. In this instance, nurses can be instrumental in altering the institutional structure to accommodate the self-control goals of clients.

Self-management encompasses more than just adherence to a treatment regimen; it also takes into account the psychological and social management of living with a chronic illness. Chronic illnesses vary in the extent to which they intrude into the psychological and social worlds of individuals. The ideal outcome of empowerment is self-management of chronic illness through the reinforcement of self-determination and control (Aujoulat, d'Hoore, & Deccache, 2007). To this end, self-management interventions for persons with chronic conditions need to be developed to assist clients to better manage their illnesses and to take increasing responsibility for their disease. Healthcare professionals must take into account the shifting nature of chronic conditions and offer self-management strategies appropriate for the problems and issues that may be encountered at a particular phase of the illness. Granger and colleagues (2006) propose the use of trajectory theory to ensure interventions remain client centered and are relevant to the particular illness phase the client is experiencing or may encounter in the future. Further, healthcare professionals must be aware that some persons with chronic illness may not have the physical or mental abilities necessary for self-management. Assessment of the client to determine if self-management is attainable, realistic, and desired is necessary.

Difficulty in managing the often complex treatment schedules of chronic illnesses has led to the development of self-management interventions (SMIs). The key feature of these SMIs is the drive to increase clients' involvement and control in their treatment, and to improve the subsequent impact on their lives (Newman et al., 2004). The skills necessary for clients to develop a SMI are problem solving and goal setting. Even with these skills in place, most persons with chronic illnesses are likely to encounter barriers to care that create major challenges in compliance with SMIs. Those who experience increased barriers are less likely to adhere to plans of care. Such barriers may include time constraints, knowledge deficits, limited social support, inadequate resources, limited coping skills, poor client–provider relationship, and low self-efficacy. Patient-centered, collaborative nursing strategies reinforce client strengths and ameliorate the impact of these barriers. As part of this effort, the nurse becomes a partner with the client to facilitate collaboration in the development of a realistic self-management program and to identify resources and support systems to reach the goal of self-management. Conversely, failure of the nurse to identify or adequately estimate barriers to and resources for self-management will negatively impact adherence to the treatment regimen (Nagelkerk, Reick, & Meengs, 2006).

CONTROL

Aujoulat and colleagues (2008) suggest that "the process of relinquishing control is as central to empowerment as is the process of gaining control" (p. 1228). Perceived control is an antecedent to function, acts as a mediator between social support and psychological well-being, and is useful for effective disease self-management (Jacelon, 2007). This concept is related to better adjustment to chronic illness. Nurses need to be aware of two dimensions of perceived control (Rotter, 1966): (1) one can believe one is personally able to control one's outcomes or (2) one can believe that more powerful others control one's outcomes. With the latter belief, vicarious control is perceived as being exerted by physicians, parents, God, or family. To assist the client in achieving optimal functioning, the nurse must assess the client's belief about the source of control, whether within self or from others.

When the professional nurse exerts too much control, the client may totally relinquish control and put his or her life in the hands of the professional to the detriment of the client's own empowerment (Delmar et al., 2006). Client power is a fundamental element in the client–provider relationship because clients, due to their chronic illness, may become dependent on, and therefore subordinate to, healthcare professionals (Efraimsson et al., 2003). Independence, self-control, and self-responsibility are important elements for increasing patient empowerment. The ability to ask for assistance may be an indicator of self-control and self-management (Delmar et al., 2006).

SELF-DETERMINATION

Self-determination is a basic human right of individual choice and control. It ensures that an individual has the autonomy and support to make decisions and to reach personal goals. Self-determination must be balanced with safety and risk to the client and family. When supported, however, it can successfully restore the power of choice to the client.

Fostering self-control is integral to promoting wellness in persons with chronic illness, and this control is central to self-determination. To live a self-determined life, clients must have the knowledge and resources to deal with illness-related issues as they arise (McCann & Clark, 2004). Good choices are the result of good options from which to choose. Nurses can give persons with chronic illness adequate and appropriate knowledge as a foundation for making such good choices (Delmar et al., 2006). To manage self-control and live with dignity requires support from both healthcare professionals and significant others in the decision-making process. Other people can help provide knowledge and expertise as a foundation for

making the right choice. Clients with significant physical or mental impairments may be unable to engage in social discourse and may require additional resources to promote self-management. The nurse should provide the client with appropriate and relevant resources and work with the client and his or her family to obtain connections and referrals to appropriate community-based services.

ESTABLISHING A SENSE OF MASTERY

Powerlessness is reduced and empowerment is facilitated by the development of a sense of mastery. Mastery entails helping clients focus on how they can affect their chronic conditions and foster a sense of control in an otherwise uncontrollable illness course. Intervention techniques encourage clients to identify strengths and shift the focus away from uncontrollable aspects of chronic illness, such as use of a wheelchair or dialysis treatments, to the controllable aspects, such as decision making or self-care activities, which can imbue patients with a sense of mastery over their condition (Cvengros, Christensen, & Lawton, 2005). WHO (2003) has published guidelines for healthcare professionals that encourage them to facilitate client identification of strategies to reduce barriers to mastery and facilitate integration of self-care into daily activities.

Knowledge

Knowledge is power. Information about all aspects of chronic illness management is essential to restore power and control for persons with chronic illness and their families. For example, information about complex medical and treatment regimens is essential for empowerment. Further, information about the social and cultural impact of a chronic illness on one's life must be addressed to facilitate effective strategies to deal with loss, adjust to changes, and make alterations in daily life.

Over their lifetimes, persons with chronic illness and their families must shoulder the burden of coordinating medical information and treatment regimens. Information must be tailored to meet the needs of the individual client relative to the disease course. The client may not be able to effectively assimilate information at the time of the diagnosis of a chronic illness; therefore, information should be provided to the client and his or her family at a follow-up visit to ensure understanding of information and available services (Barker-Collo et al., 2006). Diagnosis of a chronic disease is an overwhelming and confusing period for clients and their families; consequently, the expectation that clients will be able to fully assimilate all information given to them about the chronic illness at the time of diagnosis is unrealistic.

Knowledge about community resources is essential for clients and families to assist them in restoring power and achieving effective chronic disease management. Therefore, it is incumbent upon the healthcare professional to maintain current information about available, accessible, appropriate, and affordable community resources and services. In collaboration with the client and family members, the nurse should recommend appropriate referrals for community resources. Community resources may include support groups, which can promote empowerment through the expression of shared experiences.

The digital age provides numerous opportunities for information sharing and gathering for persons with chronic illness. The Internet provides boundless sources of information to persons with chronic illness who are seeking health information and enables clients to independently obtain information, thereby promoting a sense of power and control. Sources of information on the Internet range from professional organizations to individuals who share the same chronic condition.

In addition, social media and other social tools such as texting are becoming important tools for information sharing about chronic conditions. Social networks are used with increasing frequency to disseminate information and connect healthcare clients with healthcare professionals, reducing the barriers of time and distance. Peer-to-peer social networks facilitate sharing of experiences and personal knowledge about a chronic condition. Online communication and Internet support groups have become not only sources of information for individuals with chronic illness, but also sources of social support (Laschinger et al., 2010; Van Uden-Kraan, Drossaert, Taal, Seydel, & van de Laar, 2009). Research has shown that women are more likely to use the Internet for health information and illness-related support than are their male counterparts (Pandey, Hart, & Tiwary, 2003).

HEALTH NAVIGATION

Formalized patient navigation using healthcare professionals arose from the need to assist persons with cancer through the complexities of the healthcare system (Harold P. Freeman Patient Navigation Institute, 2012). In response to this need, healthcare professionals were trained to navigate individuals with cancer through the cancer care continuum (National Cancer Institute, 2012). Patient navigation moves beyond advocacy to identify barriers and challenges to healthcare access and focuses on individual well-being. In this process, clients are guided through the bureaucracy of the healthcare system by a nurse advocate to complete a specific diagnostic procedure or therapeutic task. Navigation through the complexities of the healthcare system reduces barriers to healthcare access and treatment. Patient navigators also mobilize appropriate resources for the client. In a study of low-income women of color with breast abnormalities, patient navigation was shown to improve the timeliness of diagnosis, compliance with follow-up treatment (Psooy, Schreuer, Borgaonkar, & Caines, 2004), and diagnostic resolution follow-up by healthcare professionals (Ell, Vourlekis, Lee, & Xie, 2007). Furthermore, patient navigation has proved successful in reducing barriers to care and improving health outcomes in persons with HIV infection (Bradford, Coleman, & Cunningham, 2007).

While not a new concept, patient navigators today may be healthcare professionals as well as community or lay health workers.

Lay health workers are used to lead self-care management programs for people with chronic conditions. A growing body of evidence supports the effectiveness of community health workers as patient navigators to assist in the management of chronic illness (Foster, Taylor, Eldridge, Ramsay, & Griffiths, 2007) as well as to address determinants of health (Hunter, de Zapien, Papenfuss, Fernandez, Meister, & Giuliano, 2004).

Cultural and linguistic concordant interventions and services are a hallmark of successful patient navigation programs. Transformacion Para Salud, a culturally sensitive patient navigation program, was developed and implemented by community health workers to deliver health care, preventive services, and health education to an underserved population for self-management of chronic disease. Improvements in clinical and behavioral outcomes were observed in those who participated in this program (Esperat et al. 2012).

Patient navigators promote self-determination in their clients through empowerment. Although patient navigators are charged with helping clients obtain necessary healthcare services, clients must be afforded the right to choose regarding their individual welfare. The role of patient navigators reveals the essential elements of nursing functions such as liaison and resource coordinator. Patient navigators also have potential utility for serving at-risk women who have a high incidence of powerlessness (Ell et al., 2007).

ADVOCACY

In addition to patient navigation, advocacy is an important tool for increasing empowerment in clients with chronic illness. Advocacy activities seek to redistribute power and resources to people (individuals or groups) who demonstrate a need. Although the ideal of nursing advocacy is to empower clients within the healthcare system, institutional, social, political, economic, and cultural constraints often prevent clients from accessing health care. When such constraints are present, an advocate is necessary to facilitate procurement of the necessary services. The manner in which the nurse advocate intercedes to increase the client's power depends on the underlying values and beliefs held by the nurse regarding the advocate role. No one wants to be dependent on others, to inconvenience others, or to be a burden to others. Dignity and respect are linked with individual independence. The nurse must take care to ensure the client still holds the authoritative position in his or her own life and is able to maintain responsibility and self-determination. Even when these elements are present, situations may arise in which clients need help from an advocate to regain dignity and integrity.

MOTIVATIONAL INTERVIEWING

Motivational interviewing (MI) promotes client power and control. This clinical approach has been used to effectively address health and substance use–related conditions in many cultures (Morse, Schiff, Levit, Cohen-Moreno, Williams, & Neumark, 2012), and is now widely used as a tool for health behavior change. MI is a client-centered, nonjudgmental approach with a focus on interpersonal relationships that enhances intrinsic motivation to change and promotes client autonomy and self-responsibility in health behavior change. It explores and seeks to resolve ambivalences in behavior, using change talk to evoke and reinforce client behavior change. This client-centered approach provides the client with necessary information and lets the client decide what to do with that information. In some instances, clients may prefer a more directive approach, in which the healthcare professional provides information as well as recommendations that are in accordance with the client's perspectives. In such a case, the healthcare professional preserves the client's autonomy while providing a structure for the internalization of recommendations for behavior change (Deci & Ryan, 2012).

In one study, focus groups were conducted with African American women with type 2 diabetes, aged 21–50 years, to obtain their views on motivational interviewing. These women were asked to talk about their perceptions about

MI after viewing an example on a DVD. While the women reported MI consultation as effective health communication, the client-centered approach was negatively perceived. These women preferred a more traditional paternalistic approach—that is, healthcare professional–directed interaction of good counseling (Miller, Marolen, & Beech, 2010). Nevertheless, MI can facilitate autonomy in decision making by clients with chronic illnesses.

DECISION MAKING

When clients make their own decisions and act on them, there may be a difference between the client's choices and those that would have been made by family members or healthcare professionals. Consequently, clients may not only experience disapproval from others regarding their decisions, but also may encounter resistance when attempting to implement them. In the example discussed earlier in this chapter, Sara made a decision to interrupt her chemotherapy to connect with her past despite protests from her oncology nurse. This example provides the foundation for further discussions among healthcare professionals engaged in client-empowered health care. How much control belongs to the client, to the healthcare professional, and to family members? How do control issues affect the nurse–client, nurse–family, and client–family relationships? What are the guiding principles in this approach to nursing care of clients with chronic illness?

Healthcare professionals must provide clients with all the information they need to make a decision. Providing information about all aspects of the illness and about all services and resources available is essential to ensure informed decisions. As clients come to know the nature and meaning of their illnesses, their power tends to be restored and their vulnerability is reduced.

ANTICIPATORY GUIDANCE

Anxiety is triggered by uncertainty about the future. With chronic diseases, uncertainty of the illness trajectory suggests the need for the nurse to offer anticipatory guidance to persons with such illnesses. Anticipatory guidance is based on identifying expected future needs and can begin weeks, months, or years before any actual help is required. Future needs can have a profound effect on clients' lives because major life decisions can be influenced by them. Clients need a coach to help them chart an anticipated course throughout their chronic illness (Courts et al., 2004). Anticipating future dependency needs, for example, allows clients with progressive chronic illnesses to express their own wishes and preferences for care options. Even though informed anticipation lacks certainty, it facilitates greater rational future planning for clients and their families, minimizing the potentially difficult decisions that must be made during a time of crisis.

CULTURAL/LINGUISTIC COMPETENCE AND CULTURAL HUMILITY

Cultural competence is a process that evolves over time. The culturally competent healthcare professional must first identify and understand his or her own cultural values, beliefs, and practices to begin to know and understand the values and beliefs of his or her healthcare clients. Cultural competency enables healthcare professionals to provide services that are respectful of and responsive to the health beliefs, practices, and cultural and linguistic needs of diverse patients. Linguistic competency ensures effective communication and conveyance of information that is readily understood by diverse audiences, including those with limited English proficiency, those with low or nonexistent literacy skills, and those with disabilities including hearing and vision deficits (National Center for Cultural Competency, 2014).

It is imperative for nurses to explore potential differences and similarities among clients and their beliefs to ensure culturally competent care (Leininger & McFarland, 2002). Leininger (1995) asserts, "Clients who experience nursing care that fails to be reasonably congruent with the client's beliefs, values, and care life ways will show signs of cultural conflicts, noncompliance, stresses, and ethical or moral concerns" (p. 45). When nurses acknowledge and incorporate the client's cultural perspective into care activities and the plan of care, the environment of communication and understanding increases feelings of power and control in the client and family.

Healthcare professionals are called upon to learn the traditional cultural practices and beliefs of their clients and to develop culturally appropriate treatment plans and health education strategies. Nonetheless, cultural knowledge alone is not enough. Cultural humility is a viewpoint that addresses the issue of power and privilege in healthcare settings and relationships. It acknowledges the limitations that healthcare professionals bring to a healthcare relationship and honors and respects the client's expertise in cultural lifeways, values, and beliefs. Cultural humility meets the healthcare client where he or she is at any point in the illness trajectory; in demonstrating this trait, the healthcare professional suspends judgment and imposition of personal or professional values, beliefs, and practices. Cultural humility is a lifelong process that requires the healthcare professional to engage in ongoing self-awareness and self-critique to ensure that each healthcare encounter is client centered, with the client being viewed as the expert and a collaborator, and reflects respectful attitudes toward diverse points of view (Miller, 2009).

Outcomes

Outcomes associated with powerlessness in clients with chronic conditions can be measured from three perspectives: self, relationships with others, and client behaviors.

From the first perspective, changes in self are evaluated by measures such as increased self-confidence and self-esteem, which facilitate coping with and management of chronic illness. While self-management of chronic illness is optimal, self-care strategies can be complex and exhaust physical and mental reserves in persons with chronic conditions. Interventions that focus on emotional responses to chronic illness including feelings of powerlessness are essential to address disease acceptance and management. The client must monitor and make adjustments in the management of the chronic illness, just as a driver of a car turns the wheel, monitors speed, and applies the brakes while driving a car. Self-management presumes the client is given the opportunity to communicate effectively, seek information, collect data, analyze options, and make decisions. Information and resources must be available to the client with a chronic condition when the need arises, as opposed to when it may be convenient for the healthcare professional to provide information to the client. Healthcare professionals must recognize the limits of professional knowledge for self-management of chronic illness and respect the inherent expertise and primary authority of the client in matters pertaining to living with a chronic illness. In doing so, healthcare professionals become consultants and resource brokers within the context of shared and collaborative care (Thorne, 2006).

Evidence-Based Practice Box

The increased costs of chronic illnesses in United States serve as an urgent call to develop a cost-effective approach to improve chronic disease self-management, especially among vulnerable populations. An emerging role for professionals and paraprofessionals is the patient navigator. Transformacion Para Salud (TPS), a patient navigation model for chronic disease self-management, was a two-year demonstration program that sought to develop culturally sensitive interventions to facilitate patient behavior changes. The TPS project was based on the transformation for health (TFH) conceptual framework. TFH conceptualizes a transcendent process wherein people overcome oppressive conditions that lead to the defeat of the human spirit. Paulo Freire, a Brazilian educational philosopher, proposed that individual people or groups must achieve transformational power; it cannot be

(continues)

given to them. In the TPS program, TFH guided the training of certified community health workers (CHWs) to deliver health care, preventive services, and health education to underserved populations to promote chronic disease self-management. Patients involved in the TPS intervention showed improvements in clinical and behavioral outcomes after 12 months of intervention. Use of CHWs in the patient navigator role was found to be a cost-effective method to improve access to quality primary healthcare services as well as to facilitate chronic disease self-management.

TPS provides a new paradigm to facilitate behavior change among people with chronic diseases through the use of a trained patient navigator. TFH is a powerful framework that can be used in healthcare practice to empower individuals with chronic illness for behavior change and effective disease management. The concept of patient navigators is a growing and evolving role for both professional and paraprofessional providers. The use of *promotora* navigators appears to be a cost-effective method to facilitate behavior changes in those with chronic illness. The addition of these community health workers to the interdisciplinary healthcare team suggests one useful mechanism to improve access to quality, cost-effective primary healthcare services, particularly for chronic disease management.

Source: Esperat, M. C., Flores, D., McMurry, L., Feng, D., Song, H., Billings, L., & Masten, Y. (2012). Transformacion Para Salud: A patient navigation model for chronic disease self-management. *Online Journal of Issues in Nursing, 17*(2), 2. http://nursingworld.org /MainMenuCategories/ANAM

The second outcome that can be measured to demonstrate a change in powerlessness is relationships with others. Changes in relationships include improved relationships with family, friends, and healthcare professionals. Relationships are reciprocal in nature. That is, family, friends, and healthcare professionals must play active roles in providing social support and positive interaction with the client with chronic illness. Positive relationships have a powerful impact on the health and well-being of healthcare clients. Client–professional partnerships improve self-efficacy, symptom control, and functional status (Yu et al., 2008). Relationships with others who share a similar chronic illness experience can help individuals with chronic illness to reconcile themselves to the illness and develop a realistic view of the future (Delmar et al., 2005).

The last measurable outcome of reduced powerlessness is behavior. Clients with chronic illness experience transformation when empowered. Empowerment shapes illness perspectives and the approach to involvement in self-care (Dowling, Murphy, Cooney, & Casey, 2011). Positive changes in behavior can result in increased treatment-regimen adherence, better management of symptoms, and decreases in feelings of powerlessness.

Recommendations for Further Conceptual and Data-Based Work

Chronic illness research with a focus on empowerment interventions is essential not only at the micro level but also at the macro level. Policy development to address issues such as determinants of health, literacy, care transition resources, and other salient issues is essential to mitigate issues related to powerlessness in persons with chronic illness. Healthcare professionals within all dimensions of health care must provide the leadership and expertise to initiate policy initiatives to create significant and needed change in healthcare delivery for chronic illness management.

Continued development of knowledge and understanding of the experiences and needs of individuals with serious, chronic, progressive, and largely uncontrollable illnesses is essential to the development of effective strategies for greater perception of power and control. As we move away from the medical model and toward a sociological model of care, client and family empowerment are essential. The process of empowerment interventions at the social level would benefit clients with chronic illness, their families, and healthcare professionals.

CASE STUDY 12-1

Susan is a 54-year-old mother with two daughters, aged 11 and 9. She and her husband, Sam, live in an affluent neighborhood in an urban setting in the Midwest. Sam is an executive of a corporation, and Susan is a full-time mother after having had a successful career as an accounting executive. After years of being drug free, Susan is once again using prescription opiates. This time, she started to use drugs to ease the gnawing pain in her hip. Not only did the opiates ease her pain, but they also elevated her mood and helped her get through the tedium and stress of her day.

This is not Susan's first encounter with prescription opiate addiction. In college, she sustained significant injuries from a fall from her bike. She continued to take opiates after her broken bones healed and her pain subsided. After years of prescription drug use, Susan went into rehabilitation and resumed a drug-free life. Life was good. She married Sam and they welcomed their daughters into their lives. Susan was drug free during her pregnancies and deliveries of her daughters and during the early years of their childhood. It was after the piercing pain from kidney stones on Labor Day weekend necessitated a trip to the emergency room that she passed into the familiar darkness of prescription opiate addiction.

After months of physician shopping and drug seeking, Susan entered rehabilitation with the goal of returning home sober to care for her family and home. Susan's addiction to prescription opiates, however, has become all consuming. She is unable to meet the needs and demands of her household and her family. She has isolated herself from her friends and extended family. She is depressed and angry. Sam has assumed the daily household routines and ensures the girls maintain their school work and continue in their extracurricular and social activities. He takes the girls away for the weekends, further isolating Susan. Susan tried to cut back and stop taking her prescription pills, only to find she is feeling sick, irritable, and powerless. Susan is overwhelmed with the reality that her addiction to prescription opiates is a chronic disease that will persist throughout her lifetime. She is overcome with emotion and anxiety about her future and the future of her family.

Despite long periods of sobriety, Susan has relapsed again into opiate use. Will she ever be able to maintain her role as a mother and wife? Will she die from her addiction like so many women she has known during her periods of recovery? Will she ever achieve and maintain sobriety?

Discussion Questions

1. Discuss the determinants of health and vulnerability in relation to Susan's chronic disease of addiction.
2. Identify and discuss the problems and issues Susan and her family face with chronic drug addiction.
3. How do theoretical perspectives of power and powerlessness guide a plan of care for Susan?
4. If you were the case manager, which nursing interventions would you implement to restore power and control to Susan? How would you prioritize her plan of care?

CASE STUDY 12-2

Stan is a 73-year-old male who has been married to Sylvia for 20 years. They live in the small rural community where both were born and raised. The couple shared and enjoyed numerous hobbies, including gardening, horseback riding, and bowling. Stan regularly played card games with a group of his lifelong friends.

Two years ago, Stan had a cerebral vascular accident (CVA) resulting in temporary paralysis. After months of physical therapy, Stan regained his physical strength and abilities. Six months ago, Stan had another CVA that left him paralyzed on the right side of his body and unable to physically care for himself. Despite all rehabilitation therapies, he needs assistance with all his activities of daily living. His cognitive abilities are keen but he is unable to communicate verbally. While Sylvia was able to care for Stan in their home, she was not strong enough to assist Stan outside their home and into their automobile. Unable to leave his home, Stan is powerless to engage in his social activities or his hobbies. He feels isolated, frustrated, and helpless. He fears he will suffer another stroke, leaving him even more vulnerable and powerless.

Discussion Questions

1. Identify and discuss the issues Stan and Sylvia encounter in managing Stan's chronic condition.
2. Discuss interventions to restore power and promote empowerment for Stan.
3. Incorporate theoretical underpinnings into a plan of care for Stan and Sylvia that diminishes powerlessness.

STUDY QUESTIONS

1. Using the theoretical perspectives presented in this chapter, design nursing interventions to reduce powerlessness in persons with chronic illness.
2. Compare and contrast social determinants of health and vulnerability in the context of chronic illness.
3. Critique the potential strengths and limitations of nursing interventions to reduce powerlessness.
4. Discuss the relationship between chronic illness and powerlessness.
5. Compare and contrast the concepts of power and powerlessness in relation to chronic illness.
6. Discuss the factors that promote powerlessness in clients with chronic illness.
7. Propose policy directions to restore power in persons with chronic conditions.

References

Aday, L. (2001). *At risk in America* (2nd ed.). San Francisco, CA: Jossey-Bass.

Anthony, J. S. (2007). Self-advocacy in health care decision-making among elderly African Americans. *Journal of Cultural Diversity, 14*(2), 88–94.

Aujoulat, I., d'Hoore, W., & Deccache, A. (2007). Patient empowerment in theory and practice: Polysemy or cacophony? *Patient Education and Counseling, 66*(1), 13–20.

Aujoulat, I., Luminet, O., & Deccache, A. (2007). The perspective of patients on their experience of powerlessness. *Qualitative Health Research, 17,* 772–785.

Aujoulat, I., Marcolongo, R., Bonadiman, L., & Deccache, A. (2008). Reconsidering patient empowerment in chronic illness: A critique of models of self-efficacy and bodily control. *Social Science & Medicine, 66*(5), 1228–1239.

Bandura, A. (1989). Human agency in social cognitive theory. *American Psychologist, 44,* 1175–1184.

Barker-Collo, S., Cartwright, C., & Read, J. (2006). Into the unknown: The experiences of individuals living with multiple sclerosis. *Journal of Neuroscience Nursing, 38*(6), 435–446.

Beach, M. C., Sugarman, J., Johnson, R. L., Arbelaez, J. J., Duggan, P. S., & Cooper, L. A. (2005). Do patients treated with dignity report higher satisfaction, adherence, and receipt of preventive care? *Annals of Family Medicine, 3,* 331–338.

Beal, C. C. (2007). Loneliness in women with multiple sclerosis. *Rehabilitation Nursing, 32*(4), 165–171.

Bradford, J. B., Coleman, S., & Cunningham, W. (2007). HIV system navigation: An emerging model to improve HIV care access. *AIDS Patient Care and STDs, 21,* S49–S58.

Burack, O., Weiner, A., Reinhardt, J., & Annunziato, R. (2012). What matters most to nursing home elders: Quality of life in the nursing home. *Journal of the American Medical Directors Association, 13*(1), 48–53.

Charmaz, K. (1983). Loss of self: A fundamental form of suffering in the chronically ill. *Sociology of Health & Illness, 83*(2), 168–195.

Cooper, J. M., Collier, J., James, V., & Hawkey, C. J. (2010). Beliefs about personal control and self-management in 30–40 year olds living with inflammatory bowel disease: A qualitative study. *International Journal of Nursing Studies, 47,* 1500–1509.

Courts, J. F., Buchanan, E. M., & Werstlein, P. O. (2004). Focus groups: The lived experience of participants with multiple sclerosis. *Journal of Neuroscience Nursing, 36*(1), 42–47.

Cvengros, J. A., Christensen, A. J., & Lawton, W. J. (2005). Health locus of control and depression in chronic kidney disease: A dynamic perspective. *Journal of Health Psychology, 10*(5), 677–686.

Deci, E. L., & Ryan, R. M. (1985). *Intrinsic motivation and self-determination in human behavior.* New York, NY: Plenum.

Deci, E. L., & Ryan, R. M. (1991). A motivational approach to self: Integration in personality. In R. Dienstbier (Ed.), *Nebraska symposium on motivation: Perspectives on motivation, 38* (pp. 237–288). Lincoln, NE: University of Nebraska Press.

Deci, E. L., & Ryan, R. M. (2000). The "what" and "why" of goal pursuits: Human needs and the self-determination of behavior. *Psychological Inquiry, 11*(4), 227–268.

Deci, E. L., & Ryan, R. M. (2012). Self-determination theory in health care and its relations to motivational interviewing: A few comments. *International Journal of Behavioral Nutrition and Physical Activity, 9,24.* doi: 10.1186/1479-5868-9-24

Delmar, C., Bøje, T., Dylmer, D., Forup, L., Jakobsen, C., Møller, … Pedersen, B.D. (2006). Independence/dependence: A contradictory relationship? Life with a chronic illness. *Scandinavian Journal of Caring Sciences, 20*(3), 261–268.

Delmar, C., Bøje, T., Dylmer, D., Jakobsen, C., Moller, M., Sonder, H., & Pederson, B. D. (2005). Achieving harmony with oneself: Life with a chronic illness. *Scandinavian Journal of Caring Science, 19,* 204–212.

Dennis, N. L., Larkin, M., & Derbyshire, S. W. G. (2013). "A giant mess": Making sense of complexity in the accounts of people with fibromyalgia. *British Journal of Health Psychology, 18,* 763–781.

Dowling, M., Murphy, K., Coone, A., & Casey, D. (2011). A concept analysis of empowerment in chronic illness from the perspective of the nurse and the client living with chronic obstructive pulmonary disease. *Journal of Nursing and Healthcare of Chronic Illness, 3,* 476–487.

Eanes, S. P. D. (2003). An exploration of dignity in palliative care. *Palliative Medicine, 17*(3), 263–269.

Efraimsson, E., Rasmussen, B. H., Gilje, F., & Sandman, P. (2003). Expressions of power and powerlessness in discharge planning: A case study of an older woman on her way home. *Journal of Clinical Nursing, 12,* 707–716.

Ell, K., Vourlekis, B., Lee, P.-J., & Xie, B. (2007). Patient navigation and case management following an abnormal mammogram: A randomized clinical trial. *Preventive Medicine, 44,* 26–33.

Esperat, M. C., Flores, D., McMurry, L., Feng, D., Song, H., Billings, L., & Masten, Y. (2012). Transformacion Para Salud: A patient navigation model for chronic disease self-management. *Online Journal of Issues in Nursing, 17*(2), 2. http://nursingworld.org/MainMenuCategories/ANAM

Falk, S., Wahn, A. K., & Lidell, E. (2007). Keeping the maintenance of daily life in spite of chronic heart failure. A qualitative study. *European Journal of Cardiovascular Nursing, 6,* 192–199.

Foster, G., Taylor, S. J. C., Eldridge, S., Ramsay, J., & Griffiths, C. J. (2007). Self-management education programmes by lay leaders for people with chronic conditions. *Cochrane Database of Systematic Reviews, 4,* CD005108.

Franklin, L. L., Ternestedt, B. M., & Nordenfelt, L. (2006). Views on dignity of elderly nursing home residents. *Nursing Ethics, 13*(2), 130–146.

Freeman, K., O'Dell, C., & Meola, C. (2003). Childhood brain tumors: Children's and siblings' concerns regarding the diagnosis and phase of illness. *Journal of Pediatric Oncology Nursing, 20*(3), 133–140.

Glaser, B. G., & Strauss, A. L. (1968). *Time for dying.* Chicago, IL: Aldine.

Goffman, E. (1963). *Notes on management of spoiled identity.* Englewood Cliffs, NJ: Prentice Hall.

Granger, B. B., Moser, D., Germino, B., Harrell, J., & Ekman, I. (2006). Caring for patients with chronic heart failure: The trajectory model. *European Journal of Cardiovascular Nursing, 5,* 222–227.

Green, B. L., Lewis, R. K., Wang, M. Q., Person, S., & Rivers, B. (2004). Powerlessness, destiny, and control: The influence on health behaviors of African Americans. *Journal of Community Health, 29*(1), 15–27.

Hägglund, D., & Ahlström, G. (2007). The meaning of women's experience of living with long-term urinary incontinence is powerlessness. *Journal of Clinical Nursing, 16*(10), 1946–1954.

Hansson, L., & Björkman, T. (2005). Empowerment in people with a mental illness: Reliability and validity of the Swedish version of an empowerment scale. *Scandinavian Journal of Caring Sciences, 19,* 32–38.

Harold, P. Freeman Patient Navigation Institute. (2012). Our model. http://www.hpfreemanpni.org/our-model/

Hay, M. C. (2010). Suffering in a productive world: Chronic illness, visibility, and the space beyond agency. *American Ethnologist, 37*(2), 259–274.

Healthy people 2020. (n.d.). http://www.healthypeople.gov/2020/default.aspx

Huffman, M. (2007). Health coaching: A new and exciting technique to enhance patient self-management and improve outcomes. *Home Healthcare Nurse, 25*(4), 271–275.

Hughes, J., Wood, E., & Smith, G. (2009). Exploring kidney patients' experiences of receiving individual peer support. *Health Expectations, 12,* 396–406.

Hunter, J. B., de Zapien, J. G., Papenfuss, M., Fernandez, M. L., Meister, J., & Giuliano, A. R. (2004). The impact of a *promotora* on increasing routine chronic disease prevention among women aged 40 and older at the U.S.–Mexico border. *Health Education & Behavior, 31*(4 suppl), 18S–28S.

Institute of Medicine (IOM). (2001). *Crossing the quality chasm: A new health system for the 21st century.* Washington, DC: National Academies Press.

Institute of Medicine (IOM), Committee on Health Literacy. (2004). *Health literacy: A prescription to end confusion.* Washington, DC: National Academies Press.

Jacelon, C. S. (2007). Theoretical perspectives of perceived control in older adults: A selective review of the literature. *Journal of Advanced Nursing, 59*(1), 1–10.

Jacobson, N. (2009). Dignity violation in health care. *Qualitative Health Research, 19*(11), 1536–1547.

Johansson, A., Anderzen-Carlsson, A., Åhlin, A., Andershed, B., & Sköndal, E. (2012). Fathers' everyday experiences of having an adult child who suffers from long-term mental illness. *Illness in Mental Health Nursing, 33,* 109–117.

Johnson, D. (1967). Powerlessness: A significant determinant in patient behavior? *Journal of Nursing Education, 6*(2), 39–44.

King, J., & Taylor, M. C. (2010). Adults living with limited literacy and chronic illness: Patient education experiences. *Adult Basic Education and Literacy Journal, 4*(1), 24–33.

Laschinger, H. K. S., Gilbert, S., Smith, L. M., & Leslie, K. (2010). Towards a comprehensive theory of nurse/patient empowerment: Applying Kanter's empowerment theory to patient care. *Journal of Nursing Management, 18,* 4–13.

Leininger, M. L. (1995). *Transcultural nursing: Concepts, theories, research and practice.* Columbus, OH: McGraw-Hill College Custom Series.

Leininger, M. L., & McFarland, M. R. (2002). *Transcultural nursing: Concepts, theories, research and practices* (2nd ed.). New York, NY: McGraw-Hill.

McCann, T., & Clark, E. (2004). Advancing self-determination with young adults who have schizophrenia. *Journal of Psychiatric and Mental Health Nursing, 11,* 12–20.

McCubbin, M. (2001). Pathways to health, illness and well-being: From the perspective of power and control. *Journal of Community and Applied Social Psychology, 11,* 75–81.

Merriam-Webster. (2014a). Power. http://www.merriam-webster.com/dictionary/power

Merriam-Webster. (2014b). Powerlessness. http://www
.merriam-webster.com/dictionary/powerlessness

Miller, J. F. (Ed.). (1983). *Coping with chronic illness: Overcoming powerlessness.* Philadelphia, PA: F.A. Davis.

Miller, J. F. (Ed.). (1992). *Coping with chronic illness: Overcoming powerlessness* (2nd ed.). Philadelphia, PA: F. A. Davis.

Miller, J. F. (Ed.). (2000). *Coping with chronic illness: Overcoming powerlessness* (3rd ed.). Philadelphia, PA: F.A. Davis.

Miller, S. (2009). Cultural humility is the first step to becoming global care providers. *Journal of Obstetric, Gynecologic, & Neonatal Nursing, 38*(1), 92–93.

Miller, S. T., Marolen, K. N., & Beech, B. M. (2010). Perceptions of physical activity and motivational interviewing among rural African-American women with type 2 diabetes. *Women's Health Issues, 20*(1), 43–49.

Mishel, M. H. (2014). Theories of uncertainty in illness. In M. J. Smith & P. R. Liehr (Eds.), *Middle range theory for nursing* (3rd ed., pp. 53–86). New York, NY: Springer.

Moden, L. (2004). Power in care homes. *Nursing Older People, 16*(6), 24–26.

Mok, E., Martinson, I., & Wong, T. K. (2004). Individual empowerment among Chinese cancer patients in Hong Kong. *Western Journal of Nursing Research, 26*(1), 59–75.

Moller, A. C., Deci, E. L., & Ryan, R. M. (2006). Choice and ego-depletion: The moderating role of autonomy. *Personality and Social Psychology Bulletin, 32*(8), 1024–1036.

Morse, D. S., Schiff, M., Levit, S., Cohen-Moreno, R., Williams, G. C., & Neumark, Y. (2012). A pilot training program for a motivational enhancement approach to hepatitis C virus treatment among individuals in Israeli methadone treatment centers. *Substance Abuse and Misuse, 47*, 56–66.

Nagelkerk, J., Reick, K., & Meengs, L. (2006). Perceived barriers and effective strategies to diabetes self-management. *Journal of Advanced Nursing, 54*(2), 151–158.

National Cancer Institute. (2012). What are patient navigators? http://crchd.cancer.gov/pnp/what-are.html

National Center for Cultural Competency (2014). *Foundations of Cultural and Linguistic Competence.* http://ncc.georgetown.edu/foundations/index.html

National Center for Health Statistics. (2010). *Health United States 2010: With chartbook on trends in the health of Americans.* Hyattsville, MD: Author. http://www.cdc.gov/nchs/data/hus/hus10.pdf#056

Newman, S., Steed, L., & Mulligan, K. (2004). Self-management interventions for chronic illness. *Lancet, 364*(9444), 1523–1537.

Niven, C. A., & Scott, P.A. (2003). The need for accurate perception and informed judgment in determining the appropriate use of the nursing resource: Hearing the patient's voice. *Nursing Philosophy, 4*, 201–210.

Oosterveld-Vlug, M. G., Roeline, H., Pasman, W., van Gennip, I. E., Muller, M. T., Willems, D. L., & Onwuteaka-Philipsen, B. D. (2014). Dignity and the factors that influence it according to nursing home residents: A qualitative interview study. *Journal of Advanced Nursing, 70*(1), 97–106.

Pandey, S. K., Hart, J. J., & Tiwary, S. (2003). Women's health and Internet: Understanding emerging trends and implications. *Social Science and Medicine, 56*, 179–191.

Paterson, B. L. (2001). The shifting perspectives model of chronic illness. *Journal of Nursing Scholarship, 33*, 21–26.

Paterson, B. L. (2003). The koala has claws: Applications of the shifting perspectives model in research of chronic illness. *Qualitative Health Research, 13*(7), 987–994.

Phelan, J. C., Link, B. G., & Tehranifar, P. (2010). Social conditions as fundamental causes of health inequalities: Theory, evidence, and policy implications. *Journal of Health and Social Behavior, 51*(1 suppl), S28–S40.

Pihl-Lesnovska, K., Hjortswang, H., Ek, A. C., & Frisman, G. H. (2010). Patients' perspective of factors: Influencing quality of life while living with Crohn's disease. *Gastroenterology Nursing, 33*(1), 37–44.

Psooy, B. J., Schreuer, D., Borgaonkar, J., & Caines, J. S. (2004). Patient navigation: Improving timeliness in the diagnosis of breast abnormalities. *Canadian Association of Radiologists Journal, 55*(3), 145–150.

Rånhein, M., & Holand, W. (2006). Lived experience of chronic pain and fibromyalgia: Women's stories from daily life. *Qualitative Health Research, 16*(6), 741–761.

Rotter, J. P. (1966). Generalized expectancies for internal versus external control of reinforcement. *Psychological Monographs, 80*, 1–28.

Ryan, R. M., & Deci, E. L. (2000). Self-determination theory and the facilitation of intrinsic motivation, social development, and well-being. *American Psychologist, 55*(1), 68–78.

Ryan, R. M., Patrick, H., Deci, E. L., & Williams, G. C. (2008). Facilitating health behaviour change and its maintenance: Interventions based on self-determination theory. *European Health Psychologist, 10*, 2–5.

Shi, L., & Singh, D. A. (2011). *The nation's health* (8th ed.). Sudbury, MA: Jones and Bartlett.

Shi, L., & Stevens, G. D. (2010). *Vulnerable populations in the United States* (2nd ed.). San Francisco, CA: Jossey-Bass.

Skuladöttir, H., & Halldorsdóttir, S. (2008). Women in chronic pain: Sense of control and encounters with health professionals. *Qualitative Health Research*, *18*, 891–901.

Skuladóttir, H., & Halldorsdóttir, W. (2011). The quest for well-being: Self-identified needs of women in chronic pain. *Scandinavian Journal of Caring Science*, *25*(1), 81–91.

Strandmark, M. K. (2004). Ill health is powerlessness: A phenomenological study about worthlessness, limitations and suffering. *Scandinavian Journal of Caring Science*, *18*, 135–144.

Sutton, R., & Treloar, C. (2007). Chronic illness experiences, clinical markers and living with Hepatitis C. *Journal of Health Psychology*, *12*(2), 330–340.

Tang, S. T., & Lee, S. C. (2004). Cancer diagnosis and prognosis in Taiwan: Patient preferences versus experiences. *Psycho-oncology*, *13*, 1–13.

Thorne, S. (2006). Patient–provider communication in chronic illness: A health promotion window of opportunity. *Family and Community Health*, *29*(1S), 4S–11S.

Thorne, S., Paterson, B., & Russell, C. (2003). The structure of everyday self-care decision making in chronic illness. *Qualitative Health Research*, *13*(10), 1337–1352.

van Gennip, I. E., Pasman, H. R. W., Oosterveld-Vlug, M. G., Willems, D. L., & Onwuteaka-Philipsen, B. D. (2013). The development of a model of dignity in illness based on qualitative interviews with seriously ill patients. *International Journal of Nursing Studies*, *50*(8), 1080–1089.

Van Uden-Kraan, C. F., Drossaert, C. H. C., Taal, E., Seydel, D. R., & van de Laar, M. A. F. J. (2009). Participation in online patient support groups endorses patients' empowerment. *Patient Education and Counseling*, *74*, 61–69.

Walker, C. (2010). Ruptured identities: Leaving work because of chronic illness. *International Journal of Health Services*, *40*(4), 629–643.

Wilkinson, R., & Marmot, M. (2003). *Social determinants of health: The solid facts* (2nd ed.). Copenhagen, Denmark: World Health Organization. http://www.euro.who.int/__data/assets/pdf_file/0005/98438/e81384.pdf

World Health Organization (WHO). (2003). *Adherence to long-term therapies: Evidence for action.* Geneva, Switzerland: Author. http://www.who.int/chp/knowledge/publications/adherence_report/en/

Yu, D. S. F., Lee, D. T. F., Kwong, A. N. T., Thompson, D. R., & Woo, J. (2008). Living with chronic heart failure: A review of qualitative studies of older people. *Journal of Advanced Nursing*, *61*(5), 474–483.

Zickmund, S., Ho, E., Masuda, M., Ippolito, L., & LaBrecque, D. (2003). "They treated me like a leper": Stigmatization and the quality of life of patients with hepatitis C. *Journal of General Internal Medicine*, *18*, 835–844.

Chapter 13

Culture

Susan K. Rice

Introduction

Concepts of health and illness are deeply rooted in culture, race, and ethnicity and influence an individual's perceptions and behavior. Culture "encompasses a broader range of commonalities and differences between groups of people and communities than do the terms race or ethnicity" (Schim, Doorenbos, Benkert, & Miller, 2007, p. 104).

Defining Terms

A thorough literature search of multiple disciplines and professions fails to produce a consensus definition for the term *culture*. In fact, "a definition of culture reflects the priorities and interests of the professional group that creates it as much as it does some objective standard definition" (Bonder & Martin, 2013, p. 2). For nursing, whose development was based on a multidisciplinary foundation, the ability to define culture clearly is especially problematic.

Although clear definitions of culture and related terms have not emerged over time, some definitions of culture have stood the test of time and continue to be cited in current literature. Spector referenced the historic Fejos (1959) definition of culture: "the sum total of socially inherited characteristics of a human group that comprises everything which one generation can tell, convey, or hand down to the next; in other words, the nonphysically inherited traits we possess" (as cited in Spector, 2013, p. 21). Schim and others in 2007 cited the historic definitions of culture of Tylor (1871/1958) and Leininger (1991). Tylor defined culture as "that complex whole which includes knowledge, belief, arts, morals, law, custom, and many other capabilities and habits acquired by man as a member of society." Leininger (1991) defined culture as "the learned and transmitted values, beliefs, and practices that provided a critical means to establish culture care patterns from the people" (p. 36).

Table 13-1 offers examples of definitions of culture from nursing and related literature. These definitions, which expand the definition of culture beyond race and ethnicity, share commonalities of sharing or integration of learned values, beliefs, and norms in patterns of behaviors.

According to Spector (2013), "all facets of human behavior can be interpreted through the lens of culture, and everything can be related to and from this context" (p. 23). Culture has been identified as shared, learned, dynamic, and evolutionary (Schim et al., 2007). This evolution was described by Dreher and MacNaughton (2002): "People live out their lives in communities, where circumstances generate conflict, where people do not always follow the rules, and where cultural norms and institutions are massaged and modified in the exigencies of

Table 13-1 Culture

Author	Definition
Office of Minority Health, 2014	The thoughts, actions, customs, beliefs, values, and institutions of racial ethnic, religious, or social groups.
National Prevention Information Network, 2014	Integrated patterns of human behavior that include the language, thoughts, communications, actions, customs, beliefs, values, and institutions of racial, ethnic, religious, or social groups.
Giger, 2013	Patterned behavioral response that develops over time as a result of imprinting the mind through social and religious structures and intellectual and artistic manifestations.
Helman, 2007	A set of guidelines (both explicit and implicit) that individuals use to view the world and tell them which behaviors are appropriate.
Racher & Annis, 2007	Integrated lifestyle, the learned and shared beliefs, values, worldviews, knowledge, artifacts, rules, and symbols that guide behavior of a particular group of people.
Leininger, 1991 (as cited in Schim et al., 2007)	The learned and transmitted values, beliefs, and practices that provided a critical means to establish culture care patterns from the people.
Fejos, 1959 (as cited in Spector, 2013)	The sum total of socially inherited characteristics of a human group that comprises everything which one generation can tell, convey, or hand down to the next; in other words, the nonphysically inherited traits we possess.

daily life" (p. 184). It is within these communities that people learn from others in the culture and then share this learning with others through the generations. Within these communities, the environment provides a key to the culture learning that occurs for people in the culture. According to Spector (2013), people "learn from the environment how to see and interpret that they see" (p. 22). It is within this cultural group that shaping occurs based on shared values, beliefs, norms, and practices (Giger, 2013).

Myths of Culture and Diversity

There is documented confusion and discrepancies surrounding the use of the many terms related to culture. Given that confusion and discrepancies, it might seem as though there would be ample literature to support that there are myths common to culture and diversity. Although a growing body of literature has

focused on culture and diversity, a comprehensive review of nursing and related literature does not support the idea that myths common to culture and diversity exist. However, in 1996, Masi identified cultural myths and misconceptions, which could be barriers to developing cultural competence. Srivastava (2007) further described these myths and identified the need to examine and challenge such cultural myths as a way to develop cultural competence.

Although these myths are not commonly cited in the literature, the ideas contained within these myths will seem strikingly familiar to nurses in practice. These myths, as described here, can easily be extended beyond traditional cultural groups and are very relevant to subgroups. For nurses caring for people with chronic illness, the myths at times seem more like common knowledge that need to be countered often in the healthcare setting.

MYTH #1: THE MYTH OF EQUALITY

The myth of equality "refers to the view that fairness means equal treatment for all" (Srivastava, 2007, p. 42). This myth implies that equal treatment for all people is an acceptable goal in achieving culturally competent care. In providing care to all people, it is important to understand that *equality* in care does not mean the *same* care. *Equity*, not equality, "refers to equality with respect to opportunity, access, and outcome, and the notion of giving each person his or her due" (p. 43). In people with chronic illness, this myth is especially important so that people with chronic illness have an opportunity to maximize their successful outcomes. For people with chronic illness, it is essential for healthcare professionals to move beyond the myth of equality and to assure equity in opportunities and access to health care for all patients.

Case Example Madge, a 60-year-old nurse, has provided care to patients with chronic illness for more than 35 years and relates her frustrations with the myth of equality. In her practice, which consists of primarily low-income, inner-city elderly patients, there is a constant "battle" with the administration over access to care for her patients. Madge tells the story that the administration's answer to her questions about access is "All patients can have an equal opportunity to come to the clinic at open hours during the days Monday to Friday." According to Madge, "They do not get that my patients cannot get there during the day. Someone needs to hear that these patients need hours to meet their needs with their limited resources—like weekends, or after hours, or alternative sites. They are not like everyone else. They don't live in a 9-to-5, Monday-to-Friday world. We need to enter their world to be able to help them."

MYTH #2: THE MYTH OF SAMENESS

The assumption of this myth is based on the concept of ethnic matching, which matches people and healthcare professionals of the same ethnic background (Srivastava, 2007). The myth of sameness "suggests that clients receive the best care from health care providers of their own background" (p. 43). This myth follows from a narrow definition of culture focusing on race and ethnicity, rather than the broader concept of culture supported in this chapter. To extend this myth of sameness, the assumption is that a person who shares a chronic illness would be more effective in providing health care to a person with chronic illness. The myth of sameness is not consistent with the focus of care based on the individual needs and does not support optimal outcomes for the patient.

Case Example Tyra, a 35-year-old African American nurse in an acute care setting, conveyed her frustration over the myth of sameness. Tyra identifies herself as the "cultural expert" of her nursing unit and frequently is the nurse assigned to African American patients on her nursing unit. The charge nurse told Tyra that this assignment is made "because you understand what they are going through." Tyra laughs as she recounts being raised from birth by her adoptive Caucasian professional parents with three Caucasian siblings in an affluent suburb of a different state. Tyra adds, "I guess they just see me for the color of my skin and not for who I really am."

MYTH #3: CULTURAL DIFFERENCES ARE A PROBLEM

Traditionally there has been a negative view in health care of the issues of culture and diversity, with a focus on cultural differences and resulting problems (Srivastava, 2007, p. 45). Health care has often viewed culture as a barrier, resulting in a healthcare focus on limitations, with the outcome being avoidance behavior by patients. By embracing culture in health care, Srivastava suggests an alternative approach of focusing on cultural considerations as a way to improve the relevance and meaning for the person.

For people with chronic illnesses, the concept of embracing cultural differences could lead to a focus on improved patient outcomes rather than a focus on limitations based on differences for people with chronic illness.

Case Example   Jennifer, a 42-year-old family nurse practitioner, relates a learning experience about embracing differences as a way to focus on improved outcomes rather than on limitations. Jennifer recalls her first experience with children with disabilities, when she was working as a student volunteer with children with special needs in a local ice skating program. As a volunteer, Jennifer skated for months with a young child with autism and watched the child blossom on the ice and advance to a higher group later in skating. One day as a student, she met the same child in a clinic during her clinical student experiences. As Jennifer tells the story, "When I saw him in the clinic, I was shocked. I never thought of him as having limitations on the ice. I just saw him as a child who loved to skate and dreamed of riding on the Zamboni to clear the ice. I am so glad I saw him first outside the clinic because I did not focus on his limitations or differences. I only thought of him as Bill and what we could do to make him skate better."

MYTH #4: EVERYTHING MUST BE ACCEPTABLE

According to Srivastava, a cultural myth has existed that all cultural values must be accepted. Masi (1996) suggests that respecting an individual's cultural value not be confused with acceptance. For example, according to Masi, although society states that child abuse is unacceptable, the definition of child abuse may vary among individuals from different cultures. A practice known as "scratching the wind," where bruises are caused by cupping and scratches are created by running a coin on the skin, is used to relieve fevers and illness in some cultures. Respecting

this cultural value does not mean acceptance of this practice. However, the cultural context of the practice needs to be understood by the healthcare professional (Srivastava, 2007). Clearly, the standards of practice need to be followed closely to provide the optimal outcome for the person.

This myth can be extended for people with chronic illness. In providing health care to this population, the healthcare professional needs to respect the values and understand the cultural context of people with chronic illness, rather than focusing on the acceptance of all values.

MYTH #5: GENERALIZATIONS ARE UNACCEPTABLE

Another myth suggests that generalizations about a culture are unacceptable because they result in stereotyping individuals (Srivastava, 2007). In reality, generalizations are often a necessary starting point to understand groups of individuals because they may indicate trends and patterns. These generalizations may help a healthcare professional initiate a conversation with a patient. In contrast, stereotypes close down conversation and knowledge development (p. 47).

Healthcare professionals who are caring for patients with chronic illness need to understand the trends and patterns among people with chronic illness. By first understanding generalizations that apply to this group of people, the healthcare professional has a starting point in understanding the needs of the individual patient, ultimately resulting in improved care for the patient.

MYTH #6: FAMILIARITY EQUALS COMPETENCE

Cultural diversity is an issue now being addressed in health care through the increasing focus on cultural competence for healthcare professionals. Srivastava (2007) cautions that familiarity with diversity does not equal competence. In fact, "familiarity with difference paradoxically makes the difference invisible" (p. 48). Srivastava further identifies that cultural competence does not come from travel, but rather from increased knowledge and understanding based on the desire to learn about and from cultures (p. 48).

This myth can be extended to people with chronic illness. It is not sufficient for healthcare professionals to simply become familiar with people with chronic illness. Ultimately, the healthcare professional must have a desire to learn about and from people with chronic illness. It is only when the healthcare professional gains increased knowledge and understanding about and from people with chronic illness that the provider can provide competent care.

Case Example   James, a 51-year-old emergency department nurse, has worked in the same emergency department for more than 30 years and has spent most of that time as a charge nurse on the night shift. James readily shares stories about his experiences in his job. When asked about cultural diversity and its role in his job, James laughs and reports, "Yep. Cultural diversity is the buzzword, and the people way above me say we all have to have it. We all took the dog-and-pony show training about cultural diversity and how it is the focus here. But I sure don't see it in real life in practice. The big guys in charge say the right words and put the policies in place that meet the government regulations. But I see the reality. The reality is people are hurting and come in here for help. Time after time after time, we see the same people. We implement the same protocols for all people and send them out the door, and they come back. We need to listen to the patients and understand where they are coming from so we can really help them. We can't just say the right words. We have to do it with our actions."

Impact

Racial and Ethnicity Classification

Just as there are many definitions of culture and culturally related terms, so there are also many ways to define racial and ethnic classification. In 1997, the Office of Management and Budget (OMB) identified the following categories to be used by federal programs when reporting data: American Indian or Alaska Native; Asian; black or African American; Hispanic or Latino; Native Hawaiian or other Pacific Islander; and white. American Indian or Alaska Native refers to people of North and South America and those who maintain tribal affiliations (Wallman, 1998). Since that time, other categories have been identified by federal agencies for reporting data. According to the Office of Minority Health (2014), a division of the U.S. Department of Health and Human Services, the minority categories now include African Americans, American Indians/Alaska Natives, Asian Americans, Hispanic/Latinos, and Native Americans and Pacific Islanders. The Agency for Healthcare Research and Quality (AHRQ, 2013), also a division of the U.S. Department of Health and Human Services, identifies the categories of black, Asian, American Indian/Alaska Native, non-Hispanic white, and Hispanic white. In 2007, the Department of Education added the category of "two or more races" for the purpose of collecting and maintaining racial and ethnic data from students and staff, which has been in use since 2010.

For the purpose of recording data related to the population of the United States, race and ethnicity are markers that are monitored through the federal reports generated by the U.S. Census Bureau, a department of the U.S. Department of Commerce. For example, the U.S. Census Bureau collects data on race and ethnicity as a foundation for its U.S. Census report. **Table 13-2** describes the racial categories that were used in the 2010 U.S. Census.

Changing Demographics

The U.S. Census (2010a) reported that the United States had a population of 308.7 million people in 2010, with approximately 35% of this population defined as racial and ethnic

Table 13-2 DEFINITIONS OF RACE CATEGORIES USED IN THE 2010 U. S. CENSUS

Race Category	Definition
White	Refers to a person having origins in any of the original peoples of Europe, the Middle East, or North Africa.
Black or African American	Refers to a person having origins in any of the black racial groups of Africa.
American Indian or Alaska Native	Refers to a person having origins in any of the original peoples of North and South America (including Central America) and who maintains tribal affiliation or community attachment.
Asian	Refers to a person having origins in any of the original peoples of the Far East, Southeast Asia, or the Indian subcontinent, including, for example, Cambodia, China, India, Japan, Korea, Malaysia, Pakistan, the Philippine Islands, Thailand, and Vietnam.
Native Hawaiian or Other Pacific Islander	Refers to a person having origins in any of the original peoples of Hawaii, Guam, Samoa, or other Pacific Islands.
Some other race	Includes all other responses not included in the white, black or African American, American Indian or Alaska Native, Asian, and Native Hawaiian or other Pacific Islander race categories described above. Respondents reporting entries such as multiracial, mixed, interracial, or a Hispanic or Latino group (e.g., Mexican, Puerto Rican, Cuban, or Spanish) in response to the race question are included in this category.

Source: Reproduced from U.S. Census Bureau (2010a). Retrieved from http://quickfacts.census.gov/qfd/meta/long_RHI525211.htm.

minorities. Currently four states—Hawaii, New Mexico, California, and Texas—as well as the District of Columbia have minority populations that exceed 50% of their total population, with Texas being the newest addition to this small list of states. Although culture extends beyond race and ethnicity, race and ethnicity play a critical role in the consideration of provision of access to healthcare services in this country.

The North American healthcare system(s) is based on Western culture, including the dominant biomedical model. Given the increasingly diverse society, this narrow view continues to limit the ability of healthcare professionals to provide culturally competent care. This is especially true in light of the projected changing demographics of the U.S. population. As people age, the potential for having one or more chronic diseases increases significantly, so the need to look at the demographics of aging Americans is paramount. Of critical importance are the changing demographics related to race and ethnicity of the aging population.

For example, non-Latino older adults currently account for approximately 83.5% of the older adult U.S. population. Projections for 2050 indicate that this percentage will decrease significantly. Given these projections, a culturally competent workforce will be essential for assessing the complex needs and providing individualized care to meet the needs of individuals from many racial and ethnic groups. **Table 13-3** compares the current and projected distribution of the aging U.S. population for people of various races and Hispanic origin.

Table 13-3 Projected Distribution of the Population, Age 65 and Older, by Race and Hispanic Origin: 2010, 2030, and 2050

	2010	2030	2050
White	14.2	20.7	21.0
Non-Hispanic white	16.1	24.8	25.5
Black	8.6	15.2	18.5
American Indian and Alaska Native	7.4	14.5	16.8
Asian	9.3	16.5	21.9
Native Hawaiian and other Pacific Islander	6.5	13.2	17.9
Two or more races	5.1	7.2	7.8
Hispanic	5.7	10.0	13.2

Note: Data are middle-series projections of the population. Hispanics may be of any race. Reference population: These data refer to the resident population. These data refer to the resident population, U.S. Census Bureau 2008.
Source: Data from U.S. Census Bureau (2010b). Retrieved from http://www.census.gov/prod/2010pubs/p25-1138.pdf295.

Health Disparities

Although the focus of this chapter is culture and its influence on individuals with chronic illness, health disparities that occur with individuals from different cultures must be noted as well. Race, ethnicity, and culture sharply divide the health and health care of the population in the United States. Although such disparities have been noted for some time, the Institute of Medicine report titled *Unequal Treatment* (Smedley, Stith, & Nelson, 2003) was a landmark publication that put these disparities in the forefront. This report demonstrated that racial and ethnic disparities in health care, with a few exceptions, are consistent across a range of illnesses and healthcare services.

Currently in the United States, there are continuing disparities in health care among people of different cultures, races, ethnicities, and socioeconomic status (AHRQ, 2013). The National Healthcare Quality Report (NHQR) and the National Healthcare Disparities Report (NHDR), which are produced by AHRQ, report national data on the quality and disparities in health care in the United States. In the 2012 report, the combined summary of the NHQR and the NHDR identified three themes:

1. Healthcare quality and access are suboptimal, especially for minority and low-income groups.
2. Overall quality is improving, access is getting worse, and disparities are not changing.
3. Urgent attention is warranted to ensure continued improvements in the following areas:
   - Quality of diabetes care, maternal and child health care, and adverse events
   - Disparities in cancer care
   - Quality of care among states in the South

Another important national document that addresses health disparities is *Healthy People 2020*. This document has four overarching goals, two of which address health disparities:

- Achieve health equity, eliminate disparities, and improve the health of all groups
- Promote quality of life, healthy development, and healthy behaviors across all life stages

For healthcare professionals, there is a paramount need to incorporate appropriate strategies in all healthcare settings and to allocate resources in ways recognizing the patterns and lifeways of people of all cultures. Nurses are in a position, based on their educational preparation of viewing patients holistically, to rise to leadership positions in advocating for the cultural needs of their patients. These efforts to address racial, ethnic, and other disparities in health care require nurses to employ creative interventions to assure culturally competent care for these populations.

Interventions

Cultural Competence

Throughout the literature, becoming culturally competent is seen as the first step in decreasing and eventually eliminating documented health disparities. There are continuing efforts to document the status of healthcare disparities and the progress made at the local, state, national, and international levels. To address these ongoing disparities, there must also be increasing efforts at all levels to provide culturally competent care that addresses the individual needs of people of all cultures.

Defining Cultural Competence

The plethora of definitions of culture and related terms contribute to the multiplicity of definitions and descriptions of cultural competency. **Table 13-4** lists some of the more common definitions found in the literature.

Culture has been identified as "an individual concept, a group phenomenon, and an organizational reality" (Schim et al., 2007, p. 104). Although being culturally competent is important on an individual basis, becoming so as an organization is important as well. The National Center for Cultural Competence (NCCC, 2014) at Georgetown University has identified six reasons why organizations should incorporate cultural competence into policy:

1. To respond to the current and projected demographic changes in the United States
2. To eliminate long-standing disparities in the health status of people of diverse racial, ethnic, and cultural backgrounds

Table 13-4 Cultural Competency

Author	Definition
National Prevention Information Network, 2014	Integration and transformation of knowledge about individuals and groups of people into specific standards, policies, practices, and attitudes used in appropriate cultural settings to increase the quality of services, thereby producing better outcomes.
Office of Minority Health, 2014	Cultural and linguistic competency is a set of congruent behaviors, attitudes, and policies that come together in a system, in an agency, or among professionals that enables effective work in cross-cultural situations.
Spector, 2013	Provision of health care across cultural boundaries that takes into account the context in which the patient lives, as well as the situations in which the patient's health problems arise.
Andrews & Boyle, 2012	Services that are respectful and responsive to the cultural and linguistic needs of patients.
Campinha-Bacote, 2007	The ongoing process in which the healthcare professional continuously strives to achieve the ability and availability to work effectively within the cultural context of the patient (individual, family, and community).
Schim, Doorenbos, Benkert, & Miller, 2007	Specific cognitive, affective, and psychomotor skills that are necessary for the facilitation of cultural congruence between provider and patient.
Giger, 2013; Giger & Davidhizar, 2004	A dynamic, fluid, continuous process whereby an individual, system, or healthcare agency finds meaningful and useful care delivery strategies based on knowledge of the cultural heritage, beliefs, attitudes, and behaviors of those to whom they render care.

3. To improve the quality of services and health outcomes
4. To meet legislative, regulatory, and accreditation mandates
5. To gain a competitive edge in the market place
6. To decrease the likelihood of liability/malpractice claims (Cohen & Goode, 2003)

Cultural Awareness and Sensitivity

Throughout the literature, many terms are commonly used to describe the knowledge and behaviors necessary for addressing cultural diversity and resulting health disparities. The terms *cultural awareness* and *cultural sensitivity* are examples of two widely encountered terms in these areas. With the ongoing confusion about the definition of culture, it is not surprising that these culturally related terms also lack clear definitions. In fact, these terms are oftentimes confused with the term *cultural competence*.

Purnell (2008) explains cultural awareness as an appreciation of the external signs of culture, whereas cultural sensitivity is one's personal attitude toward others of different cultures (p. 6). According to Schim and colleagues (2007), cultural awareness deals with knowledge and cultural sensitivity deals with attitude. A basic understanding of the meaning and use of these terms is important to be able to differentiate these terms from cultural competence. So as to address the documented ongoing health disparities in the United States, policies and standards at all levels need to move beyond cultural awareness and cultural sensitivity. To be able to make an impact on these well-established health disparities, cultural competence needs to be the minimal standard and expectation at all levels.

Culturally and Linguistically Appropriate Standards

Cultural competence for systems and organizations may be seen as existing on a continuum (Racher & Annis, 2007; Srivastava, 2007). The Cultural Competence Continuum was developed by NCCC to capture this idea; it features six levels, spanning from cultural destructiveness at level 1 to cultural proficiency at level 6, the highest level. When an organization is culturally proficient, it holds culture in high esteem and uses this perspective to guide its work (Racher & Annis, 2007, p. 263).

On April 24, 2013, the U.S. Department of Health and Human Services' (DHHS) released 15 revised national standards for culturally and linguistically appropriate services (CLAS) as a means to address and correct inequities in the provision of health care to culturally and ethnically diverse groups (**Table 13-5**). These standards were organized by the themes: principal standard (Standard 1); governance, leadership, and workforce (Standards 2–4); communication and language assistance (Standards 5–8); and engagement, continuous improvement, and accountability (Standards 9–15).

Culturally Competent Care

Nurses have the ability to function in leadership roles at all levels as they embrace the challenges of moving the United States forward in addressing healthcare disparities so as to improve outcomes for their culturally diverse patients. To provide culturally competent care, it is essential to have theoretical frameworks and standards of practice guiding nursing practice; such underpinnings will maximize the outcomes for clients of all cultures. Many different nursing theoretical frameworks can be used as a foundation for providing culturally competent care. Also, nurses can incorporate the national CLAS standards and transcultural nursing standards into their care to improve patient outcomes.

NURSING THEORETICAL FRAMEWORKS

Currently, a variety of models, theories, and frameworks are available to assist nurses in providing appropriate care for diverse populations. The website of the Transcultural Nursing

Table 13-5 CLAS Standards

Principal Standard

Standard 1   Provide effective, equitable, understandable, and respectful quality care and services that are responsive to diverse cultural health beliefs and practices, preferred languages, health literacy, and other communication needs.

Governance, Leadership, and Workforce

Standard 2   Advance and sustain organizational governance and leadership that promotes CLAS and health equity through policy, practices, and allocated resources.

Standard 3   Recruit, promote, and support a culturally and linguistically diverse governance, leadership, and workforce that are responsive to the population in the service area.

Standard 4   Educate and train governance, leadership, and workforce in culturally and linguistically appropriate policies and practices on an ongoing basis.

Communication and Language Assistance

Standard 5   Offer language assistance to individuals who have limited English proficiency and/or other communication needs, at no cost to them, to facilitate timely access to all health care and services.

Standard 6   Inform all individuals of the availability of language assistance services clearly and in their preferred language, verbally and in writing.

Standard 7   Ensure the competence of individuals providing language assistance, recognizing that the use of untrained individuals and/or minors as interpreters should be avoided.

Standard 8   Provide easy-to-understand print and multimedia materials and signage in the languages commonly used by the populations in the service area.

Engagement, Continuous Improvement, and Accountability

Standard 9   Establish culturally and linguistically appropriate goals, policies, and management accountability, and infuse them throughout the organization's planning and operations.

Standard 10   Conduct ongoing assessments of the organization's CLAS-related activities and integrate CLAS-related measures into assessment measurement and continuous quality improvement activities.

Standard 11   Collect and maintain accurate and reliable demographic data to monitor and evaluate the impact of CLAS on health equity and outcomes and to inform service delivery.

Standard 12   Conduct regular assessments of community health assets and needs, and use the results to plan and implement services that respond to the cultural and linguistic diversity of populations in the service area.

Standard 13   Partner with the community to design, implement, and evaluate policies, practices, and services to ensure cultural and linguistic appropriateness.

Standard 14   Create conflict- and grievance-resolution processes that are culturally and linguistically appropriate to identify, prevent, and resolve conflicts or complaints.

Standard 15   Communicate the organization's progress in implementing and sustaining CLAS to all stakeholders, constituents, and the general public.

Source: Data from Office of Minority Health. (2014). National standards for culturally and linguistically appropriate services in health and health care: A blueprint for advancing and sustaining CLAS policy and practice. Retrieved from http://minorityhealth.hhs.gov/templates/browse.aspx?lvl=2&lvlID=15

Society (www.tcns.org) provides information about six transcultural nursing theories and models. Models include those developed by Margaret Andrews and Joyceen Boyle; Josepha Campinha-Bacote; Joyce Giger and Ruth Davidhizar; Madeline Leininger; Larry Purnell; Rachel Spector; Marianne Jeffreys; and Marilyn Ray. Three of these models are described here, with the primary focus being on Leininger's cultural care diversity and universality theory.

Giger-Davidhizar Transcultural Assessment Model The Giger-Davidhizar model was developed initially in 1991, with a metaparadigm that included five concepts: (1) transcultural nursing and culturally diverse nursing, (2) culturally competent care, (3) culturally unique individuals, (4) culturally sensitive environments, and (5) health and health status based on culturally specific illness and wellness behaviors (Giger, 2013, p. 5).

This model is built upon concentric concepts, with the client—a unique cultural being—positioned in the center. The next circle contains concepts of religion, culture, and ethnicity. The outermost circle includes six cultural concepts: (1) communication, (2) space, (3) social organization, (4) time, (5) environmental control, and (6) biological variation (Giger & Davidhizar, 2004; Giger, 2013). Communication refers to all human interaction and behavior, both verbal and nonverbal. Space refers to the distance between individuals when they interact, communicate, or reside together. Time can be past, present, or future oriented. How individuals view this concept is often uncovered through their style of communication. Individuals who focus on the past attempt to maintain tradition, whereas those focused on the present do not formulate goals. Environmental control refers to the ability of the individual to control nature and to plan and direct factors in the environment that affect them. If persons come from cultural groups where there is external control, they may adopt a fatalistic view, ultimately resulting in the belief that seeking health care is useless. Biological differences, especially genetic variations, exist between individuals. These biological differences among various racial groups are often less well understood (Giger & Davidhizar, 2004).

Purnell Model for Cultural Competence Purnell's model for cultural competence is graphically represented in a model that includes both the macro and micro concepts. The metaparadigm concepts of this model include (1) global society, (2) community, (3) family, (4) person, and (5) conscious competence (Cultural Competence Project, 2014).

This model is graphically depicted as four concentric circles, each representing a macro concept. The outer circle represents global society. The second circle is the community and is defined as a group of people who have common interests, but do not necessarily live in the same geographic area. It is the physical, social, and symbolic characteristics of the community that enable its members to feel connected, rather than a common geography (Purnell, 2008, p. 21). The third circle represents the family, which is made up of two or more individuals who are emotionally connected, and who may or may not live together. The fourth circle represents the person, who is continually adapting to his or her community (Cultural Competence Project, 2014).

The Purnell model's organizing framework comprises 12 micro concepts, or domains, that are interconnected and common to all cultures, and that have implications for health and health care. To assess the ethnocultural attributes of the community, family, or person, each of the following domains needs to be addressed: (1) overview and heritage; (2) communication; (3) family roles and organization; (4) workforce issues; (5) biocultural ecology; (6) high-risk behaviors; (7) nutrition; (8) pregnancy and childbearing practices; (9) death rituals; (10) spirituality; (11) healthcare practices; and (12) healthcare practitioners (Cultural Competence

Project, 2014). Since the domains are all inter-connected in Purnell's model for cultural competence, no single domain stands alone.

Transcultural Nursing   Transcultural nursing had its beginnings in the 1950s with Madeleine Leininger. Through her work over more than 50 years, as well as the efforts of other theorists, transcultural nursing has evolved as a specific and unique specialty. Transcultural nursing is defined as "a formal area of study and practice focused on comparative human-care (caring) differences and similarities of the beliefs, values and patterned lifeways of cultures to provide culturally congruent, meaningful, and beneficial health care to people" (Leininger & McFarland, 2002, p. 6).

Leininger and McFarland (2002) summarized eight factors that led to the development of and need for transcultural nursing:

1. Increase in immigration and migration of people across the world
2. Implicit expectation that nurses and other healthcare providers need to know, understand, respect, and respond appropriately to care for others of diverse cultures
3. Increase in the use of technologies in caring or curing, with different responses and effects on clients of diverse cultures
4. Increased signs of cultural conflicts, cultural clashes, and cultural imposition practices between nurses and those from diverse cultures
5. Increase in the number of nurses who travel and work in different places in the world
6. Anticipated legal defense suits against nurses resulting from cultural negligence, cultural ignorance, and cultural imposition practices in working with diverse cultures
7. Rise in gender and the issues and rights of special groups
8. Growing trend to care with and for people, whether well or ill, in their familiar or particular living and working environments (Leininger & McFarland, 2002, pp. 13–18)

The factors that led to the development of transcultural nursing continue to be the factors still present today as continued reminders that there is a critical need for preparing transcultural nurses to provide culturally competent care to culturally diverse populations.

The Transcultural Nursing Society (TCNS), founded in 1974 by Leininger, is a worldwide organization for nurses and others interested in and prepared to advance transcultural nursing. The mission of TCNS is "to enhance the quality of culturally congruent, competent, and equitable care that results in improved health and well-being for people worldwide" (www.tcns.org). The society provides a forum to bring nurses together worldwide with common and diverse interests to improve the care for culturally diverse people. The goals of the society include the following:

- To advance cultural competencies for nurses worldwide
- To advance the scholarship (substantive knowledge) of the discipline
- To develop strategies for advocating social change for cultural competent care
- To promote a sound financial nonprofit corporation (www.tcns.org)

Cultural values, beliefs, and practices impact health and illness and inform and guide the client and the client's family in the choices and patterns of health care. Care is universal; however, patterns of care vary among and between cultural groups regarding healthcare beliefs and behaviors (Leininger, 2002; Leininger & McFarland, 2002, 2006). Leininger's culture care diversity and universality theory provides a theoretical framework for healthcare professionals to discover the differences and similarities between and among cultural groups related to their cultural values, beliefs, and practices. The meanings and uses of these diversities and universalities among the cultures of the world need to be uncovered and understood (Leininger & McFarland, 2002, p. 78).

The social structure of the client and his or her family—such as their characteristics vis-à-vis economics, religion, and worldview—influence cultural care meanings, expressions, and patterns in different cultures (Leininger & McFarland, 2002, p. 78). Embedded within these structures are generic (folk) care practices, which are separate and distinct from professional care practices (Leininger, 1997; Leininger & McFarland, 2002). This theoretical tenet is particularly instructive for healthcare professionals. For example, an individual with chronic pain may rely on the home remedies taught by an elder in the family or use a variety of herbs and compounds that have been obtained from a traditional healer to manage pain. The healthcare professional must be vigilant in the belief and use of generic care practices, and incorporate those into the plan of care. The last theoretical tenet of Leininger's theory provides three modes of nursing decisions and actions for culturally congruent care: (1) culture care preservation and maintenance, (2) culture care accommodation and/or negotiation, and (3) culture care restructuring and/or repatterning (Leininger, 2002; Leininger & McFarland, 2002, 2006).

For example, Mrs. Huerta has degenerative arthritis. Her mother was a traditional healer in the village where she grew up. As a young child, Mrs. Huerta learned the healing ways and practices from her mother. Now, as an elderly woman, she continues to use these traditional methods to manage her chronic pain. When Mrs. Huerta was admitted to the acute care setting, she brought with her remedies, which have brought her comfort and relief in the past. Leininger's three modes of nursing decisions and action are informative and directive for the nurse to provide culturally competent care to Mrs. Huerta: (1) The nurse can incorporate these home remedies into the care within the acute setting; (2) the nurse can talk with Mrs. Huerta; or (3) in the event the home remedies Mrs. Huerta is taking are known to be unsafe or contraindicated with her present care regimen, the nurse can explore alternative comfort and pain relief strategies with Mrs. Huerta. In this way, the client's cultural care values, beliefs, and practices are honored and maintained. Therefore, Leininger advocates that healthcare professionals develop cultural holding knowledge so that they can provide culturally competent care; such knowledge will also enable them to minimize the potential for culturally inappropriate care that has the potential for harm and pain to the healthcare client and his or her family.

STANDARDS FOR CULTURAL COMPETENCE IN NURSING PRACTICE

A task force of the Expert Panel for Global Nursing and Health of the American Academy of Nursing, along with members of the Transcultural Nursing Society, has developed a set of standards for cultural competence in nursing practice (**Table 13-6**). The aim of this project was to define standards that can be universally applied by nurses around the world in the areas of clinical practice, research, education, and administration, especially by nurses involved in direct patient care.

Key to Culturally Competent Care: Communication

Communication is the crux of cultural care. It is important for nurses to be aware of appropriate body stance and proximities, gestures, languages, listening styles, and eye contact when communicating with clients, as different cultural groups—nearly 3,000 worldwide—vary widely in their ideas regarding these aspects of communication (Narayanasamy, 2003). Differences in language between the client and the healthcare professional may impede detection of health needs, treatment, and patient care. For nursing interventions to be effective,

Table 13-6 STANDARDS OF PRACTICE FOR CULTURALLY COMPETENT CARE

Standard	Description
Standard 1. Social Justice	Professional nurses shall promote social justice for all. The applied principles of social justice guide nurses' decisions related to the patient, family, community, and other healthcare professionals. Nurses will develop leadership skills to advocate for socially just policies.
Standard 2. Critical Reflection	Nurses shall engage in critical reflection of their own values, beliefs, and cultural heritage to have an awareness of how these qualities and issues can affect culturally congruent nursing care.
Standard 3. Knowledge of Cultures	Nurses shall gain an understanding of the perspectives, traditions, values, practices, and family systems of culturally diverse individuals, families, communities, and populations they care for, as well as a knowledge of the complex variables that affect the achievement of health and well-being.
Standard 4. Culturally Competent Practice	Nurses shall use cross-cultural sensitive skills in implementing culturally congruent nursing care.
Standard 5. Cultural Competence in Healthcare Systems and Organizations	Healthcare organizations should provide the structure and resources necessary to evaluate and meet the cultural and language needs of their diverse clients.
Standard 6. Patient Advocacy and Empowerment	Nurses shall recognize the effect of health care policies, delivery systems, and resources on their populations and shall empower and advocate for their patients as indicated. Nurses shall advocate for the inclusion of their patients' cultural beliefs and practices in all dimensions of their health care.
Standard 7. Multicultural Workforce	Nurses shall actively engage in the effort to ensure a multicultural workforce in healthcare settings. One measure to achieve a multicultural workforce is through strengthening of recruitment and retention efforts in the hospital and academic settings.
Standard 8. Education and Training in Culturally Competent Care	Nurses shall be educationally prepared to promote and provide culturally congruent health care. Knowledge and skills necessary for assuring that nursing care is culturally congruent shall be included in global healthcare agendas that mandate formal education and clinical training, as well as required as ongoing, continuing education for all practicing nurses.
Standard 9. Cross-Cultural Communication	Nurses shall use culturally competent verbal and nonverbal communication skills to identify clients' values, beliefs, practices, perceptions, and unique healthcare needs.
Standard 10. Cross-Cultural Leadership	Nurses shall have the ability to influence individuals, groups, and systems to achieve outcomes of culturally competent care for diverse populations.

(Continues)

Table 13-6 TANDARDS OF PRACTICE FOR CULTURALLY COMPETENT CARE (CONTINUED)

Standard	Description
Standard 11. Policy Development	Nurses shall have the knowledge and skills to work with public and private organizations, professional associations, and communities to establish policies and standards for comprehensive implementation and evaluation of culturally competent care.
Standard 12. Evidence-Based Practice and Research	Nurses shall base their practice on interventions that have been systematically tested and shown to be the most effective for the culturally diverse populations whom they serve. In areas where there is a lack of evidence of efficacy, nurse researchers shall investigate and test interventions that may be the most effective in reducing the disparities in health outcomes.

Source: Douglas, M. K., et al. (2011). Standards of Practice for Culturally Competent Nursing Care: 2011 Update, *Journal of Transcultural Nursing 22*(4), p. 318, copyright © 2011 by SAGE Publications. Reprinted by Permission of Sage Publications.

it is imperative that nurses give attention to all aspects of the client's care as well as the communication process involving them.

Giger and Davidhizar (2004) have developed guidelines for communication, which are provided in **Table 13-7**. Although these are general guidelines, they provide a basis or a starting point. Although all of the guidelines are important, perhaps the most important one is to assess your own personal beliefs about persons from different cultures. It is difficult to understand others' beliefs if you do not have an awareness of your own, and how they may influence your attitudes toward others.

Communication can be difficult between cultures because of misunderstandings, inability to speak a language, or the use of technical terminology. Each culture has patterns for word choice, inflection, gestures and facial expressions, eye movement and eye contact, volume and speed of speech, use of silence, directness, and the degree of emotion. Nonverbal cues also affect communication. The amount of personal space, social space, and public space often differ between cultures, and one should always note another person's comfort zone.

Assessment: The First Step of the Nursing Process

As the initial step in the nursing process, it is critical that healthcare professionals understand certain cultural behaviors related to their physical assessment. Simple things like eye contact and touch can affect an individual's response to the healthcare professional and determine what can and cannot be done regarding the individual's health care. Giger (2013) has identified some basic cultural variations that may be seen in health assessment (**Table 13-8**). Again, as with all cultures, there is uniqueness in each individual, and these behaviors should be seen as general guidelines only.

Providing Culturally Congruent Care

In a classic 2007 article on culturally congruent care, Schim and colleagues apply the puzzle metaphor to four cultural care terms and see the finished puzzle with four constructs (p. 105). These constructs include cultural diversity, cultural awareness, cultural sensitivity, and cultural competence.

1. Cultural diversity: varies in quality and quantity across place and time; is dynamic, ever changing.

Table 13-7 GUIDELINES FOR RELATING TO PATIENTS FROM DIFFERENT CULTURES

1. Assess your personal beliefs surrounding persons from different cultures.
   - Review your personal beliefs and past experiences.
   - Set aside any values, biases, ideas, and attitudes that are judgmental and may negatively affect care.
2. Assess communication variables from a cultural perspective.
   - Determine the ethnic identity of the patient, including generations in the United States.
   - Use the patient as a source of information when possible.
   - Assess cultural factors that may affect your relationship with the patient and respond appropriately.
3. Plan care according to the communicated needs and cultural background.
   - Learn as much as possible about the patient's cultural customs and beliefs.
   - Encourage the patient to reveal cultural interpretation of health, illness, and health care.
   - Be sensitive to the uniqueness of the patient.
   - Identify sources of discrepancy between the patient's and your own concepts of health and illness.
   - Communicate at the patient's personal level of functioning.
   - Evaluate effectiveness of nursing actions and modify nursing care plan when necessary.
4. Modify communication approaches to meet cultural needs.
   - Be attentive to signs of fear, anxiety, and confusion in the patient.
   - Respond in a reassuring manner in keeping with the patient's cultural orientation.
   - Be aware that in some cultural groups, discussion with others concerning the patient may be offensive and impede the nursing process.
5. Understand that respect for the patient and communicated needs are central to the therapeutic relationship.
   - Communicate respect by using a kind and attentive approach.
   - Learn how listening is communicated in the patient's culture.
   - Use appropriate active listening techniques.
   - Adopt an attitude of flexibility, respect, and interest to help bridge barriers imposed by culture.
6. Communicate in a nonthreatening manner.
   - Conduct the interview in an unhurried manner.
   - Follow acceptable social and cultural amenities.
   - Ask general questions during the information-gathering stage.
   - Be patient with a respondent who gives information that may seem unrelated to the health problem at hand.
   - Develop a trusting relationship by listening carefully, allowing time, and giving the patient your full attention.
7. Use validating techniques in communication. Be alert for feedback that the patient is not understanding.
   - Do not assume meaning is interpreted without distortion.
8. Be considerate of reluctance to talk when the subject involves sexual matters.
   - Be aware that in some cultures sexual matters are not discussed freely with members of the opposite sex.
9. Adopt special approaches when the patient speaks a different language.
   - Use a caring tone of voice and facial expression to help alleviate the patient's fears.
   - Speak slowly and distinctly, but not loudly.
   - Use gestures, pictures, and play acting to help the patient understand.
   - Repeat the message in different ways if necessary.
   - Be alert to words the patient seems to understand and use them frequently.
   - Keep messages simple and repeat them frequently.
   - Avoid using medical terms and abbreviations that the patient may not understand.
   - Use an appropriate language dictionary.
10. Use interpreters to improve communication.
   - Ask the interpreter to translate the message, not just the individual words.
   - Obtain feedback to confirm understanding.
   - Use an interpreter who is culturally sensitive.

Source: This material was published in *Transcultural nursing: Assessment and intervention,* 6th ed., Giger, J., p. 13, Copyright Mosby 2013.

Table 13-8 Behaviors Related to Health Assessment

Cultural Group	Belief/Practice	Nursing Implication
African Americans	Dialect and slang terms require careful communication to prevent error.	Question the client's meaning.
Mexican Americans	Eye behavior is important. An individual who looks at and admires a child without touching the child has given the child the "evil eye."	Always touch the child you are examining.
American Indians	Eye contact is considered a sign of disrespect.	Recognize that the client may be attentive and interested even though eye contact is avoided.
Appalachians	Eye contact is considered impolite or a sign of hostility. Verbal pattern may be confusing.	Avoid excessive eye contact.
American Eskimos	Body language is very important. Individual seldom disagrees publicly with others. May nod yes to be polite, even if not in agreement.	Monitor own body language.
Jewish Americans	Orthodox Jews consider excess touching offensive, particularly from members of the opposite sex.	Establish whether client is an Orthodox Jew and avoid excessive touch.
Chinese Americans	Individual may nod head to indicate yes or shake head to indicate no. Excessive eye contact indicates rudeness. Excessive touch is offensive.	Ask questions carefully and clarify responses. Avoid excessive eye contact and touch.
Filipino Americans	Offending people is to be avoided at all cost; nonverbal behavior is very important.	Monitor nonverbal behaviors.
Haitian Americans	Touch is used in conversation. Direct eye contact is used to gain attention and respect.	Use direct eye contact when communicating.
East Indian Hindu Americans	Women avoid eye contact as a sign of respect.	Be aware that men may view eye contact by women as offensive. Avoid eye contact.
Vietnamese Americans	Avoidance of eye contact is a sign of respect. The head is considered sacred; it is not polite to pat the head. An upturned palm is offensive in communication.	Limit eye contact. Touch the head only when mandated and explain clearly before proceeding to do so. Avoid hand gesturing.

Source: This material was published in *Transcultural nursing: Assessment and intervention,* 6th ed., Giger, J., p. 13, Copyright Mosby 2013.

2. Cultural awareness: cognitive construct; a reality to be contemplated and a corresponding capacity for processing knowledge.
3. Cultural sensitivity: affective or attitudinal construct; attitude about their own person and others.
4. Cultural competence: behavioral construct; the action that is taken in response to diversity, awareness, and sensitivity.

Schim and colleagues suggest that there is one piece missing from their puzzle model—namely, the client, whether that entity is an individual, a family, or a community. The client "layer" of the puzzle, although essential, is not visualized in the current model (p. 106). This missing piece, the person, expands cultural competence to cultural congruence.

Leininger was the first to use the term *culturally congruent care*, and Schim and colleagues' model builds on Leininger's work and definition. Culturally congruent care is defined by Leininger as follows:

> *Those cognitively based assistive, supportive, facilitative, or enabling acts or decisions that are tailor made to fit with individual, group, or institution cultural values, beliefs, and lifeways in order to provide or support meaningful beneficial and satisfying health care or wellbeing services. (Leininger, 1991, p. 49)*

As the United States continues to identify and document the health disparities that are present for culturally diverse populations, including people with chronic illnesses, it is essential for the focus of the country to move beyond identification and documentation. Nurses are in a position to push for improved outcomes for their patients by advocating for all patients to be at the center of plans of care at all levels. Only when the patient is the focus will care be moved to the level of culturally congruent care, resulting in improved outcomes for the patient.

Evidence-Based Practice Box

A vast literature points to the increasing number of individuals with type 2 diabetes in the United States. There is a documented greater incidence of type 2 diabetes among people with racial/ethnic minority backgrounds than among people of non-Hispanic white backgrounds. People with uncontrolled blood glucose levels are at risk for associated health problems, including increased levels of blood pressure, weight, and stress. For these at-risk populations, health disparities have been well documented. The study described here is one such example.

Study Measures: Patient Demographic and Medical Information Questionnaire (Patient DMIQ), Adherence to Treatment Measure (DMT), and Strain Questionnaire (SQ).

Study Theory: Health self-empowerment theory. This theory asserts that "to engage in health promoting behaviors or a health promoting lifestyle, one must have related self-motivation, self-efficacy, and self-responsibility and knowledge, use self-praise of efforts and achievement of the target/behaviors/lifestyle, and use coping skills for managing stress and depression" (p. 304).

Participants: There were 120 participants in this study, including 70% African Americans and 22.3% Hispanic/Latinos. The study participants were divided between an intervention group and a wait-list control group.

Significant Findings: The post-test program participants of the intervention group were found to have decreased levels of body mass index (BMI), diastolic blood pressure, and physical stress.

Nursing Implications: The findings of this study support the need for culturally sensitive, empowerment-focused, community-based health programs for adults with type 2 diabetes. The study also supports the need for additional research in this area.

Source: Tucker, C. M., Lopez, M., Campbell, K., Marsiske, M., Daly, K., Nghiem, K., Marsiske,….. Patel, A. (2014). The effects of a culturally sensitive, empowerment-focused, community-based health promotion program on health outcomes of adults with type 2 diabetes. *Journal of Health Care for the Poor & Underserved., 25*(1), 292–307.

CASE STUDY 13-1: MIDDLE EASTERN CULTURE

K.T., an 82-year-old female patient of Middle Eastern descent, was admitted to the surgical intensive care unit (SICU) during the previous shift. K.T. was transferred to the unit from the emergency department, where staff began treatment for a severe exacerbation of her chronic condition, congestive heart failure. You arrive for your shift and are the charge nurse for the day. At the door to the unit you are greeted by Mary, K.T.'s nurse, who demands that you "deal with the family." Mary tells her story about the previous shift, where the family did not seem to care about the very structured rules of the SICU. According to Mary, "We can't get them to listen and they won't follow the rules. Rules are rules, but they don't seem to get that. They are demanding and telling us how to do our job. We can't get them to leave and they are interfering with us doing our job. You have to deal with them because we all have tried and gave up. And by the way, K.T. is stable and we did ..." (leading into the rest of the report on the health status of K.T.).

Discussion Questions

1. As the charge nurse, where do you begin with dealing with this situation? What is your first step in the process? (Hint: What are the steps of the nursing process?)
2. Who is your priority at this time? (Hint: Who or what is the central focus of culturally congruent care?)
3. How does the Middle Eastern culture affect this scenario?
4. How does a family with a member with chronic illness affect this scenario?
5. How could this situation have been handled in a different way to avoid the situation escalating to this level?

CASE STUDY 13-2: AMISH CULTURE

A.Y., an 8-year-old Amish boy, has recently been transferred as a patient to the rehabilitation unit where you are a nurse on the evening shift. You have been a nurse on this unit for 10 years and have a familiarity with the Amish culture, given the large number of Amish people living in the region of the hospital. A.Y. was struck by a car one evening, while riding in an unlit family buggy on one of the narrow country roads. A.Y. experienced multiple trauma and has been hospitalized for two months. You are assigned for the first time to A.Y. and are receiving report from the previous nurse, Mike, who has worked on this unit for less than a year. Mike starts his report: "Well, you may not have had A.Y., but you have seen it before and here it is again: a buggy without lights, and the poor car doesn't see the buggy and hits the buggy. I don't understand it, do you? They can't drive cars, but A.Y.'s family rides here every day in a car. They can't have lights on the buggy, but A.Y. can be in a hospital with lights. It would sure help if they did what was best for the children.

(continues)

CASE STUDY 13-2: AMISH CULTURE (Continued)

It is really tough to keep seeing these poor kids coming in time and time again with these traumas. You have been here a lot longer than I have. What can we do to help these kids? I just want the kids to be safer."

Discussion Questions

1. How do you respond to Mike's question, "What can we do to help these kids?"
2. Review the beliefs of the Amish culture, especially related to their beliefs about electricity and transportation.
3. Who is your priority at this time? (Hint: Who or what is the central focus of culturally congruent care?)
4. How do you work with Mike and the other nurses on the unit to deal with this ongoing issue?
5. What role does culture play in this ongoing situation?
6. How will culture affect this child's rehabilitation plan and discharge plan?

STUDY QUESTIONS

1. Identify one historical definition and one current definition of culture. Compare and contrast the two definitions of culture.
2. Review the six myths of culture and diversity. Identify one clinical example that is relevant to each of the six myths.
3. Identify one cultural group as defined by the U.S. Census Bureau. Review the literature and identify five health concerns for this cultural group. For one health concern, find three current journal articles that discuss this health concern for this cultural group.
4. Review the National CLAS Standards and the themes for the standards. Describe how the primary standard is related to the other standards.
5. Compare and contrast the terms *culture*, *cultural sensitivity*, *cultural awareness*, and *cultural competence*. How does culturally congruent care relate to these terms?
6. Describe the role of culture for individuals, family, and community.
7. Identify and describe one theorist with a transcultural nursing theory. Describe the parts of the model of this theory. How can this model be applied to nursing practice in a clinical setting?
8. Review the Standards for Culturally Competent Care. How are these standards similar to the National CLAS Standards? How are they different?

Internet Resources

Association of Asian Pacific Community Health Organizations (AAPCHO): http://www.aapcho.org

Centers for Disease Control and Prevention: http://www.cdc.gov

Centers for Disease Control and Prevention, National Center for Health Statistics: http://www.cdc.gov/nchs/

Centers for Disease Control and Prevention, National Prevention Information Network (NPIN): http://www.cdcnpin.org

Cultural Competence Project: http://www.ojccnh.org/project/index.shtml

Culture, Health and Literacy: http://www.healthliteracy.worlded.org/docs/culture/materials/websites_009.html

Diversity Rx, Improving Health Care for a Diverse World: http://www.diversityrx.org

EthnoMed, Integrating Cultural Information into Clinical Practice: http://www.ethnomed.org

Georgetown University Center for Child and Human Development, National Center for Cultural Competence: http://www11.georgetown.edu/research/gucchd/nccc

Cultural Competence Project: http://www.ojccnh.org/project/index.shtml

Diversity Data: http://diversitydata.sph.harvard.edu/

Hablamos Juntos, Language Policy and Practice in Health Care: http://www.hablamosjuntos.org/signage/symbols/default.symbols.asp

Healthcare Communities: http://www.healthcarecommunities.org/

International Multicultural Institute (iMCI): http://www.nmci.org

National Institute on Minority Health and Health Disparities: http://www.nimhd.nih.gov

National Institutes of Health: http://www.nih.gov

Office of Minority Health: http://www.minorityhealth.hhs.gov

Office of Minority Health, National Culturally and Linguistically Appropriate Services (CLAS) Standards in Health and Health Care: http://www.minorityhealth.hhs.gov/templates/browse.aspx?lvl=2&lvlID=15

Provider's Guide to Quality and Culture: http://erc.msh.org/mainpage.cfm?file=1.0.htm&module=provider&language=English

Transcultural Nursing Society: http://www.tcns.org

University of North Carolina at Chapel Hill, Minority Health Project to Eliminate Health Disparities: http://www.minority.unc.edu

U.S. Census Bureau: http://www.census.gov

U.S. Department of Health and Human Services: http://www.hhs.gov

References

Agency for Healthcare Research and Quality (AHRQ). (2013). *National healthcare disparities report 2012* (AHRQ Pub. No. 13-0002). Rockville, MD: U.S. Department of Health and Human Services.

Andrews, M. M., & Boyle, J. S. (2012). *Transcultural concepts in nursing care* (6th ed.). Philadelphia, PA: Wolters Kluwer/Lippincott, Williams, & Wilkins.

Bonder, B., & Martin, L. (2013). *Culture in clinical care: Strategies for competence* (2nd ed.). Thorofare, NJ: Slack.

Campinha-Bacote, J. (2007). Delivering patient-centered care in the midst of a cultural conflict: The role of cultural competence. *Online Journal of Issues in Nursing, 16*(2), 1. doi: 10.3912/OJIN.Vol16No02Man05

Cohen, E., Goode, T., & Dunne, C. (2003). *Policy brief 1: The rationale for cultural competence*. Washington, DC: National Center for Cultural Competence, Georgetown University Center for Child and Human Center.

Cultural Competence Project. (2014). Theories and models. http://www.ojccnh.org/project/theories-models.shtml

Department of Education. (2007). Final guidance on maintaining, collecting, and reporting racial and ethnic data to the U.S. Department of Education. http://www2.ed.gov/legislation/FedRegister/other/20074/101907c.html

Douglas, M. K., Pierce, J. U., Rosenkoetter, M., Pacquiao, D., Callister, L.C., Hattar-Pollara, M., … Purnell, L. (2011). Standards of practice for culturally competent nursing care: 2011 update. *Journal of Transcultural Nursing, 22*(4), 317–333.

Dreher, M., & MacNaughton, N. (2002). Cultural competence in nursing: Foundation or fallacy? *Nursing Outlook, 50*, 181–186.

Giger, J. (2013). *Transcultural nursing: Assessment and intervention* (6th ed.) St. Louis. MO: Elsevier.

Giger, J., & Davidhizar, R. (Eds.). (2004). *Transcultural nursing: Assessment and intervention* (4th ed.). St. Louis, MO: Mosby.

Healthy people 2020. (2014). http://www.healthypeople.gov/2020/default.aspx

Helman, C. G. (2007) *Culture, health and illness* (5th ed.). London, UK: Hodder Arnold.

Leininger, M. (Ed.). (1991). *Culture care diversity and universality: A theory of nursing.* New York, NY: National League of Nursing.

Leininger, M. (1997). Overview of the theory of culture care with the ethnonursing research method. *Journal of Transcultural Nursing, 8*(2), 32–53.

Leininger, M. (2002). Culture care theory: A major contribution to advance transcultural nursing knowledge and practices. *Journal of Transcultural Nursing, 13,* 189–192.

Leininger, M. M., & McFarland, M. R. (2002). *Transcultural nursing: Concepts, theories, research & practice* (2nd ed.). New York, NY: McGraw-Hill.

Leininger, M. M., & McFarland, M. R. (2006). *Culture care diversity and universality: A worldwide nursing theory* (3rd ed.). Sudbury, MA: Jones and Bartlett.

Masi, R. (1996). Inclusion: How can a health system respond to diversity. In A. S. Zieberth (Ed.), *Pinched: A management guide to the Canadian health care archipelago* (pp. 147–157). Nepean, ON: Pinched Press.

Narayanasamy, A. (2003). Transcultural nursing: How do nurses respond to cultural needs? *British Journal of Nursing, 12*(3), 185–194.

National Center for Cultural Competence. (2014). The compelling need for cultural and linguistic competence. http://www11.georgetown.edu/research/gucchd /nccc/foundations/need.html

National Prevention Information Network. (2014). Cultural competence. http://www.cdcnpin.org/scripts /population/culture.asp

Purnell, L. (2008). Transcultural diversity and healthcare. In L. Purnell & B. Paulanka (Eds.), *Transcultural health care: A culturally competent approach.* Philadelphia, PA: F. A. Davis.

Racher, F. E., & Annis, R. C. (2007). Respecting culture and honoring diversity in community practice. *Research*

and *Theory for Nursing Practice: An International Journal, 21*(4), 255–270.

Schim, S., Doorenbos, A., Benkert, R., & Miller, J. (2007). Culturally congruent care: Putting the puzzle together. *Journal of Transcultural Nursing, 18*(2), 103–110.

Smedley, B. D., Stith, A. Y., & Nelson, A. R. (2003). *Unequal treatment: Confronting racial and ethnic disparities in health care.* Washington, DC: National Academies Press.

Spector, R. (2013). *Cultural diversity in health and illness* (8th ed.). Upper Saddle River, NJ: Pearson Prentice Hall.

Srivastava, R. H. (2007). Understanding cultural competence in health care. In R. H. Srivastava (Ed.), *The healthcare professional's guide to clinical cultural competence* (pp. 3–27). Toronto, ON: Mosby Elsevier.

Transcultural Nursing Society. (2014). http://www .tcns.org

Tucker, C. M., Lopez, M., Campbell, K., Marsiske, M., Daly, K., Nghiem, K., … Patel, A. (2014). The effects of a culturally sensitive, empowerment-focused, community-based health promotion program on health outcomes of adults with type 2 diabetes. *Journal of Health Care for the Poor & Underserved, 25*(1), 292–307.

U.S. Census Bureau. (2010a). Race. http://quickfacts .census.gov/qfd/meta/long_RHI525211.htm

U.S. Census Bureau. (2010b). The next four decades: The older population in the United States: 2010 to 2050. http://www.census.gov/prod/2010pubs/p25-1138.pdf

U.S. Department of Health and Human Services (2014). Think Cultural Health. https://www .thinkculturalhealth.hhs.gov/Content/clas.asp

Wallman, K. K. (1998). Data on race and ethnicity: Revising the federal standard. *American Statistician, 52,* 1, 31–33.

Chapter 14

Self-Management

Raeann LeBlanc and Cynthia Jacelon

Introduction

"Self-management is a dynamic process in which individuals actively manage chronic illness" (Schulman-Green et al., 2012, p. 136). It is more than compliance or adherence to health prescriptions; it is a strategy for living with chronic disease. Self-management implies that the individual with the chronic condition engages in daily management by making informed decisions regarding health and life choices. Coaching and consultation from healthcare professionals support effective self-management.

Although chronic illness can affect individuals of any age, older adults are disproportionately afflicted with chronic illness. By 2030, one in eight individuals will be older than 65 years of age (National Institute of Aging [NIA], 2011), and the oldest old—those individuals age 85 and older—represent the fastest-growing segment of the U.S. population. With increasing age, the likelihood of experiencing multiple chronic health problems also increases (NIA, 2012; Vogeli et al., 2007). In 2005, 21% of Americans (roughly 63 million people) had more than one chronic condition or impairment expected to last a year or longer. Approximately 80% of older adults have one chronic condition, and 50% have at least two chronic health problems (Centers for Disease Control and Prevention [CDC], 2011). It was estimated that in 2009, 326 million primary care office visits were made by adults with multiple chronic conditions. These visits accounted for 37.6% of all medical visits by adults (Ashman & Beresovsky, 2013).

Multimorbidity, meaning the co-occurrence of acute and chronic conditions, also increases as one ages (Boyd, 2010). According to a systematic review by Marengoni et al. (2011), the prevalence of multimorbidity in older persons ranges from 55% to 98% and "all studies [in this review] pointed out the prevalence of multimorbidity among the older adult population is much higher than the prevalence of the most common diseases of the older adults such as heart failure and dementia" (pp. 431–432).

Multiple factors account for an individual's ability to self-manage complex symptoms and chronic diseases. Strategies for self-management include self-monitoring, managing medications, exercise plans, diet, and healthy lifestyle behaviors.

Definitions of Self-Care, Self-Management, and Disease Management

The terms *self-care*, *self-management*, and *disease management* are often used interchangeably. Although the goals of these strategies are similar, including promotion of health, reduction of complications, and prevention of disability while living with chronic illness, the terms actually have quite distinct meanings. Self-care is a concept that is related to living a healthy lifestyle (Schulman-Green et al., 2013). Disease management focuses on interventions initiated by healthcare professionals and treatments based on standards of care often outlined in disease-specific algorithms (Creer & Holroyd, 2006).

Self-management is more poorly understood. Ryan and Swain (2009) found that differences in understanding of the meaning of self-management have slowed the translation of self-management research into practice. Clarity of this term is essential for effective research translation. Self-management emphasizes the client's involvement in defining health management problems. Self-management is intentional and "involves the use of specific processes, can be affected by specific programs and interventions, and results in specific types of outcomes" (Ryan & Swain, 2009, p. 218).

Disease management programs emphasize individual aspects of care in the successful management of chronic illness and traditionally have targeted a specific chronic disease (Fortin, Lapointe, Hudon, & Vanasse, 2005). For example, there are many evidence-based programs for management of single diseases such as diabetes, chronic obstructive pulmonary disease (COPD), and heart failure. These interventions have demonstrated successful outcomes (Barlow, Sturt, & Hearnshaw, 2002). However, simply adding one single-disease approach to others in the case of individuals with multiple chronic conditions is not effective. Individuals with comorbid conditions need to understand the management of the interactions between disease states, balance priorities, and simplify complex regimens to be able to self-mange and prevent complications effectively. With multiple chronic conditions, a person needs to manage his or her general state of health as well as the chronic illness(es) with their overlapping self-management needs.

Using a client-centered approach in self-management programs, instead of the disease-based approach used in disease management programs, is needed for individuals to successfully manage multiple conditions (Boyd, 2010). According to the website Improving Chronic Illness Care (2006), self-management is defined as the decisions and behaviors a person living with chronic illness engages in that affect the individual's health outcomes. Collaborating with family, clinicians, and communities supports individuals in managing their health more effectively.

The Environment of Self-Management

Self-management is not limited to the outpatient or community setting, although the majority of self-management programs do focus on individuals in the community. Indeed, self-management programs are expanding across a variety of settings. For example, self-management programs are emerging among persons living in nursing homes (Park, Chang, Kim, & Kwak, 2012) and among those experiencing homelessness (Morrison, 2007). It is important for nurses working in any setting to consider the self-management skills of the person living with chronic illness and to promote a client-centered and client-involved approach that encourages the skills and attitudes that foster self-management.

During hospitalization and transitions of care, promotion of self-management—including educational needs, self-regulation, self-efficacy, social support, planning, motivation, and self-monitoring—is a fundamental aspect of collaboration between the nurse and the client. Case management follow-up provides essential resources for the client to continue to self-manage. Nurses are key individuals in maintaining client access to care and self-management support across care settings.

In the community, the home has particular meanings among individuals as a space of healing and health care; when the home becomes the location for receiving health and social services, however, both the meaning of home and the means of managing oneself when supportive management is needed change (Dyck, Kontos, Angus, & McKeever, 2005; Lindahl, Lide'n, & Lindblad, 2011). Levels of independence, privacy, and power in determining individual needs also change when self-management of illness requires a modification in one's role to that of receiving care and support while also trying to maintain as much independence as is possible (Hertz & Anschutz, 2002; Lindahl et al., 2010). No matter where an individual is living, the person who is self-managing one or more chronic conditions must manage symptoms, medications, equipment, medical specialty appointments, and activities of daily living while making personal meaning out of the experience (Corser & Dontje, 2011).

Policy Incentives for Self-Management of Chronic Disease

Healthy People 2020 (U.S. Department of Health and Human Services [HHS], 2013) outlines the federal government's health goals for the United States. Of the 42 topic areas covered by this initiative, several relate to specific chronic diseases (arthritis, osteoporosis and chronic back conditions, chronic kidney disease, dementias [including Alzheimer's disease], diabetes, heart disease and stroke, HIV, mental health disorders, respiratory diseases, substance abuse, hearing and other sensory or communication disorders). Other topics—including access to health care, particularly primary care—are also important in caring for persons with chronic illness. The related topics addressed by *Healthy People 2020* are health indicators that emphasize the need to better manage chronic illness to improve the health of the nation.

In 2009, the American Recovery and Reinvestment Act funded the Communities Putting Prevention to Work: Chronic Disease Self-Management Program. This initiative is led by the U.S. Administration on Aging (AOA) in collaboration with the Centers for Disease Control and Prevention and the Center for Medicare and Medicaid Services (CMS). Utilizing local agencies, health departments, and community partners, the program delivers the Chronic Disease Self-Management Program (CDSMP) and enables older Americans with chronic diseases to learn how to manage their conditions and take control of their health, with special attention being paid to low-income, minority, and underserved populations (AOA, 2013).

Other incentives seek to help persons living with chronic illness remain within the community, aided by home-based community services and agency support through self-management programs, and care assistance to prevent costly institutionalized long-term care or hospitalization (Kaye, 2012). For example, for the frailest populations in the United States, the Medicaid Home Care Waiver program offers a choice to children and adults to receive their care at home, instead of in long-term institutional care facilities, through a host of medical, social services, and self-management support (Kaye, 2012). In concordance with this imperative, many individuals and families are choosing to remain at home for their care (Spencer, Patrick, & Steele, 2009).

Middle-Range Theories of Self-Management

Middle-range nursing theories offer an understanding of the theory of self-management by conceptualizing nursing care as based on relationships and coaching, and providing guidelines for collaborative decision making. The three theories discussed here are the *theory of self-care of chronic illness* (Riegel, Jaarsma, & Strömberg, 2012); Ryan and Sawin's (2009) *individual and family self-management theory*; and Grey, Knafl, and McCorkle's (2006) *self-management and family management framework*, which includes updates by Schulman-Green and colleagues (2012).

The basis of the *theory of self-care of chronic illness* is the idea that "if health care professionals better understand the processes used by clients in performing self-care, they can use this information to identify where clients struggle" (Riegel et al., 2012, p. 195). Three key concepts inform this theory: self-care maintenance, self-care monitoring, and self-care management. Processes that underline self-management include decision making and reflection. In addition, several factors affect the complex process of self-management, including self-care, one's experience and skill, motivation, cultural beliefs and values, confidence, habits, functional and cognitive abilities, support from others, and access to care. The *theory of self-care of chronic illness* includes seven propositions:

1. There are core similarities in self-care across different chronic illnesses.
2. Previous personal experience with illness increases the quality of self-care.
3. Clients who engage in self-care that is purposive but unreflective are limited in their ability to master self-care in complex situations. Reflective self-care can be learned.
4. Misunderstandings, misconceptions, and lack of knowledge all contribute to insufficient self-care.
5. Mastery of self-care maintenance precedes mastery of self-care management because self-care maintenance is less complex than the decision making required for self-care management.
6. Self-care monitoring for changes in signs and symptoms is necessary for effective self-care management because one cannot make a decision about change unless it has been noticed and evaluated.
7. Individuals who perform evidence-based self-care have better outcomes than those who perform self-care that is not evidence based (Riegel et al., 2012, pp. 199–200).

According to Ryan and Sawin's *Individual and Family Self-Management Theory* (IFSMT), self-management encompasses "dynamic phenomena consisting of three dimensions: context, process and outcomes" (p. 9). The IFSMT acknowledges the complexity of self-management that occurs within the context of social arrangements (individually, in families, and in dyads) and across developmental levels. Instead of seeing self-management on an individual level, the IFSMT understands self-management on both family and individual levels (**Figure 14-1**). This theory addresses the complexity of self-management in the three previously mentioned dimensions of context, process, and outcomes.

The framework for self and family management of chronic conditions is designed to provide a structure for understanding factors influencing the ability of individuals and their families to manage chronic illness (Grey et al., 2006; Tanner, 2004). The components of this framework are self-management, risk and protective factors including condition factors, individual factors, psychosocial characteristics, family factors, and the environment (**Figure 14-2**).

Self- and family management of chronic illness is defined as the decisions and activities that individuals make on a daily basis to manage their chronic health problems (Grey et al., 2006; Improving Chronic Illness Care, 2007; Ryan & Sawin, 2009). In further work on the model, Schulman-Green and colleagues (2012) identified three processes of self-management. The first process, "focusing on illness needs," includes the activities the individual uses to take care of the body and treatments pertaining to the disease process—in other words, disease management. The second process is "activating resources"; in employing these processes, the individual engages in procuring assistance and support for family, friends, and community. The third process, "living with a chronic illness," is where the individual places the chronic illness within the context of living and growing as a human—that is, the process of illness management.

For some individuals, particularly those who are older or have cognitive deficits, engaging

Figure 14-1 Individual and Family Self-Management Theory

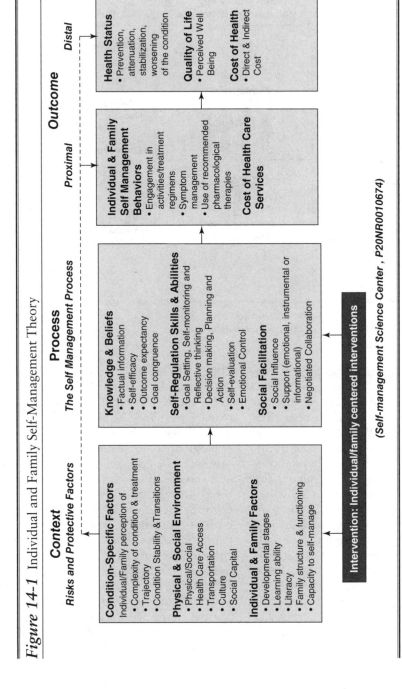

Source: Ryan, P., & Swain, K. J. (2009). The individual and family self-management theory: Background and perspectives on context process and outcomes. *Nursing Outlook*, 57, 217–225; Ryan, P. (2009). The integrated theory of health behavior change: Background and intervention development. *Clinical Nurse Specialist*, 23(3), 161–170. http://www4.uwm.edu/nursing/about/centers-institutes/self-management.cfm

---

Figure 14-2 Self-Management and Family Management Framework

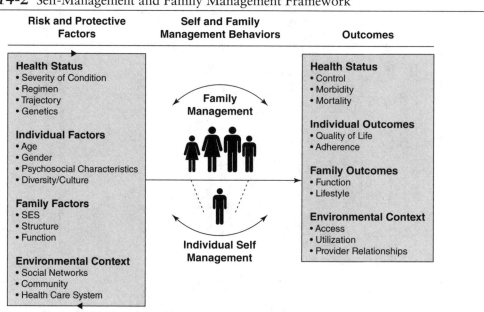

in self-management is an ongoing challenge
(Tanner, 2004). The nurse, in turn, is challenged to help the client manage at the level
of his or her ability (Jacelon, Furman, Rea,
Macdonald, & Donoghue, 2011). The concept
of self-management extends the responsibility
of individuals with chronic illness beyond compliance and adherence to managing an ongoing
condition within the context of their daily lives.
In home care, it is imperative that the nurse
consider both the client's ability to self-manage
and the family's ability to support the individual's self-management (Grey et al., 2006).

The ability of individuals and families to
manage chronic illness depends on the severity of the condition, the treatment regimen, the
course of the disease, individual and family characteristics, and the environment in which individuals will manage their disease (Grey et al.,

2006). The severity of the illness from the perspective of the individual may not be the same
as the nurse's perception. The implications for
management may be affected by the meaning
of the illness to the individual and family. The
etiology of the condition (e.g., a lifestyle disease such as emphysema as a result of smoking
or a genetically determined disease) will affect
the ability for self-management. The implications for the family in these situations may be
guilt or concern for the susceptibility of other
family members. The treatment regimen for a
chronic illness may be complex, requiring significant lifestyle adjustments. Individual factors
such as the person's age, psychosocial situation,
functional ability, self-perceived ability to manage the illness, education, and socioeconomic
status all contribute to the individual's ability
for self-management. Careful assessment by the

nurse is imperative in providing care. Once an assessment is complete, the nurse is in a position to coach the individual or family in managing the illness.

In the model of self-management and family management, outcomes can include decreased symptoms as well as improved individual and family outcomes such as better disease management, improved quality of life, or improved self-efficacy (Grey et al., 2006). The main goal of the model is to help the individual improve his or her health, using the broadest definition of health possible. The nurse should support the self and family's self-management, teach them the skills needed to improve health, and coach the individual and family on incorporating those activities into their daily lives.

The Meaning of Self-Management

Understanding how older adults living in the community manage their health and make meaning of this experience with supportive care is essential in delivering efficient, cost-effective, appropriate, and respectful care. It is critical to understand this process from the perspective of the older adult. Effective self-management does not happen all at once. Indeed, in a longitudinal study of self-management, Audulv, Asplund, and Norbergh (2012) found that clients assimilated the process of self-management in stages. Immediately after diagnosis of a chronic illness, the individual engaged in seeking effective self-management strategies. This step was followed by considering costs and benefits, creating routines and plans of action, and negotiating self-management that fits one's life.

How health care is provided and how incentives are determined in delivering care in the community are based on healthcare policy. Personal choice and the meanings of maintaining self-care and managing chronic illness at home among older adults are understood from within the societies in which those individuals live, how formal and informal care services are provided (or not), and through healthcare policy and payer systems.

A Balancing Act

The theme of a balancing act and making adjustments on multiple levels emerged in the research of several authors (Crist, 2005; Ebrahimi, Wilhelmson, Moore, & Jakobsson, 2012; Jacelon, 2010; Kralik, Koch, Price, & Howard, 2004; Nicholson, Meyer, Flatley, & Homan, 2013). A balancing act was the most dominant theme in explaining and finding meaning in living at home and maintaining the care of oneself in the face of changing aspects of chronic illness, frailty, debility, and dependence on others.

Kralik and colleagues' (2004) descriptive study used written autobiography and interviews among nine older adults with a mean age of 60 years. This relatively young sample included six women and three men with osteoarthritis. In the study, participants understood self-management as a multidimensional and complex process "where the purpose was to create order from the disorder imposed by illness" (p. 262). The individuals in this study learned about their response to illness as a process through daily life experiences and adjusted their lives and identity by exploring their limitations. Finding balance emerged as the meaning of self-management, as perceived by people living with chronic illness. Living with the pain of arthritis also affected the participants' sense of self-esteem, identity, and helplessness, which was contrasted with, and balanced by, the strong and common theme of striving to maintain independence. Although participants knew they needed help with certain activities, and sought this assistance, they focused on what they could do for themselves to recover a sense of value.

Jacelon (2010) used the theoretical framework of symbolic interaction "to understand the meaning older adults attributed to their self-care activities" (p. 16). Unstructured interviews, participant logs, and researcher logs identified the overarching theme as "maintaining the balance" among 10 older adults aged 75 to 98 years who managed chronic illness at home. The study participants' function was either primarily independent or required assistance with instrumental activities of daily living, such as shopping, cooking, and housekeeping. Participants maintained balanced activity, attitude, autonomy, health, and relationships in their daily lives. This balance included participating in complex activities in maintaining health, such as monitoring health, keeping track of medication, and adjusting to health status changes.

Similarly, in Kralik and colleagues' study (2004), self-management held a unique place and meaning in the lives of community-dwelling older adults that was broader than the management of their disease(s). Instead, managing illness was seen as part of a larger fabric of self-care strategies that accommodated the prescribed healthcare requirements. These strategies were balanced in ways that sought to maintain independence and autonomy in the individual.

Nicholson et al. (2013) utilized a narrative approach in understanding the experience over time of 15 frail older adults aged 86 to 102 years. This study challenged the negative meaning in which frailty is often viewed and stereotyped. Instead, the meaning of maintaining care at home and being frail was understood as one of potential for capacity in which new meanings and self-identity emerged. A sense of meaning flowed from states of imbalance when there was loss in physical, social, and psychological health. Contrasting this was the ability to create new connections and realize well-being beyond that of functional incapacity. Nicholson et al.'s study challenges the current understandings of frailty in older adults at home, instead holding that affected individuals experience both loss and capacity to create connections to themselves and to others in maintaining this capacity

"of relating to their ordinary world in a different way" (p. 1179).

Two studies explored separate aspects of receiving care from family caregivers and formal caregivers. From and colleagues (2007) sought to understand how older adults' self-management and health was understood in the context of being dependent on healthcare services in their home, while Crist's (2005) study focused on the meaning of receiving care from family members. In both studies, older adults negotiated their autonomy within the context of dependence on others while maintaining their balance in health and place in the community.

From et al. (2007) studied 19 older adults aged 70 to 94 years, all of whom required assistance in their home from care providers. Experiences of health and illness were described as negative and positive polarities of the subcategories of autonomy versus dependency, togetherness versus being ignored, tranquility versus disturbance, and security versus insecurity. In addition to identifying the overall sense of finding balance between health and illness, the participants in this study did not focus specifically on their diseases or current health problems. Instead, they identified strategies to adjust in daily life. One important implication from this study was the importance of the continuity of caregivers in maintaining this balance, developing trust and security, and ensuring the caregiver's ability to honor self-determination of the older adult.

Receiving care specifically from family members was the focus of Crist's (2005) study. Through the use of interviews and observations, older adults were asked to describe their experience of receiving care from family members as part of their overall self-management. The theme of maintaining the balance between receiving the care they needed and maintaining their autonomy was prominent. Additionally, all nine older adults were comfortable with and accepted family care. Balance was supported by positive relationships with the family caregiver, who encouraged personal growth. The assistance the older adult received was not seen as task oriented, but rather as an inherent part of being in a relationship. Despite receiving variable levels of family care, the older adults viewed themselves as leading autonomous lives (Crist, 2005).

Ebrahimi et al. (2012) described frail elders, who had differing self-perceived health, and highlighted how harmony and balance were achieved in everyday life when the older adults were able to adjust to the demands of day-to-day living in the context of their resources and capabilities. This included being active decision makers and being validated as capable persons. Such a finding is consistent with the goal of human beings to maintain harmony and balance as an experience of self-care and health.

In all of these studies, researchers identified the theme of maintaining balance as essential to self-management. Such a balancing act requires adjustments to complex social, psychological, and physical changes. Balance is achieved through the acceptance of receiving assistance from others while maintaining autonomy and independence to the fullest extent possible. These studies demonstrate the importance of the relationships older adults have with formal and family caregivers and indicate how supportive social interactions promote balance in health and self-care management capacity.

Home as a Self-Care Space

The home as an environment that supports self-care has not been well studied in the literature, although it is often cited as a preferred location for care among older adults (Spencer et al., 2009). In describing the experiences of African Americans, ages 60 to 89 years, with hypertension and cognitive difficulty, Klymko, Artinian, Price, Abele, and Washington (2011) used a semi-structured interview process that focused on the participants' management of their hypertension.

The environment of home was considered a safe place and provided emotional support that promoted self-management. Participants in this study found home and their connection to home to be something that allowed them to emotionally and mentally care for themselves (Klymko et al., 2011, p. 207). These individuals maintained adequate blood pressure control despite their cognitive challenges. Maintaining self-care was challenging, but home was a supportive location that was meaningful in promoting health.

Self-Determination and Shifting Identities

Self-determination is the ability to control one's own life and make decisions based on one's values (Holmberg, Valmari, & Lundgren, 2012). Self-identity is challenged with changes in health status and the need to depend on others for certain aspects of care. This can threaten one's ability to make decisions and choices. Self-determination is an important aspect of how people choose to care for themselves and the role one takes or does not take in managing one's health and making self-care decisions.

Three studies sought to understand the meaning of self-management, self-care, and maintaining care at home with assistance among older adults with explicit vulnerabilities. Clark and colleagues (2008) contrasted 12 socioeconomically challenged older adults with incomes at or below the poverty level with 12 older adults with private health insurance, and asked each group to describe their perceptions of self-management. Racial diversity was achieved by the equal representation of black and white men and women in both samples.

The in-depth interviews suggested that among the socioeconomically challenged group, the meaning and significance of self-management was limited to taking medications and maintaining physician appointments. In contrast, the more financially secure older adults assumed a broader meaning, which considered the possibility of health promotion and being engaged in mental and physical activities, all as part of positive expectations for their health and aging processes.

Using a case study design focusing on life history interviews and participant observations, Donlan (2011) explored the meaning of receiving community-based care in six frail Mexican American elders; men and women were equally represented in the sample. Findings from these interviews revealed the significance of cultural identity that attributed meaning to the context of care being received from community-based care providers. These cultural themes included Latino familism, respect for the aged, gender identity, and religious belief systems. The themes of the study demonstrated that participants identified the meaning of self-care management with family. Participants in this study shared how having an identity as old or frail was not valued by society at large, but contrasted this view with their Hispanic culture, which did value older adults. Maintaining self-care, managing illness, and retaining a positive identity were self-determined by receiving concordance of care within their Hispanic culture.

Nicholson et al.'s (2013) narrative study highlighted how loss of self-determination was a challenge to study participants' self-identity and was often provoked by receiving formal care services in the home or through challenges with family caregivers who themselves were experiencing a decline in health status. All narratives in this study referenced challenges to social identity and position in the world due to declining functional ability and chronic illness.

Breiholtz, Snellman, and Fagerberg (2013) studied 12 frail older adults and described how as frail elders became more dependent on caregivers' help, the older adults' opportunity to self-determine was greatly challenged. This challenge compromised their self-identity and was very stressful. Unlike the theme of recovery toward balance and acceptance found in other studies, a theme of loss and resignation was apparent in this investigation.

These diverse studies highlight how increased vulnerability and threats to self-identity impact self-determination and expectations of health. Social determinants of health, including socioeconomic status and cultural identity, also affect perceived self-determination and ability to self-manage chronic illness. Individual experiences of dependency on family members and outside agencies can compromise choices and self-care agency, which in turn may dismantle one's social identity.

Self-Realization as Self-Transformation

Self-realization is understood as the knowledge of the self that can motivate an individual to change or transform. Awareness of one's needs and desires is part of self-realization and part of self-care management. The theme of self-transformation was noted in the qualitative studies of Dunn and Riley-Doucet (2007) and Söderhamn, Dale, and Söderhamn (2013). Söderhamn et al.'s work revealed an important understanding of self-realization in the ability to actualize self-care and manage complex illness. In their study of actualizing self-care management, actions were taken to improve, maintain, or restore health and well-being among community-dwelling older adults. Motivational themes included carrying on, being of use to others, self-realization, and a sense of confidence in managing the future. In addition to illuminating how older adults find meaning and motivation to manage their care, this study offered the lesson that older people who are able to actualize self-care resources can be valuable for other older adults who may need social contact and practical assistance both as peers and as role models.

The exploration of the phenomenon of maintaining holistic well-being throughout life by Dunn and Riley-Doucet (2007) elucidated how older adults view self-care activities within a holistic framework. In this study, 28 older adults were organized into four focus groups.

Two of these four groups included racial and ethnic diversity representation. Self-realization of how self-care activities impacted the participants' physical, psychological, social, and spiritual health was revealed. Faith and spirituality, positive energy, support systems, wellness activities, and affirmative self-appraisal described the context of health. Activities to promote self-care and support self-management included prayer, exercise, altruism, and belief in God, and were essential to maintaining health in older adult's lives.

Self-realization and transformation are important to self-care management because of how these dynamic personal understandings motivate individuals to act in certain ways that promote health and care for themselves. In both the studies by Dunn and Riley-Doucet (2007) and Söderhamn et al. (2013), the participants strived for an understanding of self and an awareness of what influenced their physical, social, psychological, and spiritual health. Transformation was supported by freedom of choice and finding ways internally (prayer, altruism, belief, self-confidence, desire to live) and externally (being useful to others) to care for one's self.

These qualitative studies add to our understanding of self-care and self-management because of their broad view of meanings for older adults living at home. Self-care is part of self-management of disease, as well as management of the social arrangements, attitudes, and opportunities to grow from these experiences in self-realization. Self-care management and the integrity of self-identity can be thwarted by caregivers due to a lack of sensitivity, other competing stressors (e.g., low socioeconomic status), and caregiver relationships in which the older adult's self-determination is impeded.

One salient point highlighted by this review of the literature is that older adults living in the community with multiple medical diagnoses, disease management needs, and self-care needs do not view the meaning of their health and self-care as specifically the self-management of disease(s), nor is illness the central tenet of their health. Rather, managing illness is a process that intermingles with other areas of care and meaning. In fact, it appears that social support and management of relationships determine well-being and, therefore, health and ability to manage illness. Areas of disease self-management, such as taking medications and monitoring health, are only a part of the essential activities that allow older adults to maintain stability in health and at home.

Meaning is found in the relationships and activities that support balance, self-determination, and security in daily life. Meaning, as revealed in this literature review, is less about disease management and more about a larger holistic sense of self and home as multidimensional. Self-care management seeks to maintain these balances and polarities that are in danger of being disrupted by illness, reliance on others for care, and older adults' attitudes in the face of loss. As summarized by Kralik et al. (2004), these studies suggest that clinicians need to reevaluate what represents self-management because the current "prescriptive" approach— one of "adherence" to a particular set of medical treatments and physical monitoring—has little meaning to people living with chronic illness and the means by which they actually manage their lives (p. 265).

These studies suggest that healthcare professionals should pay more attention to the social lives of older adults and not limit the understanding of health to merely managing a set of diagnoses. These studies also offer new insight into functional status and dependency, which is often based on mental or functional disability, and reveal the resourcefulness that older adults demonstrate in caring for themselves and others. Supportive care systems can preserve a sense of meaning and promote autonomy over dependence in promoting health. Understanding the value of a broader, more holistic sense of self as highlighted in this review is integral.

In an additional study addressing the self-management needs of vulnerable older adults, Haslbeck, McCorkle, and Schaeffer (2012) looked at research focusing on self-management among older adults living alone late in life. Their integrated review reflects the challenges of chronic illness self-management within the context of difficult living situations, isolation, lack of support, and limited resources while dealing with multiple chronic conditions that need to be actively managed and adjusted. This research also highlights how the majority of studies focus on older women's challenges in living with chronic illness—comparatively little information is available on older men living alone and their self-management processes. Haslbeck at al. (2012) call for future research to address this disparity. The authors concluded that shifting resources toward the community and home is necessary, as home is the primary setting in which self-management occurs; they also noted that self-management interventions must be individually tailored, because a one-size-fits-all approach is ineffective.

Nursing Interventions

Kawi (2012) organized interventions to support self-management into three categories. First are strategies to support patient-centered attributes. such as involving patients as partners, providing education tailored to clients' specific needs, and individualizing patient care. The second category of interventions includes healthcare professional attributes such as possessing adequate knowledge, skills, and attitudes to promote self-management. The third category of interventions includes organizational attributes such as an organized system of care employing an inter-professional team and appropriate social support (p. 108). Each of these categories is apparent in the interventions discussed here.

Interprofessional collaborative care is essential in the management of chronic illnesses, and nurses as leaders are key in asserting a direct relationship with clients to promote the management of chronic illness over time while respecting the goals and readiness of the client. Holman and Lorig (2004) highlighted elements of chronic disease management that change the way the healthcare system must respond. Chronic illness management calls for an ongoing partnership between healthcare professionals and their clients. It is important for healthcare professionals to understand that the client knows the most about the consequences of mismanagement of disease and to take advantage of that knowledge. The client and the healthcare professional must share complementary knowledge and authority in the healthcare process to achieve the desired outcomes of improved health, ability to cope, and reduction in healthcare spending (p. 239). The following nurse-led interventions highlight innovative approaches to promoting client self-management of chronic disease and are included here as examples: coaching, medication management, and group visits.

Coaching as a Technique to Enhance Self-Management and Family Management

In the chronic care model (CCM), one key component is self-management support (Wagner, 1998). Nurses are in an excellent position to coach the client and family in the management of the chronic illness. Coaching is a strategy in which the nurse uses a combination of education, collaborative decision making, and empowerment to help clients manage their health needs (Butterworth, Linden, & McClay, 2007; Huffman, 2007, 2009). Health coaching may also include active listening, questioning, and reflecting (Howard & Ceci, 2013). This intervention has its roots in substance abuse counseling and has been found to be a relatively short-term, successful strategy. Health coaching is a client-centered approach to care in which the focus is on the issues and barriers to self-management.

To use health coaching, the nurse begins by asking the client what he or she is most concerned about. In this way, the nurse can capitalize on the client's interest in resolving or managing a particular problem. The next step is to validate the client's feelings about his or her capacity to manage the problem. Following this, the nurse might help the client develop solutions to the problem by asking which strategies the client has used in the past and which strategies he or she might like to try (Huffman, 2007).

Medication Self-Management

One aspect of self-management of chronic illness is the management of medications. Care providers monitor therapeutic and side effects of the medication as well as client management of complex therapeutic plans of care. Self-management of medications from the client's perspective requires organization, tracking, self-monitoring (e.g., blood sugar, weight, vital signs), and record keeping. Self-organization of medication regimens, either independently or with support, may require using technologies such as medication planners and cueing systems. Effective self-management implies that the client will report concerns or complications such as side effects, adverse effects, or lack of therapeutic improvement at the client's regular meetings with healthcare professionals.

Medication self-management includes the processes of accessing medications, obtaining refills, and negotiating costs. It also includes routine follow-up for medical appointments, laboratory monitoring, advocating for medication list review, and possible medication reductions in cases of complex polypharmacy. Seeking out and engaging in education vis-à-vis adjusting to changes in medication regimens is required as well.

As identified in the theory of self-care of chronic illness (Riegel et al., 2012), there is a need for both critical thinking and reflection in this process. Social supports, family, and healthcare professional interactions may all influence the outcomes of medication safety and chronic illness management. The nurse's role in supporting client self-management of medications occurs within the context of interprofessional collaboration with the pharmacist, insurers, case managers, and physicians, as well as directly with the client in ongoing assessment, communication, behavioral and psychosocial support, and education.

A Model of Medication Self-Management

In a qualitative nursing study of 19 older adults aged 64 to 96 years, who were taking an average of 8.68 medications each day, Swanlund, Scherck, Metcalfe, and Jesek-Hale (2008) identified themes in the successful self-management of medications that included "successful self-managing of medications, living orderly, and aging well" (p. 241). The processes identified in this study required high levels of organization to successfully self-manage medications and included establishing habits, adjusting routines, tracking, simplification, valuing medications, collaborating to manage, and managing costs (p. 241).

The theme of living orderly was how participants incorporated medications into their day-to-day activities and included organizing daily routines and making order out of complexity despite physical limitations (Swanlund et al., 2008). Attitude was also linked to successful self-management of medications and was part of aging well, being active, and maintaining a self-perception as being healthy. **Figure 14-3** summarizes this model of medication self-management.

Nursing Care Coordination, Technology, and Medication Self-Management

In a randomized clinical trial to test the efficacy of using nursing care coordination and technology with the health status outcomes of frail older adults in medication self-management,

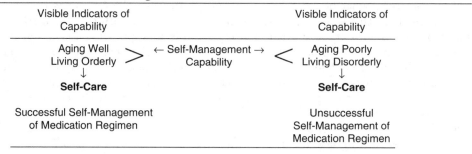

Figure 14-3 Medication Self-Management Model

Source: Data from Swanlund, S., Scherck, K., Metcalfe, S., & Jesek-Hale, S. (2008). Keys to successful self-management of medications. *Nursing Science Quarterly, 21*(3), 238-246.

Marek et al. (2013) recruited 414 older adults who had difficulty in managing their medications. A team of advanced practice nurses and registered nurses coordinated care for 12 months for the two intervention groups. All participants received a pharmacy screen; the control group received no intervention beyond this pharmacy screen. The two intervention groups received nurse care coordination related to self-management. One intervention group received an additional medication dispensing machine (an automatic medication dispensing technology known as MD.2) or a medication planner (a pre-filled medication box).

The study was guided by the IFSMT theoretical framework and viewed self-management as a complex and dynamic phenomenon incorporating context, process, and proximal and distal outcomes (Ryan & Swain, 2009). The range of the mean age of participants was 78.2–79.6 years; the majority of participants in each group were female and primarily white. Results of this intervention study showed that care coordination led by nurses had a beneficial effect on the health status outcomes of cognitive function, depressive symptoms, functional status, and quality of life (Marek et al., 2013). The medication planner and nursing care coordination were effective in supporting client self-management and improved clinical health outcomes.

Advanced Practice Nurse–Led Group Visits

A salient aspect of supporting self-management focuses on the psychosocial aspects of behavior change to promote health and wellness. It is also essential to collaborate with clients and provide encouragement and support to increase self-confidence and self-efficacy. *Strategies to Support Self-Management in Chronic Conditions: Collaboration with Clients* is an evidence-based practice guideline created by Registered Nurses Association of Ontario, Canada, and published by the Agency for Healthcare Research and Quality (AHRQ, 2010). These strategies include the "Five A's Behavioral Change Approach." Nurses utilize the "Five A's"—of assess, advise, agree, assist, and arrange—to improve outcomes in patients with chronic illness and incorporate multiple self-management strategies. The following strategies are addressed with the "Five A's":

- Establishing rapport
- Screening for depression
- Establishing a written agenda for appointments
- Assessing the client's readiness for change
- Combining effective behavioral and psychosocial strategies with self-management education processes

- Encouraging monitoring methods and self-management techniques (e.g., diaries, logs, personal health records)
- Establishing goals, action plans, and monitor progress
- Motivational interviewing
- Follow-up (AHRQ, 2010)

In addressing self-management needs that incorporate these areas of psychosocial support, a strategy that is gaining popularity is the group visit (GV). Advanced practice nurses are in an ideal position to promote self-management strategies through group visits in primary care. Because clients with specific chronic illnesses may have similar needs, group visits can be efficient methods of clinical intervention and action. In addition, group visits may provide psychosocial support, peer connections, and motivation.

Simmons and Kapustin (2011) reviewed studies focusing on the group visit for clients living with type 2 diabetes mellitus. Nine studies were reviewed. The average group size was 8–20 and lasted for 2 hours. Simmons and Kapustin's review of the evidence revealed that group visits yielded positive client satisfaction, improved perception of continuity of care by clients, increased knowledge about diabetes, improved quality of life, and increased self-monitoring. Clients reflected more positive attitudes regarding a group visit for self-management of their diabetes as compared to a routine office visit.

Four studies in this review revealed positive financial impact through a decrease in emergency department visits and an increase in healthcare provider productivity. Group visits may be reimbursed per insurance standards. Improvement in client outcomes was also apparent in several studies in the form of decreases in HgbA$_{1c}$, improved lipid management, and improved documentation of American Diabetes Association health screening indicators such as foot examinations.

Group visits often include interprofessional collaboration between teams of healthcare professionals and clients. Although data are still relatively limited regarding the incorporation of group visits into primary care, Simmons and Kapustin's (2011) review does suggest positive outcomes and the need for more research in this area of practice implementation.

In addition to group visits, other technological innovations can be added to stay connected with clients and support their chronic illness experience both independently and in group formats. Email reminders, virtual education platforms, telemonitoring, and online support groups are all options for individuals living with a chronic illness who require ongoing self-management support and are ideal ways to incorporate the "Five A's" while fostering connections.

Advanced practice nurses are ideal leaders of these programs because of their knowledge of chronic disease; implementation of evidence-based practice; systems leadership for quality improvement; and abilities to apply client care technology for the improvement of health, prevent complications, work well in interprofessional teams for improved client outcomes, and utilize advanced nursing skills including those that are client centered and provide psychosocial support (American Association of Colleges of Nursing, 2006).

Ethical Considerations in Self-Management

It is important to acknowledge the ethical issues that are largely based on structural issues within the U.S. healthcare system in the implementation of self-management programs for persons living with chronic illness. The fundamental imperative of self-management is the positive outcome from increased client involvement in care, which offers the client the personal benefits of agency, self-efficacy, and empowerment while improving health outcomes. These are ethical aims. However, as Redman (2007) notes, some very important ethical issues remain unaddressed. Redman (2007) identifies four central ethical issues in the move toward client self-management of chronic illness:

1. Access is far from guaranteed. Availability of appropriate preparation so that clients and families are sufficiently competent at self-management is necessary to avoid harm.
2. The appropriate philosophy of client empowerment that has accompanied part of the self-management movement rings hollow if the process makes the client responsible without assuring the means of self-management or competent medical care.
3. There is the assumption that education is noninvasive, not requiring formal informed consent.
4. The potential for widening the gap between the "haves" and the "have-nots" in health care is very real, as the "have-nots" struggle with low literacy, the resulting inability to self-educate, and lack of access to educational materials and teachers matched to their learning needs (Redman, 2007, pp. 245–246).

Addressing these four ethical considerations requires providing uniform access to quality self-management support and competent care, addressing healthcare disparities, and acknowledging that harm may be related to educational interventions and inadequate support for self-management while still maintaining the expectation for clients to self-manage their conditions. Among these ethical issues, there may also be a tendency to blame persons living with chronic illness who are doing poorly or whose chronic illness is complicated by other comorbidities and/or psychosocial issues.

Outcomes

In addressing the needs of persons living with multiple chronic conditions, the Department of Health and Human Services (2010) published a framework with four goals:

- Goal 1: Foster healthcare and public health system changes to improve the health of individuals with multiple chronic conditions.
- Goal 2: Maximize the use of proven self-care management and other services by individuals with multiple chronic conditions.
- Goal 3: Provide better tools and information to healthcare, public health, and social services workers who deliver care to individuals with multiple chronic conditions.
- Goal 4: Facilitate research to fill knowledge gaps about and interventions and systems to benefit individuals with multiple chronic conditions.

Grey, Knafl, and McCorkle (2006) describe effective self- and family management of chronic illnesses as being measured by several outcomes across a range of general domains, including condition outcomes, individual outcomes, family outcomes, and environmental outcomes.

Condition Outcomes

Improved condition outcomes are the main goals of chronic disease self-management. The outcomes of improved health, prevention of complications of chronic illness, and prevention of worsening chronic conditions are key measures of effective self-management. For example, improved $HgbA_{1c}$ levels in persons living with diabetes, improved peak-flow measurements in persons living with asthma, and improved functional mobility in persons living with arthritis are all measurable condition outcomes that are associated with evidence of improved health and a result of improved self-management. Likewise, decreased hospitalization and emergency department use are measures of improved management of chronic conditions.

Individual Outcomes

Individual outcomes are related to quality of life and well-being for the individual and his or her family. Quality of life is important to living with chronic illness and functioning well in the management of chronic conditions. Outcomes related to quality of life include positive behavioral change, self-confidence, and self-efficacy. Well-being and health are subjective experiences and defined by the individual.

Family Outcomes

Family outcomes reflect the relationship within the family system and indicate how management of chronic conditions and self-management outcomes are influenced by this system. Enhanced family self-management focuses on the well-being of the family and its function.

Environmental Outcomes

Environmental outcomes extend the outcomes of quality of life, health condition, individual well-being, and family well-being to the larger environment, such as the healthcare system. Environmental outcomes reflect how improved self-management by clients and families impacts the cost of health care and healthcare utilization.

Proximal Versus Distal Outcomes

In their IFSMT model, Ryan and Swain (2009) described outcomes as being either proximal or distal outcomes of effective self-management. For example, the proximal outcomes of self-management are specific to the conditions, risk factors, and management of the condition. Distal outcomes are related to the success of the proximal outcomes and include costs associated with health care.

According to Ryan and Swain (2009, p. 10), outcomes fall into three primary categories: health status, quality of life, and cost of health. Cost of health includes both direct costs—that

is, the monetary cost to manage a healthcare issue (e.g., medications, healthcare visits, durable medical equipment)—and indirect costs—that is, loss of productivity, absenteeism from work, lost leisure time, and disability (DeLong, Culler, Saini, Beck, & Chen, 2008).

Client-Reported Outcome Measures

To assess the results from client-reported outcome measures (also known as patient-reported outcome measures [PROMs]) in chronic disease self-management, a framework has been developed by Santana and Feeny (2014). This framework provides insight into clinically effective outcomes. PROMs range from distal to proximal, and include proximal outcome measures in the domain of communication as outcomes of client–clinician communication, client–family communication, clinician–clinician communication, and clinician–family communication. The proximal outcome of client engagement includes shared decision making. Client management, client satisfaction, clinician satisfaction, client adherence, and client condition outcomes are all interrelated and measurable. This framework can be used to develop interventions to improve the care of persons living with and managing chronic conditions and to evaluate these interventions after they are implemented (Santana & Feeny, 2014).

National Study of Chronic Disease Self-Management

Ory and colleagues (2013) investigated how the Chronic Disease Self-Management Program (CDSMP) affected health outcomes, individual outcomes, and healthcare cost utilization over a 6-month time frame. The CDSMP is an evidence-based program that has been disseminated through aging-service networks nationally across 22 states through the Administration on Aging (AOA, 2013);

it is funded by the American Recovery and Reinvestment Act.

This study used a pre–post longitudinal design and assessed 903 participants from 17 states (English and Spanish speaking) at 6 months. Primary and secondary outcomes of participants in the CDSMP were followed. Primary outcomes included role management, emotional management, and medical management. Specifically, social role and activity limitations, depression, and communication with physicians all improved significantly from baseline at the 6-month follow-up point. Secondary outcomes included self-assessed health status, health-related behaviors, and healthcare utilization over the past 6 months. Significant improvements were noted in increased physical activity and less healthcare utilization (i.e., decreased emergency room visits and hospitalization).

Conclusion

Self-management of chronic illness combines the elements and behaviors of client self-care with the management of disease and encourages clients to be active agents in managing their illnesses. Self-management is achieved through a use of strategies such as self-monitoring and organization of medications and treatments. Effective self-management occurs in partnership with others. Clients, families, communities, and healthcare professionals influence an individual's confidence, motivation, and ability to manage complex illnesses daily.

Self-management requires both critical thinking and reflection. Ultimately, nurses and healthcare professionals need to understand that clients are the experts in their disease "when they are able to achieve a level of self-agency that does not rely on healthcare professionals taking the lead role in management" (Koch, Jenkin, & Kralik, 2004, p. 490). Self-management of chronic illness is a shift away from the medical paradigm and is a relationship-based, client-centered model of care.

Evidence-Based Practice Box

A 12-month parallel randomized controlled trial was used to evaluate an online disease management system that supported clients with uncontrolled type 2 diabetes. The sample included 415 clients with type 2 diabetes with baseline glycosylated hemoglobin (HgbA$_{1c}$) values of 7.5% or greater. Most of the clients (382 people) completed the study. The setting for the study included primary care sites from a large, integrated group practice that shared electronic health records.

The intervention included the following elements: wirelessly uploaded home glucometer readings with graphical feedback; comprehensive client-specific diabetes summary status report; nutrition and exercise logs; insulin record; online messaging with the client's health team; a nurse care manager and a dietitian who provided advice and medication management; and personalized text and video educational "nuggets" dispensed electronically by the care team. The HgbA$_{1c}$ level was the primary outcome variable.

Compared with clients who received the usual care, the intervention group had significantly reduced HgbA$_{1c}$ levels at 6 months. At 12 months, the differences were not significant. In post hoc analysis, significantly more intervention-group clients had improved diabetes control (more than a 0.5% reduction in HgbA$_{1c}$) than usual-care clients.

The implications are that a nurse-led, multidisciplinary health team can manage a population of clients with diabetes in an online disease management program. Clients demonstrating continuous engagement through sustained uploading of glucose readings achieved better results.

Source: Tang, P. C., Overhage, J. M., Chan, A. S., Brown, N. L., Aghighi, B., Entwistle, M. P.,... Young, C. Y. (2013). Online disease management of diabetes: Engaging and Motivating Clients Online With Enhanced Resources-Diabetes (EMPOWER-D), a randomized controlled trial. *Journal of the American Medical Informatics Association, 20,*(3), 526–534.

CASE STUDY 14-1

You are a nurse working in a busy primary care office and are in charge of a telephonic health intervention program to provide disease self-management to clients with multiple chronic conditions. The first self-management goal is to address medication self-management. You are preparing for your first call to a middle-aged gentleman who is living with poorly controlled diabetes, hypertension, hyperlipidemia, and newly diagnosed chronic obstructive pulmonary disease.

Discussion Questions

1. How do you begin your telephone call to introduce yourself and the self-management program?
2. The patient admits to not taking his medication regularly, especially his insulin, because he finds it difficult to take time during the day to monitor his blood sugar. How would you respond to this statement?
3. Which type of strategies will you use to assess this client's readiness to change his behavior?
4. Which questions will you ask to better understand his family and social supports and their influence on his disease self-management?

CASE STUDY 14-2

As an advanced practice registered nurse (APRN), you are writing a proposal to your practice manager in a busy internal medicine large group practice; the proposal seeks to begin diabetes group visits (DGVs) for clients with type 2 diabetes mellitus. Your plan is to start your DGVs within the next 2 months. You have already mentioned this potential project to several of your clients, and there is great deal of interest. The practice manager is reluctant to approve this new method in delivering health care, as this is not something the practice has done before. The manager would prefer you to continue seeing your clients individually. She sees no benefit in group visits and is not ready to support this practice innovation.

Discussion Questions

1. Which evidence would you use to support client outcomes of DGVs?
2. How would you explain how DGVs would impact your productivity and reimbursement?
3. Describe how the group visit is an effective model for the care for all chronic illnesses.
4. Which other innovations or uses of technology might also be an adjunct to the care of persons living with chronic illness to support and improve self-management?

STUDY QUESTIONS

1. How would you describe a chronic disease self-management program to a person and his or her family living with a newly diagnosed chronic disease?
2. Discuss factors that make disease self-management programs successful.
3. What are the three dimensions of self-management according the IFSMT?
4. Why is it necessary to think critically and be reflective to self-manage one's chronic illness?
5. Which types of activities do persons need to be able to do to self-manage chronic illness?
6. Which strategies might a nurse use in leading a chronic disease self-management program for persons and their families living with multiple chronic conditions?

Internet Resources

Primary care resources and supports (PCRS) for chronic disease management: http://improveselfmanagement.org

Stanford University School of Medicine, Chronic Disease Self-Management Program: http://clienteducation.stanford.edu/programs/cdsmp.html

National Council on Aging, Chronic Disease Self-Management Fact Sheet: http://www.ncoa.org /improve-health/center-for-healthy-aging/content-library/CDSMP-Fact-Sheet.pdf

Institute for Health Improvement (IHI), Self-Management Toolkit for People with Chronic Conditions and Their Families: http://www.ihi.org/knowledge/Pages/Tools/SelfManagementToolkitforClientsFamilies.aspx

Acknowledgment

The author would like to thank Judith E. Hertz for her work on the chapter entitled *Self-Care* in the eighth edition.

References

Administration on Aging (AOA). (2013). American Recovery and Reinvestment Act Communities putting prevention to work: Chronic disease self-management program. http://www.aoa.gov/AoA_programs/HPW/ARRA/index.aspx

Agency for Healthcare Research and Quality (AHRQ). (2010). Strategies to support self-management in chronic conditions: Collaboration with clients. Registered Nurses' Association of Ontario. http://www.guideline.gov/content.aspx?id=34758&search=self+management

American Association of Colleges of Nursing. (2006). The essentials of doctoral education for advanced nursing practice. http://www.aacn.nche.edu/publications/position/DNPEssentials.pdf

Ashman, J. J., & Beresovsky, V. (2013). Multiple chronic conditions among US adults who visited physician offices: Data from the national ambulatory medical care survey, 2009. *Prevention of Chronic Disease, 10.* doi: http://dx.doi.org/10.5888/pcd10.120308

Audulv, A., Asplund, K., & Norbergh, K-G. (2012). The integration of chronic illness self-management. *Qualitative Health Research, 22*(3), 332–345.

Barlow, J. H., Sturt, J., & Hearnshaw, H. (2002). Self-management interventions for people with chronic conditions in primary care: Examples from arthritis, asthma and diabetes. *Health Education Journal, 61*(4), 365–378.

Boyd, C. F. M. (2010). Future of multimorbidity research: How should understanding of multimorbidity inform health system design? *Public Health Reviews, 32*(2), 6.

Breitholtz, A., Snellman, I., & Fagerberg, I. (2013). Older people's dependence on caregivers' help in their own homes and their lived experiences of their opportunity to make independent decisions. *International Journal of Older People Nursing, 8*(2), 139–148. doi: 10.1111/j.1748-3743.2012.00338.x

Butterworth, S. W., Linden, A., & McClay, W. (2007). Health coaching as an intervention in health management programs. *Disease Management of Health Outcomes, 15*(5), 299–307.

Centers for Disease Control and Prevention (CDC). (2011). Healthy aging: Chronic disease prevention and health promotion. http://www.cdc.gov/chronicdisease/resources/publications/AAG/aging.htm

Clark, D. O., Frankel, R. M., Morgan, D. L., Ricketts, G., Bair, M. J., Nyland, K. A., & Callahan, C. M. (2008). The meaning and significance of self-management among socioeconomically vulnerable older adults. *Journals of Gerontology Series B: Psychological Sciences & Social Sciences, 63B*(5), S312–S319.

Corser, W., & Dontje, K. (2011). Self-management perspectives of heavily comorbid primary care adults. *Professional Case Management, 16*(1), 6–15. doi: 10.1097/NCM.0b013e3181f508d0

Creer, T. L., & Holroyd, K. A. (2006). Self-management of chronic conditions: The legacy of Sir William Osler. *Chronic Illness, 2*(1), 7–14.

Crist, J. D. (2005). The meaning for elders of receiving family care. *Journal of Advanced Nursing, 49*(5), 485–493. doi: 10.1111/j.1365-2648.2004.03321.x

DeLong, L. K., Culler, S. D., Saini, S. S., Beck, L. A., & Chen, S. C. (2008). Annual direct and indirect health care costs of chronic idiopathic urticaria: A cost analysis of 50 non-immunosuppressed clients. *Archives of Dermatology, 144*(1), 35–39.

Donlan, W. (2011). The meaning of community-based care for frail Mexican American elders. *International Social Work, 54*(3), 388–403. doi: 10.1177/0020872810396258

Dunn, K. S., & Riley-Doucet, C. (2007). Self-care activities captured through discussion among community-dwelling older adults. *Journal of Holistic Nursing, 25*(3), 160–169.

Dyck, I., Kontos, P., Angus, J., & McKeever, P. (2005). The home as a site for long-term care: Meanings and management of bodies and spaces. *Health & Place, 11*(2), 173–185.

Ebrahimi, Z., Wilhelmson, K., Moore, C. D., & Jakobsson, A. (2012). Frail elders' experiences with and perceptions of health. *Qualitative Health Research, 22*(11), 1513–1523.

Fortin, M., Lapointe, L., Hudon, C., & Vanasse, A. (2005). Multimorbidity is common to family practice: Is it commonly researched? *Canadian Family Physician, 51*, 244–245.

From, I., Johansson, I., & Athlin, E. (2007). Experiences of health and well-being, a question of adjustment and compensation: Views of older people dependent on community care. *International Journal of Older People Nursing, 2*(4), 278–287.

Grey, M., Knafl, K., & McCorkle, R. (2006). A framework for the study of self-and family management of chronic conditions. *Nursing Outlook, 54*(5), 278–286.

Haslbeck, J. W., McCorkle, R., & Schaeffer, D. (2012). Chronic illness self-management while living alone in later life: A systematic integrative review. *Research on Aging, 34*(5), 507–547.

Hertz, J. E., & Anschutz, C. A. (2002). Relationships among perceived enactment of autonomy, self-care, and holistic health in community-dwelling older adults. *Journal of Holistic Nursing, 20*(2), 166–186.

Holman, H., & Lorig, K. (2004). Client self-management: A key to effectiveness and efficiency in care of chronic disease. *Public Health Reports, 119*(3), 239.

Holmberg, M., Valmari, G., & Lundgren, S. M. (2012). Patients' experiences of homecare nursing: Balancing the duality between obtaining care and to maintain dignity and self-determination. *Scandinavian Journal of Caring Sciences, 26*(4), 705–712.

Howard, L. M., & Ceci, C. (2013). Problematizing health coaching for chronic illness self-management. *Nursing Inquiry, 20*(3), 223–231.

Huffman, M. (2007). Health coaching: A new and exciting technique to enhance client self-management and improve outcomes. *Home Healthcare Nurse, 25*(4), 271–274.

Huffman, M. (2009). Health coaching: A fresh, new approach to improve quality outcomes and compliance for clients with chronic conditions. *Home Healthcare Nurse, 27*(8), 491–496.

Improving Chronic Illness Care. (2006). The chronic care model: Self management support. http://www.improvingchroniccare.org/index.php?p=Self-Management_Support&s=22

Jacelon, C. S. (2010). Maintaining the balance: Older adults with chronic health problems manage life in the community. *Rehabilitation Nursing, 35*(1), 16–22.

Jacelon, C. S., Furman, E., Rea, A., Macdonald, B., & Donoghue, L. C. (2011). Creating a professional practice model for post acute care: Adapting the chronic care model for long-term care. *Journal of Gerontological Nursing, 37*(3), 53–60.

Kawi, J. (2012). Self-management support in chronic illness care: A concept analysis. *Research and Theory for Nursing Practice: An International Journal, 26*(2), 108–125.

Kaye, H. S. (2012). Gradual rebalancing of Medicaid long-term services and supports saves money and serves more people, statistical model shows. *Health Affairs, 31*(6), 1195–1203.

Klymko, K. W., Artinian, N. T., Price, J. E., Abele, C., & Washington, O. G. (2011). Self-care production experiences in elderly African Americans with hypertension and cognitive difficulty. *Journal of the American Academy of Nurse Practitioners, 23*(4), 200–208. doi: 10.1111/j.1745-7599.2011.00605.x

Koch, T., Jenkin, P., & Kralik, D. (2004). Chronic illness self-management: Locating the 'self'. *Journal of Advanced Nursing, 48*(5), 484–492.

Kralik, D., Koch, T., Price, K., & Howard, N. (2004). Chronic illness self-management: Taking action to create order. *Journal of Clinical Nursing, 13*(2), 259–267. doi: 10.1046/j.1365-2702.2003.00826.x

Lindahl, B., Lide'n, E., & Lindblad, B. M. (2011). A meta-synthesis describing the relationships between clients, informal caregivers and health professionals in home-care settings. *Journal of Clinical Nursing, 2*, 3–4.

Marek, K. D., Stetzer, F., Ryan, P. A., Bub, L. D., Adams, S. J., Schlidt, A., ... O'Brien, A. M. (2013). Nurse care coordination and technology effects on health status of frail older adults via enhanced self-management of medication: Randomized clinical trial to test efficacy. *Nursing Research, 62*(4), 269–278.

Marengoni, A., Angleman, S., Melis, R., Mangialasche, F., Karp, A., Garmen, A., ... Fratiglioni, L. (2011). Aging with multimorbidity: A systematic review of the literature. *Ageing Research Review, 10*(4), 430–439. doi: 10.1016/j.arr.2011.03.003

Morrison, S. (2007). Self-management support: Helping clients set goals to improve their health. National Health Care for the Homeless Council. http://www.nhchc.org/wp-content/uploads/2011/09/SelfManagementSupport052907.pdf

National Institute of Aging (NIA). (2011). Why population aging matters: A global perspective. http://www.nia.nih.gov/health/publication/why-population-aging-matters-global-perspective/endnote-data-aging-world

Nicholson, C., Meyer, J., Flatley, M., & Holman, C. (2013). The experience of living at home with frailty in old age: A psychosocial qualitative study. *International Journal of Nursing Studies, 50*(9), 1172–1179.

Ory, M. G., Ahn, S., Jiang, L., Lorig, K., Ritter, P., Laurent, D. D., ... Smith, M. L. (2013). National study of chronic disease self-management: Six-month outcome findings. *Journal of Aging and Health, 25*(7), 1258–1274.

Park, Y. H., Chang, H., Kim, J., & Kwak, J. S. (2012). Client-tailored self-management intervention for older adults with hypertension in a nursing home. *Journal of Clinical Nursing, 22*(5), 710–722.

Redman, B. K. (2007). Responsibility for control: Ethics of client preparation for self-management of chronic disease. *Bioethics, 21*(5), 243–250.

Riegel, B., Jaarsma, T., & Strömberg, A. (2012). A middle-range theory of self-care of chronic illness. *Advances in Nursing Science, 35*(3), 194–204.

Ryan, P., & Sawin, K. J. (2009). The individual and family self-management theory: Background and perspectives on context, process, and outcomes. *Nursing Outlook, 57*(4), 217–225.

Santana, M. J., & Feeny, D. (2014). Framework to assess the effects of using patient-reported outcome measures in chronic care management. *Quality of Life Research, 23*(5), 1505–13.

Schulman-Green, D., Jaser, S., Martin, F., Alonzo, A., Grey, M., McCorkle, R., ... Whittemore, R. (2012). Processes of self-management of chronic illness. *Journal of Nursing Scholarship, 44*(2), 136–144.

Simmons, C., & Kapustin, J. F. (2011). Diabetes group visits: An alternative to managing chronic disease outcomes. *Journal for Nurse Practitioners, 7*(8), 671–679.

Söderhamn, U., Dale, B., & Söderhamn, O. (2013). The meaning of actualization of self-care resources among a group of older home-dwelling people: A hermeneutic study. *International Journal of Qualitative Study of Health Well-Being, 8*, 20592. http://dx.doi.org/10.3402/qhw.v8i0.20592 doi:10.3402/qhw.v8i0.20592

Spencer, S. M., Patrick, J. H., & Steele, J. C. (2009). An exploratory look at preferences for seven long-term care options. *Seniors Housing & Care Journal, 17*(1), 91–99.

Swanlund, S., Scherck, K., Metcalfe, S., & Jesek-Hale, S. (2008). Keys to successful self-management of medications. *Nursing Science Quarterly, 21*(3), 238–246.

Tang, P. C., Overhage, J. M., Chan, A. S., Brown, N. L., Aghighi, B., Entwistle, M. P., ... Young, C. Y. (2013). Online disease management of diabetes: Engaging and Motivating Clients Online With Enhanced Resources-Diabetes (EMPOWER-D), a randomized controlled trial. *Journal of the American Medical Informatics Association, 20*(3), 526–534.

Tanner, E. (2004). Chronic illness demands for self-management in older adults. *Geriatric Nursing, 25*(5), 313–317.

U.S. Department of Health and Human Services (HHS). (2010). Multiple chronic illness framework goals. http://www.hhs.gov/ash/initiatives/mcc/goals /framework-goals.html

U.S. Department of Health and Human Services (HHS), Office of Disease Prevention and Health Promotion. (2013). *Healthy people 2020*. Washington, DC. http:// www.healthypeople.gov/2020/default.aspx. doi: 10.1001/archdermatol.2007.5

Vogeli, C., Shields, A., Lee, T., Gibson, T., Marder, W., Weiss, K., & Blumenthal, D. (2007). Multiple chronic conditions: Prevalence, health consequences, and implications for quality, care management, and costs. *Journal of General Internal Medicine, 22*, 391–395.

Wagner, E. H. (1998). Chronic disease management: What will it take to improve care for chronic illness? *Effective Clinical Practice, 1*(1), 2–4.

Part II

Impact of the System

Chapter 15

Client and Family Education

Elaine T. Miller

Introduction

For most clients and their families, chronic illness creates a life-changing event, uniquely affecting them as they deal with the long-term nature of the illness, the added demands on their lives, and its impact on their physical, psychological, economic, social, and spiritual being. Even more importantly, chronic illnesses do not always have a similar predictable trajectory of presentation and management (e.g., heart disease, cancer, stroke, diabetes, arthritis, asthma, hypertension). These diseases also do not discriminate according to age, race, gender, socioeconomic status, culture or ethnicity, or learning capability. Moreover, the client's and family's response and resources to cope with chronic illnesses may vary tremendously, requiring healthcare professionals (HCPs) to be attuned to each client's and family's particular strengths/limitations, needs, expectations, resources, and personal goals.

In the United States, chronic illness is the leading cause of death and disability, consuming 75% of all healthcare dollars spent each year and lowering quality of life for millions of people (Centers for Disease Control and Prevention [CDC], 2013a). The vast majority of chronic diseases (e.g., stroke, heart disease, hypertension, pulmonary, hypertension), however, could be prevented or better managed by adopting a more client-centered,

interprofessional, evidence-based approach that fosters client and family involvement, client self-management, and continuous quality improvement (Dwamena et al., 2012; Jacobs, Jones, Gabella, Spring, & Brownson, 2012; Wensing & Kersnik, 2012). For instance, Auger, Kenyon, Feudtner, and Davis (2014), in their systematic review of 14 research studies, discovered that targeted education and feedback along with coordinated postdischarge support can reduce subsequent emergency room visits and readmissions of chronically ill children with asthma or cancer.

Increasingly, research supports the notion that maximizing the client's and family's coping abilities for chronic illness and improving their knowledge, attitudes, and behaviors, in conjunction with HCPs providing a more unified approach and subsequent monitoring, management, and evaluation of care outcomes, are central in the care delivery process (Cameron, 2013; Kyung, Fritschi, & Kim, 2012). Given that many clients and their families are likely to experience more than one chronic illness in their lifetime, it is critical for HCPs to be cognizant of the potential interplay of diverse chronic illnesses that may influence the client's and family's responses to further losses, such as those associated with incontinence, fatigue, diminishing cognitive function, or mobility.

It is well documented that educating clients and their families is critical to successful coping with chronic illnesses and overall long-term quality of life. In addition, the family frequently serves as the client's primary support system, affecting the client's decision making about health, willingness and ability to seek health care, and adherence to recommended healthcare recommendations (e.g., taking prescribed medication, following a diet, having a recommended procedure or test) (Delisel, 2013; Falvo, 2011). Although there are often some commonalities, each client and family situation has its distinctive characteristics that require HCPs to approach every situation carefully and systematically, without making assumptions about the client's and family's resources, capability to learn, and ability to achieve educational outcomes. In addition, HCPs must continually assess the factors influencing the client's and family's educational needs, their resources (e.g., social support, financial, geographic), the teaching and learning approach, and evaluation of short- and long-term outcomes. Another central element in this educational process is identifying what clients and their families want to learn, establishing their priorities in terms of their educational needs, and engaging in mutual goal setting, so that clients, families, and HCPs are working together to achieve common short-term as well as long-term goals.

Because numerous factors contribute to the success or failure of client and family education related to chronic illness, this chapter presents an overview of the fundamental elements that should be considered and clarifies the state of evidence-based knowledge pertaining to client and family education related to chronic illnesses. Even though much is known about client and family education, the literature and research do not suggest simple solutions or approaches that will optimize this educational process in all situations. Moreover, the nature of the chronic disease(s) as well as specific attributes of the learner(s), such as age, gender, race/ethnicity, culture, socioeconomic status, motivation, self-efficacy, general health literacy, reading ability,

psychological conditions (e.g., depression, bipolar disorder), sensory deficits (e.g., low-level vision, hearing impairment, learning capability), and/or learning disabilities, will significantly influence how the HCP approaches and evaluates the success of each client and family educational encounter. The primary focus of this chapter is the adult learner. However, a basic distinction is described regarding key learning differences between adults and children. Finally, because this chapter purports to present only a broad overview of key issues affecting client and family educational processes regarding chronic illnesses, it is highly recommended that additional evidence-based resources be obtained that more specifically target the chronic illness and client population of concern, recognizing that research and the associated findings continue to expand the science of what is known.

The Teaching–Learning Process

The teaching–learning process is characterized by multifaceted, dynamic, and interactive exchanges that are fundamental to client–family education and nursing practice. Teaching involves a deliberative, intentional act of communicating information to individuals in response to their identified educational needs and with the objective of achieving a desired outcome (Bastable, 2014, Falvo, 2011; McDonald, 2014). Learning, by comparison, assists the individual to acquire new knowledge, skills, and/or attitudes that can be measured (Bastable, 2014; McDonald, 2014). As the HCP reflects on the purpose of the educational activity, more than 40 major evidence-based teaching–learning theories offer ways to assess the learning situation, identify educational objectives, design the educational intervention(s), and determine educational outcomes. For example, perhaps you have a newly diagnosed client with hypertension who needs to learn how to take her medication as prescribed, lose 25 pounds, eat a more healthy diet, and more effectively manage her work- and family-related stress.

A variety of frameworks should be considered. Perhaps social cognitive theory would be appropriate, or humanistic learning theory, or even constructionist theory? A general listing of the major possibilities can be obtained at http://www.learning-theories.com

Before moving forward to illustrate how teaching–learning theories can affect the design of educational experiences for a diverse population of clients/families living with chronic illnesses, it is recommended HCPs consider a shift in thinking from content- or teacher-centered teaching to learner-centered teaching. **Table 15-1** describes the essential differences between these two paradigms when framed within the context of client/family education.

When reviewing the various teaching–learning theories, it becomes readily apparent that each theory offers a different orientation regarding what is most important and what should be the HCP's focus of attention when educating individuals with chronic illness and their families. Every theory has a particular perspective in terms of the purpose of education, assessment of learning needs, structuring of the teaching and learning process according to the theory's assumptions, concepts and relationship statements of the selected theory, measurement of concepts, and evaluation of the success of the educational activity in the short and long term. Moreover, when contemplating a particular teaching–learning theory, it is always advisable to go to the literature and determine if evidence exists, to assess the quality of the evidence, and to determine how the present teaching–learning situation fits (e.g., client/family population, context, preferred outcomes) with previous research. In addition, have any best practices been established, or is the evidence limited or not rigorously performed? Collectively, all of this information then guides how educators operationalize the theory to the specific client/family learning situation.

Table 15-1 Client Centered versus Educator Centered Teaching

Client/Family (Learner) Centered	HCP Educator (Teacher) Centered
Focus on the client/family and the educator, with collaborative educational goal setting	Focus on the HCP performing the teaching
Client/family actively interact and are involved with the HCP educator	HCP educator talks and the client/family listen
Client/family has consistent two-way communication with the HCP educator, who monitors progress along with the client/family; each party provides feedback and collaborates on revising the educational plan and outcomes	HCP educator monitors and corrects the client/family: one-way communication
Emphasis of the interaction is to communicate knowledge and address continuing and emerging issues in the client/family's real-life situation	Acquisition of knowledge is the focus but may not be specifically tailored to the particular client/family issues or problems
Client/family evaluate their short- and long-term learning outcomes, as does the educator	Learning is determined by the educator
Educational environment is cooperative, collaborative, and supportive	Educational environment is more individualistic and nonparticipatory

For example, when the behaviorist framework is applied, learning is envisioned as resulting from the connections between the stimuli in the environment and the individual's responses (Skinner, 1974). Within this framework, the educator would identify environmental or supportive actions (e.g., educational booklets pertaining to hypertension and lifestyle changes, hospital educational cable channel, location of exercise facilities or walking paths in neighborhood, local support groups, praise when progress in weight reduction occurs) enabling the particular client to follow the prescribed antihypertensive medication regimen and lifestyle changes that would foster weight reduction.

Social cognitive theory, in contrast, involves role modeling as a central concept and offers a different approach to teaching clients and their families to perform the same task (Bandura, 1986). In this identical client/family situation when applying social cognitive theory, the HCP would discuss strategies to foster long-term adherence with taking antihypertensive medication as prescribed, making appropriate menu choices that fit with the recommended diet plan, and identifying a realistic exercise routine that could contribute to weight loss of 1–2 pounds per week. In this theory, feedback is very important, so the HCP would make sure it is given in a manner that enhances the confidence of the client and perhaps revise the recommended plan and actions based on progress in achieving the mutually established plan and outcome by the client/family and educator.

Meanwhile, if Maslow's hierarchy of needs (one of the best-known humanistic frameworks; Maslow, 1962) is applied to this identical scenario, the educator would first need to fulfill lower-level physiologic needs before reviewing strategies that would enable the client to correctly take the prescribed antihypertensive medications as well as consume a balanced diet and increase regular exercise to facilitate long-term weight loss. When using this framework, mutual goal setting and

feedback are not normally included, but they could be if the educator used this framework and superimposed a learner-centered teaching–learning approach.

Finally, the constructionist learning theory offers yet another viable theoretical perspective to guide the HCP's educational encounter. It emphasizes that learners are actively creating meaning as they learn. When viewed from this constructionist orientation, learning is perceived as contextual, not only requiring time, social contact, and motivation, but also creating meanings that foster learning over time (Hein, 1991). With regard to learning how to take medications as prescribed, the constructionist theory provides a framework to connect the client's understanding/meaning of why it is essential to take antihypertensive medications as prescribed, how to manage any side effects, and the client's motivation to learn, and then applies this knowledge to a regular life pattern and promotion of long-term health. What is imperative when applying constructionist theory to this scenario is being attuned to the client and/or family and their perceptions and meanings associated with the medication, lifestyle changes, and what is feasible in their life situation over the short and long term.

In conjunction with the numerous teaching–learning theories that guide the HCP's client/family educational encounters, it is valuable to contemplate several basic assumptions underpinning these interactions. According to Petty (2006), learning involves "an active process of making sense and creating a personal interpretation of what has been learned" (p. 8), rather than simply being an exact interpretation of what has been taught. What occurs is more than a storing of personal interpretations of facts and ideas; it is "also linking them in a way that relates ideas to other ideas, and to prior learning, and so creates meaning and understanding" (p. 8). According to this perspective, learners create meaning that is more easily applied to solve problems, make judgments, and assist clients and their families to perform the numerous tasks associated with living with one or more chronic illnesses. Evidence is steadily expanding to support the constructivism perspective and its positive outcomes (Muijs & Reynolds, 2005; Rhee, Zwar, & Kemp. 2013). In addition, results from multiple meta-analyses of educational research reinforce the pivotal influence that feedback and reinforcement exert on individual teaching as well as group teaching (Petty, 2006).

In summary, theoretical frameworks offer alternative ways to approach a teaching–learning situation involving clients and their families. Because myriad theoretical frameworks exist, it is important that HCPs determine what is most relevant to each specific situation, examine available evidence-based research pertaining to that framework (preferably evidence published in the last 5 years), then translate that framework to the particular client/family interactions and systematically evaluate the efficacy of using that perspective to direct their educational interventions.

Significance of Client and Family Teaching to Practice and Healthcare Costs

Practice standards from the American Nurses Association (ANA), the American Association of Colleges of Nursing (AACN), the National League for Nursing (NLN), specialty nursing practice standards, and other national documents consistently identify health teaching as a fundamental component of nursing practice (AACN, 2008; ANA, 2010; Camica et al., 2014; Lindell et al., 2005; NLN, 2003). Even in the early writings of Florence Nightingale, teaching was recognized as a prominent nursing activity (Nightingale, 1992). In addition, all state nurse practice acts include teaching within the scope of nursing practice responsibilities and identify teaching as essential in promoting optimal health and disease management of clients and their families.

The underlying premise of *Healthy People 2010* and *Healthy People 2020* (U.S. Department of Health and Human Services [DHHS], 2010) is that an individual's health is almost inseparable from the health of the larger community and is profoundly influenced by the collective beliefs, attitudes, and behaviors of this community. Throughout this comprehensive national health promotion and disease prevention roadmap, there is a recurrent theme emphasizing the improvement of "the availability and dissemination of health related information" (*Healthy People 2010,* n.d., p. 17) pertaining to the leading health indicators of our society. Central to accomplishing these health objectives is education of all stakeholders (e.g.., clients, families, HCPs, the overall community). *Healthy People 2020* further emphasizes how disparities in income and education are associated with increased occurrence of illness and death and places greater importance on targeting community-based health educational programming.

For instance, *Healthy People 2020* focuses on systematic and targeted health promotion education and preventive actions for adults who are most at risk for long-term health problems/diseases. In addition, the 2020 edition emphasizes the coordination and targeting of health promotion education and other activities beginning in preschool and continuing through high school. *Healthy People 2020* concentrates on health problems such as unintentional injury, violence, dental caries, unhealthy dietary patterns, tobacco use and addiction, and alcohol and drug use—all factors that have ramifications for long-term chronic health issues.

In addition to *Healthy People 2020*'s emphasis on evidence-based, coordinated, targeted, and individualized client and family education, The Joint Commission's (2012) *2012 Hospital Accreditation Standards* identify specific critical educational standards that must be achieved by organizations seeking accreditation. The Joint Commission (2012) standards include the following items:

PC.02.03.01 The hospital provides client education and training on each client's needs and abilities.

- The hospital performs a learning needs assessment for each client, which includes the client's culture and religious beliefs, emotional barriers, desire and motivation to learn, physical or cognitive limitations, and barriers to communication.
- The hospital provides education and training to the client based on assessed needs.
- The hospital coordinates the client education and training provided by all disciplines involved in the patient's care, treatment, and services.
- Based on the client's condition and assessed needs, the education and training provided to the client by the hospital include any of the following:
  - An explanation of the plan of care, treatment, and services
  - Basic health and safety information
  - Information on the safe and effective use of medications
  - Nutrition information (e.g., supplements) and modified diets
  - Discussion of pain, risk for pain, the importance of effective pain management, the pain assessment process, and methods for pain management
  - Information on oral health
  - Information on safe and effective use of medical equipment or supplies provided by the hospital
  - Habilitation or rehabilitation techniques to help the client reach maximum independence
- Evaluate the client's understanding of the education and training
- Provide education on how to communicate concerns about client safety issues that occur before, during or after care is received

Several additional Joint Commission standards reference the need for client education:

- NPSG.03.05.01: Reduce the likelihood of client harm associated with the use of anti-coagulant therapy.
- NPSG.03.06.01: Maintain and communicate accurate client medication information.
- NPSG.0703.01: Implement evidence-based practices to prevent healthcare-associated infections due to multidrug-resistant organisms in acute care hospitals.
- NPSG.07.04.01: Implement evidence-based practices to prevent central line–associated bloodstream infections.
- NPSG.07.05.01: Implement evidence-based practices to prevent surgical site infections.
- PC.02.03.03: The client's personal hygiene is maintained.
- PC.010.03.03: The hospital defines its client behavior management policies.
- PC.01.03.05: The hospital's use of behavior management procedures adheres to the client's plan of care, treatment, and services and organizational policy.
- PC.03.01.03: The hospital provides the client with care before initiating operative or other high-risk procedures, including those that require the administration of moderate or deep sedation anesthesia.

The Joint Commission education standards further specify that clients and families assume an active role in this process and have responsibilities just as the educator does. In instances where clients do not understand the information, they are to indicate this fact and must take responsibility for self-management of their needs when capable (e.g., medication, safety, nutrition, pain). Moreover, the educator is expected to consistently and comprehensively assess the client's and family's learning needs and barriers affecting the educational outcomes. According to The Joint Commission, the educational activities must be coordinated, tailored according to the client's and family's needs/abilities, and evaluated to determine whether learning has occurred.

Data from the CDC highlight the pivotal role that education has in clients' self-management of chronic illness. For instance, the CDC (2005) reports that for each $1.00 invested in diabetic education to assist clients in self-managing their diabetes and preventing hospitalizations, healthcare costs are reduced by $8.76. With regard to heart disease and stroke, the CDC further emphasizes that much of the burden associated with these two diseases can be eliminated by reduction of major risk factors such as high blood pressure, high cholesterol, tobacco use, limited physical activity, and poor nutrition. By targeting client and family education to those modifiable risk factors, the likelihood of heart disease and stroke can be significantly diminished and personal and financial costs reduced. The CDC's (2013b) Chronic Disease Cost Calculator permits determination of state-level estimates of medical expenditures and absenteeism costs for arthritis, asthma, cancer, cardiovascular diseases, depression, and diabetes.

The 2010 passage of the Patient Protection and Affordable Care Act (ACA) into law is anticipated to reduce the number of uninsured individuals in the United States by 31 million people by 2019, at a net cost of $938 billion over 10 years, while reducing the deficit emerging from escalating healthcare costs by $124 billion during that same time period (Kaiser Foundation, 2010). Among the benefits of this law are the following:

- Insurance for people with preexisting conditions
- Coverage for preventive care and screenings such as immunizations and screening for conditions such as cancer and diabetes
- More spending on care—at least 80% of a customer's premium dollars need to be for direct medical care and efforts to improve quality care

- All insurance plans must include mental health and substance abuse services by 2014
- Persons with Medicare have an annual wellness visit that includes a personalized prevention plan that identifies health risk factors and treatment options

A main feature of these changes and others included within this legislation is the focus on prevention and management of chronic health conditions. As a result, identifying evidence-based, effective, timely, and targeted educational interventions will be pivotal to achievement of the desired short- and long-term health outcomes in settings ranging from acute care to long-term care. In addition, with the passage of the ACA, there is a growing demand to perform research and thereby expand the evidence base that underpins nurses' educational interventions and attainment of the preferred client and family outcomes. When contemplating how to choose and develop such written educational materials, Pierce (2010) provides valuable recommendations that should be considered.

Further acknowledgment of the escalating importance internationally of healthcare education is illustrated by the Institute of Medicine's (IOM) Global Forum on Innovation in Health Professional Education. This IOM forum was created in 2013 to encourage multinational and interprofessional stakeholders to engage in discussion of contemporary issues in health professional education and to cultivate new educational ideas and approaches through global, interprofessional collaborative partnerships between university-based health institutions that are seeking to implement recommendations from either the 2010 Lancet Commission report or the Future of Nursing report. The four innovation collaborators are located in Canada, India, South Africa, and Uganda (http://www.iom.edu/Activities/Global/InnovationHealthProfEducation.aspx).

Major Learning Considerations of Children, Young and Middle-Age Adults, and Older Adults

It is essential that the educator consider the differences associated with working with children, younger adults, and older persons (Bastable, 2014; Mauk, 2014) when designing and executing educational activities for clients and their families. The science and art of teaching children (pedagogy) involves a distinctive approach and level of understanding compared to the teaching of younger adults (andragogy) and the teaching of older adults (gerogogy). Like the other perspectives, gerogogy must accommodate the physical, cognitive, psychosocial, and spiritual elements observed during this phase of growth and development. Older adults are very capable of learning and adapting to new situations, but when structuring their educational interventions consideration needs to be given to establishing rapport, developing personalized goals, cueing, positive reinforcement, pacing with rest periods, rehearsing, time for questions and internalizing of information, flexibility, relaxed environment, and easily read materials or resources for hearing-impaired individuals (Mauk, 2014; Miller & Harris, 2013).

Evaluating the Quality of Research and Evidence to Guide Educational Interventions

When developing educational interventions for clients and their families, it is essential to first determine the quality of the evidence that forms the basis for the planned actions. Evidence-based practice (EBP) refers to a problem-solving approach used in practice that combines three components: the best available evidence, the HCP's clinical expertise, and the client's values and preferences (Melnyk & Fineout-Overholt, 2010). A meta-analysis and systematic review of randomized controlled trials (RCTs) is recognized as the highest level of evidence (Melnyk & Fineout-Overholt, 2010).

Unfortunately, a sizable portion of the currently available evidence falls short of this standard, with lower levels of evidence—such as single randomized trials, nonrandomized studies, consensus opinion of experts, and case studies—still being very prevalent. As a result, educators must carefully scrutinize the rigor and level of the available evidence to determine its applicability to each educational situation and always consider the unique client/family and teaching situation attributes.

Research is constantly evolving and affecting how we look at the teaching and learning environment and modalities. The Pew Research Center's Internet and American Life Project (Brenner & Stone, 2013), for instance, discovered that almost three fourths (72%) of U.S. adults use online social networking sites, up from 67% in 2012. Younger adults are widely recognized as avid adopters of this technology, but this study discovered that 6 out of 10 Internet users aged 50–64 accessed social networking sites and adults aged 65 and older have tripled their use in the last four years (from 13% in 2009 to 43% in 2013). Freeman (2012) further revealed that more than 90% of those persons aged 18–24 trust the health information they find on social media. A 2012 PriceWaterhouseCoopers (PwC) survey found that one third of consumers now use social media sites such as Facebook, YouTube, Twitter, and other online forums.

Fortunately, healthcare organizations and educators are starting to recognize the power of social media sites. Moreover, educators and nurses in particular have a professional responsibility to cultivate in clients and families an appreciation of the importance of identifying and accessing reputable healthcare information sources (e.g., CDC, National Institutes of Health, Cochrane Library, PubMed, World Health Organization) and of finding the most up-to-date evidence. Gremeaux and Coudeyre's (2010) systematic review focused on the accuracy of Internet sites for chronic disease management, with the authors concluding that Internet sites must be improved.

Assessment of the Learner

Evidence indicates that the assessment process associated with the teaching–learning experience of the client and family is frequently not given the proper attention that it deserves (McDonald, 2014). It is imperative that an individualized client and family assessment occur, and that this information then be incorporated into the client- and/or family-centered learning objectives, planning, implementation, and evaluation of the outcomes of each educational encounter. Because it is assumed that the client and family dealing with the chronic illness are equal partners with the HCP, the following are critical questions to ask the client and family:

- Which information do you want provided? Recognize that the client and family may identify different needs and that these needs may differ from what the educator views as most important. If such a discrepancy occurs, make sure each of the client/family needs is addressed. In addition, working on what the client and/or family member considers vital will facilitate rapport and lead to a more collaborative and respectful exchange.
- Are there any new skills that you want to learn or ones you want to review?
- What are the specific educational goals for the client and family? You may need to give an example (e.g., correctly identify signs/symptoms of hypoglycemic reactions, know what to do when an insulin reaction occurs, and how to correctly give an insulin injection). Do not assume that just because a client has had, for instance, diabetes for 5 years, the person is well informed, has accurate information, and does what the client says he or she does. It is best to observe the client perform an activity from beginning to end—for example, from washing the hands prior to drawing up the insulin (correct amount, type), to administering the injection correctly, to rotating injection sites.

- Is the focus of the education on knowledge acquisition, improved attitude, or confidence in ability to perform an activity and/or a particular behavior (e.g., administer an injection or change a dressing correctly, safely transfer the client from a bed to a chair)?
- Of the goals identified, which are the most important? Once again, the client and family may differ markedly in their specific goals and priorities. Listen carefully to both of them.
- What does the client perceive as factors that will affect the client's ability to achieve these educational goals? How will any barriers be overcome?
- Does the client feel confident using the information provided? If not, how might the HCP assist the client in increasing confidence and ability to use this information?

When clients and family members are providing answers, the HCP must be an astute listener, nonjudgmental, and capable of developing individualized and attainable client and/or family goals, and must reflect back to the client and family an understanding of what has been heard (Bastable, 2014; Miller et al., 2010). While collecting the relevant client and family data, the HCP needs to be organized, perform the assessment in a timely manner, and be aware of the readability of assessment materials. In addition, the client with chronic illness often has associated limitations that affect the assessment (e.g., easily fatigued and diminished hearing and/or vision and/or comprehension). Packer and colleagues (2012) further emphasize that when clients with low socioeconomic status have a positive attitude and are encouraged to participate in either generic or disease-specific educational programing, health improves.

Influences on Teaching and Learning

This section identifies a variety of factors that may influence the teaching–learning process.

The list of factors presented here is not all inclusive. Each individual with chronic illness is unique and his or her teaching–learning may be influenced by other factors.

Family Structure and Function

Families can vary significantly in structure and function. The chronic illness of a family member often precipitates changes in the family structure and function, as do changes associated with marriage, raising children, or death of a family member. When a family has a member with a chronic illness, the family's response to this change and its capacity to adapt and make decisions can influence their receptiveness to education. When the client and family experience high anxiety, that factor can markedly interfere with their ability to receive and comprehend information, maintain normal patterns of family functioning, and use appropriate coping skills. Because culture and lifestyle affect the development of family norms and beliefs, differences in these client/family and HCP factors can affect the dynamics of the educational process (Deng, Zhang, & Chan, 2013; Rankin, Stallings, & London, 2005; Rivers, August, Sehovic, Green, & Quinn, 2013; Smith, Roth, Okoro, Kimberlin, & Odedina, 2011). Once these beliefs and values are identified, they can be addressed through individualized teaching. It is imperative, therefore, that the family structure, function (e.g., roles, resources, strengths, and weaknesses), and norms be considered in the assessment and educational planning process.

According to the 2012 Joint Commission standards, the family is to be included in client teaching (e.g., fall-reduction strategies, reporting concerns related to care and safety). Because the client's family may be large with members having varying roles and functions, the HCP must determine the primary family member who should receive the relevant education. Just as in the case of the client, the HCP needs to assess the primary family caregiver's role, expectations, learning needs/goals, learning style,

fears, concerns, cognitive and physical abilities, and present knowledge pertaining to the client's healthcare needs (Bastable, 2014; Miller et al., 2010). Moreover, the client and the family member may need to receive similar information, reinforcement, and feedback related to their knowledge and/or skill performance. In many instances, the family member is the single most important factor in determining the success or failure of the teaching plan (Haggard, 1989).

Culture

When working with clients and their families, culture can dramatically affect how educational activities are structured, delivered, and evaluated. The client's and family's culture represents a fundamental component of their lives; culture includes integrated patterns of human behavior such as language, thoughts, communications, actions, customs, beliefs, values, and institutions of racial, ethnic, religious, and social groups (Office of Minority Health, 2013). A fundamental first step for the HCP is becoming culturally sensitive, which refers to the process of becoming aware of one's own biases and prejudices about another culture or ethnic group. Cultural competence—a higher level of knowledge—denotes educational interventions reflecting knowledge, understanding, respect, and acceptance of the client's and/or family's culture (Bastable, 2014).

For a successful educational encounter to occur, HCPs, clients, and families must bridge these cultural differences through the use of effective interpersonal communication. The establishment of a common understanding between HCPs and clients and their families is facilitated by the HCP performing the following tasks:

- Explore and respect the client/family's beliefs, values, and effectiveness of communication by determining whether the HCP truly comprehends the client/family's stated meaning of the chronic illness, preferences, support systems, resources, and needs.

- Identify what will build rapport and trust. Potential sources of information to assist in this process include other colleagues, family members of the client, community groups, and reputable websites.
- Determine whether there are any common views or interests.
- Identify the HCP's own biases and assumptions.
- Maintain and convey an unconditional positive regard. Be an excellent listener, be open and nonjudgmental, and use consistent perception checks to assess comprehension of what has been communicated.
- Become knowledgeable of the culture and health disparities/discrimination of the particular client/family's culture. Websites listed at the end of this chapter can provide a starting point for resources from reputable sources.
- Use interpreter services when needed.

Cultural differences make each client and family situation unique, but some essential considerations also apply across communication, interactions, and the ultimate delivery of any educational activity. For example, Deng, Zhang, and Chan (2013) examined the general barriers to adherence of Chinese immigrants in the United States to a specific diet; the researchers discovered that with respect to nutritional interventions for type 2 diabetes, acceptance and adherence over the long term depended on overall health literacy as well as the cultural acceptability of the recommended diet. When planning these interventions, it is important to appreciate traditional Chinese families' filial piety. Respect for elders is highly valued in Chinese American families, but less so in American culture. As a result, Chinese elders may perceive less family support, especially for diabetes management practices. In addition, lower socioeconomic status was identified as leading to loss of respect, depression, burden on

family caregivers, and barriers to activities such as physical activity. Moreover, within the family, interpersonal harmony was an important value, leading Chinese Americans to not express negative emotions in front of their family.

In an effort to reduce health disparities and improve education of those most at risk for heart failure, Nundy and colleagues (2013) performed a study to assess the feasibility and acceptability of text message–based interventions in a largely African American population as well as the program's effects on self-management. Participants in this study, all of whom had heart failure, received automated text messages. These messages provided self-care reminders and education on diet, symptom recognition, and healthcare navigation. Results indicated that there was observable client satisfaction and improved heart failure self-management. However, an identified barrier affecting more widespread participation of clients was the lack of access to mobile phones.

Recognizing that culture has been linked to some cancer-related beliefs and practices, Kreuter and associates (2003) examined the effects of culture on responses to cancer education materials. In a convenience sample of 1,227 African American women, it was determined that responses to culturally tailored materials were no different than to other materials, regardless of the women's cultural characteristics. However, for all types of educational materials, women with higher religiosity and racial pride paid more attention to the educational materials. In this study, it appeared that selected cultural attributes (e.g., religiosity and racial pride) moderated responses to tailored health education materials.

In an integrative review that focused on Hispanic adults and their beliefs about type 2 diabetes, Hatcher and Whittemore (2007) identified several findings that should be considered when developing educational interventions for this population. After reviewing 15 research studies, these authors concluded that generally,

Hispanic adults' understanding of the etiology of diabetes comprised an integration of biomedical causes (e.g., heredity) and traditional folk beliefs. Given this knowledge of the importance of heredity and folk beliefs in how Hispanics viewed diabetes, Hatcher and Whittemore recommended it as a starting point to clarify misconceptions and develop individualized plans of teaching and care. Results from this synthesis of the research literature highlight the necessity of obtaining specific knowledge of how race and culture can affect the structure, implementation, and evaluation of educational outcomes.

In their systematic review and qualitative meta-synthesis of evidence, Brundisini and colleagues (2013) argue that rurality contributes to the vulnerability of clients and families living with chronic disease and that this has cultural ramifications. In particular, these researchers identified three major themes that should be considered: rural culture, geography, and availability of HCPs. Many rural communities are characterized by self-reliance, a sense of community belonging, and unwillingness to seek health care at a distance from the local community. Moreover, the geographic distance from needed services poses challenges related to access to care and worsened transportation problems, especially in adverse weather conditions. In addition, limited access to HCPs contributes to clients' increased sense of vulnerability. When care is available locally, however, clients appreciate the long-term relationship with clinicians and personalized care and are less inclined to feel marginalized, especially if their health literacy is low.

Table 15-2 identifies additional resources to facilitate cultural competence with diverse client and family populations.

Gender and Learning Styles

When planning teaching and learning experiences for clients and their families, the educator must consider how learning styles affect perception, processing, storage, recall of information and the approach to learning activities. Chaudhary, Dullo, and Tanden (2011) revealed that both male and female college students prefer multimodal ways of learning. In particular, males were more inclined to like information structured in a rational manner and achievement oriented. By comparison, females preferred learning situations that had personal relevance and were more socially and performance oriented. Thus, these researchers' findings suggest that the educator must assess the learning preferences of their subjects. In another study assessing 204 African American women's knowledge of stroke, Miller and Harris (2013) identified that 61% of these women's information came from television, 57% from their primary healthcare professional, and the remainder from family/friends and the Internet, in that order.

With the increased usage of online courses and Web-based educational materials, research is revealing that there is a variation in learning styles of online students and students who take face-to-face courses (Garland & Martin, 2005). Moreover, gender is related to learning style and engagement. In Garland and Martin's study involving 7 online courses and 168 students (102 female and 66 male), there was a significant relationship with regard to male students' preference for an abstract conceptualization mode of learning and the number of times they accessed the communication area of Blackboard, an online course management system. Female students, meanwhile, were more highly motivated to perform required class activities than male students. The researchers emphasize that faculty who are constructing online courses need to be aware of how discussions, chats, and groups are influenced by gender, while keeping in mind that postings may be intimidating to some female students. Garland and Martin further stress the need for additional studies that investigate not only the relationship between online learning, learning style, and gender, but also the importance of considering gender

Table 15-2 CULTURAL COMPETENCE RESOURCES FOR CLIENT–FAMILY EDUCATION

Center for Human Diversity: provides consulting and training in cultural competence, diversity, and customer service	http://www.centerforhumandiversity.org
The Joint Commission: "Advancing Effective Communication, Cultural Competence, and Patient-and Family-Centered Care: A Roadmap for Hospitals"	http://www.jointcommission.org/Advancing_Effective_Communication
Kaiser Family Foundation: monthly update on health disparities (2013)	http://www.kff.org/minorityhealth/report.cfm
Knowledge Path: electronic resource guide to racial and ethnic disparities in health that includes information on (and links to) websites, electronic and print publications, webcasts, and databases	http://www.mchlibrary.info/KnowledgePaths/kp_race.html
National Center for Cultural Competence: increase the capacity of health and mental health programs to design, implement, and evaluate culturally and linguistically competent service delivery systems (there is also a Spanish version)	www11.georgetown.edu/research/gucchd/nccc/
National Mental Health Information Center, U.S. Department of Health and Human Services, Substance Abuse and Mental Health Services Administration (SAMHSA)	http://www.samhsa.gov/prevention/
Network for Multicultural Health Research on Health and Healthcare	http://www.multiculturalhealthcare.net/
Office of Minority Health	http://minorityhealth.hhs.gov/
Rural Assistance Center for Minority Health, U.S. Department of Health and Human Services: Rural Initiative Center's resource on issues of minority health in rural communities	http://www.raconline.org/info_guides/minority_health/
Working Together to End Racial and Ethnic Disparities: One Physician at a Time: AMA toolkit designed to help physicians eliminate healthcare disparities	http://www.ama-assn.org/ama1/pub/upload/mm/433/health_disp_kit.pdf

equity in building and designing online courses and educational programs.

In another study involving Women-to-Women (WTW), an online health education program, Cudney, Sullivan, Winters, Paul, and Orient (2005) were interested in determining issues for and solutions preferred by a sample of 50 middle-aged women with cancer, diabetes, multiple sclerosis, or rheumatoid arthritis who lived in rural communities. The problems identified included difficulties carrying out self-management programs, negative fears/ feelings, poor communication with HCPs, and disturbed relationships with family and friends. Self-identified solutions pertained to problem-solving techniques that were tailored to their rural lifestyle. Although most women indicated that their health promotion problems were not easily solvable, they continued to identify feasible ways to self-manage their chronic illnesses (e.g., small achievable goals, taking one day at a time, taking responsibility for being informed, improving communication with HCPs, being proactive in family relationships, being able to say "no"). Results from this study affirm the importance of performing research to expand the best available evidence to guide practice.

Just as gender differences need to be assessed, many educators indicate that determination of the individual's learning style is equally important. The presumed method by which an individual learns best is defined as one's learning style. The difficulty is that more than 80 learning style models have been developed, albeit with limited scientific evidence to support any of them (Coffield, Moseley, Hall, & Ecclestone, 2004; Stahl, 2002). Despite the controversy over the presence and quality of the evidence, it is still worthwhile to ask clients and families which approach to learning they prefer (e.g., spoken word, reading, writing, doing, or interacting). Armed with this information, the HCP can then more effectively plan the teaching interventions. Moreover, age, intelligence, motor skills, degree of impairment, anxiety, and past experiences can significantly affect an individual's ability to learn (Rankin et al., 2005). Along with the aforementioned factors, educational activities must be adapted to clients' and families' favored style of learning and preferences regarding what they need to learn.

Readiness to Learn, Self-Efficacy, and Readiness to Change

Once the learning needs of the client and family are identified, determination of their readiness to learn and self-efficacy are important next steps. Readiness to learn refers to the time when learners are receptive to learning, whereas self-efficacy indicates that they have confidence in their capability of attaining a particular goal (Bastable, 2014). For learning to occur, clients and family members must be ready to learn and possess average to high self-efficacy.

Readiness to learn manifests in a variety of areas, such as physical readiness, emotional readiness, experiential readiness, and knowledge readiness (Lichtenthal, 1990). More specifically, physical readiness can be affected by the client's ability to perform the task, the task's complexity,

environmental conditions that keep the client's attention and interest, the client's health status, and gender (Bastable, 2014; Lichtenthal, 1990). Research supports the contention that women are more receptive to medical care and less likely to take risks associated with their health compared with men (Bertakis, Rahman, Helms, Callahan, & Robbins, 2000).

Emotional readiness to learn, in contrast, has been demonstrated to be affected by anxiety level, strength of one's support system, motivation, state of mind, and developmental stage (Bastable, 2014). Previous positive as well as negative learning experiences can dramatically affect experiential readiness of clients and family members. Therefore, HCPs planning an educational activity should identify any previous learning successes and failures and prior ways of coping with similar situations, and understand the potential influence of culture and human motivation. Finally, readiness to learn new knowledge can be influenced by what the client or family member already knows, the individual's cognitive ability, any learning disabilities, and general learning style (Bastable, 2014; Mauk, 2014; Muijs & Reynolds, 2005; Rankin et al., 2005).

While assessing clients and family members for readiness to learn, self-efficacy must also be determined. In the research literature, a strong sense of self-efficacy—that is, confidence in one's ability to achieve a behavior—has repeatedly been demonstrated to have significant positive influence on accomplishing a health-promoting behavior change in individuals with chronic illness (Coleman & Newton, 2005; Osborne, Wilson, Lorig, & McColl, 2007; Tung & Lee, 2006).

Readiness to change is another increasingly familiar term applied to chronic illness and reduction of unhealthy behaviors. Although readiness to change has varied definitions, the best known emerges from the transtheoretical model of change (TTM), which involves intentional decision making and was developed to promote effective interventions to facilitate positive behavioral change. TTM reflects an integration of constructs from other theories and describes how individuals modify problem behaviors such as smoking, limited exercise, and overeating to acquire a more positive behavior (Prochaska & DiClemente, 1983; Prochaska, DiClemente, & Norcross, 1992; Prochaska & Velicer, 1997). The central organizing construct is stages of change, but the model also includes other variables (e.g., self-efficacy, processes of change, decisional balance, and temptation). TTM focuses on stage-focused interventions pertaining to the individual's readiness to change an unhealthy behavior (e.g., smoking, limited exercise). Within TTM, there are five stages of readiness to change: pre-contemplation, contemplation, preparation, action, and maintenance. Measurement instruments for these stages with demonstrated reliability and validity can be obtained at the Cancer Prevention Research Center (2008) website.

Developmental Stage

Chronologic age provides a basic indication of clients' and family members' projected physical, cognitive, and psychological state of development. When planning a teaching–learning activity for a client and family member, consideration of the client's or family member's developmental stage is pivotal, along with past learning experiences, stress level, physical and emotional health, personal motivation, environmental conditions, and available support systems (Bastable, 2014).

Within the literature, several prominent developmental theorists have shaped how HCPs view life stages (Erikson, 1968; Piaget, 1951, 1976). In contrast with childhood, where learning is student centered, adult learning tends to be more problem centered, with the primary emphasis on how to apply new knowledge and skills to immediate problems (Bastable, 2006). Adults tend to be more resistant to change, which is why establishing mutual goals and an action plan with HCPs markedly improves the achievement of educational outcomes (Miller, 2003; Rankin et al., 2005).

Table 15-3 provides a brief overview of the developmental stages of adults, the major attributes of such learners, and the most applicable

---

Table 15-3 LINKING DEVELOPMENTAL STAGE WITH LEARNER CHARACTERISTICS AND TEACHING STRATEGIES

Developmental Stage	Learner Characteristics	Recommended Teaching Strategies
Young adulthood (18–39 years)	Peak body function Self-directive Independent in learning Making decisions about career, education, social roles Competency-based learner If has a chronic illness, tends to want to learn as much as possible to remain independent and lead as normal a life as possible	Immediate application Active participation Learning needs to be convenient, self-paced, and blend of visual and written Group interaction Organized materials and presentation Use past experiences as a resource for learning Provide practical answers to their problems Give opportunity for immediate application of teaching Seek credible/evidence-based information

(Continues)

Table 15-3 Linking Developmental Stage with Learner Characteristics and Teaching Strategies (Continued)

Developmental Stage	Learner Characteristics	Recommended Teaching Strategies
Middle age (40–64 years)	Well-developed sense of self Usually at career peak Concerned about physical changes Reexamines goals and values Confident in abilities Tends to want to reduce unsatisfying aspects in life May be experiencing midlife crises	Maintain independence and perhaps reestablish what constitutes normal life patterns Assess prior positive and negative learning experiences Identify potential stressors Provide information that fits to life problems and/or concerns; use past experiences as a resource for learning Provide practical answers to their problems Give opportunity for immediate application of teaching
Older adult (65 years and older)	Cognitive changes Decreased ability to think abstractly Reduced short-term memory Increased reaction time Focus on past life experiences Motor and sensory losses Auditory and visual changes Hearing loss especially with high-pitched tones, consonants, and rapid speech Decreased peripheral vision Decreased risk taking	Use concrete examples Build on past experiences Make information relevant Allow time for processing and responses Use verbal interactions and coaching Encourage active involvement Keep explanations brief (20–40 minutes) Speak distinctly and slowly Minimize distractions while teaching Avoid shouting—if working with a large group, a microphone may be needed Use large font in handouts Avoid glare (optimize lighting) Provide a safe environment Keep teaching sessions short Provide rest periods Rooms where conducted should be neutral temperature (not too hot or cold)

Sources: Bastable, S. B. (2014). *Essentials of patient education.* Burlington, MA: Jones & Bartlett; Mauk, K. L. (Ed.). (2014). *Gerontological nursing: Competencies for care.* 3rd ed. Burlington, MA: Jones and Bartlett; Rankin, S. H., Stallings, K. D., & London, F. (2005). *Patient education in health and illness* (5th ed.). Philadelphia, PA: Lippincott.

teaching strategies. A common misconception is that older adults cannot learn. In fact, when older adults are provided information at a slower rate, material being taught is relevant, and positive feedback is received, they are very capable of learning new knowledge and skills (Bastable, 2014; Mauk, 2014). Because depression, grief, and loneliness are not restricted to older adults, these factors can markedly affect any client's or family member's ability to concentrate on content being presented. HCPs, moreover, must be continually aware of other potential cognitive and physical limitations (i.e., pain, fatigue, diminished vision, reduced hearing) that might affect the ability of clients and family members to learn. **Table 15-4** lists recommended

Table 15-4 HELPFUL RESOURCES TO FACILITATE TEACHING AND LEARNING OF OLDER ADULTS

Organization	Website
American Society on Aging	http://www.asaging.org
Association for Gerontology in Higher Education	http://www.aghe.org
John A. Hartford Foundation Institute for Geriatric Nursing	http://www.hartfordign.org
National Center for Education Statistics	http://www.nces.ed.gov
National Institute on Aging	http://www.nia.nih.gov
National Council on Aging	http://www.ncoa.org
Osher Lifelong Learning Institute	http://www.olli.gmu.edu

resources that can help HCPs identify how to optimally structure and evaluate educational activities involving older adults.

Health Literacy

According to the Patient Protection and Affordable Care Act (ACA), Title V, health literacy is defined as the degree to which an individual has the capacity to obtain, communicate, process, and understand basic health information and services to make appropriate health decisions. This definition is almost identical to the one in *Healthy People 2020* except that the word "communicate" was added to the legislative definition (CDC, 2013a). Unfortunately, an estimated 9 out of 10 adults have difficulty using everyday health information that is readily available in healthcare facilities, media, and communities (Kutner, Greenberg, Jin, &

Paulsen, 2006). (Tools to assess the readability of educational materials and individuals' reading comprehension are identified in **Table 15-5**.) Based on the evidence, if clients do not receive clear health information and understand its importance, clients are more likely to skip medical tests, come to the emergency room more often than needed, and have greater difficulty in managing their chronic health conditions such as asthma, hypertension, heart disease, and diabetes (Rudd, Anderson, Oppenheimer, & Nath, 2007).

To address these concerns and improve health literacy, healthcare professionals, community members, legislators, and other stakeholders must work together. Through collaborative and coordinated efforts, targeted action plans need to be developed that are based on a systematic and comprehensive assessment of the health knowledge of citizens from different socioeconomic groups, ethnic and cultural backgrounds, and geographic regions to build and maintain the resources needed.

System Factors That Influence the Teaching and Learning Process

To ensure an optimal client, family, and HCP educational situation, certain elements need to be in place. System factors that can significantly contribute to positive educational outcomes include the following (Edwardson, 2007; Nobel, 2006; Rankin et al., 2005):

- Preparation of the HCP in terms of knowledge of the educational content and teaching capabilities
- Cultural competence and knowledge related to all of the other factors that help to personalize the educational approach (i.e., age, developmental stage, and cognitive and physical status related to the chronic illness)
- Required resources for effective teaching (e.g., equipment/technology; materials—booklets, figures).

Table 15-5 Tools to Access Readability of Educational Materials and Individuals' Reading Comprehension

Measurement Tools to Assess Readability of Educational Materials	Measurement Tools to Assess an Individual's Reading Comprehension
Flesch Formula In use more than 70 years to assess news reports, adult educational materials, and government publications. Based on a count of two basic language components: average sentence length in words and average word length measured in syllables per word of selected samples of text (Flesch, 1948; Spadero, 1983). Helpful Web sources to assist with these calculations: http://www.readabilityformulas.com/flesch-reading-ease-readability-formula.php http://www.csun.edu/~vcecn006/read1.html	*Wide Range Achievement Test (WRAT)* A word-recognition screening test that typically takes about 5 minutes to complete. It assesses the client's ability to recognize and pronounce a list of words out of context to determine reading skills. It has two levels of testing: Level 1 is for children 5–12 years and Level 2 is for individuals older than 12 years of age (Doak, Doak, & Root, 1996). Helpful Web source: http://www4.parinc.com/Products/Product.aspx?ProductID=WRAT4
Fog Formula Assesses the reading level of materials from fourth grade to college level. One of the easier tools to use, with the calculation based on the average sentence length and percentage of multisyllabic words based on a sample of 100 words (Bastable, 2006; Spadero, 1983). Helpful Web sources: http://www.readabilityformulas.com/gunning-fog-readability-formula.php http://www.thelearningweb.net/fogindex.html	*Rapid Estimate of Adult Literacy in Medicine (REALM)* Tests the client's ability to read medical and health-related vocabulary (an advantage over the WRAT), takes less time, and has easy scoring (Duffy & Snyder, 1999). Although the test has validity, it offers less precision and reliability than other word tests (Hayes, 2000). In the test, 66 medical and health-related words are placed in three columns ranging from short and easy to more difficult. Clients are to begin reading the words from the top and go down. The total number of correctly pronounced words is the raw score that is then converted to a grade range (Doak et al., 1996). Helpful Web source: http://library.med.utah.edu/Patient_Ed/workshop/handouts/realm_test.pdf
SMOG Formula A formula that has been used primarily to evaluate the grade-level readability of patient educational materials and can measure reading level with as little content as 10 sentences. This formula determines readability from grades 4 to college level, and is based on the number of multisyllable words (three or more syllables) within a set number of sentences (McLaughlin, 1969). Helpful Web source: http://www.readabilityformulas.com/smog-readability-formula.php	*Test of Functional Health Literacy in Adults (TOFHL)* A newer measurement tool to assess clients' literacy skills that uses actual hospital materials (i.e., appointment slips, informed consent documents, and prescription labels). The test consists of two parts: reading comprehension and numeracy (Bastable, 2006). It has demonstrated validity and reliability, takes approximately 20 minutes to administer, and has an English and Spanish version (Quirk, 2000). Helpful Web source: http://education.gsu.edu/csal/TOFHLA.htm

- Time limitations that permit updating teaching plans, using evaluation tools, and developing/updating educational protocols
- Coordinating educational activities that are consistent with discharge plans and other important client and family information that needs to be communicated
- Succinct and timely documentation of what was taught, when, and the outcome, so that others can build on and reinforce prior teaching
- If client and family education is not valued by the system and rewards are not given for educational excellence and positive outcomes
- If there are inadequate record-keeping and reimbursement policies that reimburse HCPs fully for direct, hands-on illness interventions, but poorly for client/family education and interventions via telephone and computer

The following strategies (Bastable, 2014; Falvo, 2011; Mayer & Vallaire, 2007; McDonald, 2014; Petty, 2006) may serve as a starting point when assessing and educating clients and families with low literacy:

- Materials should not be above fifth-grade level and should be culturally appropriate.
- Keep sentences short, limiting them to 20 words or fewer if possible.
- Speak and write using short words with only one or two syllables whenever possible. Rely on common words that are easily recognized by most individuals.
- Put the most important information first and limit the focus to what the client and family member need to know.
- Clearly and simply define technical words or ones that are unfamiliar (e.g., "fasting blood glucose," "hypertension"), or replace them with simpler words ("high blood pressure" for "hypertension").
- Remember that persons with low literacy skills may require more time to read and absorb the materials.

- Visual presentation ("A picture is worth a thousand words") can be especially helpful to someone with low literacy skills.
- Avoid abbreviations (e.g., MI, FBS, I and O).
- Use consistent words throughout the presentation (e.g., don't switch from "diet" to "menu" to "dietary prescription").
- Organize information into "chunks" that facilitate recall. Use numbers only when necessary and realize that statistics are usually confusing and meaningless for the low-health-literate client and family member.
- Keep the number of items in a list to no more than seven.
- Keep teaching sessions short and preferably no longer than 10–15 minutes.
- Use the teach-back method with clients to ensure that they understand their care routine and warning signs if there is a problem (i.e., signs of a wound infection or urinary tract infection, signs of a stroke or heart attack—not myocardial infarction). Never ask, "Do you understand?" Ask the patient to explain the processes or state the signs of an infection, stroke, or heart attack. These perception checks are an important part of the teaching–learning process and enable the HCP to assess whether learning is occurring as planned. In addition, these perception checks allow the HCP to redirect activities if the client and/or family educational outcomes are not being achieved as planned.
- Have written materials reviewed by a literacy expert to determine the grade reading level. Also, ask the client and family member questions to determine their specific ability to read and comprehend what is described. Do not assume that the teaching materials address all of the client's and family's concerns; instead, ask if there is something missing or whether they have questions about anything that is not included in the materials provided. Remember, too, that blending

written materials with auditory interactions enhances learning and retention of information.

- Present information one step at a time to pace instruction and allow clients and family members to understand each step and ask questions before moving on to the next step.

In conjunction with the system challenges just identified, HCPs must consider other diverse attributes (i.e., age, gender, culture, developmental stage, literacy, and functional status) that make each client and family educational encounter unique.

What is the best available evidence that will help shape these interventions? Townsend, Bruce, Hooten, and Rome (2006) assert that HCPs do not always recognize the tensions and ambiguities permeating clients' experiences, particularly those who have multiple chronic illnesses. Results of their research revealed that clients with chronic illness utilize multiple techniques to manage their symptoms, and frequently feel pressure to manage "well" and have a "normal life" for both their families and HCPs.

Despite the lack of current strong evidence that might support the various aspects of HCPs' educational interventions, research in this area continues to expand, as do the meta-analyses and systematic reviews that synthesize the evidence and identify additional areas to be explored. To more comprehensively document the specific contribution of nursing to the education and self-care of clients with chronic illness, Edwardson (2007) recommends two focus areas for research. First, researchers should measure the outcomes of client and family education and have this information included in both the clinical and administrative databases. Whenever possible, the client and family educational process and outcomes should be separated according to type of education, objectives, timing, dose (i.e., strategies, length), and so forth. Second, systematic reviews and meta-analyses suggest that inpatient education followed

by some form of postdischarge intervention may be the most promising approach to reduce hospitalizations (Gonseth, Castillion, Banegas, & Artalejo, 2004). However, for this care system to succeed, databases from ambulatory care, acute care, and after-care services need to be linked to monitor symptoms, monitor adherence to treatment prescription, and modify treatment plans as needed (Edwardson, 2007).

Educational Interventions for the Client and Family

As indicated in previous sections of this chapter, multiple factors must be carefully assessed and considered in the development of an educational plan for clients with chronic illness and their families. Because of the variance in how these elements are manifested, the goals mutually established by the client, family, and HCP; associated interventions; and outcomes need to be uniquely planned, implemented, and evaluated. In most instances, nurses are the principal HCPs who participate in this ongoing educational process and provide the continuity of care for clients and families with chronic illness.

Development of the Teaching Plan

The teaching plan provides the overall blueprint or outline for instruction that clearly defines the relationship among the behavioral objectives, instructional content, teaching strategies, time frame for teaching, and methods of evaluation (Bastable, 2014). All aspects work together to achieve a predetermined goal that should be mutually agreed upon by the client and family and the HCP. Three domains of learning should be addressed: cognitive (knowledge), psychomotor (physical activities), and affective (attitudes or emotions). When constructing teaching plans to address these learning domains for specific chronic illnesses, HCPs should also refer to published practice standards such as those from the Agency for Healthcare

Research and Quality (AHRQ), specialty nursing groups, and disease-specific organizations such as the American Heart Association, which have developed their own evidence-based guidelines. The specific teaching plan includes the following aspects: purpose of the teaching plan; goal(s)—that is, broad statement(s) of what is to be achieved; objective(s), which need to be specific and measurable; content covered to achieve each objective; teaching strategies; time required; and evaluation methods to determine if the learning has occurred. Key aspects of the

teaching plan are described next, followed by a specific example.

Teaching Strategies

Knowing how to use varied teaching strategies to achieve educational objectives can make client and family education more interesting, challenging, and effective for HCPs and learners (Rankin et al., 2005). A general overview of widely used teaching strategies and their predominant characteristics is presented in **Table 15-6**. For the client with chronic illness,

Table 15-6 General Overview of Common Teaching Strategies

Teaching Strategy	Learning Domain	Learner Role	Teacher Role	Strength	Weakness
Lecture	Cognitive	Passive	Presents information	Cost-effective; targeted to larger groups	Not individualized
Group discussion	Cognitive; affective	Active, if learner participates	Directs and focuses discussion	Share emotions and ideas	Shy or dominant members affect participation; may lose focus
One-to-one teaching	Cognitive; affective; psychomotor	Active	Presents information and encourages individualized learning	Tailored to client or family member's needs and goals	Great diversity; labor intensive; learner isolated
Demonstration	Cognitive	Passive	Modeling of skill or behavior	Preview of skill or behavior, can ask questions	Need individual or small group to visualize
Return demonstration	Psychomotor	Active	Individualized feedback to refine skill performance	Immediate feedback	Labor intensive; anxiety may affect actions
Gaming	Cognitive; affective	Active if client/family participates	Oversees pacing; debriefs	Stimulates learners' enthusiasm and participation	May be too competitive; overstimulating

(Continues)

Table 15-6 GENERAL OVERVIEW OF COMMON TEACHING STRATEGIES (CONTINUED)

Teaching Strategy	Learning Domain	Learner Role	Teacher Role	Strength	Weakness
Simulation	Cognitive; psychomotor	Active	Designs situation; facilitates learning; debriefs	Practice a reality situation in a safe setting	Labor intensive; equipment costs/access; scheduling issues
Online learning	Cognitive; affective	Passive, but can be active if client/family participates in group discussions, problem solving, group projects	Usually designs program/class; presents information; provides active learning exercises, discussions, case studies, and group projects	Learners usually at a distance; flexibility when accessing learning content and activities; learners need to be motivated; feedback provided is usually individualized and immediate	Need equipment to access; lack of personal contact; accessibility; all feedback may not be instantaneous
Computer-assisted instruction	Cognitive; affective	Active	Purchases or designs program; expected to provide feedback to student	Individualized instruction; learner controls pace of the learning; can program to receive feedback; valuable modality if hearing impaired, learning disability, or aphasic	Must have equipment and software

Sources: Bastable, S. B., Gramet, P., Jacobs, K., & Sopezk, D. (2010). *Essentials of patient education.* Sudbury, MA: Jones & Bartlett; Miller, E. (2014) *Theoretical Basis for Clinical Reasoning (29NURS8002), Online Course Manual.* Cincinnati, OH: University of Cincinnati, College of Nursing; Wantland, D. J., Portillo, C. J., Holzemer, W. L., & Slaughter, R. (2004). The effectiveness of Web-based vs. non-Web-based interventions: A meta-analysis of behavioral change outcomes. *Journal of Medical Internet Research, 6*(4), 40–71.

the research strongly supports that combining multiple teaching methods during several educational sessions consistently produces more positive client outcomes than single teaching methods and events (Bastable, 2006; Beranova & Sykes, 2007; Edwardson, 2007; Joanna Briggs Institute, 2006). However, the HCP must also remain cognizant of the system factors contributing to the success and/or failure of the teaching and learning process.

A pivotal aspect of any client and family teaching event is preparing measurable objectives that can be achieved in the time frame specified. For example, the client with diabetes may need to learn the signs and symptoms of a hypoglycemic reaction. An appropriate measurable objective could be "Ms. Jones will state four signs/symptoms of a hypoglycemic reaction by the end of this 12-hour shift."

Increasingly, more clients with chronic illness and their family members are receiving education regarding disease management from Web-based sources, with the young to middle-aged population being the biggest consumers (Beranova & Sykes, 2007; Lee, Yeh, Liu, & Chen, 2007; Stone, 2014). Research from a survey published by the Pew Research Center's Internet and American Life Project and the California Healthcare Foundation found that 80% of Internet users look online for health information, making it the third most popular online pursuit, after email and use of a search engine (Fox, 2011). For clients with chronic illness, use of the Internet provides a means to encourage behavior change that requires knowledge sharing, education, and greater understanding of the condition. Results of a meta-analysis comparing Web-based and non–Web-based education of adults with chronic illness (mean age 41.2 years) from 1996 to 2003 revealed that substantial evidence that Web-based interventions improve behavioral change outcomes (Wantland, Portillo, Holzemer, & Slaughter, 2004). The specific positive outcomes identified were increased knowledge of nutritional status, increased knowledge of asthma treatment, increased exercise time, slower health decline, and 18-month weight-loss maintenance. Web-based interventions that were relevant and individually tailored were associated with more and longer website visits. Wantland and associates further discovered that sites with chat rooms increased social support scores of the users. They caution, however, that the long-term effects on individual persistence with the chosen therapies and the cost-effectiveness of the Web-based

therapies and hardware and software development demand ongoing evaluation.

LEARNING CURVE

The learning curve describes how long it takes a learner to acquire an attitudinal and/or psychomotor skill. It also encompasses the level of difficulty in achieving this change (Bastable, 2014). Individual learning curves are characterized by irregularity. Fluctuations in performance can be attributed to factors such as interest, ability to focus, energy, ability, situational circumstances, and favorable or unfavorable conditions within the learning environment (Gage & Berliner, 1998). In the case of a client with chronic illness, learning to walk again following a stroke may take time and create frustration, as expectations do not match physical capability. Because learning may not always occur in a linear fashion, HCPs must recognize this fact and assist clients and their families when they experience anger, discouragement, or depression associated with achievement not progressing as anticipated. In addition, research supports that retention of learning is enhanced when there are opportunities to see, hear, observe demonstrations, discuss, and practice as well as teach others (Bastable, 2014; Mauk, 2014; Muijs & Reynolds, 2005; Petty, 2006).

EVALUATION

Evaluation of educational outcomes is a critical step in the teaching and learning process. It encompasses a systematic and continuous activity that involves collecting and using information to determine whether the educational objectives have been achieved. This outcome evaluation is labeled summative evaluation, but formative evaluation is also possible. Formative evaluation occurs during the actual teaching process while the implementation is still on-going. Formative evaluation permits the HCP to adjust or change aspects of the implementation process that may improve the quality or delivery of the educational program or session. For instance, the HCP may decide to use a Web-based program and face-to-face demonstration of a task with clients and their families. On the basis of immediate negative feedback regarding a client's unfamiliarity with computers and reluctance to use such a program, the HCP may decide to replace this Web-based education with a small-group discussion involving the client and family.

When performing any type of evaluation, it is important to identify which outcome is being measured, how and when the data will be collected, and then how those data will be interpreted. For example, assume the HCP and the client have established the following outcome objective: "Client will state three signs/symptoms of hypoglycemia by the end of a 12-hour shift." Determination of achievement of this objective is straightforward. Yet, sometimes barriers occur that hinder the evaluation process. Barriers that can be particularly problematic include lack of clarity regarding what is being evaluated, lack of ability to perform the evaluation, and fear of punishment or low self-esteem (Bastable, 2014). With regard to lack of ability, the HCP may not know how to construct a short test to determine if the client and family have a basic understanding of diabetes or may not feel comfortable orally quizzing them to assess their learning. In other situations, clients may be too ill to learn the information, perform a new task, or respond as they anticipate the HCP wants them to.

In many settings, practice guidelines or protocols identify how formative and summative evaluations are to be conducted and which information needs to be documented. Data from the evaluation process, especially as it applies to the teaching and learning process for the client and family, can be extremely valuable as the chronic illness progresses and additional knowledge,

attitudinal, and psychomotor skills need to be developed.

Example of a Teaching Plan

The teaching plan provided in **Table 15-7** was developed for the following case situation. Your client is Nettie Campbell, who is 35 years old, is a single parent of two little girls (ages 4 and 7), and was just diagnosed with hypertension and a transient ischemic attack (TIA). Ms. Campbell is 15 pounds overweight and works as an accountant in a large firm. She has been experiencing lots of stress related to the adoption of a new accounting system in the organization where she works. Her company provides good health insurance, but Ms. Campbell worries about her ability to work full-time given her present health condition and her need to juggle all of the demands of being a single parent. Her family tries to be helpful to her, but they all work and can provide assistance only on the weekends. Ms. Campbell has been referred to you for education pertaining to her medications, signs and symptoms of stroke and TIA, treatment-seeking plan if stroke or TIA symptoms occur, and weight and stress reduction.

The specific approach to this client will consider such elements as gender, culture, learning curve, importance of feedback, and reinforcement. Given the content and objectives of this specific teaching plan, it is recommended that *not all* of this teaching occur at the same time. Instead, the teaching plan pertaining to the first three objectives could be performed first, and then teaching of the fourth objective might occur later in the day. During this second educational session, review the key points associated with the first teaching episode. Furthermore, make sure that each teaching session is not interrupted and that there is adequate time to permit questions from the client and family, who should also be present if at all possible.

Table 15-7 Sample Teaching Plan for Nettie Campbell

Objectives	Content (Topics)	Time Frame	Teaching Strategy	Evaluation Method
Ms. Campbell will be able to: 1. State the purpose of Lasix, the importance of taking her medication as prescribed (time, dose), and major side effects. *Cognitive domain of learning* It is recommended that there are two or three different instances where a review covers taking medication correctly and keeping follow-up appointments.	a. Describe the purpose of Lasix. b. Importance of taking as prescribed. c. Taking blood pressure consistently. d. Need to monitor potassium regularly.	4 minutes	One-to-one teaching presentation. Review a poster listing hypertensive management and how her treatment fits the standard treatment plan for hypertension. Give a booklet that is culturally appropriate and at her reading level. Ask Nettie if she has any questions regarding the medication and side effects. If client has difficulty getting the content correct, repeat teaching as well as discuss other strategies that may facilitate retention of the information.	Use several vignettes and then ask the client to state the purpose of Lasix, how frequently to take it each day, and key side effects. Need a 100% correct response. Ask the immediate action to take when each side effect is present. Must get all correct.
2. Nettie will demonstrate what is to be done when a stroke or TIA is suspected. *Psychomotor domain of learning*	a. Review the signs/ symptoms of a stroke and/or TIA. b. Demonstrate what to do when stroke or TIA is suspected—call 911. c. Help client and family identify user-friendly educational materials that they can review now and as needed to educate other family members who may witness a TIA or stroke.	5 minutes	One-to-one teaching presentation. Review the AHA/ASA FAST video (http://www.strokeassociation.org/STROKEORG/WarningSigns/Stroke-Warning-Signs-and-Symptoms_UCM_308528_SubHomePage.jsp#). Then demonstrate what to do. Assess leaning to determine if the client and/or her family have any questions.	Have the client verbally state the signs/symptoms of stroke and TIA. Then have the client demonstrate what to do.

(Continues)

Table 15-7 SAMPLE TEACHING PLAN FOR NETTIE CAMPBELL (CONTINUED)

Objectives	Content (Topics)	Time Frame	Teaching Strategy	Evaluation Method
3. Nettie will verbalize confidence in identifying signs/symptoms of stroke and TIA and in knowing what to do when either is suspected. *Affective domain of learning*	Indicate that the client is capable of identifying the signs/symptoms and sharing this information with family, especially members with whom she has close contact and who could potentially be present if a stroke or TIA occurs.	2 minutes	One-to-one teaching and blend of brief discussion, reinforcement, and feedback. Talk about where to keep the list of signs/symptoms so the client has easy access for self and significant others. Importance of keeping a phone handy.	Have the client rate on a scale of 0 (no confidence) to 10 (complete confidence) her ability to identify signs/symptoms of stroke or TIA and engage in immediate treatment-seeking behavior.
4. Nettie will establish with the advanced practice nurse a realistic exercise plan to lose 10 pounds within the next 3 months. *Psychomotor domain of learning.*	Mutual goal setting and identify priorities. Importance of exercise in weight reduction and how best to exercise over time and as part of a daily routine. Potential activities that can be performed to lose weight.	5 minutes	Discuss what Nettie wants to do or prefers as part of her increase in exercise plan. Discuss what is feasible given that she works full-time and has two small children. Review exercise possibilities in her home and work environments. Discuss how she can find the time to regularly incorporate exercise in her daily routine.	Nettie will state what her plan is for the next 3 months regarding her realistic weight-reduction plan. Every 2 weeks Nettie will communicate with the advanced practice nurse to determine how this plan is progressing and which adjustments, if any, are needed.
5. Nettie will identify two realistic actions she can take in the next week to reduce her stress level. *Cognitive domain and also psychomotor domain (exercise)*	Review the association between stress and hypertension, and the client's potential inability to have the energy to exercise. Identify causes of stress in her home and work situations. Identify feasible and preferably evidence-based strategies to reduce stress.	5 minutes	Explore realistic activities to reduce long- and short-term stress. Perhaps keep a log of relaxing and stressful activities and what is helpful in reducing stress. Discuss activities that are helpful and fun in reducing stress.	Have Nettie state every 2 weeks how she would rate her stress, with 10 being high and 0 being absent. State which activities are stress reducing at work and home and how the client is eliminating or reducing those that are stressful.

Outcomes

Education serves as an essential vehicle to provide the client and family with the knowledge, skills, and confidence needed to address the many facets associated with living with a chronic illness. Although numerous factors contribute to the success or failure of this educational process, HCPs—and nurses, in particular—play a fundamental role as part of their scope of practice and other national standards such as *Healthy People 2020* and Joint Commission benchmarks.

Research evidence on healthcare education continues to expand, with such findings guiding the assessment of all learners, teaching plan development, and ultimate educational outcomes. Teaching and learning is a complex process and requires consideration of many elements, such as family structure and function, culture, gender, learning styles, readiness to learn/change, self-efficacy, developmental stage, literacy, socioeconomic status, resources, and learning capability. In addition, as HCPs partner with clients and their families during this educational process, it is critical that the HCPs assess their educational objectives and redirect their actions when needed. Because more than 50% of the U.S. population has at least one chronic illness, the teaching and learning process is paramount to clients attaining greater quality of life and adapting to the frequently dynamic nature of most chronic diseases.

Another central element that is sometimes overlooked is the mutual goal setting that occurs among the client, family, and HCP. When all of these parties work together, clients are much more inclined to achieve the planned educational objectives, whether they are targeted at knowledge, attitudes, and/or behaviors pertaining to the chronic health problem.

Evidence-Based Practice Box

Purpose and background: Client education is an important intervention in the management of heart disease. This article is a systematic review of the literature that examined the educational interventions implemented for clients with heart failure and assessed their related outcomes.

Methods: Randomized controlled trials from 1998–2008 in CINAHL, MEDLINE, EMBASE, PsychINFO, and the Cochrane Library were reviewed by using the following search terms: *patient education, educational intervention, self-care* in combination with *heart failure*. Two reviewers independently examined 1,515 abstracts.

Results: A total of 2,686 patients in 19 studies met the inclusion criteria for this literature review. The initial intervention for all reported studies was typically a one-to-one educational intervention. Seven of these studies had a theoretical framework for their educational intervention. Of the studies reviewed, 15 revealed that the educational intervention had a significant positive effect on at least one of the desired outcomes.

Conclusions: Even though improvements in educational outcomes were observed, the study samples varied considerably. It was also difficult in this systematic review to determine the most effective educational strategy because of the variance in delivery methods, duration of the interventions, and the outcomes evaluated. A client-centered approach to education based on an educational theory and evaluated consistently with that framework is recommended.

Source: Boyde, M., Turner, D., Thompson, D. R., & Stewart, S. (2010). Educational interventions for patients with heart failure: A systematic review of randomized controlled trials. *Journal of Cardiovascular Nursing, 26*(4), E27–E35.

CASE STUDY 15-1

Marco Sanchez is a 43-year-old man who has a history of obesity (body mass index [BMI] > 30) and smoking since age 15. Six months ago, he was diagnosed with type 2 diabetes. He is now taking NPH insulin every 12 hours. Given that Marco is a truck driver and travels cross-country from California to New York each week, following his diet is frequently problematic. He lives with his wife and four young children, who range in age from 9 months to 10 years.

Discussion Questions

1. What appear to be the primary educational objectives for Marco?
2. Which additional assessment data would assist in establishing educational objectives and structuring your related interventions?
3. Which teaching method(s) would be most appropriate? What is your rationale for this decision?
4. Briefly describe your teaching plan. What would it consist of in terms of objective(s), content, timeline, and teaching strategies?
5. Which valuable and evidence-based contributions can the advanced practice nurse make in the teaching–learning situation?

STUDY QUESTIONS

1. Which level of evidence provides the greatest confidence in the applicability of research findings to practice?
2. What are the pros and cons of three teaching strategies that can be used to educate an individual with a chronic illness?
3. What are the differences between pedagogy, andragogy, and gerogogy? How might these differences influence your approach to teaching?
4. What are major factors that should be considered when planning an educational session for a client with chronic illness?
5. How might the approach to an educational intervention differ if the client is a male compared to a female?
6. How might cultural and ethnic/race differences affect how you structure and evaluate the outcomes of a specific educational intervention?
7. How would you specifically assess the literacy of a client and his or her family?
8. What is the difference between a formative evaluation and a summative evaluation?
9. Describe how *Healthy People 2020* and/or Joint Commission standards affect the importance of educational interventions in your practice.

References

American Association of Colleges of Nursing (AACN). (2008). *The essentials of baccalaureate education for professional nursing.* Washington, DC: Author.

American Nurses Association (ANA). (2010). *Nursing: Scope and standards of practice* (2nd ed.). Washington, DC: Author.

Auger, K. A., Kenyon, C. C., Feudtner, C., & Davis, M. M. (2014). Pediatric hospital discharge interventions to reduce subsequent utilization: A systematic review. *Journal of Hospital Medicine, 9*(4), 251–260.

Bandura, A. (1986). *Social foundations of thought and action: A social cognitive theory.* Englewood Cliffs, NJ: Prentice Hall.

Bastable, S. B. (2006). *Essentials of patient education.* Sudbury, MA: Jones and Bartlett.

Bastable, S. B. (2014). *Nurse as educator: Principles of teaching and learning for nursing practice* (4th ed.). Burlington, MA: Jones & Bartlett Learning.

Bastable, S. B., Gramet, P., Jacobs, K., & Sopezk, D. (2010). *Essentials of patient education.* Sudbury, MA: Jones and Bartlett.

Beranova, E., & Sykes, C. (2007). A systematic review of computer based software for educating patients with coronary heart disease. *Patient Education and Counseling, 66*(1), 21–28.

Bertakis, K., Rahman, A., Helms, L. J., Callahan, E., & Robbins, J. (2000). Gender differences in the utilization of health care services. *Journal of Family Practice, 49*(2), 147–152.

Boyde, M., Turner, D., Thompson, D. R., & Stewart, S. (2010). Educational interventions for patients with heart failure: A systematic review of randomized controlled trials. *Journal of Cardiovascular Nursing, 26*(4), E27–E35.

Brenner, J., & Stone, A. (2013). 72% of online adults are social networking site users. Pew Research Center's Internet & American Life Project. http://www.pewinternet.org/Reports/2013/social-networking-sites.aspx/

Brundisini, F., Giacomini, M., DeJean, D., Vanstone, M., Winsor, S., & Smith, A. (2013). Chronic disease patients' experiences with accessing health care in rural and remote areas: A systematic review and qualitative meta-synthesis. *Ontario Health Technology Assessment Series, 13*(15), 1–33.

Cameron, V. (2013). Best practices for stroke patient and family education in the acute care setting: A literature review. *Medsurg Nursing, 22*(1), 51–55.

Camica, M., Black, T., Farrell, J., Waites, K., Wirt, S., Lutz, B. & Association of Rehabilitation Nurses Task Force (2014). The essential role of the rehabilitation nurse in facilitation care transition: A white paper by the Association of Rehabilitation Nurses. *Rehabilitation Nursing, 39*(1), 3–15.

Cancer Prevention Research Center. (2008). Measures. http://www.uri.edu/research/cprc/measures.htm

Centers for Disease Control and Prevention (CDC). (2005). Preventing diabetes and its complications. http://www.cdc.gov/nccdphp/publications/factsheets/prevention/pdf/diabetes.pdf

Centers for Disease Control and Prevention (CDC). (2013a). Chronic disease prevention and health promotion. http://cds.gov/chronicdisease/chronicdisease/overview/index.htm

Centers for Disease Control and Prevention (CDC). (2013b). Chronic disease cost calculator version 2. http://www.cdc.gov/crhonicdisease/resources/calculator/index.htm

Chaudhary, R., Dullo, P. & Tanden, R. W. (2011). Gender difference in both learning styles and performance of first year medical students. *Pakistan Journal of Physiology, 7*(2), 42–45.

Coffield, F., Moseley, D., Hall, E., & Ecclestone, K. (2004). Learning styles and pedagogy in post-16 learning: A systematic and critical review. http://www.pedagogy.ir/images/pdf/learning-styles-pedagogy.pdf

Coleman, M., & Newton, K. (2005). Supporting self-management in patients with chronic illness. *American Family Physician, 72*(8), 1503–1510.

Cudney, S., Sullivan, T., Winters, C., Paul, L., & Orient, P. (2005). Chronically ill rural women: Self-identified management problems and solutions. *Chronic Illness, 1,* 49–60.

Delisel, D. R. (2013). Care transitions programs: A review of hospital-based programs targeted to reduce readmissions. *Professional Care Management, 18*(6), 273–283.

Deng, F., Zhang, A., & Chan, C. B. (2013). Acculturation, dietary acceptability, and diabetes management among Chinese in North America. *Frontiers in Endocrinology, 4,* 108. doi: 10.3389/fendo.2013.00108

Doak, C. C., Doak, L. G., & Root, J. H. (1996). *Teaching patients with low literacy skills* (2nd ed.). Philadelphia, PA: Lippincott.

Duffy, M. M., & Snyder, K. (1999). Can ED patients read your patient education materials? *Journal of Emergency Nursing, 25*(25), 294–297.

Dwamena, F., Holmes-Rovner, M., Gaulden, C.M., Jorgenson, S., Sadigh, G., Sikorskii, A., ….. Olumu, A. (2012). Interventions for providers to promote a patient-centered approach in clinical consultations.

Cochrane Database Systematic Review, 12, CD003267. doi: 10.1002/14651858.CD003267.pub2

Edwardson, S. (2007). Patient education in heart failure. *Heart and Lung: The Journal of Critical Care, 36*(4), 244–252.

Erikson, E. H. (1968). *Identity: Youth and crisis.* New York, NY: Norton.

Falvo, D. R. (2011). *Effective patient education: A guide to increased adherence* (2nd ed.). Sudbury, MA: Jones and Bartlett.

Flesch, R. (1948). A new readability yardstick. *Journal of Applied Psychology, 32*(3), 221–233.

Fox, S. (2011). Health topics. Pew Internet Project and California Healthcare Foundation. http://www .pewinternet.org/Reports/2011/HealthTopics.aspx

Freeman, K. (2012). How social media, mobility are playing a bigger part in healthcare. http:// mashable.com/2012/12/18/social media-mobile-healthcare/

Gage, N. L., & Berliner, D. C. (1998). *Educational psychology* (6th ed.). Boston, MA: Houghton Mifflin.

Garland, D., & Martin, B. (2005). Do gender and learning style play a role in how online courses should be designed? *Journal of Interactive Online Learning, 4*(2), 67–81.

Gonseth, J., Castillion, G. P., Banegas, J. R., & Artalejo, F. R. (2004). The effectiveness of disease management programmes in reducing hospital re-admission in older adults with heart failure: A systematic review and meta-analysis of published reports. *European Heart Journal, 25*(18), 1570–1590.

Gremeaux, V., & Coudeyre, E. (2010). The Internet and therapeutic education in patients: A systematic review of the literature. *Annals of Physical and Rehabilitation Medicine, 53*(10), 669–692.

Haggard, A. (1989). *Handbook of patient education.* Rockville, MD: Aspen.

Hatcher, E., & Whittemore, R. (2007). Hispanic adults' beliefs about type 2 diabetes: Clinical implications. *Journal of the American Academy of Nurse Practitioners, 19*(10), 536–545.

Hayes, K. S. (2000). Literacy for health information of adult patients and caregivers in a rural emergency department. *Clinical Excellence for Nurse Practitioners, 4*, 35–40.

Healthy people 2010: Understanding and improving health (2nd ed.). Washington, DC: U.S. Government Printing Office.

Hein, G. E. (1991). Constructivist learning theory. Institute of inquiry. http://www.exploratorium.edu/ifi /resources/constructivistlearning.html

Institute of Medicine (IOM), Committee on Health Professions Education Summit. (2003). *Health professions education: A bridge to quality.* Quality Chasm Series. Washington, DC: National Academies Press.

Jacobs, J. A., Jones, E., Gabella, B. A., Spring, B., & Brownson, R. C. (2012). Tools for implementing an evidence-based approach in public health practice. *Preventing Chronic Disease, 9*, 110324. http://dx.doi .org/10.58888.pcd9.110324

Joanna Briggs Institute. (2006). Educational interventions for mental health consumers receiving psychotropic medication. *Best Practice, 10*(4), 1–4.

The Joint Commission. (2012). 2011 *Hospital accreditation standards.* Oakbrook, Terrace, IL: Author.

Kaiser Foundation. (2010). *Focus on health reform.* Menlo Park, CA: Author.

Kreuter, M., Steger-May, K., Bobra, S., Booker, A., Holt, C., Lukwago, S., & Skinner, C.S. (2003). Sociocultural characteristics and responses to cancer education materials among African American women. *Cancer Control: Journal of the Moffitt Cancer Center, 10*(5), 69–80.

Kutner, M., Greenberg, E., Jin, Y., & Paulsen, C. (2006). *The health literacy of America's adults: Results from the 2003 National Assessment of Adult Literacy.* NCES 2006-483. Washington, DC: U.S. Department of Education, National Center for Education Statistics.

Kyung, C. A., Fritschi, C., & Kim, M. J. (2012). Nurse-led empowerment strategies for hypertensive patients with metabolic syndrome. *Contemporary Nurse, 42*(1), 118–128.

Lee, T., Yeh, Y., Liu, C., & Chen, P. (2007). Development and evaluation of a patient-oriented education system for diabetes management. *International Journal of Medical Informatics, 76*, 655–663.

Lichtenthal, C. (1990). *A self-study model of readiness to learn.* Unpublished manuscript.

Lindell, D., Aucoin, J. W., Adams, C. E., Connolly, M. A., Devaney, S., Love, A., ... Ortelli, T.A. (2005). *The scope of practice for academic nurse educators.* New York, NY: National League for Nursing.

Maslow, A. H. (1962). *Towards a psychology of being.* New York, NY: John Wiley and Sons.

Mauk, K. L. (Ed.). (2014). *Gerontological nursing: Competencies for care* (3rd ed.). Burlington, MA: Jones & Bartlett Learning.

Mayer, G. G., & Vallaire, M. (2007). *Health literacy in primary care: A clinician's guide.* New York, NY: Springer.

McDonald, M. E. (2014). *The nurse educator's guide to assessing learning outcomes* (3rd ed.). Burlington, MA: Jones & Bartlett Learning.

McLaughlin, G. H. (1969). SMOG-grading: A new readability formula. *Journal of Reading, 12*, 639–646.

Melnyk, B. M., & Fineout-Overholt, E. (2010). *Evidence-based practice in nursing and healthcare* (2nd ed.). Philadelphia, PA: Lippincott.

Miller, E. (2003). Readiness to change and brief educational interventions: Successful strategies to reduce stroke risk. *Journal of Neuroscience Nursing, 35*(4), 215–222.

Miller, E. (2014). *Theoretical basis for clinical reasoning (29NURS8002): Online course manual.* Cincinnati, OH: University of Cincinnati, College of Nursing.

Miller, E., & Harris, A. (2013, February 5). *Delay in treatment seeking of African American when a stroke is suspected.* Presentation at International Stroke Association, Las Vegas, NV

Miller, E., Murray, L., Richards, L., Zorowitz, R., Bakas, T., Clark, P., & Billinger, S. (2010). A comprehensive overview of nursing and interdisciplinary rehabilitation care of the stroke patient. AHA Scientific Statement from the American Heart Association on behalf of the American Heart Council on Cardiovascular Nursing and the Stroke Council. *Stroke, 41*, 2402–2448. doi: 10.1161/STR.obO13e3181e7512b

Muijs, D., & Reynolds, D. (2005). *Effective teaching: Evidence and practice* (2nd ed.). Thousand Oaks, CA: Sage.

National League for Nursing (NLN). (2003). Innovation in nursing education: A call to reform (Position statement). http://www.nln.org/aboutnln /PositionStatements/innovation082203.pdf

Nightingale, F. (1992). *Notes on nursing: What it is and what it is not.* Philadelphia, PA: Lippincott.

Nobel, J. (2006). Bridging the knowledge–action gap in diabetes: Information technologies, physician incentives and consumer incentives converge. *Chronic Illness, 2*, 59–69.

Nundy, S., Razi, R. R., Dick, J. J., Smith, B., Mayo, A., O'Connor, A., & Meltzer, D.O. (2013). A text messaging intervention to improve heart failure self-management after hospital discharge in a largely African-American population: Before–after study. *Journal of Medical Internet Research, 15*(3), e53. doi: 10.2196/jmir.2317

Office of Minority Health. (2013). *Office of Minority Health and health equity.* Atlanta, GA: Centers for Disease Control and Prevention.

Osborne, R., Wilson, T., Lorig, K., & McColl, G. (2007). Does self-management lead to sustainable health benefits in people with arthritis? A 2-year transition study with 452 Australians. *Journal of Rheumatology, 34*(5), 1112–1117.

Packer, T. L., Ghahari, S., Melling, L., Parsons, R., & Osborne, R. H. (2012). Self-management programs conducted within a practice setting: Who participates, who benefits, and what can be learned? *Patient Education & Counseling, 87*(1), 93–100.

Petty, G. (2006). *Evidence based teaching: A practical approach.* Oxford, United Kingdom: Nelson Thornes.

Piaget, J. (1951). *The origin of intelligence in children.* New York, NY: International Universities Press.

Piaget, J. (1976). *Behavior and evolution.* Richmond, CA: McCutchen.

Pierce, L. L. (2010). How to choose and develop written educational materials. *Rehabilitation Nursing, 35*(3), 99–105.

PriceWaterhouseCoopers. (2012). *Social media "likes" healthcare: From marketing to social business.* http://www .pwc.com.us/en/health-industries/publicatoins/health-care-social-media.jhtml.

Prochaska, J. O., & DiClemente, C. C. (1983). Stages and processes of self-change of smoking: Toward an integrative model of change. *Journal of Consulting and Clinical Psychology, 51*, 390–395.

Prochaska, J. O., DiClemente, C. C., & Norcross, J. C. (1992). In search of how people change: Applications to addictive behavior. *American Psychology, 47*(9), 1102–1114.

Prochaska, J. O., & Velicer, W. F. (1997). The transtheoretical model of health behavior change. *American Journal of Health Promotion, 12*, 38–48.

Quirk, P. A. (2000). Screening for literacy and readability: Implications for the advanced practice nurse. *Clinical Nurse Specialist, 14*(1), 26–32.

Rankin, S. H., Stallings, K. D., & London, F. (2005). *Patient education in health and illness* (5th ed.). Philadelphia, PA: Lippincott.

Rhee, J., Zwar, N., & Kemp, L. (2013). Advance care planning and interpersonal relationships: A two way street. *Family Practice, 30*(2), 219–226.

Rivers, D., August, E. M., Sehovic, I., Green, B. L., & Quinn, G. P. (2013). A systematic review of the factors influencing African Americans' participation in cancer clinical trials. *Contemporary Clinical Trials, 34*(2), 13–32.

Rudd, R. E., Anderson, J. E., Oppenheimer, S., & Nath, C. (2007). Health literacy: An update of public health and medical literature. In J. P. Comings, B. Garner, & C. Smith. (Eds.), *Review of adult learning and literacy* (Vol. 7, pp. 175–204). Mahwah, NJ: Lawrence Erlbaum Associates.

Skinner, B. F. (1974). *About behaviorism.* New York, NY: Merrill.

Smith, W., Roth, J., Okoro, O., Kimberlin, C., & Odedina, F. (2011). Disability in cultural competency pharmacy education. *American Journal of Pharmaceutical Education, 75*(2), 1–9.

Spadero, D. C. (1983). Assessing readability of patient information materials. *Pediatric Nursing, 4*, 274–278.

Stahl, S. A. (2002). Different strokes for different folks? In L. Abbeduto (Ed.), *Taking sides: Clashing on controversial issues in educational psychology* (pp. 98–107). Guilford, CT: McGraw-Hill.

Stone, K. (2014). Enhancing preparedness and satisfaction of caregivers of patients discharged from an inpatient rehabilitation facility using an interactive website. *Rehabilitation Nursing, 39*(2), 76-85. doi: 10.1002/rnj.123.

Townsend, C., Bruce, B., Hooten, M., & Rome, J. (2006). The role of mental health professionals in multidisciplinary pain rehabilitation programs. *Journal of Clinical Psychology, 62*(11), 1433–1443.

Tung, W. C., & Lee, I. F. (2006). Effects of an osteoporosis educational programme for men. *Journal of Advances in Nursing, 56*(1), 26–34.

U.S. Department of Health and Human Services (DHHS). (2010). Healthy people 2020. http://www.healthypeople.gov/2020/default.aspx

Wantland, D. J., Portillo, C. J., Holzemer, W. L., & Slaughter, R. (2004). The effectiveness of Web-based vs. non–Web-based interventions: A meta-analysis of behavioral change outcomes. *Journal of Medical Internet Research, 6*(4), 40–71.

Wensing, M., & Kersnik, J. (2012). Improving the quality of care for patients with chronic diseases: What research and education in family medicine can contribute. *European Journal of General Practice, 18*, 238–241.

Chapter 16

Health Promotion

Alicia Huckstadt

Introduction

Chronic diseases are among the most preventable healthcare problems in the United States (Centers for Disease Control and Prevention [CDC], National Center for Chronic Disease Prevention and Health Promotion [NCCDPHP], 2012), with 75% of all U.S. healthcare dollars going to the treatment of these diseases (CDC, 2013). Health-promoting behaviors strongly influence whether one prematurely succumbs to disease or whether one postpones and possibly avoids major diseases. Yet, all too often health promotion is viewed as insignificant as healthcare systems scramble to treat heart disease, cancer, and other diseases that are frequently diagnosed only when they have reached advanced stages. Only recently has national attention been directed toward understanding the underlying cause of disease and determining how health promotion may change the course of disease. The once-believed single causation theory of morbidity has now been largely replaced by multifactorial causation theories and chronicity of conditions. As a consequence of improved recognition and management of disease processes, better sanitation, immunizations, and other health measures, the longevity of Americans has increased. In the early 1900s, the life expectancy was the late 40s in the United States; it has now increased to the upper 70s for both genders. Diseases that once brought sudden death have been surpassed by chronic disease in terms of prevalence. In short, Americans are living longer, but not necessarily healthier, lives. Seven out of 10 deaths among Americans each year are from chronic diseases, and one out of two Americans has at least one chronic illness (CDC, NCCDPHP, 2012).

Societal influences and individual lifestyle choices have negatively influenced health. According to two important early research articles describing the actual causes of death (nongenetic) in the United States, smoking has remained the leading cause of death in this country since 1990 (McGinnis & Foege, 1993; Mokdad, Marks, Stroup, & Gerberding, 2004). Poor diet, physical inactivity, alcohol consumption, microbial agents, toxic agents, motor vehicle crashes, incidents involving firearms, sexual behaviors, and illicit use of drugs follow smoking as actual causes of death. In a subsequent editorial, McGinnis and Foege (2004) suggested that diet/physical activity patterns are now greater contributors to mortality than tobacco and that their effects on death rates are increasing rapidly. However, these authors acknowledge that tobacco remains in the top three actual causes, with diet/physical activity patterns, tobacco, and alcohol all accounting for a sizable proportion of preventable deaths in the United States.

According to the CDC's NCCDPHP (2013), cigarette smoking remains the nation's leading cause of death, with about one of every five deaths (450,000 deaths) each year resulting from this cause. Smoking causes deaths from lung and other cancers, chronic lung disease, heart disease, and stroke. Exposure to secondhand smoke causes premature death and disease in other persons who do not smoke. Smokeless tobacco use may also cause cancer and other conditions, although epidemiologic studies are less clear on this correlation (Colilla, 2010).

Following closely behind tobacco use as a major health risk is obesity. The prevalence of obesity among U.S. adults shows upward trends and the number of overweight children has been increasing. One of every three adults and almost one in five children are obese (CDC, NCCDPHP, 2012). As researchers study this condition, they are discovering that long-term obesity is linked to avoidable hospitalizations and substantial risk for health complications (Schafer & Ferraro, 2007). Obesity is associated with increased risk of diabetes, stroke, heart disease, some cancers, hypertension, osteoarthritis, gallbladder disease, and disability (CDC, NCCDPHP, 2009). Rillamas-Sun et al. (2013) examined 36,611 women from the Women's Health Initiative observational study and clinical trials and found that abdominal and overall obesity were significant, potentially modifiable factors associated with disability, major chronic disease, and death.

The CDC (2012) has maintained that four modifiable health-risk behaviors—smoking, poor diet, physical inactivity, and excessive alcohol consumption—are the major underlying causes of much of the illness, suffering, and early death related to chronic illness. These factors and the other modifiable behavioral risk factors listed previously are believed to be the genesis of heart disease, malignant neoplasm, cerebrovascular disease, diabetes mellitus, and other chronic diseases. Indeed, half of all deaths in the United States may be attributed to a limited number of largely preventable health behaviors and exposures (Mokdad et al., 2004). The United States spends more on health care than any other nation, yet the average life expectancy of its citizens is far below that of many other developed countries that spend less on health care each year (CDC, NCCDPHP, 2009). The escalating healthcare costs, disease, and deaths associated with these factors make health promotion essential for all.

Defining Health Promotion in Chronic Illness

Health promotion is a multidimensional concept that focuses on maintaining or improving the health of individuals, families, and communities. Minimizing preventable health risk factors such as tobacco use, inadequate diets, and physical inactivity would substantially decrease the development and severity of many chronic diseases and conditions (Cory et al., 2010).

Health promotion for individuals with chronic or disabling conditions is commonly defined as efforts to create healthy lifestyles and a healthy environment to prevent secondary conditions, including teaching individuals to address their healthcare needs and increasing opportunities to participate in usual life activities. These secondary conditions may include the medical, social, emotional, mental, family, or community problems that an individual with a chronic or disabling condition is likely to experience. Environmental factors that encompass healthy living include the policies, systems, social contexts, and physical surroundings that facilitate an individual's participation in activities, including work, school, leisure, and community events (*Healthy People 2020*, 2011).

Health-promoting activities can be implemented at the public level or the personal level, and may involve passive or active strategies (Greiner & Edelman, 2010). Passive strategies, such as those used in food industry sanitation, decrease infectious agents in foods and improve public health. National, state, and local public and private agencies are given the responsibility to develop passive strategies to promote health for their constituents. Active strategies, such as engaging in better personal nutrition or activity regimens, depend on the individual and/or family becoming involved (Edelman & Mandle, 2010). Although both types of strategies are essential, this chapter focuses primarily on active strategies for individuals with chronic illness and their families.

Health promotion applies to all individuals, regardless of age or disability. The goal of health promotion is to increase the involved person's control over his or her health and to improve it. Leddy (2006) adds that health promotion seeks to mobilize strengths to enhance health, wellness, and well-being.

Health promotion in chronic illness involves engaging in individual behavioral change to ensure positive lifestyle activities, accepting one's condition and making the necessary adjustments, decreasing the risk of secondary disabilities and preventing further disease, and striving for optimal health. Behavioral change becomes possible when environmental and political policies support the provision of resources necessary for such change (Aro & Absetz, 2009).

Health promotion in chronic illness is important in maintaining and enhancing the function of the individual. It is also critical to prevent exacerbations of some conditions. Often families direct their energies toward the illness rather than health. It has been recognized for many years that illness and its cascade of effects alter family dynamics, usual roles, and patterns of life. Managing medicines, conserving physical and mental energy, keeping appointments with healthcare professionals, adjusting finances, and learning new resources likely will require substantial effort on the part of the client and family. These new stressors often overtax the individual, and activities to maintain a healthy lifestyle may consequently be ignored. For example, preventive health screening for other conditions may be forgotten by the client and the healthcare professional. Nevertheless, health-promoting behaviors remain critical in the management

of chronic conditions and are often the essential aspect in ensuring successful management. Individuals with chronic illness may develop comorbidities that could be avoided or minimized with early detection. Disease-specific preventive care needs and related physical, social, emotional, and spiritual well-being are components of health promotion for those with and without chronic illness. McWilliam, Stewart, Brown, Desai, and Coderre (1996), in their early phenomenological study exploring health and health promotion in a sample of 13 participants with chronic illness, found "a dynamically changing and evolving endeavor that encompassed four components: fighting and struggling, resigning oneself, creatively balancing resources, and accepting" (p. 5).

Undoubtedly, chronic illness presents numerous challenges to health promotion. The potential for these activities and overall health remains largely untapped in many individuals with chronic illness. Creating new ways of accomplishing health promotion often remains an unfulfilled goal for nurses and their clients with chronic illness. Efforts must go beyond the individual's chronic illness and limitations to include a holistic approach that focuses on personal goals, evidence-based care tailored to the individual, and a willingness to adjust the plan as needed. Determining individuals' perceptions of their condition, their goals, and available resources, and supporting their efforts to achieve health promotion, is an ongoing process. Leddy (2006) emphasizes that health promotion develops an individual's strengths and environmental resources to find solutions rather than focusing solely on illness repair. Chronicity presents challenges to all involved and, in many cases, may take precedence over other health considerations.

Nurses are ideally suited to promote the health of individuals and their families. The holistic, caring perspective held by nurses provides opportunities to promote strengths at a time when others may perceive only threats to health. The consequences of failure to promote health are devastating. Additional morbidity, deaths, and financial strain for individuals, families, and society weigh heavy on the healthcare system. Rising healthcare costs and an aging population compound the problem. Sustained increases in out-of-pocket healthcare spending for Medicare recipients makes health care less affordable for all but individuals with the highest income (Neuman, Cubanski, Desmond, & Rice, 2007). Newer legislation such as the Patient Protection and Affordable Care Act (ACA) includes no-cost preventive health care but has yet to demonstrate improved outcomes (U.S. Department of Health and Human Services [DHHS], 2013a).

Issues and Impact

National Documents

One of the issues of health promotion and disease prevention is compliance with national documents. Launched more than 30 years ago with the publication of *Healthy People: The Surgeon General's Report on Health Promotion and Disease Prevention* (1979), and the subsequent documents *Healthy People: Objectives for the Nation* (1980), *Healthy People 2000: National Health Promotion and Disease Prevention Objectives*, *Healthy People 2010*, and *Healthy People 2020*, the 10-year *Healthy People* initiatives build on one another and address selected areas of health promotion with a vision for achieving improved health for all Americans. Each document was developed through a broad consultative process, made use of the best scientific knowledge available, and was designed to measure outcomes over time.

HEALTHY PEOPLE 2020

The *Healthy People* documents identify a comprehensive set of 10-year health objectives focusing on disease prevention and health promotion that the United States should achieve as a nation. The vision for *Healthy People 2020* is a society where all people live long, healthy lives. The mission

of this initiative is to (1) identify nationwide health improvement priorities; (2) increase public awareness and understanding of the determinants of health, disease, and disability and the opportunities for progress; (3) provide measurable objectives and goals that are applicable at the national, state, and local levels; (4) engage multiple sectors to take actions to strengthen policies and improve practices that are driven by the best available evidence and knowledge; and (5) identify critical research, evaluation, and data collection needs.

The four overarching goals are (1) to attain high-quality, longer lives free of preventable disease, disability, injury, and premature death; (2) to achieve health equity, eliminate disparities, and improve the health of all groups; (3) to create social and physical environments that promote good health for all; and (4) to promote quality of life, healthy development, and healthy behaviors across all stages (*Healthy People 2020*, 2011). Topic areas for *Healthy People 2020* objectives are identified in **Table 16-1**. Each area has specific goals and potential relevance for individuals with chronic illness and their families.

One example of relevance for individuals and families with chronic illness is the topic area "Disability and Health." The specific goal for this focus area from *Healthy People 2020* is to promote the health and well-being of people with disabilities. People with disabilities are more likely to experience delays and other difficulties in receiving health screening and other health care, develop chronic diseases, use tobacco, not engage in fitness and other healthy activities, experience symptoms of psychological distress, and receive less social–emotional support. The *Healthy People 2020* objectives reinforce that individuals can have a disabling impairment or chronic condition at any point in life, but these conditions do not define individuals, their health, or their talents and abilities. The objectives highlight that people with chronic conditions should (1) be included in public health activities, (2) receive well-timed

Table 16-1 TOPIC AREAS FOR *HEALTHY PEOPLE 2020*

1. Access to Health Services	22. HIV
2. Adolescent Health	23. Immunization and Infectious Diseases
3. Arthritis, Osteoporosis, and Chronic Back Conditions	24. Injury and Violence Prevention
4. Blood Disorders and Blood Safety	25. Lesbian, Gay, Bisexual, and Transgender Health
5. Cancer	26. Maternal, Infant, and Child Health
6. Chronic Kidney Disease	27. Medical Product Safety
7. Dementias, including Alzheimer's Disease	28. Mental Health and Mental Disorders
8. Diabetes	29. Nutrition and Weight Status
9. Disability and Health	30. Occupational Safety and Health
10. Early and Middle Childhood	31. Older Adults
11. Educational and Community-Based Programs	32. Oral Health
12. Environmental Health	33. Physical Activity
13. Family Planning	34. Preparedness
14. Food Safety	35. Public Health Infrastructure
15. Genomics	36. Respiratory Diseases
16. Global Health	37. Sexually Transmitted Infections
17. Healthcare-Associated Infections	38. Sleep Health
18. Health Communication and Health IT	39. Social Determinants of Health
19. Health-Related Quality of Life and Well-Being	40. Substance Abuse
20. Hearing and Other Sensory or Communication Disorders	41. Tobacco Use
21. Heart Disease and Stroke	42. Vision

interventions and services, (3) be able to interact with their environment without barriers, and (4) be able to participate in everyday life activities. Without these opportunities, people with disabilities and chronic conditions will continue to experience health disparities compared to the general population. Health promotion activities are relevant for all individuals and may decrease or eliminate further declines in health.

Another *Healthy People 2020* topic that is relative to chronic disease is "Nutrition and Weight Status." The goal of this topic is to promote health and reduce chronic disease risk through the consumption of healthy diets and achievement and maintenance of healthy body weights. Individual behaviors, policies, and environments such as schools, worksites, healthcare organizations, and communities must work together to accomplish this goal.

Developers of the *Healthy People* documents have also considered caregiver issues as well as environmental barriers. Environmental factors affect the health and well-being of individuals with disabilities in many ways. For example, weather can hamper wheelchair mobility, medical offices and equipment may not be accessible, and shelters or fitness centers may not be staffed or equipped for people with disabilities. Compliance with the Americans with Disabilities Act (ADA) helps overcome some of these barriers.

Throughout the *Healthy People* documents, the U.S. Department of Health and Human Services identifies objectives expressed in terms of measurable targets to be achieved by the targeted year. Full achievement of the goals and objectives depends on a healthcare system that reaches all Americans and integrates personal health care and population-based public health. The vision of *Healthy People* for communities involves broad-based prevention efforts and moves beyond what happens in physicians' offices, clinics, and hospitals to those environments in which a large portion of prevention occurs—that is, to the neighborhoods, schools, and workplaces where individuals carry out their daily lives.

Four foundational health measures are used to monitor progress toward promoting health, preventing disease and disability, eliminating disparities, and improving quality of life:

- General health status such as life expectancy, healthy life expectancy, years of potential life lost, physically and mentally unhealthy days, self-assessed health status, limitation of activity, and chronic disease prevalence
- Health-related quality of life and well-being, including physical, mental, and social health-related quality of life, well-being/satisfaction, and participation in common activities
- Determinants of health, including personal, economic, social, and environmental factors that influence health status
- Disparities including measures of disparities and inequity based on race/ethnicity, gender, physical and mental ability, and geography

These determinants include biology, genetics, individual behavior, access to health services, and the environment. The *Healthy People* documents can be accessed at http://healthypeople.gov/.

GUIDE TO CLINICAL PREVENTIVE SERVICES

The Guide to Clinical Preventive Services includes the U.S. Preventive Services Task Force (USPSTF) recommendations on screening, counseling, and preventive medication topics, as well as clinical considerations for each topic. Sponsored since 1998 by the Agency for Healthcare Research and Quality (AHRQ), the USPSTF is an independent panel of experts in primary care and prevention that systematically reviews evidence of effectiveness and develops recommendations for clinical preventive services. The task force rigorously evaluates clinical research to assess the merits of preventive measures. The clinical conditions covered by its action include cancer; heart and vascular disease; injury and violence; infectious diseases; mental health conditions and substance abuse; metabolic, nutrition, and endocrine conditions; musculoskeletal conditions; obstetrics and gynecologic conditions; pediatric disorders; and vision and hearing disorders (USPSTF, 2013a).

One example of a current recommendation from this group concerns screening for lung cancer:

Annual screening for lung cancer with low-dose computed tomography in adults 55–80 years of age who have a 30 pack-year history of smoking and currently smoke or have quit within the past 15 years. Screening should be discontinued once a person has not smoked for 15 years or developed health problems that substantially limit life expectancy or the ability of willingness to have curative lung surgery. This is a Grade B recommendation. (USPSTF, 2013b)

GUIDE TO COMMUNITY PREVENTIVE SERVICES

The Guide to Community Preventive Services serves as a filter for scientific literature on specific health problems that have a large-scale impact on groups of people who share a common community setting. This guide summarizes what is known about the effectiveness, economic efficiency, and feasibility of interventions to promote community health and prevent disease. The Task Force on Community Preventive Services—an independent decision-making body convened by the DHHS—makes recommendations for the use of various interventions based on the evidence gathered in rigorous and systematic scientific reviews of published studies conducted by review teams for the guide. The findings from these reviews are published in peer-reviewed journals and made available online. The task force has published more than 100 findings across 16 topic areas, including tobacco use, physical activity, cancer, oral health, diabetes, motor vehicle occupant injury, vaccine-preventable diseases, prevention of injuries due to violence, and social environment (U.S. Guide to Community Preventive Services, 2013).

Where Does the United States Stand?

The CDC (2012) emphasizes that chronic diseases are among the most common, costly, and preventable of all health problems. Diseases such as heart disease, cancer, stroke, diabetes, and arthritis are the leading causes of death and disability in the United States. Seven out of 10 deaths among Americans each year are from chronic diseases. Almost one out of every two American adults has at least one chronic illness. Health disparities in chronic disease incidence and mortality are widespread among members of racial and ethnic minority populations.

Four modifiable health-risk behaviors—lack of physical activity, poor nutrition, tobacco use, and excessive alcohol consumption—are responsible for much of this morbidity and mortality. More than 43 million American adults smoke, and 20% of high school students were current smokers in 2007 (CDC, NCCDPHP, 2012). The 2005–2010 National Health Interview Surveys estimated that 45.3 million U.S. adults were current cigarette smokers and 78.2% of these adults smoked every day. Non-Hispanic American Indians/Alaska Natives continue to have a higher prevalence of smoking compared with other racial/ethnic groups. Smoking rates also continue to be higher among those persons with lower educational and income levels (CDC, 2011). The U.S. Surgeon General has issued a report explaining how tobacco smoke causes disease and identifying the specific pathways by which tobacco smoke damages the human body (DHHS, Office of the Surgeon General, 2013). The CDC's NCCDPHP (2012) emphasizes that lung cancer is the leading cause of cancer death, and cigarette smoking is related in almost all cases. For example, smoking causes approximately 90% of all lung cancer deaths in men and almost 80% of such deaths in women. Smoking also contributes to cancer of the larynx, mouth and throat, esophagus, bladder, kidney, pancreas, and others. Seventeen percent of U.S. adults report binge drinking—the most dangerous pattern of drinking—with an average of eight drinks being consumed per binge (CDC, NCCDPHP, 2012).

The NCCDPHP's (2013) vision is that all people live healthy lives free from the devastation of chronic diseases. The center's mission is to lead the nation's efforts to create expertise, information, and tools to support people and communities in preventing chronic diseases and promoting health for all. Its goals are as follows:

- Monitor, prevent, delay, detect, and control chronic diseases
- Conduct chronic disease research and translate those findings into practical and effective prevention strategies
- Promote social, environmental, policy, and systems approaches that support health
- Achieve equity in health by eliminating racial and ethnic disparities and achieving optimal health for all Americans
- Work with partners from all sectors of society to increase the reach and effectiveness of public health programs
- Develop a skilled, diverse, and dynamic public health workforce at the national, state, and local levels

The CDC (2013) provides important health promotion and chronic disease information including statistics, state profiles, tools, and resources. It also supports a variety of activities geared toward improving U.S. health by preventing chronic diseases and their risk factors. Program activities focus on one or more major functions: supporting states' implementation of public health programs; public health surveillance; translational research; health communication; and development of tools and resources for stakeholders at national, state, and community levels. The NCCDPHP programs and activities are helpful in recognizing that chronic disease prevention must occur in multiple sectors and across individuals' lifespans. The CDC provides online reports that describe the performance trends and progress toward meeting the NCCDPHP targets through the previous year (http://www.hhs.gov/about/FY2012budget/ fy2012_nih_online_performance_appendix-final_revised.pdf).

In 2009, no state in the nation met the *Healthy People 2010* obesity target of 15% prevalence, and the self-reported overall prevalence of obesity in that year increased 1.1% from 2007 (Sherry, Blanck, Galuska, Pan, & Dietz, 2010). These data undoubtedly give credence to the alarms sounded by healthcare professionals. The health status of the United States was aptly summarized by the previous Surgeon General, Regina Benjamin, when she called on all Americans to help reverse the trend of obese and overweight adults and children in the nation. The priority should be enhancing the health and wellness of families and communities through focusing on healthy nutrition and regular physical activity and making the healthiest choices accessible to all citizens. (Further remarks may be found at http://www .surgeongeneral.gov/library/obesityvision /obesityvision2010.pdf.)

The ACA (DHHS, 2013b) outlines preventive services that are recommended for women, children, and adults. For example, depending on your age, you may have access—at no cost—to the following preventive services:

- Blood pressure, diabetes, and cholesterol tests
- Many cancer screenings, including mammograms and colonoscopies
- Counseling on such topics as quitting smoking, losing weight, eating healthfully, treating depression, and reducing alcohol use
- Regular well-baby and well-child visits, from birth to age 21
- Routine vaccinations against diseases such as measles, polio, or meningitis
- Counseling, screening, and vaccines to ensure healthy pregnancies
- Flu and pneumonia shots

Table 16-2 identifies the 15 preventive services that are covered for adults. Having these preventive measures of the Affordable Care Act become realities for all Americans has yet to be accomplished.

ONLINE RESOURCES

The CDC's website (http://www.cdc.gov) shares the goal of helping people live longer and healthier lives. This website provides information on numerous diseases and conditions, emergency preparedness, environmental health, travelers' health, workplace safety, and other topics. One area, healthy living (http://www .cdc.gov/HealthyLiving/), is especially beneficial to consumers and healthcare professionals for health in all life stages.

The CDC website includes additional focus areas such as one emphasizing the importance of a healthy diet and eating in moderation for the general population (http://www.cdc.gov /nutrition/everyone/basics/foodgroups.html); it includes further information on nutrition, available for healthcare professionals (http://www .cdc.gov/nutrition/professionals/index.html). The National Physical Activity Plan (http:// www.cdc.gov/physicalactivity/index.html) is

---

Table 16-2 COVERED PREVENTIVE SERVICES FOR ADULTS

1. **Abdominal aortic aneurysm** one-time screening for men of specified ages who have ever smoked
2. **Alcohol misuse** screening and counseling
3. **Aspirin** use for men and women of certain ages
4. **Blood pressure** screening for all adults
5. **Cholesterol** screening for adults of certain ages or at higher risk
6. **Colorectal cancer** screening for adults older than age 50
7. **Depression** screening for adults
8. **Type 2 diabetes** screening for adults with high blood pressure
9. **Diet** counseling for adults at higher risk for chronic disease
10. **HIV** screening for all adults at higher risk
11. **Immunization** vaccines for adults—doses, recommended ages, and recommended populations vary:
    - Hepatitis A
    - Hepatitis B
    - Herpes zoster
    - Human papillomavirus
    - Influenza
    - Measles, mumps, rubella
    - Meningococcal
    - Pneumococcal
    - Tetanus, diphtheria, pertussis
    - Varicella
12. **Obesity** screening and counseling for all adults
13. **Sexually transmitted infection (STI)** prevention counseling for adults at higher risk
14. **Tobacco use** screening for all adults and cessation interventions for tobacco users
15. **Syphilis** screening for all adults at higher risk

---

a comprehensive set of policies, programs, and initiatives that aims to increase physical activity in all segments of the American population. The CDC encourages everyone to learn how to prevent disease and improve quality of life, helping to do so through providing this information. The CDC also recommends that people know their family history and understand how genes and personal history could put their health at risk.

Another website (http://healthfinder.gov/) provides a quick guide to healthy living, personal health tools, health news, locating health providers, and other information promoting health.

A variety of screening recommendations are available from reputable sources such as the American Heart Association; CDC; National Cancer Institute; National Heart, Lung, and Blood Institute; and Agency for Healthcare Research and Quality. Individuals can review the recommendations and share their history information with their healthcare professionals to determine which tests and screenings are appropriate for them. Healthy Men (http://www.ahrq .gov/patients-consumers/patient-involvement /healthy-men/index.html) is an AHRQ resource that helps men learn which preventive medical tests they need and when to get them. The website also provides the latest recommendations on screening for colorectal cancer, abdominal aortic aneurysms, and other conditions. Information on immunizations, daily healthy choices, tips on communication with healthcare professionals, understanding prescriptions, and other sources of information for men's health are included.

These websites remind people, when faced with choices that may affect their health and the lives of those they love, that it is important to remember there are options and resources to help them make healthy decisions. Related websites, such as that for the U.S. Food and Drug Administration (FDA), provide information intended to help people make better-informed decisions, for example, in taking medications (www.fda.gov/usemedicinesafely), and the Surgeon General offers information for protecting yourself from secondhand tobacco smoke (DHSS, Office of the Surgeon General, 2013). In addition, the National Prevention Strategy guides the nation in effective and attainable ways to improve health and well-being by identifying four major strategies: (1) healthy and safe community environments; (2) clinical and community preventive services; (3) empowered people; and (4) elimination of health disparities.

The attention to healthy communities is an important health promotion component that followed reports of *Steps Communities* that were funded nationwide to address six focus areas—obesity, diabetes, asthma, physical inactivity, poor nutrition, and tobacco use and exposure. These initiatives were undertaken after a survey of outcomes from non-institutionalized community members aged 18 years and older revealed that none of the communities achieved the *Healthy People 2010* objective of increasing to 91% the proportion of adults with diabetes who have at least an annual clinical foot examination. The majority of the communities also did not meet the *Healthy People* objectives for annual dilated eye examinations or hemoglobin A_{1c} measurements. Likewise, the majority of communities did not meet the goal for asthma patients not to have had any symptoms during the preceding 30 days. However, the proportions of community residents who engaged in moderate or vigorous physical activity for 30 or more minutes at least five times a week or who reported vigorous physical activity for 20 or more minutes three times a week ranged from 40.6% to 69.8%, exceeding the *Healthy People 2010* objective of 50%. The prevalence of consumption of fruits and vegetables at least five times per day ranged from 14.6% to 37.6%. Only two of the communities reached the *Healthy People 2010* objective to reduce the proportion of adults who smoke, and no communities reached the objective of increasing smoking cessation attempts by adult smokers to 75% of this population. The findings of the *Steps Communities* report reflect considerable variation in health-risk behaviors, chronic diseases, and use of preventive health screenings and other health promotion activities. The authors strongly encourage recognition of the need for preventive interventions at the community level and design and implementation of policies that promote and encourage healthy behaviors (Cory et al., 2010).

Decreasing smoking rates among adolescents and adults is a major health objective for the United States. The Institute of Medicine (IOM) has issued a blueprint for further reducing tobacco use (several measures are available at http://www.nap.edu/catalog/11795.html) and secondhand smoke exposure (http://www.iom.edu/~/media/Files/Report%20Files/2009/Secondhand-Smoke-Exposure-and-Cardiovascular-Effects-Making-Sense-of-the-Evidence/Secondhand%20Smoke%20%20Report%20Brief%202.ashx). Recently, a large meta-analysis identified smoking as a risk factor for prostate cancer, with the heaviest smokers having a 24% to 30% greater risk of death than did nonsmokers (Huncharek, Haddock, Reid, & Kupelnick, 2010).

Other national documents that provide recommendations for screening and other preventive health care are described next.

OTHER GUIDELINES

The American Heart Association (AHA) and the American College of Cardiology (ACC) have issued an updated guideline on lifestyle management to reduce cardiovascular risks that includes dietary and physical activity recommendations (Eckel et al., 2013). The AHA and ACC joined the Task Force on Practice Guidelines and The Obesity Society (TOS) to provide another guideline for the management of overweight and obese conditions in adults (Jensen et al., 2013). These guidelines are based on current literature and offer updated evidence-based information critical to health promotion, including behavioral change therapies delivered by trained interventionists, mostly healthcare professionals. The authors of these guidelines emphasize that further study is needed, including longitudinal studies that evaluate the continuing effectiveness of these lifestyle modification strategies.

Challenges

National documents and other resources illustrate that health promotion and disease prevention are essential for all Americans. The nation needs to continually work toward these goals; however, to do so requires changes in the healthcare system. The ongoing health care needed once a chronic disease has been diagnosed is only one segment of the necessary care. Many risks to health—obesity, diabetes, hypertension, heart disease, cancer, and other chronic conditions—result from failure to engage in preventive care. More closely articulated preventive, public health, and policy programs are needed to promote a healthy life. Other factors, including genetics and environmental risks, contribute to chronic illness as well.

Health promotion can and should occur before the onset of chronic illness, and as early as possible. Health promotion ideally occurs throughout one's life and in concert with chronic conditions through the end of life. A lifetime activity, it can include end-of-life planning for individuals and their significant others. Preparing for the physical and psychosocial changes that accompany death requires attention before crisis events. Preparation, dissemination, and discussion of advance directives with significant others can help set clear boundaries for honoring the wishes of clients (Rainer & McMurry, 2002).

Barriers

Reported barriers to health screening and other preventive care must be addressed. Unhealthy behaviors continue to increase in the United States, putting people more at risk for initial chronic illness and deterring health promotion practices among those with chronic illnesses. The CDC's NCCDPHP (2012) reports that more than one third of all U.S. adults do not meet the recommendations for aerobic physical activity and 23% report no leisure-time physical activity at all during the preceding year. In 2007, only 24% of U.S. adults and 22% of high school students ate five or more fruits and vegetables each day. Cigarette smoking is responsible for about 440,000 deaths in the United States each year. More deaths are caused each year by tobacco use than by all deaths from HIV/AIDS, alcohol use, motor vehicle injuries, suicide, and murder combined. Exercising regularly, eating a healthy diet, and not using tobacco can help people prevent and manage chronic diseases. Unfortunately, many people in the United States do not have easy access to healthy foods and safe, convenient places to exercise. These barriers have led to increasingly sedentary lifestyles for the majority of Americans.

Other barriers exist for health screening. Kelly and colleagues (2007) identified fear and embarrassment as commonly cited client barriers to screening for colorectal cancer. Fewer than 44% of their study population of Appalachian residents in the state of Kentucky had colorectal cancer screening consistent with guidelines. These researchers identified establishing trust and educating clients, using resources such as educational materials, and finding inexpensive and easy ways to screen as the most productive ways to overcome the barriers.

Little is known how health screening and other preventive care affect outcomes. Norman and colleagues (2007) emphasized that we do not know what survivors of diseases such as breast cancer must do to prevent recurrence. Data are needed on lifestyle changes from prediagnosis to postdiagnosis, changes over time after diagnosis, and identification of potential lifestyle risk factors.

Health promotion has not been addressed effectively in the care of clients with multiple chronic health conditions. Capella-McDonnall (2007) reported that despite the recent focus on health promotion for persons with disabilities, adults who are visually impaired have not received adequate attention in this area. Two conditions—being overweight or obese and not being physically active—are widespread problems among persons with disabilities, including those who are visually impaired.

Problems with health literacy are commonplace in our society. Health literacy is the capacity to obtain, process, and understand basic health information and services needed to make appropriate health decisions (DHHS, Office of Disease Prevention and Health Promotion, 2013). Nine out of 10 U.S. adults may lack the skills needed to manage their health and disease prevention. Poor health outcomes and less frequent use of preventive services are linked with low literacy. Individuals with low literacy are more likely to skip important preventive screening such as colonoscopies, Pap smears, and mammograms, and are less likely to receive protective measures such as flu immunizations. Persons with low literacy are more likely to have chronic illness and are less able to manage it effectively. More preventable hospitalizations and use of emergency services are found among clients with chronic illness with limited literacy skills. People with limited literacy skills often lack knowledge about the nature and causes of disease and may not understand the relationship between lifestyle factors such as smoking, lack

of exercise and inadequate nutrition, and poor health outcomes.

Other barriers to health screening and preventive care include associated costs; lack of knowledge/understanding; negative beliefs/attitudes; lack of access, especially for those with limited geographical and/or functional ability; and other factors addressed in the models, theories, and frameworks discussed next.

Models, Theories, and Frameworks

An entire body of literature has evolved around models and theories relating to health behavior change. Considerable research has demonstrated success in changing behavior in relation to smoking cessation and alcohol abuse using these theories. The most frequently used theories in 193 articles in the health behavior literature published in 10 leading public health, medicine, and psychology journals from 2000 to 2005 were the transtheoretical model, social cognitive theory, and health belief model (Painter, Borba, Hynes, Mays, & Glanz, 2008). Of the articles included in this systematic review, most (68.1%) involved research that was informed by theory; others applied theory, tested theory, and sought to develop theory. The examples that follow are theories and models that may be useful in behavioral change in chronic illness.

The transtheoretical model (TTM) developed by Prochaska, Redding, and Evers (2002) incorporates the processes and principles of change from several major theories in psychotherapy and human behavior. The model includes five stages of change: (1) pre-contemplation (no intention to change in the foreseeable future); (2) contemplation (intention to change in the next 6 months); (3) preparation (intention to take action within the next 30 days and some behavioral steps to change); (4) action (has changed behavior for less than 6 months); and (5) maintenance (has changed behavior for more than 6 months). These five stages give a temporal dimension to change and are helpful in identifying timing of change interventions. A sixth stage—termination (individual possesses total self-efficacy and is no longer susceptible to the temptation of unhealthy behavior)—is rarely used, as few individuals reach this level. In the TTM, individuals weigh the pros and cons of changing (decisional balance) and determine their confidence (self-efficacy) that they can cope with high-risk situations without relapsing to unhealthy or high-risk behavior specific to the situation.

The 10 processes of change of the TTM are activities that people use to progress through the stages of change:

1. Consciousness raising (increasing awareness of the behavior)
2. Dramatic relief (experiencing increased emotions followed by reduced effect if appropriate action is taken)
3. Self-reevaluation (assessing one's image with and without the unhealthy behavior)
4. Environmental reevaluation (assessing how one's social environment is affected by the unhealthy behavior)
5. Self-liberation (believing and committing to change)
6. Helping relationships (building support for healthy behavior change)
7. Counterconditioning (learning that healthy behaviors can replace unhealthy behaviors)
8. Contingency management (increasing reinforcement and probability that healthy behaviors will be repeated)
9. Stimulus control (removing unhealthy behavior cues and adding healthy behavior cues)
10. Social liberation (increasing social opportunities to foster behavior change) (Prochaska et al., 2002, pp. 103–104)

The TTM has been used in numerous studies, including those focusing on smoking cessation, mammography screening, alcohol avoidance, and exercise and stress management. It has been beneficial in tailoring interventions for the most appropriate stage of change.

The theory of reasoned action (TRA) and the theory of planned behavior (TPB) offer another framework for examining factors that determine behavioral change. This framework focuses on motivational factors as determinants of the person's likelihood of performing a specific behavior. The TRA provides the rationale that the person's beliefs and values determine whether the person intends to change behavior. The TPB adds that perceived behavioral control of facilitating or constraining conditions will affect intention and behavior. Beliefs affecting behavior differ widely among persons, among groups, and even in regard to specific behaviors demonstrated by the same individual. Use of these models is helpful in understanding the likelihood that individuals will perform a specific healthier behavior and can provide a framework for interventions. These theories can be used along with others to design and deliver behavioral change to improve research and practice (Montano & Kasprzyk, 2002).

The health belief model (HBM) has been one of the most widely used conceptual frameworks to explain change in health behavior and to provide a framework for interventions (Janz, Champion, & Strecher, 2002). The components of the HBM have been revised many times since its inception in the 1950s. Originally a model used to explain readiness to obtain chest X-ray screening for tuberculosis, the HBM has evolved beyond screening behaviors to include preventive actions, illness behaviors, and sick-role behavior. Today, the HBM purports that individuals will take action to prevent, screen for, or control ill health conditions if there is perceived susceptibility (persons regard themselves as susceptible to the condition), if there is perceived severity (persons believe the condition would have potentially serious consequences), if there are perceived benefits (persons believe that a course of action available to them would be beneficial in reducing either their susceptibility to or the severity of the condition), and if the perceived barriers can be overcome (persons believe that the anticipated barriers to—or costs of—taking the action are outweighed by its benefits) (Janz et al., 2002). Determining strategies to activate persons' readiness to change (cues to action) can include providing information and awareness campaigns. As with the TTM, self-efficacy is an integral concept of the HBM.

The health promotion model (HPM) integrates constructs from the expectancy–value theory and social cognitive theory, and provides a nursing perspective to depict the multidimensional nature of persons pursuing health (Pender, Murdaugh, & Parsons, 2002). The HPM purports that behavior change will occur if there is positive personal value and a desired outcome from such change. The HPM has been revised since its initial development in the early 1980s and is considered an approach-oriented or competence model. The authors report that the HPM is different from the HBM, as it eliminates the negative source of motivation (i.e., fear or threat) from the major motivating sources for health behavior change. They emphasize that elimination of the personal threat motivational factor ensures applicability of the model across the lifespan. Self-efficacy is a major construct of the HPM, and assumptions of the model require an active role of the person "in shaping and maintaining health behaviors and in modifying the environmental context for health behaviors" (Pender et al., 2002, p. 63). The HPM has been used as a framework for studies predicting general health-promoting abilities and for specific health behaviors including hearing protection, exercise, and nutrition (Pender et al., 2002).

In a recent study, researchers examined the role of perceived susceptibility in conjunction with colorectal cancer screening intention and behavior (McQueen, Vernon, Rothman, Norman, Myers, & Tilley, 2010). Perceived susceptibility is a psychosocial variable in several health promotion theories and is viewed as a motivating factor in behavioral change,

but disagreement has arisen regarding how its mechanism affects behavior. Results of this study showed perceived susceptibility was not limited to direct effects, but rather occurred independently of perceived benefits, was mediated by the change in family influence, and moderated the change in perceived barriers and self-efficacy.

Theories and models help identify important and potentially modifiable health promotion determinants primarily for people without chronic illnesses and disabilities. Unfortunately, very little research has been conducted using these theories and models to study health-promoting behaviors of people with disabilities (Chan, Chiu, Bezyak, & Keegan, 2012). Only recently have epidemiologic studies provided evidence of a strong link between mental health and physical health as it relates to chronic disease, such as by examining the individual with depression and depression's effect on hypertension, diabetes, cancer, obesity and certain risk behaviors including physical inactivity, smoking, and drinking (Perry, Presley-Cantrell, & Dhingra, 2010).

Glass, Moss, and Ogle (2012) proposed a person-centered health promotion model for older people with chronic illness. This international model integrates research from case studies and synthesizes critical literature in identifying four key elements: construct, context, process, and outcome. The model aims to minimize emotional disruptions as people with chronic illness work with healthcare professionals to reduce lifestyle risks and promote self-care.

Ongoing work on theory and relationships between variables is helping to advance the understanding of health promotion and behavioral change. Nevertheless, some sources suggest that theory development has not kept pace with the evolution of health promotion practice (Crosby & Noar, 2010). Some of this disparity relates to problems such as the following: (1) theory is not grounded in practice; (2) theory is at the individual level and simplistic without attention to the contextual nature of human behavior and environment; and (3) theory is inaccessible to practitioners who are facing increased demands to prevent disease and promote health (Crosby & Noar, 2010). Remedies that allow for greater complexity in theory development in the future are daunting, yet remain something to aspire to. Health care frequently uses broad-stroke approaches to health promotion interventions in hopes that some clients' health behaviors will change. Further development of theory will better frame questions surrounding health promotion.

Caution should accompany any such new theory development, as misleading data can exaggerate the theories' predictive accuracy (Weinstein, 2007). Often studies in health promotion are based on correlational data collected in the form of variables such as beliefs, attitudes, self-efficacy, intentions, diet, nutrition, preventive measures, and other human behaviors. While these studies may provide descriptive information, correlations do not infer causation. Theory development needs to be carefully designed. The resulting theories must be tested in practice-based contexts, allow cross-cultural transfer, be more inclusive of environmental changes, and effectively serve health promotion practice (DiClementi, Crosby, & Kegler, 2009).

Interventions

Chronic diseases account for the vast majority of deaths that occur in the United States each year. Although chronic diseases are among the most common and costly health problems, they are also among the most preventable. Adopting healthy behaviors such as eating nutritious foods, being physically active, and avoiding tobacco use can prevent or control the devastating effects of these diseases. Developing effective health promotion interventions requires an understanding of the barriers and facilitators of behavior in people with chronic illness and disabilities (Chan et al., 2012).

Nurses have been leaders in health promotion since the time of Florence Nightingale, whose pioneering work with the use of statistics demonstrated the positive effect of improved sanitation on the health of injured soldiers. Nurses have also led the healthcare profession in recognizing that health is a state of physical and mental wellness and that it is impossible to separate the former from the latter. (Calloway, 2007, p. 105)

Olshansky (2007) emphasizes that nurses are the most appropriate healthcare professionals to address health promotion. Nursing has strong role models within our profession, such as Nola Pender, who developed the HPM. Nursing literature abounds with textbooks, articles, and other publications that emphasize nursing's role in health promotion to individuals, families, communities, and populations. Yet, nurses cannot assume sameness among all persons with chronic illness, and they cannot assume resources are equally available to all. People with chronic illness may view health differently and have different goals defined within the limits of their illness.

Selected Examples of Health Promotion Interventions

A review of the literature provides examples of health promotion interventions for clients with chronic illness. Nevertheless, the discussion here illustrates that much has yet to be examined.

In an international study, Huang, Chou, Lin, and Chao (2007) analyzed survey data including the Health-Promoting Lifestyle Profile and quality of life data for 129 outpatients with systemic lupus erythematosus. These researchers found that a health-promoting lifestyle did not enhance the physical component summary of quality of life directly without an improvement in the fatigue disability, but a health-promoting lifestyle had a significant effect on the mental component summary of quality of life. Thus, although the physical aspects of the chronic condition may not improve without other physical changes, there can be improvements in psychological health.

Hope has been recommended as a health-promoting force. Hollis, Massey, and Jevne (2007) identified hope-enhancing strategies and sources to improve one's health. Blue (2007) studied 106 adults at risk for diabetes and found the theory of planned behavior to be useful in explaining their healthy eating intentions and physical activity.

Health-promoting activities such as prevention of injuries may make the difference in whether one is able to live with one or more chronic conditions. One example is preventing falls. Falls are one of the most common causes of injuries in older adults. These preventable accidents cause loss of independence, enormous financial costs, and possibly death. One evidence-based program to prevent falls is exemplified by Ory and colleagues' (2010) analysis of community-dwelling older adults who participated in a Matter of Balance/Volunteer Lay Leader model intended to reduce fear of falling and increase physical activity of participants.

MOTIVATIONAL INTERVIEWING

Motivational interviewing (MI) incorporates behavior change principles to promote healthy activities. Four guiding principles serve as the basis for motivational interviewing: (1) resist the righting reflex that helping professionals often have (i.e., the need to set things right and the assumption that patients are wrong); (2) understand and explore the patient's own motivation; (3) listen with empathy; and (4) empower the patient, encouraging hope and optimism (Rollnick, Miller, & Butler, 2008, p. 7). The literature abounds with international and national studies supporting MI as an approach to health behavior change.

Brodie and Inoue (2005) demonstrated the effectiveness of MI over a traditional exercise program in increasing reported physical activity in older adults with chronic heart failure.

Jackson, Asimakopoulou, and Scammell (2007) demonstrated, in an experimental study of 34 clients with type 2 diabetes, that MI and behavior change training significantly increased the participants' physical activity and stage of change. In their qualitative study of Canadian telephone hotline employees, Mantler, Irwin, and Morrow (2013) concluded that MI training had a positive impact on the participants' perceived competencies in facilitating behavioral change in smokers.

Thompson et al.'s (2011) systematic review of MI found strong evidence that MI is an effective approach that elicits the individual's intrinsic motivation to change behavior. Tse, Vong, and Tang (2013) studied 56 older adults with chronic pain in two Hong Kong community centers. Using a single-blind, randomized control design, these researchers found MI and physical activity were significantly more effective in improving pain reduction, physical mobility, psychological well-being, and self-efficacy in the experimental group than in the control group. Balan, Moyers, and Lewis-Fernandez (2013) demonstrated that combining MI with psychopharmacotherapy sessions could increase treatment adherence in the management of clinical psychiatric disorders.

The majority of authors who have studied or described MI agree that MI takes time and practice. Pursey (2013) reinforces the message that healthcare professionals should avoid the "righting" reflex that assumes the patient must do things a certain way. It is much more beneficial to use open questions that help clients identify a need for a change in lifestyle. Brobeck, Bergh, Odencrants, and Hildingh's (2011) qualitative study of 20 primary healthcare nurses using MI revealed that MI places several different demands on nurses. As a consequence, those nurses using MI must make an extra effort to avoid reverting to simply giving advice. Maintaining an open mind is essential to increasing MI's effectiveness and contributing to the promotion of health lifestyle practices.

The timing of MI was tested by combining the stages of change model with motivational interviewing in an international study by Noordman, de Vet, van der Weijden, and van Dulmen (2013). These researchers found that practice nurses adapt their MI skills to the patient's stage of change, but they tend to apply MI skills to patients in the preparation stage more frequently than any other stage. Thomas et al. (2012) studied 318 adults with various types of cancer pain and found MI-based coaching used by advanced practice oncology nurses was useful in helping patients to develop an appropriate plan of care to decrease pain and other symptoms.

MOTIVATING FACTORS

→ Money is a big motivating factor today

Providing performance incentives, both financial and nonfinancial, has been explored as a means to change behaviors in individuals and in communities. The following principles are helpful in guiding the development of any incentive design:

1. Identify the desired outcome.
2. Identify the behavior change that leads to the desired outcome.
3. Determine the potential effectiveness of the incentive in achieving the behavior change.
4. Link an incentive directly to the behavior or outcome.
5. Identify possible adverse effects of the incentive.
6. Evaluate changes in the behavior or outcome in response to the incentive (Haverman, 2010).

Researchers using a randomized study of 51 adults, all age 50, demonstrated that giving modest financial incentives was an effective approach for increasing physical activity among sedentary older adults (Finkelstein, Brown, Brown, & Buchner, 2008).

In a review of 26 studies (8 randomized controlled trials and 18 observational), use of pedometers significantly increased physical activity and significantly decreased body mass index and blood pressure (Bravata et al., 2007). The use of pedometers as a motivating factor with persons with chronic illness capable of using a pedometer and the long-term effects of pedometers are yet to be investigated.

Motivating factors have been identified in theories, models, and frameworks, and positive motivators such as those in the HPM are congruent with nursing philosophical bases. Creative approaches such as dance, music, movement, and imagery, coupled with motivational interviewing, may enhance the effectiveness of motivational interviewing among individuals who are attempting to make a behavioral change (Crowe & Parmenter, 2012). Challenges for the future are to continue the testing and use of such frameworks in the health-promoting activities of persons and families with chronic illness.

HEALTH COACHING

Health coaching is emerging as a new approach for preventing exacerbations of chronic illness and supporting lifestyle changes. This method partners health coaches with clients to enhance self-management strategies. It is being piloted by Medicare for clients with congestive heart failure and diabetes (Huffman, 2007).

Holland, Greenberg, Tidwell, and Newcomer (2003) described the success of the California Public Employees Retirement System (CalPERS) Health Matters program by examining a community-based health coaching program operating in Sacramento. Criteria for eligibility included having one or more qualifying chronic health conditions and being age 65 or older, among other program criteria. The Health Matters program offers a menu of disability-prevention strategies, including health coaching, patient education on the self-management of chronic illness, and fitness. The program helps link participants to existing community, health plan, and self-directed programs. It encourages their participation in the programs developed for the project.

The self-management of care model is used for lifestyle coaching programs based on collaborative goal setting and self-management health education (Rohrer, Naessens, Liesinger, & Litchy, 2010). One study examined the usefulness of self-rated health metrics in assessing telephonic coaching programs targeting weight, exercise, stress, and nutrition (Rohrer et al., 2010). While these coaching programs showed positive improvements in all of the lifestyle interventions, the self-rated health metrics were correlated with improvements only in weight loss and exercise programs. Therefore, the coaching programs were successful, but self-ratings may not demonstrate improvements in all areas.

MASS-MEDIA CAMPAIGNS

Beaudoin, Fernandez, Wall, and Farley (2007) used a mass-media campaign of high-frequency paid television and radio advertising, as well as bus and streetcar signage, to promote walking and fruit/vegetable consumption in a low-income, predominantly African American urban population in New Orleans. Over the course of the 5-month campaign, researchers observed a significant increase in message recall measures and positive attitudes toward walking and fruit/vegetable consumption. It is unknown how many persons with chronic illness were included. It is likely that many persons targeted by the campaign were at risk for future chronic illness. These efforts demonstrate population efforts to improve health that may be researched with individuals with chronic illness.

Snyder (2007) reviewed existing meta-analyses for effectiveness of health communication campaigns, and found that the average health campaign alters prevalence of the targeted behavior within the intervention community by about five percentage points. Snyder concluded that successful campaigns likely to change nutrition behaviors need to include specific behavioral goals for the intervention, identification of the target population, identification of communication activities and channels that will be used, provision of message content and presentation, and provision of techniques for feedback and evaluation.

WEB-BASED PROGRAMS

Verheijden, Jans, Hildebrandt, and Hopman-Rock (2007) found that Web-based behavioral programs often reach those who need them the least. However, obese people are more likely to participate in follow-up than those with normal body weight. The researchers proposed that Web-based programs are a non-stigmatizing way of addressing the problem and suggested that weight management is better suited for this delivery method than many other health-related areas. Although this study was based in the Netherlands, its results may have implications for other countries with similar health-promotion problems. Successful Web-based interventions improve health knowledge and are effective in changing behaviors. These Web-based interventions have been implemented primarily through interactive messaging and information dissemination but are wide open for expansion (Annang, Muilenburg, & Strasser, 2010).

CONTRACTS

Burkhart, Rayens, Oakley, Abshire, and Zhang (2007) found in their randomized, controlled trial of 77 children with persistent asthma that the intervention group who received asthma education plus contingency management, including a contingency contract, tailoring, cueing, and reinforcement, demonstrated increased adherence to asthma self-management relative to the control group, who received asthma education without the contingency management. However, in 30 trials involving 4,691 participants, Cochrane review authors concluded that there is limited evidence showing that contracts can improve patients' adherence to health-promotion programs. Large, well-controlled studies are needed before recommending the implementation of contracts in preventive health programs (Bosch-Capblanch, Abba, Prictor, & Garner, 2007).

Health Literacy

Improving the use of health information is paramount in health promotion programs. The DHHS's Office of Disease Prevention and Health Promotion (2013) has summarized the best practices for healthcare professionals who seek to improve health literacy by providing effective communications and accessible health services. **Table 16-3** outlines these practices.

Nath (2007) reviewed the literature between 1990 and mid-2006 for information

---

Table 16-3 IMPROVING HEALTH LITERACY INTERVENTIONS

When providing health information, is the information appropriate for the user?	Identify intended users of the information and services. Evaluate the users' knowledge prior to, during, and after the introduction of information and services. Acknowledge cultural differences and practice respect.
When providing health information, is the information easy to use?	Limit the number of messages. Keep it simple, and, in general, limit the information to no more than four main messages. Use plain language. Use familiar language and an active voice. Avoid jargon. (See www.plainlanguage.gov for more information.) Focus on the behavior that you want the person to change. Supplement instructions with visual images to help convey your message. Make written communication easy to read by using a large font. Use headings and bullets to break up text; limit line length to between 40 and 50 characters. Improve Internet information by using uniform navigation and organizing information to minimize searching and scrolling, including interactive features. Apply user-centered design principles and conduct usability testing.
When providing health information, are you speaking clearly and listening carefully?	Ask open-ended questions. Use a medically trained interpreter for those clients who do not speak English or have limited ability to speak or understand English. Use words and examples that make the information relevant to the person's cultural norms and values. Check for understanding using a "teach-back" method to enhance communication.
Improve the use of health services.	Improve the usability of health forms and instructions by including plain language forms in multiple languages. · Improve the accessibility of the physical environment by including universal symbols, clear signage, and easy flow through healthcare facilities. Establish a patient navigator program in which individuals can help patients access services and appropriate healthcare information.
Build knowledge to improve health decision making.	Improve access to accurate and appropriate health information. Increase self-efficacy and facilitate health decision making. Partner with educators to improve health curricula.
Advocate for health literacy in the organization.	Make the case for health literacy improvement. Identify how low health literacy affects programs. Incorporate health literacy into mission and planning. Establish accountability by including health literacy improvement in program evaluation.

on overcoming inadequate literacy in diabetes self-management and other chronic illnesses. Culturally appropriate health literacy, improved self-efficacy, improved communication, and quality computer-assisted instruction were discussed as essential elements in tailoring health education. Nurses were recommended to address barriers related to inadequate literacy by taking the following steps: (1) increasing sensitivity to the problem; (2) developing a literacy-assessment protocol; (3) creating and evaluating materials for the target populations; (4) providing clear communication; (5) including health literacy in nursing curricula; (6) fostering decision making with patients; and (7) conducting research into literacy issues.

Additional Studies

As part of an effort to use telehealth as a means to improve access to health care, students in a community setting applied self-efficacy theory to help low-income older adults with chronic health problems increase their practices of health promotion (Coyle, Duffy, & Martin, 2007). Although faculty and students favorably evaluated the activity, measurement of patient outcomes was not conducted. The effects of telehealth require further research.

Program design of health promotion efforts can significantly influence the participation of all individuals. Warren-Findlow, Prohaska, and Freedman (2003) demonstrated factors that influenced participation and retention in an exercise intervention study targeted to African American and white older adults with multiple chronic illnesses. These researchers found that eligible participants who did not enroll were more likely to be diabetic and younger than age 60. Seventy percent of the enrolled participants remained in the program after 1 year. Attrition was related to the program site, the functional status of the individual, and having a high school degree; it was not associated with chronic illness. The researchers concluded that group-specific efforts tailored for the particular

audience can be successful in recruiting and retaining participants.

Feldman and Tegart (2003) explored the issues faced by older African American women with arthritis and their motivations and struggles with health promotion. These authors' reflections provide helpful suggestions as nurses develop health promotion programs for clients with chronic illness.

Miller and Iris (2002) found that socialization and social support were central to the participation of older adults with chronic illness in a wellness program. In this study, participants recognized that chronic disease did not prohibit them from living a healthy lifestyle. The White Crane Model of Healthy Lives for Older Adults used in this study contributed to understanding the ways in which older adults view their health. This model is also thought to be helpful in developing program evaluation measures.

In another study, a diet and exercise program to reduce cardiovascular disease risk was used with employees regardless of the presence of chronic illness. Significant differences between pre- and post-intervention lipid profiles and weight measurements were reported. Self-reported levels of participation in the diet were significantly related to improvement in the employees' low-density lipoprotein (LDL) levels (White & Jacques, 2007).

The addition of health promotion to the usual care of frail older homecare clients was studied in Canada by Markle-Reid et al. (2006). The researchers found that proactively providing health promotion to older adults with chronic health needs enhanced quality of life, but did not increase the overall costs of health care. Better mental health functioning, reduction in depression, and enhanced perceptions of social support were reported in the experimental group. The researchers concluded that their findings underscore the need to provide health promotion for older clients receiving home care.

Zhang, Fung, and Ho-hong Ching (2009) randomly assigned 111 young adults aged

18–36 and 104 older adults aged 62–86 to read health pamphlets that provided identical information about healthy eating, but contained either emotional or non-emotional goals for the healthy behavior. Their study was based on socioemotional selectivity theory, which contends that as individuals get older, they perceive time as being increasingly limited; hence older individuals tend to choose emotionally meaningful goals with more immediate payoffs over future-oriented goals. Older adults in this study evaluated health messages that contained emotional goals more positively than health messages that included non-emotional, future-oriented, or neutral goals. The former messages were better remembered and led to greater behavioral changes in the older population than in the younger adults. While generalization of these results should be undertaken only with caution, the findings may suggest that healthcare professionals should emphasize emotionally meaningful benefits when disseminating health messages to older adults.

The adverse effects of obesity in individuals with chronic disease were supported when positive associations of age, gender, race/ethnicity, body mass index, and comorbidities were found with type 2 diabetes, hypertension, and hyperlipidemia (Crawford et al., 2010). African Americans had the highest prevalence of diagnosed type 2 diabetes and hypertension, while Caucasians were found to have the highest prevalence of diagnosed hypertension. The direct associations between body mass index and disease prevalence was consistent for both genders and across all racial/ethnic groups.

A shift from preventive homecare nursing functions to acute inpatient care functions has resulted in fragmented, expensive care for older adults with chronic illness, rather than the comprehensive and proactive care that is more likely to improve health outcomes. Providing the most appropriate services to older adults was the impetus for a study conducted by Markle-Reid et al. (2006). In this Canadian research, 288 older frail adults with chronic health needs, aged 75 and older, were evaluated using a two-armed, single-blind, randomized controlled trial. The model of vulnerability developed by Rogers (1997) provided the theoretical basis for the study. Participants were randomly assigned to either the usual home care or a "proactive" nursing health promotion intervention that included a health assessment combined with regular home visits or telephone contacts, health education about management of illness, coordination of community services, and use of empowerment strategies to enhance independence. Of the 288 patients randomly assigned to the two study arms at baseline, 242 completed the study (120 in the proactive nursing intervention group and 122 in the control group). The results demonstrated that proactively providing the intervention group with nursing health promotion resulted in significantly better mental health functioning ($P = 0.009$), a reduction in depression ($P = 0.009$), and enhanced perceptions of social support ($P = 0.009$), while not increasing the overall costs of health care. These findings support the need to provide nursing services for health promotion to older patients receiving home care. They imply that health promotion efforts are productive in improving health outcomes and can be cost-effective.

Many areas remain ready for further research to measure the effect of health-promoting frameworks and interventions with individuals and families with chronic illness. The earlier discussion provides a sampling of the current literature.

Guidelines

Numerous guidelines for health promotion, health screening, and preventive care are readily accessible at the National Guideline Clearinghouse website (www.guideline.gov) and other sources. Examples of some of these guidelines are discussed here.

Immunizations are among the most important discoveries in human history. Vaccines have helped save millions of lives worldwide and millions of dollars each year in unnecessary healthcare expenditures (Infectious Diseases Society of America, 2011). Nevertheless, rates of coverage are unacceptably low among both adults and children in the United States. More widespread administration of the influenza vaccine alone might save thousands of lives by providing protection for persons with chronic illness. Immunized healthcare professionals, for example, can decrease transmission of influenza to persons with chronic illness. Recommended immunization schedules and information are easily obtained from the CDC.

Several organizations provide guidelines that include health promotion for chronic conditions. Self-management education programs such as diabetes self-management education (DSME) are outlined in the diabetes national standards (Kulkarni, 2006). Nurses are encouraged to use evidence-based guidelines in their practice.

to minimize chronic illnesses and keep people healthy. Nurses and other healthcare professionals must meet the challenge of designing and evaluating effective interventions that promote health and are accessible for all people.

The desired outcome for individuals with chronic illness and their families is to maintain and improve their overall health. Health promotion activities should target the major causes of death—tobacco use, poor diet, physical inactivity, alcohol consumption, microbial agents, toxic agents, motor vehicle crashes, incidents involving firearms, sexual behaviors, and illicit use of drugs. These causes are responsible for the majority of deaths in the United States.

Measures are needed to research outcomes of health-promoting interventions across populations and disabilities. Further efforts to make activities accessible and studies to evaluate their effectiveness are encouraged. The challenge in the coming years will be to link existing and future research studies to practice.

Outcomes

Numerous free resources are available through the U.S. federal government and other organizations, many of which have been described throughout this chapter. As in many other countries, health promotion and disease prevention are paramount concerns in the costly, fragmented U.S. healthcare system. Nurses can be instrumental in promoting health within this system. Indeed, from their earliest history, nurses have recognized the importance of health promotion.

There are substantial but missed opportunities for promoting health and extending the lifespan that present an international challenge. Countries in Europe are struggling with strategies to improve the health of their aging populations as well as to control costs. Italy has one of the oldest populations in the world, with more than 20% of its population being older than age 65 (Besdine & Wetle, 2010). Italy, like the United States, must be proactive in finding ways

Evidence-Based Practice Box

Harris et al. (2012) proposed a framework for disseminating evidence-based health promotion practices and illustrated this framework in two programs: EnhanceFitness, which focused on physical activity among older adults, and American Cancer Society Workplace Solutions, which dealt with chronic disease prevention among workers. The Harris et al. framework outlines roles for researchers, disseminators, and user organizations and identifies ways to disseminate evidence-based promotions for physical activity and workplace health programs nationally.

Source: Harris, J. R., Cheadle, A., Hannon, P. A., Lichiello, P., Forehand, M., Mahoney, E., …Yarrow, J. (2012). A framework for disseminating evidence-based health promotion practices. *Preventing Chronic Disease Public Health Research, Practice, and Policy, 9*, E22. http://www.ncbi.nlm.nih.gov/pmc/articles/PMC3277406/.

CASE STUDY 16-1

L.K. is a 47-year-old female with hypertension, arthritis, and hyperlipidemia. She is married, and L.K. and her 50-year-old husband of 25 years enjoy dining out, watching television every night, and talking on the phone to their four adult children who live out of state. Her husband and younger friends have encouraged her to text on the phone, but L.K. would rather hear her children's voices. She completed the 12th grade and works as an administrative assistant in an insurance company. Both L.K. and her husband smoke approximately one pack/day, and they have maintained this habit for 20 years. Both are overweight, and neither has a physical exercise regimen, even though both were told to increase their amount of exercise at their last medical appointment. L.K.'s last fasting glucose was 120 mg/dL. She was scheduled for a mammogram last week but decided to forego the appointment, stating she had other things to do.

Discussion Questions

1. How do L.K.'s chronic illnesses impact her lifestyle?
2. Which theoretical framework or model would be useful for her health promotion program?

CASE STUDY 16-2

K.B. is a 75-year-old man with type 2 diabetes, psoriasis, and hyperlipidemia. He is proud to tell you he has a house that is paid for, a wife of 35 years, five adult children, and 10 grandchildren whom he loves dearly. K.B. did not finish high school and does not like to read. He does not use a cell phone or a computer. He enjoys a couple of beers each night and smokes two packs of cigarettes per day. He has used alcohol and smoked for the last 20 years, beginning when he was working his last years as a custodial supervisor before retirement. His last medical appointment revealed a weight of 245 lb, BMI of 32, and hemoglobin A_{1c} of 8.2.

Discussion Questions

1. What are two health literacy implications of this case?
2. Which patient strengths can be used as motivators for K.B. to change his health behavior?
3. Which theoretical framework or model may be helpful in collaboratively designing a health promotion plan for K.B.?

STUDY QUESTIONS

1. Describe the importance of health promotion for persons with chronic illness.
2. Name the three major causes of death in the United States.
3. What is the goal of health promotion?
4. Identify a theory, model, or framework useful in working with individuals with chronic illness who need to change an unhealthy behavior.
5. Discuss the effect of national documents that address health promotion and disease prevention.
6. Which interventions can nurses use to promote health in persons with chronic illness?

References

Annang, L., Muilenburg, J. L., & Strasser, S. M. (2010). Virtual worlds: Taking health promotion to new levels. *American Journal of Health Promotion, 24*(5), 344–346.

Aro, A. R., & Absetz, P. (2009). Guidance for professionals in health promotion: Keeping it simple—but not too simple. *Psychology and Health, 24*(2), 125–129.

Balan, I. C, Moyers, T. B., & Lewis-Fernandez, R. (2013). Motivational pharmacology: Combining motivational interviewing and antidepressant therapy to improve treatment adherence. *Psychiatry, 76*(3), 203–209.

Beaudoin, C. E., Fernandez, C., Wall, J. L., & Farley, T. A. (2007). Promoting healthy eating and physical activity: Short-term effects of a mass media campaign. *American Journal of Preventive Medicine, 32*(3), 217–223.

Besdine, R. W., & Wetle, T. F. (2010). Improving health for elderly people: An international health promotion and disease prevention agenda. *Aging Clinical and Experimental Research, 22*, 219–230.

Blue, C. L. (2007). Does the theory of planned behavior identify diabetes-related cognitions for intention to be physically active and eat a healthy diet? *Public Health Nursing, 24*(2), 141–150.

Bosch-Capblanch, X., Abba, K., Prictor, M., & Garner, P. (2007). Contracts between patients and healthcare practitioners for improving patients' adherence to treatment, prevention and health promotion activities. *Cochrane Database of Systematic Reviews 2007, 2*, 1–61.

Bravata, D. M., Smith-Spangler, C., Sundaram, V., Glenger, A. L., Lin, N., Lewis, R., ... Sirard, J.R. (2007). Using pedometers to increase physical activity and improve health. *Journal of the American Medical Association, 298*, 2296–2304.

Brobeck, E., Bergh, H., Odencrants, S., & Hildingh, C. (2011). Primary healthcare nurses' experiences with motivational interviewing in health promotion practice. *Journal of Clinical Nursing, 20*, 3322–3330. doi: 10.1111/j.1365-2702.2011.03874.x

Brodie, D. A., & Inoue, A. (2005). Motivational interviewing to promote physical activity for people with chronic heart failure. *Journal of Advanced Nursing, 50*(5), 518–527. doi: 10.1111/j.1365-2648.2005.03422.x

Burkhart, P. V., Rayens, M. K., Oakley, M. G., Abshire, D. A., & Zhang, M. (2007). Testing an intervention to promote children's adherence to asthma self-management. *Journal of Nursing Scholarship, 39*, 133–140.

Calloway, S. (2007). Mental health promotion: Is nursing dropping the ball? *Journal of Professional Nursing, 23*(2), 105–109.

Capella-McDonnall, M. (2007). The need for health promotion for adults who are visually impaired. *Journal of Visual Impairment & Blindness, 101*(3), 133–145.

Centers for Disease Control and Prevention (CDC). (2011). Vital signs: Current cigarette smoking among adults aged >18 years—United States, 2005–2010. *Morbidity and Mortality Weekly Report, 60*(35), 1207–1212. http://www.cdc.gov/mmwr/preview /mmwrhtml/mm6035a5.htm?s_cid=mm6035a5_w

Centers for Disease Control and Prevention (CDC). (2013). Chronic disease prevention and health promotion. http://www.cdc.gov/chronicdisease/index.htm

Centers for Disease Control and Prevention (CDC), National Center for Chronic Disease Prevention and Health Promotion. (2009). The power of prevention: Chronic disease ... the public health challenge of the 21st century. http://www.cdc.gov/chronicdisease /overview/pop.htm

Centers for Disease Control and Prevention (CDC), National Center for Chronic Disease Prevention and

Health Promotion. (2012). Four common causes of chronic disease. http://www.cdc.gov/chronicdisease/overview/index.htm

Centers for Disease Control and Prevention (CDC), National Center for Chronic Disease Prevention and Health Promotion. (2013). Tobacco-related mortality. http://www.cdc.gov/tobacco/data_statistics/fact_sheets/health_effects/tobacco_related_mortality/index.htm

Chan, F., Chiu, C. Y., Bezyak, J. L., & Keegan, J. (2012). Introduction to health promotion for people with chronic illness and disability. *Rehabilitation Counseling Bulletin, 56*(1), 3–6. doi: 10:1177/0034355212440731

Colilla, S. A. (2010). An epidemiologic review of smokeless tobacco health effects and harm reduction potential. *Regulatory Toxicology and Pharmacology, 56*(2), 197–211.

Cory, S., Ussery-Hall, A., Griffin-Blake, S., Easton, A., Vigeant, J., Balluz, L., ... Centers for Disease Control and Prevention. (2010, September 24). Prevalence of selected risk behaviors and chronic diseases and conditions—Steps communities, United States, 2006–2007. *Morbidity and Mortality Weekly Report, 50*(SS-8), 1–9.

Coyle, M. K., Duffy, J. R., & Martin, E. M. (2007). Teaching/learning health promoting behaviors through telehealth. *Nursing Education Perspective, 28*(1), 18–23.

Crawford, A. G., Cote, C., Couto, J., Daskiran, M., Gunnarson, C., Haas, K., ... Schuette, R. (2010). Prevalence of obesity, type II diabetes mellitus, hyperlipidemia, and hypertension in the United States: Findings from the GE Centricity electronic medical record database. *Population Health Management, 13*(3), 151–161.

Crosby, R., & Noar, S. M. (2010). Theory development in health promotion: Are we there yet? *Journal of Behavioral Medicine, 33*(4), 259–263.

Crowe, A., & Parmenter, A. S. (2012). Creative approaches to motivational interviewing: Addressing the principles. *Journal of Creativity in Mental Health, 7*, 124–140. doi: 10.1080/15401383.2012.684662

DiClemente, R. J., Crosby, R. A., & Kegler, M. C. (2009). Issues and challenges in applying theory in health promotion practice and research: Adaptation, translation, and global application. In R. J. DiClemente, R. A. Crosby, & M. C. Kegler (Eds.), *Emerging theories in health promotion practice and research* (2nd ed., pp. 551–568). San Francisco, CA: Jossey-Bass.

Eckel, R. H., Jakicic, J. M., Ard, J. D., Hubbard, V. S., de Jesus, J. M., Lee, I. M., ... Yanovski, S. Z. (2013). AHA/ACC guideline on lifestyle management to reduce cardiovascular risk: A report of the American College of Cardiology/American Heart Association Task Force on Practice Guidelines. *Circulation*. http://my.amricanheart.org/statements

Edelman, C. L., & Mandle, C. L. (2010). *Health promotion throughout the lifespan* (7th ed.). St. Louis, MO: Mosby.

Feldman, S. I., & Tegart, G. (2003). Keep moving: Conceptions of illness and disability of middle-aged African-American women with arthritis. *Women & Therapy 26*(1-2), 127–144.

Finkelstein, E. A., Brown, D. S., Brown, D. R., & Buchner, D. M. (2008). A randomized study of financial incentives to increase physical activity among sedentary older adults. *Preventive Medicine, 47*(2), 182–187.

Glass, N., Moss, C., & Ogle, K. R. (2012). A person-centred lifestyle change intervention model: Working with older people experiencing chronic illness. *International Journal of Nursing Practice, 18*, 379–387. doi: 10.1111/j.1440-172X.2012.02054.x

Greiner, P. A., & Edelman, C. L. (2010). Health defined: Objectives to promotion and prevention In C. L. Edelman & P. A. Mandle (Eds.), *Health promotion throughout the lifespan* (7th ed., pp. 3–26). St. Louis, MO: Mosby.

Harris, J. R., Cheadle, A., Hannon, P. A., Lichiello, P., Forehand, M., Mahoney, E., ... Yarrow, J. (2012). A framework for disseminating evidence-based health promotion practices. *Preventing Chronic Disease Public Health Research, Practice, and Policy, 9*, E22. http://www.ncbi.nlm.nih.gov/pmc/articles/PMC3277406/

Haverman, R. H. (2010). Principles to guide the development of population health incentives. *Preventing Chronic Disease Public Health Research, Practice, and Policy, 7*(5), 1–5. http://www.cdc.gov/pcd/issues/2010/sep/10_0044.htm

Healthy People 2020. (2011). Improving the healthy Americans. http:www.healthpeople.gov/2020/default.aspx

Healthy People 2010. (n.d.). http://www.healthypeople.gov/2010

Holland, S. K., Greenberg, J., Tidwell, L., & Newcomer, R. (2003). Preventing disability through community-based health coaching. *Journal of the American Geriatrics Society, 51*, 265–269.

Hollis, V., Massey, K., & Jevne, R. (2007). An introduction to the intentional use of hope. *Journal of Allied Health, 36*(1), 52–56.

Huang, H. C., Chou, C. T., Lin, K. C., & Chao, Y. F. (2007). The relationships between disability level, health-promoting lifestyle, and quality of life in outpatients with systemic lupus erythematosus. *Journal of Nursing Research, 15*(1), 21–32.

Huffman, M. (2007). Health coaching: A new and exciting technique to enhance patient self-management and improve outcomes. *Home Healthcare Nurse, 25*(4), 271–274.

Huncharek, M., Haddock, S., Reid, R., & Kupelnick, B. (2010). Smoking as a risk factor for prostate cancer: A meta-analysis of 24 prospective cohort studies. *American Journal of Public Health, 100*(4), 693–701.

Infectious Diseases Society of America. (2011). Immunization/vaccination. http://www.idsociety.org/Content.aspx?id=6346

Jackson, R., Asimakopoulou, K., & Scammell, A. (2007). Assessment of the transtheoretical model as used by dietitians in promoting physical activity in people with type 2 diabetes. *Journal of Human Nutrition and Diet, 20,* 27–36.

Janz, N. K., Champion, V. L., & Strecher, V. J. (2002). The health belief model. In K. Glanz, B. K. Rimer, & F. M. Lewis (Eds.), *Health behavior and health education theory, research, and practice* (3rd ed., pp. 45–66). San Francisco, CA: Jossey-Bass.

Jensen, M. D., Ryan, D. H., Apovian, C. M., Ard, J. D., Comuzzie, A. G., Donato, K. A., Hu, F. B., … Yanovski, S. Z. (2013). AHA/ACC/TOS guideline for the management of overweight and obesity in adults: A report of the American College of Cardiology/American Heart Association Task Force on Practice Guidelines and The Obesity Society. *Circulation.* http://my.americanheart.org/statements

Kelly, K. M., Phillips, C. M., Jenkins, C., Norling, G., White, C., Jenkins, T., … Dignan, M.. (2007). Physician and staff perceptions of barriers to colorectal cancer screening in Appalachian Kentucky. *Cancer Control: Journal of the Moffitt Cancer Center, 14*(2), 167–175.

Kulkarni, K. D. (2006). Value of diabetes self-management education. *Clinical Diabetes, 24*(2), 54.

Leddy, S. K. (2006). *Health promotion: Mobilizing strengths to enhance health, wellness, and well-being.* Philadelphia, PA: F. A. Davis.

Mantler, T., Irwin, J. D., & Morrow, D. (2013). The experience and impact of motivational interviewing-via-coaching tools on national smokers' telephone hotline employees. *International Journal of Evidence Based Coaching and Mentoring, 11*(1), 55–68.

Markle-Reid, M., Weir, R., Browne, G., Roberts, J., Gafni, A., & Henderson, S. (2006). Health promotion for frail older home care clients. *Journal of Advanced Nursing, 54*(3), 381–395.

McGinnis, J. M., & Foege, W. H. (1993). Actual causes of death in the United States. *Journal of the American Medical Association, 270,* 2207–2212.

McGinnis, J. M., & Foege, W. H. (2004). The immediate vs the important. *Journal of the American Medical Association, 291,* 1263–1264. http://www.commed.vcu.edu/IntroPH/Introduction/editorialmcginnisfeb2006.pdf

McQueen, A., Vernon, S. W., Rothman, A. J., Norman, G. J., Myers, R. E., & Tilley, B. C. (2010). Examining the role of perceived susceptibility on colorectal cancer screening intention and behavior. *Annals of Behavioral Medicine, 40,* 205–217.

McWilliam, C. L., Stewart, M., Brown, J. B., Desai, K., & Coderre, P. (1996). Creating health with chronic illness. *Advances in Nursing Science, 18*(3), 1–15.

Miller, A., & Iris, M. (2002). Health promotion attitudes and strategies in older adults. *Health Education & Behavior, 29*(2), 249–267.

Mokdad, A. H., Marks, J. S., Stroup, D. F., & Gerberding, J. L. (2004). Actual causes of death in the United States, 2000. *Journal of the American Medical Association, 291,* 1238–1245.

Montano, D. E., & Kasprzyk, D. (2002). The theory of reasoned action and the theory of planned behavior. In K. Glanz, B. K. Rimer, & F. M. Lewis (Eds.), *Health behavior and health education theory, research, and practice* (3rd ed., pp. 67–98). San Francisco, CA: Jossey-Bass.

Nath, C. (2007). Literacy and diabetes self-management. *American Journal of Nursing, 107*(6 suppl), 43–54.

Neuman, P., Cubanski, J., Desmond, K. A., & Rice, T. H. (2007). How much "skin in the game" do Medicare beneficiaries have? The increasing financial burden of health care spending, 1997–2003. *Health Affairs, 26*(6), 1692–1701.

Noordman, J., de Vet, E., van der Weijden, T., & van Dulmen, S. (2013). Motivational interviewing within the different stages of change: An analysis of practice nurse–patient consultations aimed at promoting a healthier lifestyle. *Social Science & Medicine, 87,* 60–67. http://dx.doi.org/10.1016/j.socscimed.2013.03.019

Norman, S. A., Potashnik, S. L., Galantino, M. L., DeMichele, A. M., House, L., & Localio, A. R. (2007). Modifiable risk factors for breast cancer recurrence: What can we tell survivors? *Journal of Women's Health, 16*(2), 177–190.

Olshansky, E. (2007). Nurses and health promotion. *Journal of Professional Nursing, 23*(1), 1–2.

Ory, M. G., Smith, M. L., Wade, A., Mounce, C., Wilson, A., & Parrish, R. (2010). Implementing and disseminating an evidence-based program to prevent falls in older adults, Texas, 2007–2009. *Preventing Chronic Disease Public Health Research, Practice, and Policy, 7*(6), 1–6. http://www.cdc.gov/pcd/issues/2010/nov/09_0224.htm

Painter, J. E., Borba, C. P., Hynes, M., Mays, D., & Glanz, K. (2008). The use of theory in health behavior research from 2000 to 2005: A systematic review. *Annals of Behavioral Medicine, 35,* 358–362.

Pender, N. J., Murdaugh, C. L., & Parsons, M. A. (2002). *Health promotion in nursing practice* (4th ed.). Upper Saddle River, NJ: Prentice Hall.

Perry, G. S., Presley-Cantrell, L. R., & Dhingra, S. (2010). Addressing mental health promotion in chronic disease prevention and health promotion. *American Journal of Public Health, 100,* 2337–2339. doi: 10.2105/AJPH2010.205146

Prochaska, J. O., Redding, C. A., & Evers, K. E. (2002). The transtheoretical model and stages of change. In K. Glanz, B. K. Rimer, & F. M. Lewis (Eds.) *Health behavior and health education theory, research, and practice* (3rd ed., pp. 99–120). San Francisco, CA: Jossey-Bass.

Pursey, V. A. (2013). Using motivational interviewing to encourage behaviour change. *Journal of Renal Nursing, 5,* 248–251.

Rainer, J. P., & McMurry, P. E. (2002). Caregiving at the end of life. *Journal of Clinical Psychology, 58,* 1421–1431.

Rillemas-Sun, E., LaCroix, A. Z., Waring, M. E., Kroenke, C. H., LaMonte, M. J., Vitolins, M. Z., … Wallace, R. B. (2013). Obesity and late age survival without major disease or disability in older women. http://archinte.jamanetwork.com/article.aspx?articleid=1770523. doi: 10.1001/jamainternmed.2013.12051

Rogers, A. C. (1997). Vulnerability, health and health costs. *Journal of Advanced Nursing, 26,* 65–72.

Rohrer, J. E., Naessens, J. M., Liesinger, J., & Litchy, W. (2010). Comparing diverse health promotion programs using overall self-rated health as a common metric. *Population Health Management, 13*(2), 91–95.

Rollnick, S., Miller, W. R., & Butler, C. C. (2008). *Motivational Interviewing in health care: Helping patients change behavior.* New York, NY: Guilford Press.

Schafer, M. H., & Ferraro, K. F. (2007). Long-term obesity and avoidable hospitalization among younger, middle-aged, and older adults. *Archives of Internal Medicine, 167,* 2220–2225.

Sherry, B., Blanck, H. M., Galuska, D. A., Pan, L., & Dietz, W. H. (2010, August 6). Vital signs: State-specific obesity prevalence among adults-United States, 2009. *Morbidity and Mortality Week Report, 59*(30), 951–955.

Snyder, L. B. (2007). Health communication campaigns and their impact on behavior. *Journal of Nutrition Education and Behavior, 39*(2 suppl), S32–S40.

Thomas, M. L., Elliott, J. E., Rao, S. M., Fahey, K. F., Paul, S. M., & Miaskowski, C. (2012). A randomized, clinical trial of education or motivational-interviewing–based coaching compared to usual care to improve cancer pain management. *Oncology Nursing Forum, 39*(1), 39–49. doi: 10.1188/12.ONF.39-49

Thompson, D. R., Chair, S. Y., Chan, S. W., Astin, F., Davidson, P. M., & Ski, C. F. (2011). Motivational interviewing: A useful approach to improving cardiovascular health. *Journal of Clinical Nursing, 20,* 1236–1244. doi: 10.1111/j.1365-2702.2010.035558.x

Tse, M. M., Vong, S. K., & Tang, S. K. (2013). Motivational interviewing and exercise programme for community-dwelling older persons with chronic pain: A randomized controlled study. *Journal of Clinical Nursing, 22,* 1843–1856. doi: 10.1111/j.1365-2702.2012.04317.x

U.S. Department of Health and Human Services (DHHS). (2013a). About the law. http://www.hhs.gov/healthcare/rights/index.html

U.S. Department of Health and Human Services (DHHS). (2013b). Preventive care. http://www.hhs.gov/healthcare/rights/index.html

U.S. Department of Health and Human Services (DHHS), Office of Disease Prevention and Health Promotion. (2013). Health communication, health literacy and e-health. http://health.gov/communication/Default.asp

U.S. Department of Health & Human Services (DHHS), Office of the Surgeon General. (2013). A report of the Surgeon General: How tobacco smoke causes disease: The biology and behavioral basis for smoking: Attributable disease, 2010. http://www.surgeongeneral.gov/library/reports/tobaccosmoke/index.html

U.S. Guide to Community Preventive Services. (2013). Home. http://www.thecommunityguide.org/index.html

U.S. Preventive Services Task Force (USPSTF). (2013a). About the USPSTF. http://www.uspreventiveservices-taskforce.org/about.htm

U.S. Preventive Services Task Force (USPSTF). (2013b). Screening for lung cancer. http://www.uspreventiveservicestaskforce.org/uspstf/grades.htm#brec

Verheijden, M. W., Jans, M. P., Hildebrandt, V. H., & Hopman-Rock, M. (2007). Rates and determinants of repeated participation in a Web-based behavior change program for healthy body weight and healthy lifestyle. *Journal of Medical Internet Research, 9*(1), e1.

Warren-Findlow, J., Prohaska, T. R., & Freedman, D. (2003, March). Challenges and opportunities in recruiting and retaining underrepresented populations into health promotion research. *The Gerontologist, 37–47.*

Weinstein, N. D. (2007). Misleading tests of health behavior theories. *Annals of Behavioral Medicine, 33*(1), 1–10.

White, K., & Jacques, P. H. (2007). Combined diet and exercise intervention in the workplace: Effect on cardiovascular disease risk factors. *Journal of the American Association of Occupational Health Nurses, 55*(3), 109–114.

Zhang, X., Fung, H., & Ho-hong Ching, B. (2009). Age differences in goals: Implications for health promotion. *Aging & Mental Health, 13*(3), 336–348.

Chapter 17

The Advanced Practice Registered Nurse in Chronic Illness Care

Ann Marie Hart

Introduction

Advanced practice registered nurses (APRNs), including certified nurse practitioners (CNPs), clinical nurse specialists (CNSs), certified nurse–midwives (CNMs), and certified registered nurse anesthetists (CRNAs), play an integral role in the care and well-being of individuals and families experiencing chronic illnesses. The complex nature of chronic illness, for which care focuses primarily on maximizing function and well-being as opposed to cure and recovery, is particularly suited to nursing's holistic focus (Lupari, Coates, Adamson, & Crealey, 2011; Saxe, Janson, Dennehy, Stringari-Murray, Hirsch, & Waters, 2007). APRNs are involved in every facet of chronic illness care—from making an initial diagnosis, providing early anticipatory guidance, and coordinating care to monitoring disease progression, managing medications, and problem-solving complications (e.g., adverse treatment effects, caregiver fatigue, reimbursement issues). Truly, there is no aspect of chronic illness for which APRNs are not well suited to assist and enhance the lives of individuals experiencing it.

For almost five decades, APRNs have been involved in the health and care of patients, families, and communities. In 2008, more than 250,000 APRNs were licensed to practice in the United States—slightly more than 8% of the entire population of licensed registered nurses. Approximately half of these APRNs were CNPs (U.S. Department of Health and Human Services [DHHS], Health Resources and Service Administration, 2010), 55% of whom were engaged in primary care practice (Agency for Healthcare Research and Quality [AHRQ], 2011). A recent survey confirmed that many U.S. consumers are receptive to receiving primary care from nurse practitioners (Dill, Pankow, Erikson, & Shipman, 2013). Another study documented that the number of Medicare beneficiaries receiving primary care from APRNs increased 15-fold between 1998 and 2010 (Kuo, Loresto, Rounds, & Goodwin, 2013). Clearly, APRNs have "come of age" in primary care practice. Thus, this chapter will focus on the role of APRNs in chronic illness management within the context of *primary care*.

Primary Care

Primary care is defined as the "provision of integrated, accessible health care services by clinicians who are accountable for addressing a large majority of personal health care needs, developing a sustained partnership with patients, and practicing in the context of family and community" (Donaldson, Yordy, Lohr, & Vanselow, 1996, p. 1). The role of primary care in chronic illness management cannot be over-emphasized. Primary care is widely recognized as one of the most critical aspects of health care (e.g., Halvorson, 2009; Rittenhouse, Shortell, & Fischer, 2009; Starfield, 1994; Starfield, Shi, & Macinko, 2005; World Health Organization [WHO], 2008) and has been aptly referred to as the "bedrock" of the healthcare system (Caley, 2013). Quality primary care improves rates of prevention, early detection, and effective management of many chronic illnesses (Starfield, 2012). Primary care has also been shown to result in decreased mortality and reduced hospitalizations (Chang, Stukel, Flood, & Goodman, 2011), as well as cost savings (Baiker & Chandra, 2004) and improved sense of mental and physical health (Finklestein et al., 2012).

Research has shown that primary care delivered by APRNs results in improved chronic disease outcomes—outcomes that are comparable to care delivered by physicians (Laurant, Reeves, Hermens, Branspenning, Grol, & Sibbald, 2004; Newhouse et al., 2011; Stanik-Hutt et al., 2013). Having said this, some evidence suggests that primary care of individuals with chronic illnesses could improve. Many individuals experiencing chronic illnesses are not achieving the recommended goals, and some are unaware of their illnesses. Data from the most recent (2005–2010) National Health and Nutrition Examination Survey (NHANES) indicated that 22.6% of the U.S. population continues to smoke, 31.9% do not engage in physical activity, and 34.1% are obese (Yang et al., 2012). Another analysis of the NHANES data revealed that in adults with hypertension, only 18% were aware of their elevated blood pressure. Of the 82% who were aware of their hypertension, 75% were taking antihypertensive medication; however, only 53% had achieved their target blood pressure values (Go et al., 2013). Similarly, an analysis of adults with type 2 diabetes mellitus revealed that 76% were not at goal values for $HgbA_{1c}$, blood pressure, and low-density lipoprotein cholesterol (LDL-c). Although chronic obstructive pulmonary disease (COPD) is the third leading cause of mortality in the United States (Hoyert & Xu, 2012), it is estimated that

more than half of the individuals with COPD remain unaware of this diagnosis until it is in an advanced state associated with end-stage organ damage (Guarascio, Ray, Finch, & Self, 2013; Price, Yawn, & Jones, 2010). In addition, many individuals with COPD have been misdiagnosed and are being treated for asthma, not COPD (Tinkelman, Price, Nordyke, & Halbert, 2006). Furthermore, although mental illness is frequently encountered in primary care, several studies have shown that common mental health diagnoses such as depression and anxiety are often under- and over-diagnosed by primary care clinicians (Mitchell, Rao, & Vaze, 2011; Mitchell, Vaze, & Rao, 2009; Su, Tsai, Hung, & Chou, 2011). Clearly, primary care APRNs have their work cut out for them regarding chronic illness management.

APRN Core Competencies in Chronic Illness Primary Care

Six competencies have been identified in the APRN literature that are particularly useful in discussing the role of APRNs in chronic illness primary care:

1. Leadership
2. Ethical decision making
3. Consultation
4. Collaboration
5. Evidence-based practice
6. Guidance and coaching

These six competencies have been espoused by and/or reflected in the work of multiple scholars and organizations, including, but not limited to, Cooke, Gemmill, and Grant (2008); Mantzoukas and Watkinson (2006); the National Association of Clinical Nurse Specialists (NACNS, 2009); and the National Organization of Nurse Practitioner Faculties (NONPF, 2012). They are also reflected in the American Association of Colleges of Nursing's master's degree (AACN, 2011) and doctor of nursing practice (DNP; AACN, 2006) educational essentials (**Table 17-1**

Table 17-1 THE ESSENTIALS OF MASTER'S EDUCATION IN NURSING

  I. Background for practice from sciences and humanities
 II. Organizational and systems leadership
III. Quality improvement and safety
 IV. Translating and integrating scholarship into practice
  V. Informatics and healthcare technologies
 VI. Health policy and advocacy
VII. Interprofessional collaboration for improving patient and population health outcomes
VIII. Clinical prevention and population health for improving health
 IX. Master's-level nursing practice

Source: American Association of Colleges of Nursing. (2011). *The essentials of master's education in nursing.* Washington, DC: Author.

Table 17-2 THE ESSENTIALS OF DOCTORAL EDUCATION FOR ADVANCED NURSING PRACTICE

   I. Scientific underpinnings for practice
  II. Organizational and systems leadership for quality improvement and systems thinking
 III. Clinical scholarship and analytical methods for evidence-based practice
  IV. Information systems/technology and patient care technology for the improvement and transformation of health care
   V. Healthcare policy for advocacy in health care
  VI. Interprofessional collaboration for improving patient and population health outcomes
 VII. Clinical prevention and population health for improving the nation's health
VIII. Advanced nursing practice

Source: American Association of Colleges of Nursing. (2006). *The essentials of doctoral education for advanced nursing practice.* Washington, DC: Author.

and **Table 17-2**), and are considered "core competencies" in Hamric's (2014) model of advanced practice nursing (**Figure 17-1**).

Although these core competencies underlie all APRN practice, they are by no means unique to APRNs. Nurses who have been prepared at the basic level may also demonstrate them. What distinguishes these competencies from components of basic preparation is that they are essential to (i.e., required for) APRN practice. In other words, if an APRN is not proficient in or does not consistently demonstrate all of these competencies in his or her practice, then the nurse is *not* providing advanced practice nursing care. The expectation is that these six competencies are consistently demonstrated in the APRN's routine practice. As such, these competencies serve as an excellent framework for discussing the role of the APRN in chronic illness primary care.

LEADERSHIP

In its landmark report *The Future of Nursing: Leading Change, Advancing Health*, the Institute

of Medicine (IOM, 2010) provided four key recommendations (**Table 17-3**), all of which call for nurses to improve and act upon their professional leadership skills. These recommendations are especially relevant for APRNs who are educationally prepared for advanced practice roles. Regardless of whether the APRN feels as if he or she is a "leader," the very nature of advanced practice nursing requires leadership skills. As Tracy and Hanson (2014) aptly note, "Not all APRNs are comfortable with the idea of being leaders, but leadership is not an optional activity" (p. 268).

U.S health care is currently in a state of flux. Calls for system redesign and transformation are never ending. Although legislators, insurance carriers, healthcare professionals, and other health-related entities and individuals may not agree on "how" health care should look and work, few can deny that we are spending an exorbitant amount on health care and have very little to show for it. Of the world's top 17 industrialized nations,

Figure 17-1 Hamric's Model of Advanced Practice Nursing

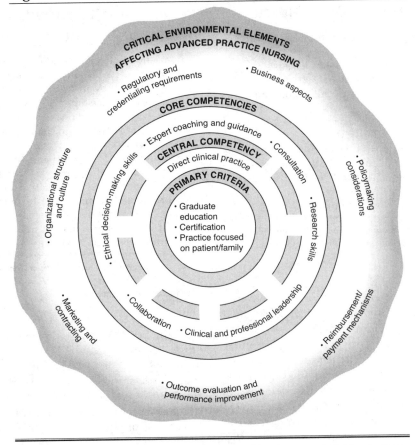

Source: Hamric, A. B. (2014). A definition of advanced practice nursing. In A. B. Hamric, C. M. Manson, M. F. Tracy, & E. T. O'Grady (Eds.), *Advanced practice nursing*, (5th ed., pp. 67–85). St Louis, MO: Elsevier Saunders.

the United States demonstrates the highest death rates from cardiovascular and other chronic diseases. It also has the lowest life expectancy for men and the second lowest life expectancy for women (Ho & Preston, 2011). With few exceptions, healthcare professionals (including primary care APRNs) are paid to be productive (i.e., see as many patients as possible), *not* to produce good outcomes. Even when individuals receive appropriate primary health care, they do not necessarily live longer or better (National Research Council [NRC] & IOM, 2013). In the words of Donald Berwick, founder of the Institute for Healthcare Improvement, "We *don't* have a health care system in this country; we have a disease management system" (Heineman & Froemke, 2013). As such, leadership opportunities for today's primary care APRNs are unlimited.

APRNs have the opportunity to demonstrate leadership in four key domains: (1) clinical

Table 17-3 KEY RECOMMENDATIONS FROM *THE FUTURE OF NURSING: LEADING CHANGE, ADVANCING HEALTH*

1. Nurses should practice to the full extent of their education and training.
2. Nurses should achieve higher levels of education and training through an improved education system that promotes seamless academic progression.
3. Nurses should be full partners, with physicians and other health professionals, in redesigning health care in the United States.
4. Effective workforce planning and policy making require better data collection and an improved information infrastructure.

Source: Reprinted with permission from *The Future of nursing: Leading change, advancing health* 2010 by the National Academy of Sciences, Courtesy of the National Academies Press, Washington, D.C.

practice environments, (2) the nursing profession, (3) the systems level, and 4) the health policy arena (Tracy & Hanson, 2014). All of these domains are applicable to APRNs who work in chronic illness primary care. The four domains are described individually here; however, chronic illness care is complex, and as such these domains frequently overlap in the real world.

Clinical Practice Environments Clinical practice is the hallmark of APRNs, and most APRNs demonstrate clinical leadership on a daily basis. Clinical practice leadership involves ensuring that all of the APRN's clients (i.e., patients, families, and communities) receive high-quality care. These patients may be the APRN's own clients, or they may represent clientele associated with the APRN's place of work (e.g., clinic, department). APRNs provide clinical leadership by acting as role models and leaders on patient care teams. They also lead on an individual basis, when patients, families, and communities meet with them for private consultation. In chronic illness management, clinical practice leadership means striving for the best care possible, even when resources and time are scarce. Clinical practice leadership requires a high degree of intellect, creativity, and autonomy. It also requires experience, knowledge of the best available research evidence and healthcare systems, and a strong set of interpersonal and collaborative skills.

Professional Leadership Professional leadership differs from clinical practice leadership in that it does not directly relate to the care of a particular individual or family. Nevertheless, because its indirect effects significantly impact patient care, its importance cannot be understated. Professional leadership involves mentorship of junior nurses and APRNs, collaboration with colleagues (both like-minded colleagues and others), and *active* participation in professional organizations. The goal of professional leadership is to ensure that all patients receive excellent clinical care; thus, along with demonstrating clinical leadership, all primary care APRNs should be engaged in some degree of professional leadership. Examples of professional organizations dedicated to primary care practice are noted in **Table 17-4**.

Table 17-4 PROFESSIONAL PRIMARY CARE ORGANIZATIONS

American Association of Nurse Practitioners: http://www.aanp.org

Institute for Healthcare Improvement: http://www.ihi.org

National Association of Pediatric Nurse Practitioners: http://www.napnap.org

National Association of Community Health Centers: http://www.nachc.org

State Primary Association: for listing, see http://www.bphc.hrsa.gov/technicalassistance/partnerlinks/associations/html

Systems Leadership Systems leadership involves leading at an organizational or delivery system level. Opportunities for quality systems leadership are available regardless of whether the APRN is responsible for an entire organization, a clinic, or a seemingly small component of an organization (e.g., patient care team, journal club, quality improvement initiative). However, true systems leadership does not occur in a vacuum, but rather requires that the APRN have a mature understanding and appreciation of the complexity of a particular system and a desire to improve it. For example, an APRN leading a patient care team demonstrates systems leadership when he or she recognizes that the seemingly unique care aspects required by a particular patient might also be needed by other patients and works within the system to ensure accessibility and equity of information, resources, and services. Entrepreneurial leadership also falls under the domain of systems leadership; it occurs when the APRN leader critically evaluates his or her opportunities and takes the initiative to practice outside of the traditional employment setting (e.g., a hospital-based or physician-run clinic).

Health Policy Leadership Health policy leadership refers to policies and laws related to patient care, public health, and nursing practice (i.e., both basic and advanced practice nursing). To be a leader in health policy, the APRN must analyze health systems data, possess advanced negotiation and communication skills, and maintain knowledge of the associated politics and stakeholders. Although not all APRNs will engage in health policy leadership, all primary care APRNs should maintain a keen interest in policies that affect primary care practice (e.g., Medicare rules and reimbursement, tort reform, state-specific Medicaid spending and APRN practice acts). In addition, all APRNs

need mechanisms for staying abreast of current health policy and practice issues (e.g., via electronic mailing lists) and should work to support those APRNs who are leaders in the health policy domain (e.g., communicate with legislators, vote).

Despite the differences that characterize clinical, professional, systems, and health policy leadership, all four of these domains build on the common concepts of mentorship, innovation, and activism (Tracy & Hanson, 2014). Thus, even though an APRN might initially pursue a career in primary care to become a clinical leader, with experience, continued education, and mentoring, the APRN may find that he or she is interested and well suited for leadership roles in nonclinical domains, using the same concepts that defined the nurse's clinical leadership. By engaging in professional, systems, and health policy leadership, the mature APRN is essentially recognizing that he or she is not the "end-all" of good patient care and has a responsibility to the future of optimal primary nursing care.

ETHICAL DECISION MAKING

The complex nature of working in primary care settings with patients and families experiencing chronic illness often gives rise to ethical dilemmas (i.e., situations where two or more moral principles are in conflict and the best course of action is not immediately apparent)—for example, inadequate pain management, abuse and neglect in the elderly or those with disabilities, decision making when patients are experiencing early dementia, end-of-life decisions when patients do not have adequate advance directives, and working with colleagues who are not competent. Another example of an ethical dilemma arising from the evidence-based practice initiative is the situation in which patient preferences differ from APRN expertise. One example is a patient with chronic back pain, who has not received adequate relief from anti-inflammatory medications and physical therapy and who desires opioid therapy, while the APRN is concerned about the risks associated with opioids and recommends pursuing an integrated approach with biofeedback, counseling, yoga, and other nonpharmacologic options.

For the APRN to develop competency in dealing with complicated ethical dilemmas, he or she must possess maturity, exhibit excellent communication and collaboration skills, and have experience working through ethical dilemmas. The APRN should also be knowledgeable regarding the traditional moral principles underlying nursing and bioethics (Beauchamp & Childress, 2012). **Table 17-5**). However, in recent decades, ethicists have become increasingly cognizant of the limitations of principlism (i.e., principle-based ethics) and have recognized the contributions offered by alternative ethical approaches such as casuistry and narrative ethics, which focus on critically examining existing dilemmas by comparing them to similar previous situations (Jecker, 2012). Other alternative ethical approaches that may assist APRNs who are providing chronic illness care include virtue- and care-based ethics, which place emphasis on the virtue (i.e., care) employed by the moral agent (i.e., APRN) as well as the relationships that may be affected by the dilemma (i.e., family members, caregivers, employers) (Armstrong, 2006; Arries, 2006; Cooper, 1991).

Primary care APRNs working with patients and families experiencing chronic illness are encouraged to familiarize themselves with the ethical references cited. They also need to be aware of the four phases that Hamric and Delgado (2014) have identified as the pathway for mastery of the ethical decision-making competency: (1) knowledge development, (2) knowledge application, (3) creation of an ethical environment, and (4) promotion of social justice within the healthcare system (**Table 17-6**). The wise APRN also recognizes that important ethical dilemmas should not be solved in isolation; rather, the APRN will develop and utilize a formal and/or informal network of mentors with whom to explore thoughts and options.

Consultation

Although primary care APRNs will often consult with other APRNs and members of the healthcare team, an essential feature of the role is that APRNs also serve as consultants to other professionals (e.g., nurses, physicians, mental health providers). There are a number of ways in which consultation may be categorized; however, in chronic illness care, APRNs primarily provide consultations related to direct patient care. They either see a patient or make specific recommendations to the consultee (i.e., basic-prepared nurse, team of nurses, or non-nursing provider) on how best to proceed with the patient's care, or they assist the consultee with formulating an effective plan of care. Regardless of whether the APRN sees the actual patient, the aim of APRN-directed consultation is to assist the consultee in providing patient care.

Acting as a consultant requires that the APRN have expertise in a particular area and be respected for this expertise. Vosit-Steller and Morse (2014, pp. 218–219) identify seven principles of professional APRN consultation

Table 17-5 Traditional Moral Principles Underlying Ethics in Health Care

Moral Principle	Description
Respect for autonomy	Duty to respect individual values and choices
Beneficence	Duty to do good
Nonmaleficence	Duty to prevent or remove harm
Justice	Duty to treat others equally

Source: Data from Beauchamp, T. L., & Childress, J. F. (2012). *Principles of biomedical ethics.* (7th ed.) New York, NY: Oxford University Press.

Table 17-6 PHASES OF DEVELOPMENT OF CORE COMPETENCY FOR ETHICAL DECISION MAKING

Phase	Knowledge	Skill/Behavior
Phase 1: Knowledge development—moral sensitivity	Ethical theories Ethical issues in specialty Professional code Professional standards Legal precedent Moral distress	Sensitivity to ethical dimensions of clinical practice Values clarification Sensitivity to fidelity conflicts Gather relevant literature related to problems identified Evaluate practice setting for congruence with literature Identify ethical issues in the practice setting and bring them to the attention of other team members
Phase 2: Knowledge application—moral action	Ethical decision-making frameworks Mediation/facilitation strategies	Apply ethical decision-making models to clinical problems Use skilled communication regarding ethical issues Facilitate decision making by using selected strategies Recognize and manage moral distress in self and others
Phase 3: Creation of an ethical environment	Preventive ethics Awareness of environmental barriers to ethical practice	Role-model collaborative problem solving Mentor others to develop ethical practice Address barriers to ethical practice through system changes Use preventive ethics to decrease unit-level moral distress
Phase 4: Promotion of social justice within the health-care system	Concepts of justice Health policies affecting specialty population	Ability to analyze the policy process Advocacy, communication, and leadership skills Involvement in health policy initiatives supporting social justice

Source: This material was published in *Advanced practice nursing: An integrative approach*, 5th ed., Hamric, A. B., & Delgado, S. A., Ethical decision making, pp.328-358, Copyright Saunders 2014

that espouse the collaborative, professional, and transparent nature of APRN consultation:

1. The consultation is usually initiated by the consultee.
2. The relationship between the consultant and the consultee is nonhierarchical and collaborative.
3. The consultant always considers contextual factors when responding to the request for consultation.
4. The consultant has no direct authority for managing patient care.
5. The consultant does not prescribe but rather makes recommendations.
6. The consultee is free to accept or reject the recommendations of the consultant.
7. The consultation should be documented.

COLLABORATION

Frequently confused with consultation or referral, collaboration goes beyond the notion of giving and receiving advice and is a fairly complex and sophisticated competency to master. Hanson and Spross's (1996) definition of collaboration continues to stand the test of time:

A dynamic, interpersonal process in which two or more individuals made a commitment to each other to interact authentically and constructively to solve problems and learn from each other to accomplish identified goals, purposes, or outcomes. The individuals recognize and articulate the shared values that make this commitment possible. (p. 232)

Due to its interpersonal nature, true collaboration cannot occur in the absence of willing partners; thus one could argue that collaboration should not be evaluated at the individual APRN level. However, components of effective collaboration—including clinical competence, interpersonal skills, respect for others, and recognition of and respect for differing values—are amenable to the individual primary care APRN's prerogative and may be improved upon and evaluated (Hanson & Carter, 2014).

In chronic illness primary care facilitated by an APRN, collaboration primarily refers to the interpersonal processes that occur between the APRN and the patient and/or family, as well as among the APRN and other members of the patient's healthcare team (e.g., psychiatric mental health nurse practitioner, home health nurse, physical therapist, social worker, specialty nurse practitioner or physician). Unlike with the care provided by "multidisciplinary" or "interdisciplinary" teams, in which the team members representing various disciplines work side by side but in different ways, truly collaborative team members are committed to one another, the patient, and the patient's family.

EVIDENCE-BASED PRACTICE

Evidence-based practice (EBP) is the "conscientious, explicit, and judicious use of current best evidence in making decisions about care of individual patients" (Sackett, Rosenberg, Gray, Haynes, & Richardson, 1996, p. 71), resulting from the integration of best research evidence with clinician expertise and patient values and preferences (Strauss, Glasziou, Richardson, & Haynes, 2011). Although EBP is now widely accepted as the "gold standard" for clinical practice in the allied

Table 17-7 STEPS OF THE EBP PROCESS

0. Cultivate a spirit of inquiry.
1. Ask a burning clinical question in PICOT format (PICOT = Patient population, Intervention or Issue of interest, Comparison intervention or group, Outcome, and Time frame).
2. Search for and collect the most relevant best evidence.
3. Critically appraise the evidence.
4. Integrate the best evidence with one's clinical expertise and patient preferences and values in making a practice decision or change.
5. Evaluate outcomes of the practice decision or change based on evidence.
6. Disseminate the outcomes of the EBP decision or change.

Source: Reproduced from Melnyk, B. M., & Fineout-Overholt, E. (2010). Making the case for evidence-based practice and cultivating a spirit of inquiry. In B. M. Melnyk & E. Fineout-Overholt (Eds.), *Evidence-based practice in nursing & healthcare: A guide to best practice* (2nd ed., pp. 3–24). Philadelphia, PA: Lippincott.

health disciplines and is operationalized using a standard process regardless of discipline (**Table 17-7**), many challenges to its use in primary care chronic illness management persist. Some recognized barriers to incorporating best research evidence in primary care practice include lack of time and access to research (Dadich & Hosseinzadeh, 2013; O'Donnell, 2004), as well as failure to place a high value on research (Dadich & Hosseinzadeh, 2013) and lack of training (O'Donnell, 2004).

Primary care clinicians do not always use best research evidence to guide their practice. For example, despite the existence of strong research-based recommendations, primary care clinicians do not always prescribe therapeutic doses of angiotensin-converting enzyme inhibitors or beta blockers for patients with congestive heart failure (Peters-Klimm et al., 2008), follow diabetes prescribing recommendations to assist in the attainment of goal $HgbA_{1c}$ levels (Kirwin, Cunningham, & Sequist, 2010), or use spirometry to assist in the diagnosis of COPD (Ghattas, Dai, Gemmel, & Awad, 2013). Although APRNs were not included in these studies, the fact that their patient outcomes have been shown to be similar to physician outcomes reflects the reality that they likely are engaging in similar practices.

To date, the EBP literature has primarily focused on how to develop compelling clinical questions, as well as how to search for and critique original research studies and systematic reviews. Very little has been published regarding how to best "integrate" patient preferences and values and clinician expertise with research findings. Although APRNs have a long history of providing patient-centered care, it is unknown how well primary care APRNs are assessing for and incorporating patient preferences and values into EBP (Burman, Robinson, & Hart, 2013). Similarly, although the development and recognition of nurse expertise has been well established and documented (e.g., Benner, 1984; De Jong et al., 2010; Foley, Kee, Minick, Harvey, & Jennings, 2002; Gorman & Morris, 1991), it is not known how to integrate this expertise into EBP. Thus, primary care APRNs need to develop methods for assessing patient values and preferences and integrating these with best research evidence and clinician expertise.

By definition, EBP does not elevate or promote the status of research evidence above clinician expertise or patient values. However, it does require a moderate degree of competency in basic statistics, research terminology, and research design; unlike clinician expertise and patient values, proficiency in these areas is not easily gained or mastered from experiential practice. Thus, it is critical that APRNs value research, master basic research skills, and utilize these skills on a routine basis.

Interpretation and Use of Research Findings and Other Evidence in Clinical Decision Making We live in exciting times, where a wealth of high-quality research exists to help inform and guide APRN practice. Although not every clinical scenario has been fully researched and a fresh set of unanswered questions arises from each new study, much of the work facing APRNs is supported by research. Indeed, it is rare for the primary care APRN working with individuals experiencing chronic illnesses not to have relevant research to draw upon. As such, it is critical for APRNs to be able to competently search for and critically evaluate the research literature, especially as it applies to their own area of clinical expertise.

Having a mechanism to remain aware of current research findings is an all-important first step toward competency in research. At present, a growing number of services exist to facilitate this endeavor. Examples include daily electronic "Smart Briefs" from the American Nurses Association, the American Academy of Nurse Practitioners (AANP), and Physician's First Watch. In addition, many other professional nursing organizations offer weekly or monthly electronic research updates to their members.

Participation in professional journal clubs is another avenue for APRNs to remain current and has the added benefit of enabling nurses to converse with others about research and explore how it applies to clinical practice. Professional journal clubs may be sponsored by a workplace organization or organized "off site" by a group of like-minded colleagues. They may follow a variety of formats, including face-to-face monthly meetings, email discussions, wikis, or blogs. Several professional organizations and journals are now hosting electronic journal clubs to subscribers—for example, the AANP Virtual Journal Club and the Cochrane Journal Club. A number of excellent publications describe the value of professional journal clubs and explain how to initiate one, and the interested reader is encouraged to review these (e.g., Deenadayalan, Grimmer-Somers, Prior, & Kumar, 2008; Dobrzanska & Cromack, 2005; Honey & Baker, 2011; Hughes, 2010; Lizarondo, Kumar, & Grimmer-Somers, 2010; Luby, Riley, & Towne, 2006).

In addition to having access to research findings related to chronic illness, APRNs must be able to critically evaluate these findings and determine whether and/or how the findings apply to practice. Simply put, critically appraising the research literature requires the ability to evaluate the validity of a single study's methodology and the meaningfulness of its findings, while simultaneously synthesizing findings from multiple studies across the literature. Obviously, there is nothing "simple" about this process. Indeed, similar to many clinical skills, research appraisal is an acquired capability that requires adequate education and experience to develop. A variety of excellent courses, workshops, and websites exist to assist APRNs with developing

the skills to be able to critically evaluate research evidence (**Table 17-8**). Having an EBP mentor or EBP team to consult with and a supportive work environment are also invaluable to the successful acquisition of EBP skills (Aitken et al., 2011; Fineout-Overholt & Melnyk, 2010).

Similarly, APRNs' practices should reflect an awareness of current research findings, which require that they have and maintain mechanisms to remain current on the latest research literature. At present, a variety of mechanisms exist to facilitate this, including daily or electronic research alerts from organizations such as the American Academy of Nurse Practitioners and Journal Watch (see Table 17-8). In addition, APRNs may be able to engage in dialogue with

Table 17-8 EXAMPLES OF USEFUL EVIDENCE-BASED RESOURCES FOR APRN PRIMARY CARE PRACTICE

Academic Center for Evidence-Based Practice: http://www.acestar.uthscsa.edu/

Agency for Healthcare Research and Quality (AHRQ): http://www.ahrq.gov/

AHRQ email updates: http://www.ahrq.gov/clinic/epcix.htm

American Association of Nurse Practitioners' Smart Brief: http://www.smartbrief.com/aanp/

American Nurses Association's Smart Brief: http://www.smartbrief.com/ana/

Center for the Advancement of Evidence-Based Practice: http://nursingandhealth.asu.edu/evidence-based-practice/index.htm

Cochrane Collaboration: http://www.cochrane.org/

Duke University Evidence-Based Practice, Center for Clinical Health Policy Research: http://clinpol.duhs.duke.edu/modules/chpr_rsch_prac/index.php?id=1

Institute for Johns Hopkins Nursing: http://www.ijhn.jhmi.edu/

Journal Watch: http://www.jwatch.org/

McMaster's University Evidence-Based Practice Center: http://hiru.mcmaster.ca/epc/

National Guideline Clearinghouse: http://www.guideline.gov/

Oregon Evidence-Based Practice Center: http://www.ohsu.edu/xd/research/centers-institutes/evidence-based-practice-center/

Prescriber's Letter: http://www.prescribersletter.com

UpToDate: http://www.uptodate.com

Vanderbilt Evidence-Based Practice Center: http://medicineandpublichealth.vanderbilt.edu/center.php?userid=1043409&home=1

other professionals, as well as patients, regarding research evidence.

Evaluation of Practice   In addition to basing care on research-based evidence, APRNs who work with individuals experiencing chronic illnesses should routinely evaluate their clinical practice and practice-related outcomes. These types of evaluations not only ensure quality, but also provide data that can be used by researchers and stakeholders (i.e., consumers, insurers, healthcare agencies) who are studying or evaluating care provided by APRNs. Evaluation of APRN practice may revolve around any number of professional aspects, including, but not limited to, scope and standards of practice, role and job descriptions, and evidence-based guidelines and national quality indicators. For example, APRNs who work with adults and children experiencing diabetes could evaluate their own practices to ensure that they are supported by (i.e., contained within) national and state scopes and standards for practice. Similarly, these APRNs could evaluate specific aspects of diabetes management for adherence rates (e.g., influenza vaccination, microalbuminuria, and retinopathy screening) and attainment of goal disease indicators (e.g., $HgbA_{1c}$, blood pressure, and lipids).

Practice evaluations may occur using a variety of mechanisms. For example, checklists can be developed to compare national and state standards to a particular agency's APRN job descriptions and evaluation criteria. In addition, APRNs may perform chart or electronic reviews of specific care practices (e.g., foot or retina evaluations in patients with diabetes) or patient outcomes (e.g., $HgbA_{1c}$ or lipid levels), albeit within the constraints of the Health Insurance Portability and Accountability Act (HIPAA, 1996).

Regardless of how or which practice parameters are evaluated, it is essential that APRNs utilize evaluative data to improve their practices. Thus it is critical that the evaluative process be understood

and supported by all participating providers (e.g., APRNs, basic-prepared nurses, technicians, and care providers). Similarly, it is important that data are reported in a clear, standardized fashion and that an established process for quality improvement/harm reduction be followed (e.g., using the principles of continuous quality improvement [Sollecito & Johnson, 2013], total quality management [Kelly, 2011], or the model for improvement endorsed by the Institute for Healthcare Improvement [Langley, Moen, Nolan, Nolan, Norman, & Provost, 2009]).

Participation in Collaborative Research   In addition to being able to interpret and apply research findings and evaluate and improve care based on research-based evidence, primary care APRNs should be able to participate and collaborate in research activities related to their area of clinical expertise. Although APRNs do not need to design and oversee research studies, they should possess general knowledge about research paradigms and phases of the research process (Burns & Grove, 2010; Polit & Beck, 2013). Perhaps most importantly, primary care APRNs need to be interested in research and earnestly desire to contribute to the research knowledge base by developing collaborative relationships with nurse scientists and others who are studying aspects of interest to APRN primary care practice.

GUIDANCE AND COACHING

In recent years, theory and technique-based guidance and coaching in primary care have received much attention—and for good reason. The evidence supporting the effectiveness of theory-based guidance and coaching in primary care is mounting, with multiple studies showing its effectiveness in chronic illnesses such as diabetes, hypertension, obesity, and tobacco addiction (Armstrong, Mottershead, Ronksley, Sigal, Campbell, & Hemmelgarn, 2011; Bredie, Fouwels, Wollersheim, & Schippers, 2011;

Chen, Creedy, Lin, & Wollin, 2012; Sjöling, Lundberg, Englund, Westman, & Jong, 2011).

On the surface, the guidance and coaching competency seems straightforward and the experienced nurse may assume he or she handles these tasks well and with "expertise." After all, most nurses and APRNs are familiar with and well versed in patient teaching and engage in it frequently during their usual patient care activities. However, upon closer examination, there is more to teaching, guidance, and coaching than meets the eye.

Although patient education, guidance, and coaching often occur together in the same patient encounter, they are quite different from one another. Patient education typically involves assisting patients to become more informed about their illness, condition, medication, procedure, options, and so on; its purpose is to enable individuals to better care for themselves. Guidance is synonymous with "advising" or "showing the way" (Spross & Babine, 2014). For example, in chronic illness primary care, the APRN might provide anticipatory guidance to a patient with asthma who in the past has used only a rescue inhaler and is now adding a twice-daily steroid inhaler. The APRN's guidance would help the client to anticipate what to expect regarding the immediacy and effectiveness of the steroid inhaler (especially when compared to the rescue inhaler) and when to anticipate needing to use the rescue inhaler.

The verb "coach" stems from the word's origins as a carriage used to facilitate the safe transmission of individual(s) from one point to another. Transferring this understanding to APRN practice, coaching is "interpersonal work that helps people who are facing personal transitions or journeys" (Spross, 2009, p. 161), such as those associated with chronic illnesses. The phenomenon of coaching is complex. In addition to establishing rapport, actively listening, and expressing empathy, expert APRN coaching requires clinical competence and creative problem solving, as well as knowledge and skill regarding how best to assist individuals who are experiencing a crisis, desiring change, or even expressing apathy toward an illness or situation.

For example, to assist a middle-aged adult female with obesity and poorly controlled type 2 diabetes who desires to lose weight and bring her $HgbA_{1c}$ into the goal range, the APRN must demonstrate expertise regarding the pathophysiology of diabetes and the complications associated with poor control. He or she must also be thoroughly familiar with current evidence regarding diabetes care parameters and treatments. In addition, the APRN should possess knowledge of and experience with efficacious diabetes education strategies, as well as theories and techniques related to behavioral change, such as the transtheoretical stages of change model (DiClemente & Prochaska, 1982; Norcross, Krebs, & Prochaska, 2011; Prochaska, 1979), the health promotion model (Pender, Murdaugh, & Parsons, 2010), and motivational interviewing (Miller & Rollnick, 1992; Rollnick, Miller, & Butler, 2008). A four-step process designed to facilitate APRN-delivered health coaching in primary care is outlined in **Table 17-9**.

Clinical Competence   To provide guidance and coaching in chronic illness primary care, APRNs must be knowledgeable regarding the illness(es) of interest and experienced enough to anticipate the informational and emotional needs of the patient and his or her family members. Going beyond asking the patient and family what they "want to know" and anticipating what they "need to know" is a critical aspect of the APRN's coaching skills and requires that the APRN be intimately familiar with the illness of interest, its progression, and its management.

Creative Problem Solving   Just as no one asks to have a chronic illness, no one asks to have the myriad problems that are often associated with chronic illness. Coaching in chronic illness care often involves assisting patients and families

Table 17-9 Steps for Applying Behavior Change Theories and Techniques in Primary Care

Preparation	Prepare for the encounter by reviewing the empirical literature related to the health behavior and patient/setting. If little is known about the patient and/or behavior beforehand, arrange to get back to the patient within a specific time frame and review the related literature prior to that meeting.
Relationship building and assessment	Work with the patient to identify the specific target and goals for behavior change. Build trust and clarify expectations for the encounter by utilizing counseling skills (i.e., open-ended questions, active and reflective listening, summarizing patient's concerns) and motivational interviewing.
Theory-based intervention	Select a theoretical approach and appropriate technique(s) to assist with understanding patient behavior and designing interventions.
Follow-up and evaluation	Using theory and literature as a guide, work with the patient to identify a follow-up and assessment strategy.

Source: Reprinted from *Journal for Nurse Practitioners. 10*(4), Thomas, J.J., Hart, A.M., & Burman, M.E. (2014). Improving health promotion and disease prevention in NP-delivered primary care, Pages 221-228, Copyright 2014, with permission from Elsevier.

who may be angry, despondent, anxious, confused, or desperate. Given these reactions, it is critical that the APRN be willing to set aside his or her routine "script" or "protocol" and be able to create a revised plan that takes into consideration the unique needs, styles, and interests of the patient or family. Examples of creative educational and coaching strategies for chronic illness management that are gaining support in the research literature include group appointments for patients with diabetes mellitus (Edelman et al., 2010); the use of lay leaders for support groups that address diabetes mellitus, hypertension, arthritis, and chronic pain (Foster, Taylor, Eldridge, Ramsay, & Griffiths, 2009); and the use of mobile phone technology for management of conditions such as diabetes and hypertension (de Johgh, Gurol-Urganci, Vodopivec-Jamsek, Car, & Atun, 2012; Yoo et al., 2009).

Summary

Hamric's (2014) six core APRN competencies—leadership, ethical decision making, consultation,

collaboration, evidence-based practice, and guidance and coaching—are critical to the quality of chronic illness primary care, regardless of whether that care is delivered directly by the APRN or delivered by RNs and other caregivers who work with APRNs. It is also important to note that meeting a competency or group of competencies is *not* a one-time goal. APRNs must continually strive to demonstrate these competencies, particularly when a change is made that significantly impacts patient care delivery, the nursing profession, and the healthcare system.

Contributions of APRNs in Chronic Illness Care

Clinical Outcomes and Patient Satisfaction

The most common chronic illnesses for which APRN primary care (primarily provided by CNPs) has been studied include diabetes, hypertension, and dyslipidemia. With rare exceptions, the data from such investigations have shown that patients who receive primary care from CNP-prepared APRNs have clinical outcomes (e.g., laboratory and blood pressure values) similar to patients who receive primary care services from physicians. Satisfaction with care has generally been found to be higher among patients seen by CNPs; however, not all studies reflect this finding and some indicate that satisfaction is higher with physician-delivered care (**Table 17-10**).

Table 17-10 SEMINAL PRIMARY CARE APRN OUTCOMES STUDIES

Study	Design	Subjects	Length of Follow-up	Primary Results
Stanik-Hutt et al. (2013)	SR of patient care provided by NPs versus MDs	37 studies representing more than 1,200 patients	Variable—not disclosed in the report	No differences in mortality, hospitalization rates, length of hospitalization stays, unexpected emergency visits, blood glucose, BP, patient satisfaction with care, and self-reports of health and functional status Better serum levels with care provided by NPs
Newhouse et al. (2011)	SR of patient care provided by NPs versus MDs	69 studies: NP = 37 CNS = 11 CNM = 21 CRNA = 0 (No data regarding number of patients represented)	Variable—not disclosed in the report	Equivalent or better outcomes across all APRNs and outcomes Same outcomes as Stanik-Hutt et al. for NPs versus MDs
Houweling, Kleefstra, van Hateren, Groenier, Meyboom-deJong, & Bilo (2011)	RCT: Adults with type 2 diabetes randomized to NP or GP	$N = 206$	14 months	No differences with regard to $HgbA_{1c}$, BP, and lipid values Subjects in NP group experienced some deterioration in QOL scores; no QOL decrease seen in GP subjects Subjects in NP group more satisfied with care than those in GP group
Dierick-van Daele, Metsemakers, Derckx, Spreeuwenberg, & Vrijhoef (2009)	RCT: Adults randomized to NP or GP	$N = 1501$	6 months	No differences in health status, medical resources utilized, or use of practice guidelines Subjects in NP group had more follow-up consultations NP consultations longer than GP consultations No differences in patient satisfaction

(Continues)

Table 17-10 Seminal Primary Care APRN Outcomes Studies (Continued)

Study	Design	Subjects	Length of Follow-up	Primary Results
Laurant et al. (2004)	SR of care provided by NPs versus MDs	16 studies	Average follow-up ≤ 12 months	No appreciable differences between patients cared for by MD or NPs with regard to health outcomes, process of care, resource utilization, or cost Patient satisfaction higher with NP care NP consultations longer than physician consultations Patient satisfaction higher with NP-led care
Lenz, Mundinger, Kane, Hopkins, & Lin (2004)	RCT: 2-year follow-up Patients originally enrolled in two groups, MD or NP	N = 406	2 years	No differences between the groups in health status, disease-specific physiologic measures, use of specialist, emergency room visits, or inpatient services No differences in patient satisfaction
Mundinger et al. (2000)	RCT with subjects randomized to NP or MD	N = 1,316	6 months; 1 year	No differences between patients cared for by NPs and MDs with regard to (1) patients' health status, (2) physiologic test results for patients with chronic conditions such as diabetes or asthma, (3) health services utilization, or (4) satisfaction after initial appointment For patients with hypertension, the diastolic value was lower for NP patients (82 versus 85 mm Hg; $p = 0.04$). Satisfaction ratings at 6 months differed for one of four dimensions measured (provider attributes), with MD rated higher (4.2 versus 4.1 on a scale where 5 = excellent; $p = 0.05$); no differences in patient satisfaction at 1 year

BP = blood pressure; CNM = clinical nurse–midwife; CNS = clinical nurse specialist; CRNA = certified registered nurse anesthetist; GP = general practitioner; MD = physician; NP = nurse practitioner; QOL = quality of life; RCT = randomized controlled trial; SR = systematic review.

Improving APRN-Delivered Primary Care for Patients with Chronic Illnesses

Despite the increase in the number of and the growing consumer support for primary care APRNs, as well as a small but impressive body of literature validating their work, there is still much to be done to improve chronic illness primary care, primarily concerning four of the six core APRN competencies: leadership, collaboration, evidence-based practice, and guidance and coaching.

Improving Leadership

One of the greatest areas for improvement in APRN chronic illness primary care is restructuring of the primary care team. The traditional "physician"- or "provider"-led primary care model (**Figure 17-2**) was developed almost a century ago when physicians were consulted and respected for knowing "best" and before the era of informed, proactive consumers. Of course, much has changed since the development of this top-down model. Patients today have ready access to quality health information, and we now recognize and value the critical role of the patient in his or her own care. We also respect the contributions of a variety of health professions, very few of which rely on a physician or other provider to dictate their patient-related activities and interaction.

The patient-centered team depicted in **Figure 17-3** has been suggested as an alternative to the traditional provider-driven model. In this model, patients and team members communicate directly with one another. Each team member is expected to practice at the highest level of his or her professional skills and is respected for his or her professional expertise. This type of innovative model is being used successfully by award-winning organizations such as Kaiser Permanente and Southcentral Foundation in Anchorage, Alaska (Bisognano & Kenney, 2012).

Improving Evidence-Based Practice

In addition to improving their ability to search for research-based evidence and to actively seek out knowledge related to integrating best research evidence with clinician expertise and patient values and preferences, APRNs should

Figure 17-2 Traditional Primary Care Team

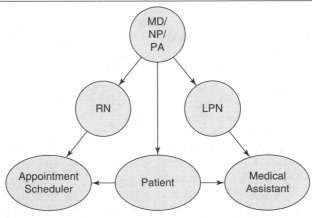

Source: Data from Bisognano, M., & Kenney, C. (2012). *Pursuing the triple aim: Seven innovators show the way to better care, better health, and lower costs,* San Francisco, CA: Jossey-Bass.

Figure 17-3 True Patient-Centered Team

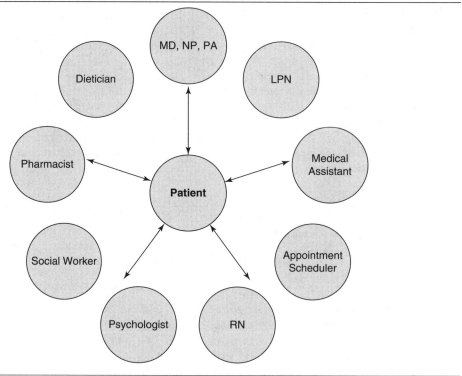

Source: Data from Bisognano, M., & Kenney, C. (2012). *Pursuing the triple aim: Seven innovators show the way to better care, better health, and lower costs.*, San Francisco, CA: Jossey-Bass.

seek to contribute to EBP by documenting and publishing evidence obtained from their own practices. They should improve their ability to ask compelling clinical questions; search for, obtain, and critically appraise best research evidence; and integrate best research with clinician expertise and patient preferences and values. It is also important for the primary care APRN to systematically document and disseminate his or her own practice findings (i.e., practice-based evidence). This methodology, which is known as the "single case experimental design" (SCED) or "*n* of 1" study, is amenable to busy clinical primary care APRNs. SCED does not require

coursework in research design and is fairly easy to learn and conduct through self-study and or consultation with nursing and other health scientists. For more information regarding SCED, see the book by Barlow, Nock, and Herson (2008).

Improving Collaboration

To improve competency in collaborative skills, APRNs are encouraged to review recent advances in collaboration and the benefits of integrated care. Over the last two decades, this concept has evolved from *multidisciplinary* collaboration, which recognizes the contributions of other disciplines; to *interdisciplinary* collaboration, in which members from different disciplines share care responsibilities for a patient; and more recently to *transdisciplinary* collaboration, where members from different disciplines are committed to engaging with and learning from one another, as well as working together across boundaries to plan and provide integrated patient services (Glittenberg, 2004; Maitland, 2010; Verdejo, 2001). When APRNs and members from other disciplines view and approach patient care from a transdisciplinary perspective, the outcomes are typically positive for patients and family members and the experience is often transformative for the involved clinicians as well (Hanson & Carter, 2014).

Integrated care models utilize the principle of transdisciplinary collaboration in providing patient care services. These models are still in their infancy and have primarily been designed for patients who are experiencing both chronic physical and mental illnesses, which are best addressed by combining primary care and behavioral health services. Preliminary studies of integrated models for patients with chronic illnesses such as diabetes, HIV infection, depression, and substance abuse have shown that integrated care models are both efficacious and cost-effective (Bogner & de Vries, 2010; Katon et al., 2010; Schouten, Niessen, van de Pas, Grol, & Hulscher, 2010). Consequently, APRNs are encouraged to pursue integrated care opportunities.

Improving Guidance and Coaching

Although APRN-delivered chronic illness primary care achieves patient outcomes similar to physician-delivered care (e.g., Newhouse et al., 2011, Stanik-Hutt et al., 2013), patient outcomes in the United States remain far below where they should be (Ho & Preston, 2011). Many chronic illnesses have a behavioral etiology and/or can be improved by lifestyle changes. Thus it has been proposed that returning to nursing's "health" roots may be a way to turn the tide and make a substantial difference in chronic illness outcomes (Burman, Hart, Conley, Brown, Sherard, & Clarke, 2009). Although most primary care APRNs are well versed in patient teaching, effective guidance and coaching require a fair amount of study and practice. Studies have shown that even when nurses and physicians undergo motivational interviewing training, they often revert to ineffective communication styles in their actual practice (Jansink et al., 2013; Noordman, van Lee, Nielen, Viek, van Weijden, & van Dulmen, 2012; Werner, Lawson, Panaite, Step, & Flocke, 2013). To deal with this dilemma, it is imperative for APRNs engaging in chronic illness primary care to commit to learning and owning effective guidance and coaching skills.

Summary and Conclusions

APRNs have a long history of providing quality primary care to individuals and families experiencing chronic illness. The quality of this care has been documented in numerous studies, and APRNs are both recognized and valued by patients and families. Despite these accomplishments, there is still much work for APRNs to do, particularly regarding leadership, collaboration, evidence-based practice, and guidance and coaching.

APRN certification and licensure do not ensure that the APRN is engaging in advanced practice nursing. What distinguishes advanced practice nursing from basic nursing is that Hamric's core competencies are *always* reflected in the APRN's practice. In this spirit, this chapter closes with the challenge offered to APRNs and APRN educators:

> *There is still much work to be done: not all APN students are educated to practice with the competencies described here; too many nurses are in APN roles without the necessary credentials or core competencies, and thus true advanced practice nursing is not demonstrated. (Hamric, Hanson, Tracy, & O'Grady, 2014, p. xiv)*

CASE STUDY 17-1

You are an APRN working with a new patient, Mary Lopez, a 65-year-old Hispanic woman, who presents to you because she hears that you are "good with train wrecks like me." Mary brings in a copy of her medical records, which show that she has a history of multiple comorbid chronic illnesses, including obesity, type 2 diabetes mellitus, essential hypertension, Parkinson's disease, stage 2 chronic kidney disease, obstructive sleep apnea, major depressive disorder, and chronic pain in her lower back and knees stemming from degenerative disc disease and osteoarthritis. She has been treated for most of these illnesses for the past decade, with the exception of the Parkinson's disease; it was diagnosed 1 year ago and has caused Mary to have a resting tremor and shuffling gait. In addition, 2 years ago, she was diagnosed with stage 1 chronic kidney disease, which has since progressed to stage 2, despite her having fairly well-controlled diabetes (HgbA$_{1c}$ levels between 6.5 and 7) and hypertension (average blood pressure readings 120/75 mm Hg). Mary's current medications include metformin 1,000 mg twice daily, insulin glargine 23 units subcutaneously at bedtime, lisinopril 10 mg every day, hydrochlorothiazide 12.5 mg every day, pravastatin 40 mg at bedtime, Sinemet (combination carbidopa and levodopa) 25/100 four times per day, fluoxetine 20 mg twice daily, MS Contin 30 mg twice daily, hydrocodone/acetaminophen 10/325 mg 1–2 times by mouth every 6 hours as needed, and Senokot-S (standardized Senna concentrate with docusate sodium 50 mg) 2 tablets twice daily. Mary also receives continuous positive airway pressure (CPAP) therapy at night. She has been on all of her medications for the last 2 years, with the exception of Sinemet, which was started after she was diagnosed with Parkinson's disease.

Mary says that she has been seeing a family practice physician in town for the last 5 years and was fairly satisfied with his care until she was diagnosed with Parkinson's disease. Since that time, her back and knee pain have worsened, but apparently her physician told her, "There is nothing more I can do to help you with your pain," and "With all of your mobility issues, we need to start transitioning you to the nursing home." Mary gets teary when she shares this information with you. She says, "I know I'm a mess, but I really love living at home and don't want to go to the nursing home."

Past Medical History

Mary has no known history of cardiac or vascular disease. Her only surgery was a cholecystectomy 10 years ago. She had a screening colonoscopy at age 50 that was normal; however, she has not had one since then due to mobility issues. There is no history of abnormal Pap smears or mammograms; however, her last Pap and mammogram were more than 3 years ago.

Family History

Mary's parents were both obese but had no health problems when they died. Her maternal grandparents lived until their 90s and died of "old age." Her paternal grandfather died of metastatic prostate cancer at age 75. Her maternal grandmother died of a "massive stroke" at age 81. Three of Mary's four siblings are also obese and have type 2 diabetes mellitus.

(continues)

CASE STUDY 17-1 (Continued)

Social History

Mary earned a bachelor's degree in secondary education with a minor in home economics when she was 23 and worked for 30 years teaching home economics (primarily cooking) to local high school students. She reports that she has "always" been overweight but was able to wear normal-size clothes and get around without difficulty until 5 years ago, when she retired. After retiring, she gained 150 pounds and started having significant pain and mobility problems, which eventually led to her disability status. She has tried multiple weight-loss regimens throughout her life but has not been successful with any of them. Mary no longer eats out, but primarily eats the food she receives from Meals on Wheels as well as some other grocery items that friends bring to her. However, she has significant mobility issues related to her pain and Parkinson's disease and continues to have a body mass index (BMI) of 56.

Mary receives Medicare and Social Security Supplemental Income benefits. She lives alone in a low-income housing apartment and receives home health services several times a week to help her with bathing and housework. She uses a walker with ambulation. She wears a "lifeline" at all times and says that she had to use it 6 months ago when she fell in the shower and could not get up. Since then, she has not attempted to bathe alone, but rather waits for the home health aide to assist her with this task.

Mary was the oldest of five children. Both of her parents died in an auto accident when she was 45. Two of her four siblings live nearby and check on her periodically; however, all of them still work and spend a lot of time caring for their grandchildren, and Mary does not want to impose upon them further. Mary also has multiple cousins in the community, and all of her siblings, cousins, and their children get together throughout the year for birthdays and religious holidays.

Mary identifies with being heterosexual, but never married and does not have an intimate partner. She has no children. She indicates that she is Roman Catholic and used to attend services at a local parish until a couple of years ago, when it became too difficult for her to drive, and she sold her car. She continues to have some friends from church who visit her and offer to take her to church. However, she goes to church and leaves her home very infrequently due to her extreme mobility problems and concern regarding falling. Mary reports infrequent alcohol use and says she has margaritas a few times a year when she gets together with her family. She denies current or past use of tobacco or other illicit drugs.

Objective

As you talk with Mary, she answers all questions appropriately. She is neatly groomed and organized, and seems to easily recall relevant facts related to her health care. Her affect is generally happy; however, she is clearly concerned about her future living arrangements and gets teary when she talks about living away from home.

(continues)

CASE STUDY 17-1 (Continued)

Discussion Questions

1. How would you assess and prioritize Mary's care needs (both today and in the future)? How does current research-based evidence fit into this?
2. Consider each of the six APRN competencies discussed in this chapter and illustrated in Figure 17-1. Which of these competencies are most challenged by this case, and how would you try to meet them as you work with Mary?
3. How would a transdisciplinary team look at Mary? Think about the available resources and providers in your own community or those whom you could consult with by telehealth. How could you provide transdisciplinary care with these individuals versus multidisciplinary or interdisciplinary care?
4. How would you assess the importance of family, culture, and spirituality in Mary's life and care?
5. Which outcomes are most important as you assess Mary's care? Identify both traditional medical outcomes and APRN-sensitive outcomes. Which outcomes are your highest priority and why?

CASE STUDY 17-2

Joe (age 67) and Maria (age 65) are a married couple who have been receiving primary care from you for the past 5 years. Both are Caucasian. Joe has essential hypertension, type 2 diabetes mellitus, and dyslipidemia. He takes the following medications: hydrochlorathiazide 25 mg QD; lisinopril 10 mg BID; metformin 100 mg BID; pravastatin 80 mg QHS; ASA 81 mg QD; and insulin gargline 25 units subcutaneous QHS. Maria has hypertension and dyslipidemia and recently had a myocardial infarction, for which she received two stents. She was also diagnosed with COPD 2 years ago, which according to the Global Initiative for Chronic Lung Disease (2014) criteria is categorized as stage 2 (low risk, more symptoms). Current medications for Maria include clopidogrel 75 mg QD; pravastatin 80 mg QHS; carvediolol 6.25 mg BID; lisinopril 10 mg BID; tiotropium 18 mcg/capsule, 2 inh of one capsule QD; fluticasone propionate 220 mcg, 2 inh BID with spacer device (rinse mouth with water afterward); and albuterol 90 mcg/inh, 2 inh QID prn.

(continues)

CASE STUDY 17-2 (Continued)

Joe and Maria have both smoked almost since they were in high school (approximately 50 years) and each has smoked two packs per day for almost 45 years. During each visit with them over the past 5 years, you have addressed smoking cessation. Specifically, you have discussed how smoking cessation can improve hypertension and the vascular risks associated with diabetes. You have also discussed how smoking cessation reduces the risk of heart disease and stroke, and how it can halt the progression of COPD. In addition, you have offered pharmacologic therapy to assist with their cessation efforts. However, every time you have brought this topic up, Joe and Maria have politely laughed and said, "We know we should quit smoking and really wish we could, but you can't change two old dogs like us."

You are now seeing Joe and Maria for the first time since Maria had her myocardial infarction. You have recently completed a motivational interviewing (Mason & Butler, 2010) workshop and are excited to try this technique with Joe and Maria. Using the four steps for behavioral change in primary care (outlined in Table 17-9), you have prepared for this meeting by (1) reviewing the most recent clinical practice guideline for tobacco cessation (DHHS, 2008); (2) deciding to use motivational interviewing as your relationship-building technique; and (3) reviewing the behavioral theory literature and deciding to use the transtheoretical stages of change model (Norcross et al., 2011; Prochaska, Norcross, & DiClemente, 2013) along with motivational interviewing for your theory-based intervention.

Discussion Questions

Prepare for this case and the first three behavioral steps outlined in Table 17-9 by reviewing the following websites: (1) DHHS's (2008) clinical practice guideline for tobacco cessation available from http://bphc.hrsa.gov/ buckets/treatingtobacco.pdf; (2) motivational interviewing techniques from http://www.motivationalinterview.org; and (3) the transtheoretical stages of change model from the University of Rhode Island, Cancer Prevention Research Center, at http://www.uri.edu/research /cprc/transtheoretical_model.html. Then discuss the following:

1. Related to tobacco cessation, Joe and Maria are in the "pre-contemplation" stage. Which specific motivational interviewing techniques would you use to facilitate their progression to the "contemplation," "action," and subsequent steps?
2. Discuss at least two ways you might follow up with Joe and Maria and evaluate their progress by using the motivational interviewing and transtheoretical stages of change models.
3. Plan for success! Assuming Joe and Maria successfully progress to the "contemplation" phase, which techniques would you implement to help them progress to the "preparation" phase? To the "action" phase? To the subsequent phases?
4. Plan for a challenge! Which techniques could you use if Joe was motivated to quit tobacco but Maria was not?

References

Agency for Healthcare Research and Quality (AHRQ). (2011, October). The number of nurse practitioners and physician assistants practicing primary care in the United States. *Primary Care Workforce Facts and Stats No. 2.* http://www.ahrq.gov/research/findings /factsheets/primary/pcwork2/index.html

Aitken, L. M., Hackwood, B., Crouch, S., Clayton, S., West, N., Carney, D., & Jack, L. (2011). Creating an environment to implement and sustain evidence-based practice: A developmental process. *Australian Critical Care, 24*(4), 244–254.

American Association of Colleges of Nursing (AACN). (2006). *The essentials of doctoral education for advanced nursing practice.* Washington, DC: Author.

American Association of Colleges of Nursing (AACN). (2011). *The essentials of master's education in nursing.* Washington, DC: Author.

Armstrong, A. E. (2006). Towards a strong virtue ethics for nursing practice. *Nursing Philosophy, 7,* 110–124.

Armstrong, M. J., Mottershead, T. A., Ronksley, P. E., Sigal, R. J., Campbell, T. S., & Hemmelgarn, B. R. (2011). Motivational interviewing to improve weight loss in overweight and/or obese patients: A systematic review and meta-analysis of randomized controlled trials. *Obesity Reviews, 12*(9), 709–723.

Arries, E. (2006). Virtue ethics: An approach to moral dilemmas in nursing. *Curationis, 28,* 64–72.

Baiker, K., & Chandra, A. (2004, April). Medicare spending, the physician workforce, and beneficiaries' quality of care. *Health Affairs,* (suppl), W4–W184.

Barlow, D. H., Nock, M. K., & Hersen, M. (2008). *Single case experimental designs: Strategies for studying behavior change* (3rd ed.). Upper Saddle River, NJ: Pearson.

Beauchamp, T. L., & Childress, J. F. (2012). *Principles of biomedical ethics* (7th ed.). New York, NY: Oxford University Press.

Benner, P. (1984). *From novice to expert: Excellence and power in clinical nursing practice.* Menlo Park, CA: Addison-Wesley.

Bisognano, M., & Kenney, C. (2012). *Pursuing the triple aim: Seven innovators show the way to better care, better health, and lower costs.* San Francisco, CA: Jossey-Bass.

Bogner, H. R., & de Vries, H. F. (2010). Integrating type 2 diabetes mellitus and depression treatment among African Americans: A randomized controlled pilot trial. *Diabetes Educator, 36,* 284–292.

Bredie, S. J., Fouwels, A. J., Wollersheim, H., & Schippers, G. M. (2011). Effectiveness of nurse based motivational interviewing for smoking cessation in high risk cardiovascular outpatients: A randomized trial. *European Journal of Cardiovascular Nursing, 10*(3), 174–179.

Burman, M. D., Hart, A. M., Conley, V., Brown, J., Sherard, P., & Clarke, P. N. (2009). Doctor of nursing practice: Reconceptualizing advanced nursing practice. *Journal of the American Academy of Nurse Practitioners, 2,* 11–17.

Burman, M. E., Robinson, B., & Hart, A. M. (2013). Linking evidence-based nursing practice and patient-centered care through patient preferences. *Nursing Administration Quarterly, 37*(3), 231–241.

Burns, N., & Groves, S. K. (2010). *Understanding nursing research: Building an evidence-based practice* (5th ed.). Philadelphia, PA: W.B. Saunders.

Caley, M. (2013). Remember Barbara Starfield: Primary care is the health system's bedrock. *British Medical Journal, 347,* f4627.

Chang, C., Stukel, T. A., Flood, A. B., & Goodman, D. C. (2011). Primary care physician workforce and Medicare beneficiaries' health outcomes. *Journal of the American Medical Association, 305*(20), 2096–2105.

Chen, S. M., Creedy, D., Lin, H. S., & Wollin, J. (2012). Effects of motivational intervention on self-management, psychological and glycemic outcomes in type 2 diabetes: A randomized controlled trial. *International Journal of Nursing Studies, 49*(6), 637–644.

Cooke, L., Gemmill R., & Grant, M. (2008). Advanced practice nurses core competencies: A framework for developing and testing an advanced practice nurse discharge intervention. *Clinical Nurse Specialist, 22*(5), 218–225.

Cooper, M. D. (1991). Principle based ethics and the ethics of care: A creative tension. *Advances in Nursing Science, 14,* 22–31.

Dadich, A., & Hosseinzadeh, H. (2013). Healthcare reform: Implications for knowledge translation in primary care. *BMC Health Services Research, 13*(1), 490.

Deenadayalan, Y., Grimmer-Somers, K., Prior, M., & Kumar, S. (2008). How to run an effective journal club: A systematic review. *Journal of Evaluation in Clinical Practice, 14,* 898–911.

De Jong, M. J., Benner, R., Benner, P., Richard, M. L., Kenny D. J., Kelley, P., ... Debisette, A. T. (2010). Mass casualty care in an expeditionary environment: Developing local knowledge and expertise in context. *Journal of Trauma Nursing, 17,* 45–58.

de Jongh, T., Gurol-Urganci, I., Vodopivec-Jamsek, V., Car, J., & Atun, R. (2012). Mobile phone messaging for facilitating self-management of long-term illnesses. *Database of Systematic Reviews, 12,* CD007459. doi: 10.1002/14651858.CD007459.pub2

DiClemente, C. C., & Prochaska, J. O. (1982). Self-change and therapy change of smoking behavior: A comparison of processes of change in cessation and maintenance. *Addictive Behavior*, 7, 133–142.

Dierick-van Daele, A. T. M., Metsemakers, J. F. M., Derckx, W. C. C., Spreeuwenberg, C., & Vrijhoef, J. J. M. (2009). Nurse practitioners substituting for general practitioners: Randomized controlled trial. *Journal of Advanced Nursing*, 65, 391–401.

Dill, M. J., Pankow, S., Erikson, C., & Shipman, S. (2013). Survey shows consumers open to greater role for physician assistants and nurse practitioners. *Health Affairs*, 32(6), 1135–1142.

Dobrzanska, L., & Cromack, D. (2005). Developing a journal club in the community setting. *British Journal of Community Nursing*, 10, 376–377.

Donaldson, M. S., Yordy, K. D., Lohr, K. N., & Vanselow, N. A. (Eds.); Institute of Medicine, Division of Health Care Services, Committee on the Future of Primary Care. (1996). *Primary care: America's health in a new era.* Washington, DC: National Academies Press.

Edelman, D., Fredrickson, S. K., Melnyk, S. D., Coffman, C. J., Jeffreys, A. S., Datta, S., ... Weinberger, M. (2010). Medical clinics versus usual care for patients with both diabetes and hypertension: A randomized trial. *Annals of Internal Medicine*, 152, 689–696.

Fineout-Overholt, E., & Melnyk, B. M. (2010). ARCC Evidence-based practice mentors: The key to sustaining evidence-based practice. In B. M. Melnyk & E. Fineout-Overholt (Eds.), *Evidence-based practice in nursing and healthcare: A guide to best practice* (2nd ed., pp. 344–351). Philadelphia, PA: Lippincott Williams & Wilkins.

Finkelstein, A., Taubman, S., Wright, B., Bernstein, M., Gruber, J., Newhouse, J. P., ... Oregon Health Study Group. (2012). The Oregon health insurance experiment: Evidence from the first year. *Quarterly Journal of Economics*, 127(3), 1057–1106.

Foley, B. J., Kee, C. C., Minick, P., Harvey, S. S., & Jennings, B. M. (2002). Characteristics of nurses and hospital work environments that foster satisfaction and clinical expertise. *Journal of Nursing Administration*, 32, 273–282.

Foster, G., Taylor, S. J. C., Eldridge, S., Ramsay, J., & Griffiths, C. J. (2009). Self-management education programmes by lay leaders for people with chronic conditions. *Cochrane Database of Systematic Reviews*, 4, CD005108. doi: 10.1002/14651858.CD005108.pub2

Ghattas, C., Dai, A., Gemmel, D. J., & Awad, M. H. (2013). Over diagnosis of chronic obstructive pulmonary disease in an underserved patient population. *International Journal of Obstructive Pulmonary Disease*, 8, 545–549.

Glittenberg, J. (2004). A transdisciplinary, transcultural model for health care. *Journal of Transcultural Nursing*, 15, 6–10.

Global Initiative for Chronic Obstructive Lung Disease. (2014). Pocket guide to COPD diagnosis, management and prevention. http://www.goldcopd.org/uploads/users/files/GOLD_Pocket_2014.pdf

Go, A. S., Mozaffarian, D., Roger, V. L., Benjamin, E. J., Berry, J. D., Borden, W. B., ... Turner, M. B. (2013). Executive summary: Heart disease and stroke statistics—2013 update: A report from the American Heart Association. *Circulation*, 127, 143–152.

Gorman, M., & Morris, A. (1991). Developing clinical expertise in the care of addicted patients in acute care settings. *Journal of Professional Nursing*, 7, 246–253.

Guarascio, A. J., Ray, S. M., Finch, C. K., & Self, T. H. (2013). The clinical and economic burden of chronic obstructive pulmonary disease in the USA. *ClinicoEconomics and Outcomes Research*, 5, 235–245.

Halvorson, G. C. (2009). *Healthcare will not reform itself: A user's guide to refocusing and reforming American health care.* New York, NY: Productivity Press.

Hamric, A. B. (2014). A definition of advanced practice nursing. In A. B. Hamric, C. M. Hanson, M. F. Tracey, & E. T. O'Grady (Eds.), *Advanced practice nursing: An integrative approach* (5th ed., pp. 67–85). St. Louis, MO: Saunders Elsevier.

Hamric, A. B., & Delgado, S. A. (2014). Ethical decision making. In A. B. Hamric, C. M. Hanson, M. F. Tracey, & E. T. O'Grady (Eds.), *Advanced practice nursing: An integrative approach* (5th ed., pp. 328–358). St. Louis, MO: Saunders Elsevier.

Hamric, A. B., Hanson, C. M., Tracey, M. F., & O'Grady, E. T. (2014). Preface. In A. B. Hamric, C. M. Hanson, M. F. Tracey, & E. T. O'Grady (Eds.), *Advanced practice nursing: An integrative approach* (5th ed., pp. xi–xv). St. Louis, MO: Saunders Elsevier.

Hanson, C. M., & Carter, M. (2014). Collaboration. In A. B. Hamric, C. M. Hanson, M. F. Tracey, & E. T. O'Grady (Eds.), *Advanced practice nursing: An integrative approach* (5th ed., pp. 299–327). St. Louis, MO: Saunders Elsevier.

Hanson, C. M., & Spross, J. A. (1996). Collaboration. In A. B. Hamric, J. A. Spross, & C. M. Hanson (Eds.), *Advanced practice nursing: An integrative approach* (pp. 229–248). Philadelphia, PA: Saunders.

Health Insurance Portability and Accountability Act (HIPAA). (1996). Public Law 104–191. http://aspe.hhs.gov/admnsimp/pl104191.htm

Heineman, M., & Froemke, S. (Directors). (2013). *Escape fire: Fight to rescue American healthcare* [DVD]. United States: Lionsgate.

Ho, J. Y., & Preston, S. H. (2011). *International comparisons of U.S. mortality*. Data analyses prepared for the National Academy of Sciences/Institute of Medicine Panel on Understanding Cross-National Health Differences among High-Income Countries. Population Studies Center, University of Pennsylvania.

Honey, C. P., & Baker, J. A. (2011). Exploring the impact of journal clubs: A systematic review. *Nurse Education Today*, *31*(8), 825–831.

Houweling, S. T., Kleefstra, N., van Hateren, K. J. J., Groenier, K. H., Meyboom-deJong, B., & Bilo, H. J. G. (2011). Can diabetes management be safely transferred to practice nurses in a primary care setting? A randomised controlled trial. *Journal of Clinical Nursing*, *20*, 1264, 1272.

Hoyert, D. L., & Xu, J. (2012). Deaths: Preliminary data 2011. *National Vital Statistics Report*, *60*(6).

Hughes, J. (2010). Developing a journal club that impacts practice. *Gastroenterology Nursing*, *33*, 66–68.

Institute of Medicine (IOM). (2010). *The future of nursing: Leading change, advancing health*. Washington, DC: National Academies Press.

Jansink, R., Braspenning, J., Laurent, M., Keizer, E., Elwyn, G., Weijden, T., & Grol, R. (2013). Minimal improvement of nurses' motivational interviewing skills in routine diabetes care one year after training: A cluster randomized trial. *BMC Family Practice*, *14*, 44.

Jecker, N. S. (2012). Applying ethical reasoning: Philosophical, clinical, and cultural challenges. In N. S. Jecker, A. R. Jonsen, & R. A. Pearlman (Eds.), *Bioethics: An introduction to the history, methods, and practice* (3rd ed., pp. 127–139). Sudbury, MA: Jones and Bartlett.

Katon, W. J., Lin, E. H., Von Korff, M., Ciechanowski, P., Ludman, E. J., Young, B., ... McCulloch, D. (2010). Collaborative care for patients with depression and chronic illnesses. *New England Journal of Medicine*, *363*, 2611–2620.

Kelly, D. L. (2011). *Applying quality management in health care: A systems approach* (3rd ed.). Chicago, IL: Health Administration Press.

Kirwin, J. L., Cunningham, R. J., & Sequist, T. D. (2010). Pharmacist recommendations to improve the quality of diabetes care: A randomized controlled trial. *Journal of Managed Care Pharmacy*, *16*(2), 104–113.

Kuo, Y., Loresto, F. L., Rounds, L. R., & Goodwin, J. S. (2013). States with the least restrictive regulations experienced the largest increase in patients seen by nurse practitioners. *Health Affairs*, *32*(7), 1236–1243.

Langley, G. J., Moen, R., Nolan, K. M., Nolan, T. W., Norman, C. L., & Provost, L. P. (2009). *The improvement guide: A practical approach to enhancing organizational performance* (2nd ed.). San Francisco, CA: Jossey-Bass.

Laurant, M., Reeves, D., Hermens, R., Branspenning, J., Grol, R., & Sibbald, B. (2004). Substitution of doctors by nurses in primary care. *Cochrane Database of Systematic Reviews*, *4*, CD001271. doi: 10.1002/14651858.CD001271.pub2

Lenz, E. R., Mundinger, M. O., Kane, R. L., Hopkins, S. C., & Lin, S. X. (2004). Primary care outcomes in patients treated by nurse practitioners or physicians: Two-year follow-up. *Medical Care Research and Review*, *61*(3), 332–351.

Lizarondo, L., Kumar, S., & Grimmer-Somers, K. (2010). Online journal clubs: An innovative approach to achieving evidence-based practice. *Journal of Allied Health*, *39*, e17–e22.

Luby, M., Riley, J. K., & Towne, G. (2006). Nursing research journal clubs: Bridging the gap between practice and research. *Medsurg Nursing*, *15*, 100–102.

Lupari, M., Coates, V., Adamson, G., & Crealey, G. E. (2011). "We're just not getting it right": How should we provide care to the older person with multi-morbid chronic conditions. *Journal of Clinical Nursing*, *20*, 1225–1235.

Maitland, M. E. (2010). A transdisciplinary definition of diagnosis. *Journal of Allied Health*, *39*, 306–313.

Mantzoukas, S., & Watkinson, S. (2006). Review of advanced nursing practice: The international literature and developing generic features. *Journal of Clinical Nursing*, *16*, 28–37.

Melnyk, B. M., & Fineout-Overholt, E. (2010). Making the case for evidence-based practice and cultivating a spirit of inquiry. In B. M. Melnyk & E. Fineout-Overholt (Eds.), *Evidence-based practice in nursing & healthcare: A guide to best practice* (2nd ed., pp. 3–24). Philadelphia, PA: Lippincott.

Miller, W. R., & Rollnick, S. P. (1992). *Motivational interviewing: Preparing people to change addictive behavior*. New York, NY: Guildford Press.

Mitchell, A. J., Rao, S., & Vaze, A. (2011). International comparison of clinicians' ability to identify depression in primary care: Meta-analysis and meta-regression of predictors. *British Journal of General Practice*, *61*(583), e72–e80.

Mitchell, A. J., Vaze, A., & Rao, S. (2009). Clinical diagnosis of depression in primary care: A meta-analysis. *Lancet*, *374*, 609–619.

Motivational interviewing. (n.d.). http://www.motivationalinterview.org

Mundinger, M. O., Kane, R. L., Lenz, E. R., Totten, A., Tsai, W., Cleary, P., ... Shelanski, M. L. (2000). Primary care outcomes in patients treated by nurse practitioners or physicians: A randomized trial. *Journal of the American Medical Association, 283*(1), 59–68.

National Association of Clinical Nurse Specialists (NACNS). (2009). *Core practice doctorate clinical nurse specialist competencies.* Philadelphia, PA: Author.

National Organization of Nurse Practitioner Faculties (NONPF). (2012). *Domains and core competencies of nurse practitioner practice.* Washington, DC: Author.

National Research Council (NRC) & Institute of Medicine (IOM). (2013). *U.S. health in international perspective: Shorter lives, poorer health.* Panel on Understanding Cross-National Health Differences among High-Income Countries, S. H. Woolf & L. Aron, (Eds.), Committee on Population Health, Division of Behavioral and Social Sciences and Education, and Board on Population Health and Public Health Practice. Washington, DC: National Academies Press.

Newhouse, R. P., Stanik-Hutt, J., White, K. M., Johantgen, M., Bass, E. B., Zangaro, G., ... Weiner, J. P. (2011). Advanced practice nurse outcomes 1990–2008: A systematic review. *Nursing Economics, 29*(5), 230–250.

Norcross, J. C., Krebs, P. M., & Prochaska, J. O. (2011). Stages of change. *Journal of Clinical Psychology, 67,* 143–154.

Noordman, J., van Lee, I., Nielen, M., Viek, H., van Weijden, T., & van Dulmen, S. (2012). Do trained practice nurses apply motivational interviewing techniques in primary care consultations? *Journal of Clinical Medicine Research, 4*(6), 383–401.

O'Donnell, C. A. (2004). Attitudes and knowledge of primary care professionals toward evidence-based practice: A postal survey. *Journal of Evaluation in Clinical Practice, 10*(2), 197–2005.

Pender, N., Murdaugh, C., & Parsons, M.A. (2010). *Health Promotion in Nursing Practice* (6th ed.). Upper Saddle River, NJ: Pearson.

Peters-Klimm, F., Muller-Tasch, T., Schellberg, D., Remppis, A., Barth, A., Holzapfel, N., ... Szecsenyi, J. (2008). Guideline adherence for pharmacotherapy of chronic systolic heart failure in general practice: A closer look on evidence-based therapy. *Clinical Research in Cardiology, 97*(4), 244–252.

Polit, D. F., & Beck, C. T. (2013). *Essentials of nursing research: Appraising evidence for nursing* (8th ed.). Philadelphia, PA: Lippincott, Williams, & Wilkins.

Price, D. B., Yawn, B. P., & Jones, R. C. M. (2010). Improving the differential diagnosis of chronic obstructive pulmonary disease in primary care. *Mayo Clinic Proceedings, 85*(12), 1122–1129.

Prochaska, J. O. (1979). *Systems of psychotherapy: A trans-theoretical analysis.* Homewood, IL: Dorsey.

Prochaska, J. O., Norcross, J. C., & DiClemente, C. C. (2013). Applying the stages of change. *Psychotherapy in Australia, 19*(2), 10–15.

Rittenhouse, D. R., Shortell, S. M., & Fischer, E. S. (2009). Primary care and accountable care: Two essential elements of delivery-system reform. *New England Journal of Medicine, 361*(24), 2301–2303.

Rollnick, S. P., Miller, W. R., & Butler, C. C. (2008). *Motivational interviewing in health care: Helping patients change behavior.* New York, NY: Guilford Press.

Sackett, D. L., Rosenberg, W. M., Gray, J. A., Haynes, R. B., & Richardson, W. D. (1996). Evidence based medicine: What it is and what it isn't. *British Medical Journal, 312*(7023), 71–72.

Saxe, J. M., Janson, S. L., Dennehy, P. M., Stringari-Murray, S., Hirsch, J. E., & Waters, C. M. (2007). Meeting a primary care challenge in the United States: Chronic illness care. *Contemporary Nurse, 26,* 94–103.

Schouten, L. M., Niessen, L. W., van de Pas, J. W., Grol, R. P., & Hulscher, M. E. (2010). Cost-effectiveness of a quality improvement collaborative focusing on patients with diabetes. *Medical Care, 48,* 884–891.

Sjöling, M., Lundberg, K., Englund, E., Westman, A., & Jong, M.C. (2011). Effectiveness of motivational interviewing and physical activity on prescription on leisure exercise time in subjects suffering from mild to moderate hypertension. *BMC Research Notes, 12*(4), 352.

Sollecito, W. A., & Johnson, J. K. (2013). *McLaughlin and Kaluzny's continuous quality improvement in health care* (4th ed.). Burlington, MA: Jones & Bartlett Learning.

Spross, J. A. (2009). Expert coaching and guidance. In A. B. Hamric, J. A. Spross, & C. M. Hanson (Eds.), *Advanced practice nursing: An integrative approach* (4th ed., pp. 259–282). St. Louis, MO: Saunders Elsevier.

Spross, J. A., & Babine, R. L. (2014). Guidance and coaching. In A. B. Hamric, C. M. Hanson, M. F. Tracey, & E. T. O'Grady (Eds.), *Advanced practice nursing: An integrative approach* (5th ed., pp. 183–212). St. Louis, MO: Saunders Elsevier.

Stanik-Hutt, J., Newhouse, R. P., White, K. M., Johantgen, M., Bass, E. B., Zangaro, G., ... Weiner, J. P. (2013). The quality and effectiveness of care provided by nurse practitioners. *Journal for Nurse Practitioners, 9*(8), 492–500; e1–e13.

Starfield, B. (1994). Is primary care essential? *Lancet, 344*(8930), 1129–1133.

Starfield, B. (2012). Primary care: An increasingly important contributor to health care effectiveness, equity, and efficiency of health care services. SESPAS report 2012. *Gaceta Sanitaria, 26*(suppl 1), 20–26.

Starfield, B., Shi, L., & Macinko, J. (2005). Contributions of primary care to health systems and health. *Milbank Quarterly, 83*(3), 457–502.

Strauss, S. E., Glasziou, P., Richardson, W. S., & Haynes, R. B. (2011). *Evidence-based medicine: How to practice and teach EBM* (4th ed.). Edinburgh, UK: Churchill Livingstone.

Su, J., Tsai, C., Hung, T., & Chou, S. (2011). Change in accuracy of recognizing psychiatric disorders by non-psychiatric physicians: Five-year data from psychiatric consultation–liaison service. *Psychiatry and Clinical Neurosciences, 65*, 618–623.

Thomas, J. J., Hart, A. M., & Burman, M. E. (2014). Improving health promotion and disease prevention in NP-delivered primary care. *The Journal for Nurse Practitioners, 10*(4), 221–228.

Tinkelman, D. G., Price, D. B., Nordyke, R. J., & Halbert, R. J. (2006). Misdiagnosis of COPD and asthma in primary care patients 40 years of age and older. *Journal of Asthma, 43*(1), 75–80.

Tracy, M. F., & Hanson, C. M. (2014). Leadership. In A. B. Hamric, C. M. Hanson, M. F. Tracey, & E. T. O'Grady (Eds.), *Advanced practice nursing: An integrative approach* (5th ed., pp. 266–298). St. Louis, MO: Saunders Elsevier.

University of Rhode Island, Cancer Prevention Research Center. (n.d.). Transtheoretical model. http://www.uri.edu/research/cprc/transtheoretical_model.html

U.S. Department of Health and Human Services (DHHS). (2008). Clinical practice guideline: Treating tobacco use and dependence: 2008 update. http://bphc.hrsa.gov/buckets/treatingtobacco.pdf

U.S. Department of Health and Human Services (DHHS), Health Resources and Service Administration. (2010). The registered nurse population: Findings from the 2008 national sample survey of registered nurses. http://bhpr.hrsa.gov/healthworkforce/rnsurveys/rnsurveyfinal.pdf

Verdejo, T. (2001). Leading into the 21st century: Changing the vision and leading toward success. *Seminars for Nurse Managers, 9*, 115–118.

Vosit-Stellar, J., & Morse, A. B. (2014). Consultation. In A. B. Hamric, C. M. Hanson, M. F. Tracey, & E. T. O'Grady (Eds.). *Advanced practice nursing: An integrative approach* (5th ed., pp. 213–236). St. Louis, MO: Saunders Elsevier.

Werner, J. J., Lawson, P. J., Panaite, V., Step, M. M., & Flocke, S. A. (2013). Comparing primary care physicians' smoking cessation counseling techniques to motivational interviewing. *Journal of Addiction Medicine, 7*(2), 139–142.

World Health Organization (WHO). (2008). Primary health care: Now more than ever. http://www.who.int/whr/2008/en/

Yang, Q., Cogswell, M. E., Flanders, W. D., Hong, Y., Zhang, Z., Loustalot, F., … Hu, F. B. (2012). Trends in cardiovascular health metrics and associations with all-cause and CVD mortality among U.S. adults. *Journal of the American Medical Association, 307*(12), 1273–1283.

Yoo, H. J., Park, M. S., Kim, T. N, Yang, S. J., Cho, G. J., Hwang, T. G., … Choi, K. M. (2009). A ubiquitous chronic disease care system using cellular phones and the Internet. *Diabetic Medicine, 26*, 628–635.

Chapter 18

Complementary and Alternative Therapies

Pamala D. Larsen

Introduction

Diseases without a cure, chronic and/or terminal, may not respond to treatment approaches of Western medicine. Often clients with chronic illness look for other options, rather than Western (allopathic) medicine, to alleviate their symptoms. For example, we have no cure for arthritis or chronic back problems, nor do we have a pain medication that an individual could take 365 days a year without side effects (Barker, 2007). Given these facts, there is motivation for individuals with these chronic diseases to try other therapies. If traditional allopathic approaches do not provide relief from suffering and improve quality of life, should healthcare professionals help individuals seek out non-allopathic treatments? What is the role of government in balancing the safety of healthcare treatments, while allowing an individual the right to access unproven alternative or complementary treatments? Addressing these questions with scientific data may lead to appropriate complementary or alternative therapies that improve the health care of patients with chronic illness.

Definitions

The terms complementary, alternative, and integrative medicine are defined by the National Center for Complementary and Alternative Medicine (NCCAM). *Alternative* refers to using a nonmainstream approach *in place of* conventional medicine. *Complementary* refers to using a nonmainstream approach *together with* conventional medicine. *Integrative medicine* is another term in the literature that combines mainstream healthcare approaches with non-conventional medicine. However, the boundaries of complementary and alternative medicine (CAM) and conventional medicine are dynamic. Over time, some CAM practices may evolve to be labeled as conventional medicine. As an example, guided imagery and massage, which were once considered complementary or alternative treatments, are now regularly used for pain management.

CAM practitioners believe that all healing is self-healing, and the role of the CAM provider is to empower patients to heal themselves, take charge of their care, and have personal responsibility for their health (Kotsirilos, Vitetta, & Sali, 2011). However, the use of CAM should respect certain boundaries. Specifically, such therapies should not be used to the exclusion of a safe, effective and superior traditional treatment (p. 12).

Currently NCCAM uses the term "complementary" rather than "integrative" on its website. That being said, the website discusses integrative medicine. Key points include the following: (NCCAM, 2013a):

- *It's happening now.* More individuals, healthcare professionals, and healthcare systems are integrating various practices with origins outside of mainstream medicine into treatment.

- *The integrative trend is growing among providers and healthcare systems.* Driving factors include marketing of integrative care by healthcare providers to consumers who perceive benefits to health or well-being from such therapies, and emerging evidence that some of the perceived benefits are real or meaningful.
- *The scientific evidence is limited.* A lack of valid and reliable data makes it difficult for consumers and healthcare professionals to make informed decisions.

Many of the research studies investigating CAM are not well designed, having methodological and/or analytical flaws. Additionally, in its reviews, the Cochrane Library has noted bias in a number of CAM studies. Because of these concerns, the research cited in this chapter has been carefully screened.

Overview of NCCAM

A national initiative established in 1991 to evaluate alternative treatments led to the establishment of the Office of Alternative Medicine (OAM) at the National Institutes of Health (NIH). In October 1998, the OAM became the National Center for Complementary and Alternative Medicine.

The mission of NCCAM is to define, through rigorous scientific investigation, the usefulness and safety of complementary and alternative medicine interventions and their roles in improving health and health care. Scientific evidence informs decision making by the public, by healthcare professionals, and by health policy makers regarding use and integration of complementary and alternative medicine (NCCAM, 2012a). NCCAM is the federal government's lead agency for examining interventions and products that are outside mainstream medicine. Its programs and organization incorporate three long-range goals (NCCAM, 2012a):

1. Advance the science and practice of symptom management

2. Develop effective, practical, personalized strategies for promoting health and well-being
3. Enable better evidence-based decision making regarding CAM use and its integration into health care and health promotion

As an institute of the National Institutes of Health, NCCAM receives its budget through NIH. The decreases seen in its funding are similar to the decreases occurring in other institutes' funding. The budget for NCCAM rose steadily from 1999 (when it became an institute) to fiscal year 2010, when the budget was $128.8 million. However, the budget for fiscal year 2013 was only $120.7 million (NCCAM, 2012a). Funding for this institute has suffered as a result of the poor U.S. economy, the federal government's debt ceiling, and the continuing squabble over the national budget.

NCCAM classifies alternative and complementary health therapies into three categories:

- Natural products
- Mind and body practices
- Other

Natural products include herbs, vitamins and minerals, and probiotics. Typically these products are sold as dietary supplements. Mind and body practices include a large group of techniques such as acupuncture, massage therapy, meditation, movement therapies, relaxation techniques, spinal manipulation, tai chi and qi gong, and yoga. The "other" category includes traditional healers, Ayurvedic medicine, traditional Chinese medicine, homeopathy, and naturopathy (NCCAM, 2013a).

Users

The data on CAM from the 2012 National Health Interview Survey (NHIS) were not yet available when this text went to press. The 2007 survey provided data from 23,393 adults to determine usage of such treatments.

At that time, nearly 4 of 10 adults (38.3%) and 11.8% of children younger than age 18 had used CAM therapies in the last 12 months (Barnes, Bloom, & Nahin, 2008). The 2007 survey included questions about 36 therapies as compared with 27 treatments in the 2002 survey, as well as expanding the number of conditions covered, from 73 in 2002 to 81 in 2007. Praying for one's own health or having others pray for one's health was not included in the 2007 survey, but was included in the 2002 survey (Barnes et al., 2008; Nahin, Barnes, Stussman, & Bloom, 2009). The most frequently cited therapies in the 2007 survey included non-vitamin, non-mineral natural products (17.7%); deep-breathing exercises (12.7%); meditation (9.4%); chiropractic or osteopathic manipulation (8.6%); massage (8.3%); and yoga (6.1%) (Barnes et al., 2008, p. 2). From 2002 to 2007, there was increased use of mind–body therapies, acupuncture, massage therapy, and naturopathy.

Research shows that CAM users are more likely to be female, aged 30–50 years, have a higher income and higher educational level, be employed full-time, and have a poorer health status. Some have suggested that there is a rural–urban split on use, with those persons living in rural environments being more likely to use CAM because of a lack of access to conventional medicine (Andrews, Adams, Segrott, & Lui, 2012; Bishop & Lewith, 2008; Tait, Laditka, Laditka, Nies, Racine, & Tsulukidze, 2013).

The AARP and NCCAM jointly surveyed older adults in 2010 about their use, intention, and communication about CAM. The survey was an extension of an earlier survey completed in 2006. Questions covered the following topics (AARP & NCCAM, 2010):

- Whether respondents had used various types of CAM sometime in the past 12 months and for what purpose
- Whether they had discussed CAM with their healthcare providers

- What they had discussed or why they had not discussed CAM with their healthcare providers
- Who initiated the discussion
- Their primary source of information about CAM
- Their current use of prescription medications

Slightly more than half (53%) of individuals aged 50 and older reported using CAM at some point in their lives, with 47% using it within the past 12 months (AARP & NCCAM, 2010, p. 3). As expected, women were more likely than men to use CAM (52% versus 43%), particularly herbal products or dietary supplements (41% versus 33%) and massage, chiropractic, or other body work (27% versus 16%). Usage appeared to peak from ages 50 to 59 and then declined with age. However, 24.2% of those aged 85 and older reported using CAM.

When asked in the survey why these older adults used CAM, the most frequent answer (77%) was for overall wellness or to treat painful conditions (73%). Of serious consequence was the fact that 67% of the older adults surveyed had not discussed CAM with their traditional healthcare provider. The primary reasons for not discussing such usage were that (1) the provider never asked and (2) patients did not know whether they should bring it up (AARP & NCCAM, 2010, p. 8). As expected in this age group, 78% of the older respondents reported taking at least one prescription medication, with 19% of the group taking five or more prescription medications. This fact, in conjunction with the high percentage of individuals not discussing CAM with their healthcare provider, certainly raises a safety concern.

In another review of the literature, Tait et al. (2013) found that older Americans used CAM because their healthcare provider recommended it; it was recommended by a friend, family member, or coworker; medical treatment did not help; or medical treatments were too expensive. These findings differ from those reported in the majority of the literature.

Johnson and colleagues (2012) used the 2007 NHIS data to determine CAM use rates among healthcare workers. Their conclusions were that individuals employed in a healthcare setting were more likely to use CAM than the general population, particularly mind–body therapies. Among employees in all healthcare settings, healthcare providers were most likely to use CAM.

Researchers have compared CAM usage in active-duty military personnel to CAM usage in civilians. Although data from the 2002 and 2007 NHIS studies are useful, they do not include active-duty military personnel. The purpose of the study by Goertz and colleagues (2013) was to assess the reported prevalence of CAM use in a globally representative sample of active-duty military personnel in the Army, Navy, Marine Corps, and Air Force and determine demographic and lifestyle factors associated with its use. Data were taken from the 2005 Department of Defense Survey of Health Related Behaviors Among Active Duty Military Personnel, which collected data from 1,011,852 participants. Through various sampling techniques, 40,000 active-duty personnel from three enlisted pay-grade groups and three officer pay-grade groups were selected. The adjusted sample size was 30,664, with officers and women being oversampled because of their smaller numbers (p. 510). Approximately 45% of active-duty military personnel reported using at least one CAM therapy within the previous 12 months. When data on prayer were omitted, the percentage fell to 36%. The eight most frequently reported types of categories were as follows (in the order of use):

1. Prayer for your own health
2. Relaxation therapies
3. Herbal medicine
4. High-dose megavitamins
5. Art/music therapy
6. Exercise/movement therapy
7. Chiropractic
8. Massage therapy

When prayer was included (as in the 2002 NHIS questionnaire), civilian usage of CAM was higher than military personnel usage (62.1% versus 55.4%; $p < 0.001$). However, when prayer for one's health was excluded (as in the 2007 NHIS questionnaire), CAM use by military personnel was significantly higher (44.5% as compared with 36.0% and 38.3% in the 2002 and 2007 NHIS surveys, respectively; $p < 0.001$) than in civilians (Goertz et al., 2013, p. 511).

One must caution when assessing these data, because patient decisions about CAM usage are not static, but dynamic. Many individuals may revisit their decision to use or not use CAM during a disease recurrence, exacerbation, flare, or metastatic disease (Balneaves, Weeks, & Seeley, 2012).

Reasons for Use

Individuals with chronic illnesses often feel frustrated with disease-focused, fragmented, time-limited traditional allopathic care. As a result, they may turn to alternative or complementary practitioners, who often take more time to listen and evaluate not just the patients' health problems, but their entire lives. Specifically, these nontraditional healthcare providers are noted for extensive clinical evaluations that focus on understanding individuals and their experiences in dealing with a chronic illness; continuity with care providers over time; active participation in care by clinicians, patients, and their family members; choice of individualized services; provision of hope; open communication and information sharing; and emphasis on the meaning and spiritual components of dealing with chronic illnesses. Self-efficacy and perceptions of control by the client are viewed as what separates the CAM provider from a traditional care provider (Bann, Sirois, & Walsh, 2010).

The most commonly reported health problems treated by CAM in the 2007 NHIS survey included musculoskeletal problems, including back pain or problems (17.1%); neck pain or problems (5.9%); joint pain or stiffness or other joint condition (5.2%); arthritis (3.5%); and other musculoskeletal conditions (1.8%) (Barnes et al., 2008, p. 4). These data were relatively unchanged from 2002. The use of CAM to treat head or chest colds showed a marked decrease from 2002 to 2007 (9.5% versus 2.0%). A small increase in CAM use was seen in treating cholesterol problems. Lastly, data from the 2007 survey were consistent with the 2002 data demonstrating that CAM use was more prevalent among women, adults aged 30–69, persons with higher levels of education, individuals who were not poor, adults living in the West, former smokers, and adults who were hospitalized within the last year (Barnes et al., 2008, p. 4).

Costs

In 2007, adults in the United States spent $33.9 billion out of pocket on visits to CAM practitioners and purchases of CAM products, classes, and materials. Of this total, practitioner costs accounted for $11.9 billion (35.2%). The remaining $22.0 billion (64.8%) was devoted to costs associated with relaxation techniques; homeopathic medicine; yoga, tai chi, and qi gong classes; and self-care costs including non-vitamin, non-mineral natural products (Nahin et al., 2009, p. 3). Approximately 75% of visits to CAM practitioners and total costs related to visits to CAM providers were associated with manipulative and body-based therapies (e.g., chiropractic or osteopathic manipulation, massage, and movement therapies) (p. 6). The $33.9 billion spent on CAM amounted to 12.6% of all other out-of-pocket medical spending ($268.6 billion) (NCCAM, 2013b).

Insurance coverage of complementary health treatments is complex and confusing, so much so that general statements about coverage are impossible. Coverage may depend on state laws, regulations, and differences among specific insurance plans (NCCAM, 2013b).

Impact

Each alternative or complementary therapy may have a positive, negative, or neutral impact on the patient. Common CAM therapies are described in this section, along with applicable research that may or may not support their use.

Natural Products

Natural products include a variety of herbal medicines (also known as botanicals), vitamins, minerals, and other "natural products." Many of these products are sold as dietary supplements. Natural products also include probiotics—live microorganisms (usually bacteria) that are similar to microorganisms normally found in the human digestive tract.

The federal government regulates dietary supplements primarily through the U.S. Food and Drug Administration (FDA). The regulations for dietary supplements are not the same as those for prescription or over-the-counter drugs. In general, the guidelines for natural products are less strict. For example, a manufacturer does not have to prove the safety and effectiveness of a dietary supplement before it is marketed. A disclaimer by the FDA also must be included on every dietary supplement label, making clear that the product "is not intended to diagnose, treat, prevent or cure any disease" (Owens, Baergen, & Puckett, 2014).

Once a dietary supplement is on the market, the FDA monitors safety and product information, and the Federal Trade Commission (FTC) monitors advertising. In 2010, an investigation by the U.S. Government Accountability Office found instances in which written sales materials for herbal dietary supplements sold through online retailers included illegal claims that the products could treat, prevent, or cure diseases such as diabetes, cancer, or cardiovascular disease (NCCAM, 2013c).

Dietary supplements were defined in a law passed by Congress in 1994 called the Dietary Supplement Health and Education Act (DSHEA). According to DSHEA, a dietary supplement is a nonfood, nondrug product taken by mouth and containing at least one identified dietary ingredient, such as a vitamin, mineral, herb or botanical, amino acid, enzyme, or metabolite (Owens et al., 2014).

Herbal supplements are one type of dietary supplement. The term "botanical" is often used as a synonym for "herbal supplement." An herbal supplement may contain a single herb or a mixture of herbs. Federal law requires that all of the herbs be listed on the product label (NCCAM, 2013d).

The NCCAM website provides a series of 48 fact sheets on herbs and botanicals. These fact sheets identify common names, sources, potential side effects and cautions, and "what the science says" about the product, as well as links to other resources (NCCAM, 2013d). Another excellent source of information is the Dietary Supplements Labels Database (2013), which provides information about the ingredients in more than 7,000 brands of dietary supplements.

Safety considerations arise when using dietary supplements. Patients need to tell their healthcare professionals if they are taking a supplement. In some instances, a prescription drug may interact poorly with a dietary supplement. For example, St. John's wort, a supplement often taken for depression, interacts with many prescription medications and makes them less effective (NCCAM, 2013c).

Many users of natural products buy their products online. Owens and colleagues (2014) conducted an online search of 13 common herbals and reviewed the top 50 websites for each. The purpose of their investigation was to review clinical claims, warnings, and other safety information. Their conclusions included the following points:

- Fewer than 8% of retail sites provided information regarding potential adverse effects, drug interactions, and other safety information.
- Only 10.5% recommended consultation with a healthcare professional.
- Fewer than 3% cited scientific literature to back up their claims.
- Patient comments and testimonials were widely used. Such comments may be viewed as making a disease claim (Owens et al., 2014, pp. 113–114).

When someone is taking a supplement, the label instructions need to be followed. Taking more of a supplement, and doing so just because the product is probably safer because it is an over-the-counter (OTC) drug, may lead to significant harm. Many dietary supplements use the term "natural" or say they come from "natural" sources—but "natural" does not mean safe. For example, the herbs known as comfrey and kava can cause serious harm to the liver (NCCAM, 2013c). Finally, users should be aware that an herbal supplement may contain dozens of compounds that may or may not be known to the producer of the supplement.

The organization known as Natural Standard was founded by healthcare providers and researchers to provide high-quality, evidence-based information about complementary and alternative medicine, including dietary supplements and integrative therapies. The grades assigned by Natural Standard reflect the level of available scientific data for or against the use of each therapy for a specific medical condition. Evidence is denoted as Grades A–F, with an A representing strong positive scientific evidence and an F denoting strong negative scientific evidence. Unfortunately, one needs a subscription to the Natural Standard to access information. Its findings on herbs and supplements have been compiled in a book, *Davis's Pocket Guide to Herbs and Supplements* (Ulbricht, 2011). This source includes information on more than 600 products and is organized like a traditional pharmacology pocket guide.

Another source of information about natural products and mind–body practices is the Natural Medicines Comprehensive Database (2014). Its website states that the database includes unbiased, scientific clinical information on complementary, alternative, and integrative therapies. Once again, a subscription is required to access the data.

PROBIOTICS

Within the last few years, probiotics have become the new darling of natural products. Originally it was thought that probiotics were an answer to supporting and supplementing the immune system. Although there may be some relationship between the two, probiotics have been used mostly in digestive disorders. Although probiotic products are more popular in Europe and Japan than in the United States, the U.S. consumer market for probiotics is growing rapidly.

Probiotics are live microorganisms (e.g., bacteria) that are either the same as or similar to microorganisms found naturally in the human body, and may be beneficial to health. Also referred to as "good bacteria" or "helpful bacteria," probiotics are available to consumers in oral products such as dietary supplements and yogurts, as well as other products such as suppositories and creams (NCCAM, 2012b). Probiotics are not regulated by the FDA.

Picturing the human body as a "host" for bacteria and other microorganisms is helpful in understanding probiotics. The body, especially the lower gastrointestinal tract, contains a complex and diverse community of bacteria. (In the body of a healthy adult, cells of microorganisms are estimated to outnumber human cells by a factor of 10 to 1.) Although we tend to think of bacteria as harmful "germs," many of them actually help the body function properly. Most probiotics are bacteria similar to the beneficial bacteria found naturally in the human gut (NCCAM, 2012b).

Probiotic research is moving forward in two ways: basic science and clinical trials to evaluate the safety and efficacy of probiotics for various medical conditions. Recent studies have produced strong evidence in favor of probiotic use in acute diarrhea and antibiotic-associated diarrhea and for atopic eczema (most commonly seen in infants) (NCCAM, 2013e).

Three systematic reviews have summarized the efficacy and safety of probiotics, although many more systematic reviews of research related to these products exist. In early 2014, the Cochrane Library listed 29 systematic reviews of probiotics (most associated with digestive disorders) and 9 protocols. Following are key points of the three major reviews of probiotic efficacy and safety:

- Overall evidence suggests a protective effect of probiotics in preventing pediatric antibiotic-associated diarrhea. The systematic review by Johnston, Goldenberg, Vandvik, Sun, and Guyatt (2011) examined 16 RCTs with 3,432 participants, 9 using a single probiotic agent and the others using 2–10 probiotic strains.
- Goldenberg and colleagues (2013) looked at the efficacy and safety for the prevention of *Clostridium difficile*–associated diarrhea in adults and children. Twenty-three RCTs demonstrated moderate-quality evidence suggesting that probiotics are both safe and effective for preventing *C. difficile*–associated diarrhea.
- There was a lack of assessment and systematic reporting of adverse events in probiotic intervention studies. The available evidence in RCTs did not indicate an increased risk from such products; however, rare adverse events were difficult to assess. Despite the abundance of literature, studies did not address specific questions on the safety of probiotic interventions with confidence (Hempel et al., 2011).

GINKGO BILOBA

Extracts of the leaves of the maidenhair tree, *Ginkgo biloba*, have long been used in China as a traditional medicine for various disorders of health. Ginkgo seeds have been used in traditional Chinese medicine for thousands of years, and cooked seeds are occasionally eaten. Extracts are usually taken from the ginkgo leaf and are used to make tablets, capsules, or teas. Occasionally, ginkgo extracts are used in skin products (NCCAM, 2013f).

Perhaps because ginkgo was one of the most frequently used herbs noted in the 2007 NHIS study, and particularly because of its widespread use by older adults, there has been a push to link the herb with a wide range of conditions. In the database pubmed.gov, entering the terms *Ginkgo biloba*, *therapeutic use*, *humans*, and *meta-analysis* turned up reviews of ginkgo use in the following conditions: intermittent claudication; macular degeneration; tinnitus; sports performance; Alzheimer's disease, cognitive impairment, and dementia; multiple sclerosis; sexual dysfunction due to antidepressant use; insulin resistance; menopause; cardiovascular events; chronic schizophrenia; and prevention of acute mountain sickness. Notably, the conditions for which ginkgo treatment was most commonly researched include dementia, memory impairment, intermittent claudication, and tinnitus (NCCAM, 2013f).

NCCAM funded perhaps the earliest and most comprehensive study of the ginkgo product EGb-761 and its relationship with dementia. The study known as the Ginkgo Evaluation of Memory Study (GEM) included 3,000 volunteers aged 75 and older located across the United States. These volunteers were followed for an average of 6 years. Results demonstrated ginkgo to be ineffective in lowering the overall incidence of dementia and Alzheimer's disease in the elderly. Additionally, its effects in slowing cognitive decline, lowering blood pressure, and reducing the incidence of hypertension were not significant compared with the group receiving a placebo (DeKosky et al., 2008).

A Cochrane review of *Ginkgo biloba* for cognitive impairment and dementia was conducted in 2009 to assess efficacy and safety of the product for dementia or cognitive decline. No significant differences were observed between the experimental groups who received ginkgo and the control groups who received a placebo. A subgroup analysis of only patients with Alzheimer's disease (925) failed to identify any consistent pattern of benefit associated with the *Ginkgo biloba*. Researchers also declared the drug to be safe based on their analysis of the 36 RCTs examined (Birks & Evans, 2009).

Age-related macular degeneration (AMD) and ginkgo have been frequently associated because of the vasoactive component of AMD and the supposed vasoactivity of *Ginkgo biloba*. A Cochrane review examined the effects of *Ginkgo biloba* extract on the progression of age-related macular degeneration. Unfortunately, only two RCTs met the criteria for inclusion in the review. The researchers were unable to answer the question posed with the review (Evans, 2013).

An original systematic review of *Ginkgo biloba* and tinnitus was conducted in 2004 and subsequently updated in 2007, 2009, and 2013. No evidence was found that ginkgo is effective in patients with a primary complaint of tinnitus (Hilton, Zimmermann, & Hunt, 2013). Similarly, in patients taking *Ginkgo biloba* for intermittent claudication, there was no difference between the experimental group and the placebo group (Nicolai et al., 2013).

Side effects of ginkgo may include headache, nausea, gastrointestinal upset, diarrhea, dizziness, and allergic skin reactions. More severe allergic reactions have occasionally been reported. Some data suggest that ginkgo can increase bleeding risk, so people who take anticoagulant drugs, have bleeding disorders, or have scheduled surgery or dental procedures should use caution and talk to a healthcare professionals if they are using ginkgo (NCCAM, 2013f).

Echinacea purpurea

Echinacea is an herb made from the leaves, flower, or root of the *Echinacea* plant. It is used as a complementary or alternative therapy to fight infections, particularly the common cold and upper respiratory infections. Some individuals take the herb to prevent a cold, while others use it to reduce symptoms (http://www.nlm.nih.gov/medlineplus/druginfo/natural/981.html#Description). However, although its use is common, its effectiveness is inconclusive. The Natural Medicines Comprehensive Database rates echinacea as "possibly effective" for the common cold. The problem with research reported for echinacea is that these scientific studies have used different types of plants and different methods of preparation; thus, it is not surprising that different studies have shown different results. If the herb is helpful as a treatment for a cold, the benefit will likely be modest at best (Natural Medicines Comprehensive Database, 2013).

The Cochrane Library completed a review of echinacea in 2006. This review sought to determine whether there was evidence that echinacea preparations are (1) more effective than no treatment, (2) more effective than placebos, or (3) similarly effective to other treatments in the prevention and treatment of the common cold. Some evidence indicated that preparations based on the aerial parts of *E. purpurea* might be effective for early treatment of colds in adults, but the results were not consistent. The RCTs that were reviewed lacked rigor (Linde, Barrett, Bauer, Melchart, & Woelkaft, 2006).

In two more recent articles, researchers investigated the risks and benefits of *E. purpurea* in the prevention of the common cold over a 4-month period, as well as examined the efficacy of this herb in the prevention of respiratory or other symptoms in air travelers. In a study that enrolled 755 healthy subjects, the experimental group received the *E. purpurea* preparation, while the control group received a placebo over a period of 4 months. Each participant kept a journal of adverse events, cold symptoms, adverse reactions, and other information, and supplied nasal secretions if an acute cold occurred. The researchers concluded that compliant prophylactic intake of *E. purpurea* over a 4-month period of time appeared to provide

a positive risk–benefit ratio (Jawad, Schoop, Suter, Klein, & Eccles, 2012).

Frequent air travelers are often affected by colds, viruses, and upper respiratory infections because they come in contact with large numbers of individuals and filtered air within airplanes that may harbor germs. In a study addressing this issue, Tiralongo and colleagues (2012) enrolled a sample of 175 adults who traveled back from Australia to America, Europe, or Africa over a period of 1–5 weeks on commercial flights. Participants took *E. purpurea* or placebo tablets on a regular basis. The researchers concluded that supplementation with standardized echinacea tablets, if taken before and during travel, may have preventive effects against the development of respiratory symptoms during travel involving long-haul flights.

Mind and Body Practices

Mind and body practices focus on interactions among the brain, mind, body, and behavior. The intent is to use the mind to affect physical functioning and, therefore, promote health. A wide range of practices are included within this category, but the main practices are meditation, yoga, acupuncture, spinal manipulation, massage therapy, movement therapies, relaxation techniques, qi gong, and tai chi (**Table 18-1**). Acupuncture is also a component of traditional Chinese medicine (NCCAM, 2013g). Use of three of these practices—deep-breathing exercises, meditation, and yoga—increased significantly in the 2007 NHIS survey compared with the 2002 NHIS survey.

ACUPUNCTURE

Acupuncture has been practiced in China and other Asian countries for thousands of years, and is considered among the oldest healing practices in the world. It has been practiced in the United States for at least 200 years (NCCAM, 2012c). The FDA approved the acupuncture needle as a medical device in 1996 (National Cancer Institute, 2011).

Table 18-1 MIND AND BODY PRACTICES

Approach	Therapeutic Method	Rationale
Acupuncture	Describes a family of procedures involving the stimulation of points on the body using a variety of techniques. The acupuncture technique that has been most often studied scientifically involves penetrating the skin with thin, solid, metallic needles that are manipulated by the hands or by electrical stimulation.	Points along channels of energy are manipulated to restore balance. Acupuncture is part of traditional Chinese medicine.
Yoga	Combines physical postures, breathing exercises, meditation, and relaxation.	Enhances stress-coping mechanisms and mind–body awareness.
Meditation	Refers to a group of techniques such as mantra meditation, relaxation, mindfulness meditation, and Zen Buddhist meditation. Uses techniques such as a specific posture, focused attention, and an open attitude toward distraction.	The practice is believed to result in a state of greater calmness and physical relaxation and psychological balance due to the person learning to focus his or her attention.
Relaxation techniques	May include deep-breathing exercises, guided imagery, progressive muscle relaxation, and biofeedback.	Designed to produce the body's natural relaxation response.
Spinal manipulation	Practiced by chiropractors, osteopathic physicians, naturopathic physicians, physical therapists, and some medical doctors. Practitioners use their hands or a device to apply a controlled force to a joint of the spine.	Adjusting spinal joints and resolving subluxations restores normal nerve function and promotes optimal health
Tai chi and qi gong	Traditional Chinese medicine practices that combine specific movements or postures, coordinated breathing and mental focus. Tai chi is often called "moving meditation."	Incorporates the Chinese concepts of yin and yang. Practicing tai chi supports a healthy balance of yin and yang, thus aiding the follow of qi (vital energy or life force)
Massage therapy	Encompasses many techniques, including rubbing, pressing, and otherwise manipulating muscles and other soft tissues of the body.	Releases muscle and soft tissue tension to ease pain

Sources: Data from NCCAM (2010a); NCCAM (2010b); NCCAM (2012c); NCCAM (2013a); NCCAM (2013h) NCCAM (2013i); NCCAM (2013j); & NCCAM (2014a)

A risk associated with acupuncture includes the quality of the practitioner. In addition, safety concerns about the needles are an ongoing issue. The FDA regulates acupuncture needles and requires them to be manufactured and labeled according to certain standards; for example, needles must be sterile, nontoxic, and labeled for single use by qualified practitioners only (NCCAM, 2012c). Overall, relatively few complications from acupuncture have been reported to the FDA. Most of the complications result from inadequate sterilization of needles and improper delivery of treatments. Each patient should have a new set of disposable needles taken from a sealed package and the sites for acupuncture should be swabbed with alcohol or another disinfectant before inserting the needles into the body. Adverse effects have been reported such as infections and punctured organs (NCCAM, 2012c).

Acupuncture has been used as a treatment for a wide variety of chronic conditions. Current systematic reviews address acupuncture as a treatment for irritable bowel syndrome and for fibromyalgia. In the review of acupuncture and irritable bowel syndrome, the researchers examined 17 RCTs (Manheimer et al., 2012). Five of the RCTs compared acupuncture with sham acupuncture; however, there was no evidence of an improvement with acupuncture. In studies comparing acupuncture, pharmacologic therapy, and no treatment, acupuncture was superior. Unfortunately, a number of studies combined acupuncture with other Chinese medicine therapy, making it difficult to tease out the effects attributable solely to acupuncture.

The review addressing use of acupuncture with fibromyalgia patients found a low to moderate level of evidence that, when compared with no treatment and standard therapy, acupuncture improved pain and stiffness in individuals with the disease (Deare et al., 2013). The effects lasted up to 1 month, but were not maintained at 6 months.

Macpherson and colleagues (2013) examined the effects of (1) acupuncture versus (2) usual care and counseling versus (3) usual care in 755 patients with moderate to severe depression. Data were collected with the Beck Depression Inventory II (BDI-II) and the Patient Health Questionnaire at three points in time—at the end of the intervention, 3 months later, and 12 months later. Differences in outcomes for acupuncture versus counseling were not significant. Both interventions were associated with significantly reduced depression at 3 months when compared to usual care alone.

Another study investigated the effects of acupuncture on the circadian rhythm of blood pressure on 33 patients with essential hypertension (Kim et al., 2012). This study was designed as a randomized, double-blind, controlled trial. Subjects were randomly assigned to either the acupuncture group or the sham acupuncture group. It was suggested that acupuncture treatment could be useful in improving the circadian rhythm of blood pressure, particularly the nighttime diastolic number.

YOGA

Yoga is a mind–body practice with historical origins in ancient Indian philosophy. One could consider it a meditative movement practice that consists of physical postures, breathing techniques, and meditation or relaxation (NCCAM, 2012d). Numerous schools of yoga exist. Hatha yoga, the version most commonly practiced in the United States and Europe, emphasizes postures (*asanas*) and breathing exercises (*pranayama*). Some of the major styles of hatha yoga are Iyengar, Ashtanga, Vini, Kundalini, and Bikram yoga (NCCAM, 2012d). Yoga was one of the top 10 CAM therapies used by patients according to the 2007 NHIS.

Studies from 1950 to 2010 were examined in one analysis that sought to evaluate the effects of yoga on older adults (Patel, Newstead, & Ferrer, 2012). Studies included in this review consisted of RCTs only. In this 60-year time period, only 18 studies were deemed eligible for analysis. Synthesis of these studies suggested that the benefits of yoga may exceed those of conventional exercise interventions. However, the effect sizes of the studies were modest at best. The authors concluded that there were mixed results regarding the relationship between yoga and depression, sleep, and bone mineral density.

Another set of authors completed a meta-analysis of the effects of yoga on psychological function and quality of life in women with breast cancer (Zhang, Yang, Tian, & Wang, 2012). The data provided little indication of how effective yoga might be when applied to this population. The studies reviewed demonstrated that yoga was mildly effective in improving quality of life, but showed no effectiveness in improving anxiety, depression, distress, sleep, and fatigue.

In a small study funded by NCCAM, researchers found that long-term practice of yoga may improve pain tolerance (Villemure, Ceko, Cotton, & Bushnell, 2013). The researchers noted that because of the cross-sectional nature of the study, no definitive causal conclusions could be made. However, based on the findings, they suggest that regular, long-term yoga practice may equip individuals with tools to deal with sensory inputs and the potential emotional reactions attached to those inputs, which may lead to structural changes in brain anatomy and connectivity.

Two Cochrane Collaboration reviews of yoga are presented here as examples of current reviews. A 2012 update of a 2002 review assessed the effect of yoga in the treatment of people with epilepsy (Ramaratnam & Sridharan, 2012). The conclusions did not change from the 2002 review. No conclusions can be made regarding this intervention's efficacy in epilepsy.

The second review addressed the effectiveness of yoga as a means of secondary prevention of mortality, morbidity, and health-related quality of life declines in patients with coronary heart disease (Lau, Kwong, Yeung, Chau, & Woo, 2012). No conclusions could be drawn due to the lack of randomized controlled trials that met the inclusion criteria for the review.

SPINAL MANIPULATION

Chiropractic dates back to Daniel Palmer's alleged healing of a deaf individual by manually aligning his spinal column (Barker, 2007, p. 15). The main emphasis of chiropractic care is the spine and its effects on the central nervous system, the autonomic nervous system, and the peripheral nervous system. Chiropractors emphasize that adjusting the spinal joints and resolving subluxations restore normal nerve function and optimal health (Freeman, 2009). Chiropractors, like many other CAM providers, believe that the body has an innate ability to heal itself, and that the primary barrier to this ability resides in subluxations within various joints (Barker, 2007).

Spinal manipulation is practiced by chiropractors, osteopathic physicians, naturopathic physicians, physical therapists, and some medical doctors. Practitioners use their hands or a device to apply a controlled force to a joint of the spine. The amount of force applied depends on the form of manipulation used. The goal is to relieve pain and improve physical functioning (NCCAM, 2013j).

A Cochrane systematic review examined 12 studies involving 2,887 participants with low back pain who were receiving combined chiropractic interventions (Walker, French, Grant, & Green, 2010). The authors concluded that combined chiropractic interventions slightly decreased pain and disability in the short term and pain in the medium term in patients with acute and subacute lower back pain. However, there is no current evidence that supports or refutes the suggestion that these interventions provide a clinically meaningful difference in pain or disability when compared with other interventions.

In their 2007 guidelines, the American College of Physicians and the American Pain Society included spinal manipulation as one of several treatment options for practitioners to consider when low back pain does not improve with self-care. More recently, a 2010 Agency for Healthcare Research and Quality (AHRQ) report noted that complementary health therapies, including spinal manipulation, offer additional options to conventional treatments, which often have limited benefit in managing back and neck pain. The AHRQ analysis also found that spinal manipulation was more effective than a placebo and as effective as medication in reducing the intensity of low back pain. However, the researchers noted inconsistent results when they compared spinal manipulation with massage or physical therapy to reduce the intensity or disability stemming from low back pain.

Researchers continue to study spinal manipulation as an intervention for low back pain:

- A 2011 review of 26 clinical trials looked at the effectiveness of different treatments, including spinal manipulation, for chronic low back pain. The authors concluded that spinal manipulation is as effective as other interventions for reducing pain and improving function.

- A 2010 review that examined various manual therapies, such as spinal manipulation and massage, for a range of conditions found strong evidence that spinal manipulation is effective for chronic low back pain and moderate evidence that it is effective for acute low back pain.
- A 2009 analysis looked at the evidence from 76 trials that studied the effects of several conventional and complementary health practices for low back pain. The researchers found that the pain-relieving effects of many treatments, including spinal manipulation, were small and were similar in people with acute or chronic pain.

- A 2008 review that focused on spinal manipulation for chronic low back pain found strong evidence that spinal manipulation works as well as a combination of medical care and exercise instruction, moderate evidence that spinal manipulation combined with strengthening exercises works as well as prescription nonsteroidal anti-inflammatory drugs combined with exercises, and limited-to-moderate evidence that spinal manipulation works better than physical therapy and home exercise (NCCAM, 2013j).

Other CAM Practices

The broad "other" category includes traditional healers and whole medical systems such as Ayurvedic medicine, traditional Chinese medicine, homeopathy, and naturopathy (**Table 18-2**).

Table 18-2 OTHER CAM THERAPIES

Approach	Therapeutic Method	Rationale
Traditional healers	Practitioners use methods based on indigenous theories, beliefs, and experiences handed down from generation to generation. An example of a traditional healer is the Native American healer/medicine man.	Theories, herbs, and beliefs have been handed down for hundreds of years and may use a combination of techniques to cure or prevent disease
Ayurvedic medicine (India)	A medical aspect based on the ancient Indian medical system known as Ayurveda, meaning knowledge (*veda*) of life (*ayu*).	Restoring a patient's normal inner balance.
Traditional Chinese medicine	All aspects of the person are interconnected and interact with the environment. Acupuncture, herbs, and nutrition are used to promote health.	Health and healing result from determining and resolving imbalances of energy flow in the body—that is, *yin* and *yang*.
Homeopathy	A medical system developed in Germany 200 years ago based on the principle of "like cures like" and "the law of minimum dose."	Very dilute solutions stimulate the body to heal itself.
Naturopathy	A medical system that has evolved from a combination of traditional practices and healthcare approaches popular in Europe during the 19th century.	Emphasizes the healing power of nature. Current practitioners may use a combination of traditional and modern therapies.

Sources: Data from NCCAM (2012e); NCCAM (2013m); Sharma & Clark (2012); & NCCAM (2013g); NCCAM (2012f).

TRADITIONAL CHINESE MEDICINE

Traditional Chinese medicine (TCM) originated in ancient China and has evolved over thousands of years. TCM practitioners use a variety of products and techniques in treating patients. These include, but are not limited to, herbal medicine, acupuncture, tai chi and qi gong, moxibustion, tui na (Chinese therapeutic massage), and dietary therapy. In general, rigorous scientific evidence is lacking that supports the effectiveness of TCM (NCCAM, 2013g).

Beliefs about TCM include the following:

- The human body is a miniature version of the larger, surrounding universe.
- Harmony between two opposing yet complementary forces, *yin* and *yang*, supports health. Disease results from an imbalance between these two forces.
- Five elements—fire, earth, wood, metal, and water—symbolically represent all phenomena.
- Qi, a vital energy that flows through the body, performs multiple functions in maintaining health (NCCAM, 2013g).

Herbal medicines used in TCM are often marketed in the United States as dietary supplements. As stated previously, the FDA does not regulate dietary supplements. Thus, some of these products may be safe, but others may not. Some reports have identified products as being contaminated with drugs, toxins, or heavy metals and not containing the listed ingredients. Additionally, the interaction between Western pharmaceuticals and Chinese herbs may have toxic results. Certain herbs, such as ephedra (ma huang), have been linked to heart attack and stroke. In 2004, the FDA banned the sale of ephedra-containing supplements in the United States, but this ban does not apply to TCM remedies (NCCAM, 2013g).

A systematic review evaluated the impact of the TCM on health-related quality of life and cost-effectiveness (Zhang, Kong, Zhang, & Li, 2012). The authors' search of the literature revealed 31 articles covering a wide range of TCM remedies that were applied to a number of different conditions. Health-related quality of life was primarily measured with SF-36–based scales, but the results of the analysis were inconclusive as to TCM's effect. Similarly, of the 10 articles that had measured cost-effectiveness, the majority reported that TCM treatments resulted in "better outcomes," albeit at a higher cost. However, the authors provided no definition of which TCM therapies were included in their study. Acupuncture and tai chi were the most-studied therapies; however, NCCAM does not consider acupuncture to be a TCM therapy, but a mind–body therapy.

A review of studies examining the use of Chinese medical herbs to mitigate the side effects of chemotherapy in colorectal cancer patients revealed no effect (Wu, Munro, Guanjian, & Liu, 2005). Few RCTs were available to be reviewed. Of the 4 trials that met the researchers' criteria, all were of low quality.

Chronic Disease and CAM

Increasing numbers of individuals with chronic disease are using complementary and/or alternative medicine. When traditional (i.e., Western) approaches to treating and managing chronic disease, whether benign or terminal, prove ineffective, individuals and their families may begin looking for alternatives. This section of the chapter focuses on the use of CAM in two conditions associated with significant morbidity and mortality in the United States: (1) cognitive function, dementia, and Alzheimer's disease and (2) cancer.

COGNITIVE FUNCTION, DEMENTIA, AND ALZHEIMER'S DISEASE

Many dietary supplements are marketed with claims that they improve cognitive function and enhance memory. To date, there has been no research to support those claims. As with other CAM therapies, more research on this topic is needed. NCCAM (2013k) lists five things that individuals should know about complementary health practices targeting cognitive function, dementia, and Alzheimer's disease:

- To date, there is no convincing evidence that any dietary supplement can prevent worsening of cognitive impairment associated with dementia or Alzheimer's disease.
- Preliminary studies of some mind and body practices, such as music therapy, suggest they may be helpful for some of the symptoms related to dementia, such as agitation and depression.
- Mindfulness-based stress reduction programs may be helpful in reducing stress among caregivers of patients with dementia.
- Complementary health approaches should not be used as a reason to postpone seeing a healthcare professional about memory loss.
- Some complementary health approaches interact with other medications and can have serious side effects (NCCAM, 2013k).

These conclusions were based on studies that examined the use of *Ginkgo biloba*, omega-3 fatty acids, B vitamins, Asian ginseng, vitamin E, grape seed extract, and curcumin (NCCAM, 2013l).

Cancer

Jain and Mills (2010) conducted a systematic review of 66 clinical studies examining the use and effectiveness of biofield therapies (Reiki, therapeutic touch, and healing touch) in individuals with a variety of chronic conditions. In their review, they noted the existence of moderate evidence (Level 2) for positive effects of these interventions on acute cancer pain. There was conflicting evidence regarding their effectiveness for longer-term pain, cancer-related fatigue, quality of life, and physiologic indicators of the relaxation response (p. 10).

Many large cancer centers offer acupuncture services as a complementary therapy, particularly to lessen the effects of chemotherapy and/or pain. However, systematic reviews of research on this therapy are few in number. Researchers from the University of Pennsylvania screened 2,151 publications, identifying 41 RCTs that met the criteria for inclusion in their review (Garcia et al., 2013). The heterogeneity of the studies meant that meta-analysis was impossible. In addition, risk of bias compromised a number of the studies. Of all of the studies, only one study, evaluating the use of acupuncture for chemotherapy-induced nausea and vomiting (CINV), was identified as having a low risk of bias and positive results (p. 954). Of the 41 studies, 16 studies had small sample sizes (60 or fewer participants). The researchers concluded that acupuncture is an appropriate adjunctive treatment for CINV; however, for other symptoms (e.g., pain, fatigue, xerostomia, hot flashes), its efficacy remains undetermined.

Complementary and alternative therapies are often used in symptom management in individuals with cancer. Boon, Olatunde, and Zick (2007) reported that 80% of their sample of 1,434 women with breast cancer used CAM for symptom management (p. 58). To better understand this statistic, Wyatt, Sikorskii, Wills, and An (2010) conducted secondary data analysis of a sample of 222 patients with Stage I and Stage II breast cancer to explore the associations among CAM use, spending on CAM therapies, demographic variables, surgical treatment, and quality of life. Overall, 58.2% of the women used CAM (specifically, the biologically-based therapies): 77 women used vitamins, 25 used audiotapes, 18 used massage, and 17 used spiritual healing. Alternative medical systems were used by 13 women. The counts for the individual therapies do not add up to the total category type sum because some women used more than one type of CAM therapy.

In a study funded by the National Cancer Institute, NCCAM, and the National Institute on Aging, researchers examined the interface between allopathic medical providers and CAM providers in a sample of older women with breast cancer (Adler, Wrubel, Hughes, & Beinfield, 2009). The qualitative study interviewed 44 women who were approximately 5 years post-diagnosis. For all but four women, the diagnosis of breast cancer was not the catalyst for CAM use. The women highly valued their simultaneous relationships with both their CAM provider and their biomedical provider. Although the study focused on the interface between different practitioners, the core results of the study reflected patient's broader beliefs related to health, illness, and aging.

Numerous studies in the literature have focused on the use of CAM to prevent cancer, treat cancer, and control cancer symptoms. In the October 2010 issue of *NCCAM Clinical Digest,* the coverage focused on "Cancer and CAM: What the Science Says." The following is a summary of the findings:

- A 2007 review of clinical trials looking at the effectiveness of multivitamin/mineral supplements for cancer prevention found that few such trials have been conducted and that the results of most large-scale trials have been mixed. According to the National Cancer Institute, the following supplements have been studied but have not been shown to lower the risk of cancer: vitamins B_6, B_{12}, E, and C; beta-carotene; folic acid; and selenium.
- A 2008 review of 20 clinical trials found no convincing evidence that antioxidant supplements prevent gastrointestinal cancer, but did uncover indications that some of these supplements might actually increase overall mortality. The review looked at beta-carotene, selenium, and vitamins A, C, and E. Selenium alone demonstrated some preventive benefits.
- Research from the National Cancer Institute indicated that higher intake of calcium may be associated with reduced risk of colorectal cancer, but concluded

that the available evidence does not support taking calcium supplements to prevent colorectal cancer.
- A 2008 review of the research concluded that some botanicals used in Ayurvedic medicine and traditional Chinese medicine may have a role in cancer treatment. However, scientific evidence on these relationships is limited, as much of the research on botanicals and cancer treatment remains in the early stages.
- It is unclear whether the use of vitamin and mineral supplements by patients with cancer is beneficial or harmful. There is a concern that some supplements might interfere with the cancer treatment (NCCAM, 2010c).

Issues

Issues concerning alternative and complementary therapies include research, safety and regulations, CAM practitioners, and collaboration between Western and Eastern healthcare providers.

Research

NCCAM (2012f) is currently in the midst of implementing its third strategic plan, *Exploring the Science of Complementary and Alternative Medicine: Third Strategic Plan 2011–2015.* The five strategic objectives within this plan are as follows:

- Advance research on mind and body interventions, practices, and disciplines
- Advance research on CAM natural products
- Increase understanding of "real world" patterns and outcomes of CAM use and its integration into health care and health promotion
- Improve the capacity of the field to carry out rigorous research
- Develop and disseminate objective, evidence-based information on CAM interventions (NCCAM, 2012f)

A number of challenges emerge when trying to design rigorous research studies to evaluate alternative and complementary therapies. Determining the correct therapy, the amount to be administered, and the population to receive the treatment is essential for testing effectiveness, but is particularly challenging when these parameters are not standardized in the practice arena. Criticisms of CAM research studies include the following points:

- Studies do not use hypothesis testing.
- Small samples are used.
- Studies do not use the randomized controlled trial methodology.
- Studies rely on subjective responses from patients rather than objective measures.
- There is a lack of standardization of CAM treatments, making replication of studies impossible and, therefore, any meta-analysis or synthesis of the treatment difficult.

Bausell (2009) reviewed 45 randomized controlled trials focusing on CAM efficiency from four high-impact journals: *New England Journal of Medicine, Journal of the American Medicine Association, Annals of Internal Medicine,* and *Archives of Internal Medicine.* Bausell's review relied on three validity criteria to select the RCTs: the existence of a placebo control, moderate attrition rates, and 50 or more participants in each group of the sample. Of the 26 trials meeting all three criteria, only two were judged to be supportive of the CAM therapy, while more than half (55.5%) of the 19 trials failed to meet one or more of the criteria reported positive results ($p < 0.001$). Of the two positive high-validity trials, one was funded and authored by the herbal company marketing the product tested, and one used a placebo control group of questionable credibility (p. 349).

In several systematic reviews generated by the Cochrane Collaboration, the reviewers noted that bias was present in the studies being examined. Although many studies may be examined in systematic reviews, Cochrane authors often note that there are few randomized controlled trials that meet the study criteria for a systematic review, let alone a meta-analysis. Walker and colleagues (2010), in their review of chiropractic and low back pain, note that of the studies they reviewed, none compared chiropractic interventions to no treatment. Kim and Zhu (2010), in their review of acupuncture and hypertension, also pointed to a lack of rigorous trials. Further, Jain and Mills (2010), in their systematic review, stated that the studies were of average quality and met minimum standards required for validity. Only 6 out of 67 studies reviewed reported an effect size.

Some individuals suggest that CAM research should not necessarily be hypothesis driven. This assumption is associated with the fact that many CAM therapies have been in use for hundreds of years; thus there is no need for hypothesis testing (Amri, Abu-Asab, Jonas, & Ives, 2011). However, that approach runs counter to evidence-based practice and the scientific process.

Using existing data sets, simply because they are "there," leaves open many questions. Although the presence of a large data set can attract research dollars, its use may be impractical owing to these questions (Sibbritt & Adams, 2012): How will CAM be defined? Is a chiropractor considered an alternative practitioner or a traditional practitioner? Is CAM self-prescribed or has the individual sought out such a practitioner?

CAM practitioners may become angry when their products fail to show any efficacy in RCTs, and often they think that a different research methodology would demonstrate positive effects. Some believe that CAM therapies should be combined with conventional approaches, as typically all treatment consists of multiple modalities, with CAM being only one of them. However, the researcher cannot tell if CAM "made a difference" if all treatments are combined (Bonnebo et al., 2012).

Bias is a recurring problem that has been noted in Cochrane reviews of CAM. Two types of bias may affect CAM research. First, publication bias may occur. This refers to a well-documented tendency for lower-tier journals to report only studies with positive results (Barker, 2007). Additionally, CAM researchers, as well as other researchers, may seek out journals that are less selective in what they publish. In other words, these journals publish most anything that is submitted to them, and they care little about the research methodology employed. Second, although it is rarely discussed outside scientific circles, cultural bias may occur, as witnessed by the fact that studies in some countries tend to produce almost nothing but positive results (Barker, 2007, pp. 170–171).

Witt (2011) points out another issue that is attendant in all research studies—those involving CAM as well as other therapies: It is still not known why some individuals respond better to a therapy than other individuals. The ideal RCT would include only "responders": studies examining acupuncture would include only patients who have already responded to acupuncture. These patients, however, would likely be able to identify a sham acupuncture versus "real" acupuncture. Unfortunately, selecting only responders would decrease the external validity of the results (Witt, 2011, p. 219).

Examples of current research project grants (RO1s) funded by NCCAM include those addressing the following topics: (1) vitamin C as a treatment for polymicrobial sepsis; (2) immunomodulatory effects of arginine supplementation in colitis and colon cancer; (3) mechanisms of meditation; and (4) safe and effective yoga prescriptions for older adults—biomechanical considerations (NIH, 2014).

Safety and Regulation of CAM

Safety depends on the specific therapy, and each complementary product or practice should be considered on its own. Mind and body practices, such as meditation and yoga, are generally considered to be safe in healthy people when practiced appropriately (NCCAM, 2013n). However, there is much that we do not know about dietary supplements. For example, little is known about the safety of these products, in part because a manufacturer does not have to prove the safety

and effectiveness of a dietary supplement before making it available to the public. Wardle and Adams (2012) suggest that there are significant safety and efficacy differences between different manufacturers' "nominally" identical CAM and even between different batches of the same CAM product (p. 212). Regulatory mechanisms focus on principles such as good manufacturing processes, but rarely extend to the other issues affecting the quality of a CAM product, such as growing and manufacturing methods related to raw materials (p. 212).

NCCAM (2013n) also warns of the possibility of product contamination. Hidden prescription drugs or other compounds have been found in some products, particularly in dietary supplements marketed for weight loss; sexual health, including erectile dysfunction; and athletic performance or body-building.

For health professionals and consumers, the NCCAM has a page on its website listing alerts and advisories, many of which involve natural products. For example, January 2014 advisories included many dietary supplements that have been determined to contain other ingredients (NCCAM, 2014b).

CAM Practitioners

For practitioner-based therapies, there is no standardized, national system for credentialing CAM practitioners. Thus, the extent and type of credentialing vary greatly from state to state. Some CAM practitioners (e.g., chiropractic) are licensed, after passing special exams, in all states plus the District of Columbia. Only 17 states and the District of Columbia license naturopathic physicians. Additionally, most states regulate massage therapists by requiring them to obtain a license (NCCAM, 2014c).

There is a great degree of variation among CAM practitioners. Patients choose a traditional healthcare professional with care, and the same can be said of a CAM practitioner. The issue remains, however: Who is identified as a CAM practitioner? Certainly, one would not assume that the clerk at a health foods store that sells a wide variety of natural products, such as dietary supplements, is a practitioner. But the truth of the matter is that these individuals often give advice to clients about the benefits of certain products. These individuals may have inaccurate or incomplete knowledge of the product, or provide claims for the product that may be false, just to make a sale (Wardle & Adams, 2012).

The National Certification Commission for Acupuncture and Oriental Medicine (NCCAOM) is a private, nonprofit organization that certifies practitioners at different levels of education and practice. NCCAOM provides information to the public about the benefits of seeking acupuncture and Oriental medicine (AOM) treatment via an NCCAOM-certified diplomate. This organization offers four certification programs: acupuncture, Chinese herbology, Oriental medicine, and Asian bodywork therapy. Currently, 43 states plus the District of Columbia require the passage of the NCCAOM examinations or NCCAOM certification as a prerequisite for licensure in these areas (NCCAOM, 2012), but each state regulatory board has established unique requirements for licensure (NCCAOM, 2012). Acupuncture.com (n.d.) provides more information about individual states' laws.

To be eligible to take the NCCAOM examination at each level, certain educational and experiential experiences are required. The Accreditation Commission for Acupuncture and Oriental Medicine (ACAOM) is the only accrediting body recognized by the United States Department of Education as an authority for quality education and training in acupuncture and Oriental medicine.

In some CAM practices, a conflict of interest may arise when the CAM practitioner is involved in the sale of a product. For example, in Australia, 98% of naturopaths have their own dispensary in their clinics. Prescribing a certain dietary supplement that the practitioner makes in his or her own dispensary could be seen as a conflict of interest (Wardle & Adams, 2012, p. 215).

Paradigm Issues

Some critics of allopathic health care have argued that physicians, out of self-interest, have convinced legislators to restrict the scope of practice of alternative and complementary healthcare providers and limit choices for individuals with chronic illnesses. They believe that because physicians work closely with hospitals, pharmaceutical companies, and payers (i.e., insurers and other sources of reimbursement), they have persuaded these organizations to avoid partnering with nontraditional healthcare providers. Therefore, according to these critics, physicians, hospitals, pharmaceutical companies, and reimbursers have influenced policy and legislation to limit these practices and, when possible, to prosecute nonphysician practitioners who offer competitive healthcare services (Boozang, 1998; Cuellar, Cahill, Ford, & Aycock, 2003).

Ultimately, this clash exists between proponents of the allopathic healthcare paradigm and proponents of the alternative and complementary healthcare paradigm. Advocates of the allopathic healthcare paradigm believe that governmental regulation is based on scientific evidence, promotes safety, and ensures that the treatment provided to persons with chronic illness is effective. Advocates of the non-allopathic healthcare paradigm believe that individuals should have access to information and treatment, the freedom to evaluate benefits and risks, and ultimately decide for themselves which form of health care they will pursue (Cuellar et al., 2003; Oguamanam, 2006).

As usage of CAM increases in the United States, would it ever be possible that a CAM provider and a traditional healthcare provider might work together to improve patient care? Even in Australia, where CAM practitioners abound and CAM is widely used among the Australian people, an integrative medicine model has proved difficult to implement in practice. Questions arise as to whether CAM approaches are being *incorporated* into care or *integrated* into care. Hunter, Corcoran, Phelps, and Leeder (2012) concluded that the biomedical model is alive and well, even if a patient has a CAM practitioner, and that the physician will continue to occupy the leadership of the healthcare team with scant attention being paid to the CAM practitioners.

Interventions

Self-Reflection

Healthcare professionals considering the role of alternative and complementary treatment in the care of individuals with chronic illnesses need to be aware of their own life experiences and feelings. Understanding one's own beliefs and biases is essential in being present with individuals with chronic illnesses and understanding their fears, concerns, motivations, and needs, without burdening them with personal biases that may inhibit them from making the wisest choices for their circumstances.

Communication

It may be difficult for a traditional healthcare professional to talk with a patient who is using CAM or is considering it. Guidelines for doing so have been developed by Schofield, Diggens, Charleson, Marigliani, and Jefford (2010). These authors performed a systematic review of the literature that discussed CAM in oncology consultations with patients and healthcare professionals over the period 1997–2007. From this review, they developed the guidelines shown in **Table 18-3**.

Selecting a CAM Practitioner

According to CAM practitioners, all healing is self-healing, and the CAM practitioner's role is to empower patients to help heal themselves. This perspective assumes that patients need to take charge of their health and have a personal responsibility for it. Practitioners should be role models for patients (Kotsirilos et al., 2011).

A person needs to be as careful when selecting a CAM practitioner as he or she is when selecting the individual who provides conventional medical care. NCCAM (2013o) provides the following helpful hints on selecting a complementary health practitioner:

1. If you need names of practitioners in your area, first check with your doctor or other healthcare provider. A nearby hospital, medical school, or state regulatory agency or licensing board may be able to assist you.

2. Find out as much as you can about any potential practitioner, including education, training, licensing (if applicable), and certifications (if applicable). Do your research. Does the type of practitioner you are seeking need a license or certification to practice in your state? There is much variation among states.

3. Find out whether the practitioner would be willing to work together with your conventional healthcare provider. Coordinated care and communication are essential to quality care.

4. Explain all of your health conditions to the practitioner, and find out about the practitioner's training and experience in working with people with your condition. Does the practitioner understand your specific needs? Certain health conditions may not be appropriate for certain CAM therapies. As an example, some yoga poses may not be safe to an individual with glaucoma.

5. Don't assume that your health insurance will cover the practitioner's services. In fact, assume that services will not be covered until you talk with your insurance provider.

6. Tell all of your healthcare providers about the CAM approaches that you are using and about all practitioners who are treating you. Full disclosure helps to better manage your health.

Table 18-3 GUIDELINES FOR HEALTH CARE PROVIDERS IN DISCUSSING CAM WITH PATIENTS

1. Understand
   a. Elicit the person's understanding of his or her situation
   b. Ask open questions about this situation
   c. Ask open questions with a psychological/existential focus to determine the person's feelings, concerns, and goals
   d. Elicit information and decision-making preferences
2. Respect
   a. Respect cultural and linguistic diversity and different belief systems
3. Ask
   a. Ask questions about CAM use at critical points in the illness trajectory
   b. Adopt an inquisitive, open-minded approach
4. Explore
   a. Explore details and actively listen
   b. Provide balanced, evidence-based advice
   c. Help respond to advice from family and friends
5. Respond
   a. Respond to the person's emotional state; encourage the person to express his or her feelings
   b. Express empathy
   c. Support the desire for hope and control
6. Discuss
   a. Discuss relevant concerns about CAM while respecting the person's belief system
   b. Safety and efficacy
   c. Financial, time, and psychological costs
   d. Trial period
7. Advise
   a. Encourage
   b. Referrals to CAM practitioners
   c. Accept
   d. Discourage
   e. Balance advice with an acknowledgment of the patient's right for self-determination and autonomy
8. Summarize
9. Document
10. Monitor

Source: Reprinted from Patient Education and Counseling, 79(2),Schofield, P., Diggens, J., Charleson, C., Marigliani, R., & Jefford, M. (2010). Effectively discussing complementary and alternative medicine in a conventional oncology setting: Communication recommendations for clinicians, Pages 143-151, Copyright 2010, with permission from Elsevier.

Evidence-Based Practice Box

Much of the recent research into complementary cancer treatments involves physical activity. Yoga is an alternative, safe, low-impact exercise that combines meditation, breathing, and exercise (p. 870). A systematic review was conducted to determine the efficacy of yoga as a treatment option for both physical health and psychosocial health. Articles were limited to the time period of 2010–2012. Thirteen studies met the inclusion criteria for review. However, similar to other studies with CAM, these studies were inconsistent in the type of yoga used and the use of control groups was limited. Additionally, different outcome measures (i.e., self-esteem, survival rate, well-being, anxiety and depression, quality of life, physical scores, fatigue and state-trait anxiety) further compounded the difficulty in comparing the results. Thus, the researchers were unable to draw any conclusions from the review.

Source: Sharma, M., Haider, T., & Knowlden, A.P. (2013). Yoga as an alternative and complementary treatment for cancer: A systematic review. *The Journal of Alternative and Complementary Medicine, 19*(11), 870–875.

Outcomes

Healthcare professionals caring for individuals with chronic illnesses need to balance an open-minded view of alternative and complementary treatments with a scientific, evidence-based perspective. Healthcare professionals are in a unique position to bridge the gap between allopathic and non-allopathic health care by melding compassion, flexibility, and commitment to scientific and clinical excellence with common sense.

If the CAM practitioner and the traditional practitioner cannot work together, make the client feel comfortable so that he or she can, at least, share with you information about seeing a CAM practitioner. As noted elsewhere in this chapter, sometimes a combination of CAM and traditional medicine presents safety concerns for the patient. Providing a safe environment for the patient may encourage the individual to confide in you about the other practitioners. The end outcome for all is safe, quality care of the patient.

CASE STUDY 18-1

Cindy, one of your closest friends, has rheumatoid arthritis (RA). Unfortunately, her physician has not been able to find the right combination of drugs to improve her health. Cindy has had to stop working at age 35 because of her symptoms, and she barely has the energy to care for her two grade-school–aged children. Her husband of 12 years helps out when he can, but he is climbing the corporate ladder "to the top" and is not always available. Cindy confides to you that she is considering several CAM therapies and is even thinking that she might get off all of her "traditional" treatment, leave her rheumatologist's care, and find a naturopath. Cindy respects your judgment as a nurse and as a friend. You feel that you cannot win no matter what you say to her about CAM.

Discussion Questions

1. What are the ethical questions that you, as a professional caregiver, struggle with in this situation?
2. How do you advise your friend wisely? What do you say to her about her proposed plan of care?
3. How can you refute her contention that her traditional medication is not working for her? What do you say to Cindy?
4. Self-reflect on your own values and beliefs associated with CAM.

CASE STUDY 18-2

Mrs. Brown is a 75-year-old woman who was admitted to your hospital for a flare-up of her heart failure. Additionally, her type 2 diabetes type is not responding well to her oral medications. As you complete your initial interview and assessment upon her admission to the hospital, you see a bag of pills of some sort in her purse. When questioned about the pills, Mrs. Brown replies, "Oh, those things... . Well, I use them to keep up my strength and make me feel better." You can tell from the bottles that they are not prescription medications, but you do not know what they are. You have a gut feeling that they are dietary supplements and wonder how they might be affecting Mrs. Brown's health. Mrs. Brown is already on seven medications for her heart failure, diabetes, and hypothyroidism.

Discussion Questions

1. How do you gain Mrs. Brown's trust to find out what the medications in her purse are? She is quite secretive about them, but you have a feeling that they may be affecting her health.
2. Would you approach Mrs. Brown's family about this issue when they come to visit? Why or why not?
3. Suppose that you have negative beliefs about dietary supplements and think they are not worth much to patients. How do you care for Mrs. Brown without your bias interfering with her care?

STUDY QUESTIONS

1. Why do individuals with chronic illnesses use CAM therapies?
2. Describe the categories of CAM as outlined by NCCAM.
3. How common is using non-allopathic therapy in the United States?
4. Why is designing a research study with CAM so challenging?
5. What are some of the safety issues associated with nontraditional treatments?
6. How does a healthcare professional's self-awareness regarding non-allopathic therapies influence his or her ability to provide unbiased care for individuals with chronic illnesses?
7. How can healthcare professionals help individuals with chronic illnesses make decisions regarding alternative and complementary treatments?
8. Describe how you might discuss with a client his or her use of CAM.

References

AARP & National Center for Complementary and Alternative Medicine (NCCAM) survey of U.S. adults 50+. (2010). Complementary and alternative medicine: What people aged 50 and older discuss with their health care providers. http://nccam.nih.gov/news /camstats/2010

Acupuncture.com. (n.d.). State laws. http://www .acupuncture.com/statelaws/statelaw.htm#top

Adler, S. R., Wrubel, J., Hughes, E., & Beinfield, H. (2009). Patients' interactions with physicians and complementary and alternative medicine practitioners: Older women with breast cancer and self-managed health care. *Integrative Cancer Therapy*, 8(1), 63–70.

Amri, H., Abu-Asab, M., Jonas, W. B., & Ives, J. A. (2011). Laboratory research and biomarkers. In G. T. Lewith, W. B. Jonas, & H. Walach (Eds.), *Clinical research in complementary therapies: Principles, problems and solutions* (2nd ed., pp. 73–98). Toronto, ON: Elsevier.

Andrews, G. J., Adams, J., Segrott, J., & Lui, C. W. (2012). The profiles of complementary and alternative medicine users. In J. Adams, G. J. Andrews, J. Barnes, A. Broom, & P. Magin (Eds.), *Traditional complementary and integrative medicine: An international reader* (pp. 11–17). New York, NY: Palgrave Macmillan.

Balneaves, L., Weeks, L., & Seeley, D. (2012). Patient decision making about complementary and alternative medicine in cancer management, context and process. In J. Adams, G. J. Andrews, J. Barnes, A. Broom, & P. Magin (Eds.), *Traditional complementary and integrative medicine: An international reader* (pp. 71–77). New York, NY: Palgrave Macmillan.

Bann, C. M., Sirois, F. M., & Walsh, E. G. (2010). Provider support in complementary and alternative medicine: Exploring the role of patient empowerment. *Journal of Alternative and Complementary Medicine*, 16(7), 745–752.

Barker, R. (2007). *Snake oil science*. Oxford, UK: Oxford University Press.

Barnes, P. M., Bloom, B., & Nahin, R. L. (2008). *Complementary and alternative medicine use among adults and children: United States, 2007*. National Health Statistics Reports, No. 12. Hyattsville, MD: National Center for Health Statistics.

Bausell, R. B. (2009). Are positive alternative medical therapy trials credible? Evidence from four high-impact medical journals. *Evaluation and the Health Professions*, 32(4), 349–369.

Birks, J., & Evans, J. G. (2009). *Ginkgo biloba* for cognitive impairment and dementia (Review). *Cochrane Database of Systematic Reviews 2009*, 1, CD003120. doi: 10.1002/14651858.CD003120.pub3

Bishop, F. L., & Lewith, G. T. (2008). Who uses CAM? A narrative review of demographic characteristics and health factors associated with CAM use. *eCAM*, 7(1), 11–28. doi: 10.1093/ecam/nen023

Bonnebo, V., Grimsgaard, S., Walach, H., Rittenbaugh, C., Norheim, A., MacPherson, H., … Aicken, M. (2012). Researching complementary and alternative treatments: The gate keepers are not at home. In J. Adams, G. J. Andrews, J. Barnes, A. Broom, & P. Magin (Eds.), *Traditional complementary and integrative medicine: An international reader* (pp. 196–203). New York, NY: Palgrave Macmillan.

Boon, H. S., Olatunde, F., & Zick, S. M. (2007). Trends in complementary/alternative use by breast cancer survivors: Comparing survey data from 1998 and 2005. *BMC Women's Health*, 30(7), 4.

Boozang, K. M. (1998). Western medicine opens the door to alternative medicine. *American Journal of Law and Medicine*, 24(2–3), 185–212.

Cuellar, N. G., Cahill, B., Ford, J., & Aycock, T. (2003). The development of an educational workshop on complementary and alternative medicine: What every nurse should know. *Journal of Continuing Education in Nursing*, 34(3), 128–135.

Deare, J. C., Zheng, Z., Xue, C. C. L., Liu, J. P., Shang, J., Scott, S. W., & Littlejohn, G. (2013). Acupuncture for treating fibromyalgia (Review). *Cochrane Database of Systematic Reviews 2013*, 5, CD007070. doi: 10.1002/14651858.CD007070.pub2

DeKosky, S. T., Williamson, J. D., Fitzpatrick, A. L., Kronmal, R.A., Ives, D.G., Saxton, J.A., ….. GEM Study Investigators. (2008). *Ginkgo biloba* for prevention of dementia: A randomized controlled trial. *Journal of the American Medical Association*, 300(19), 2253–2262.

Dietary Supplements Labels Database. (2013). http://www.dsld.nlm.nih.gov/dsld/lstProducts.jsp?list=a&db=adsld

Evans, J. R. (2013). *Ginkgo biloba* extract for age-related macular degeneration (Review). *Cochrane Database of Systematic Reviews 2013*, 1, CD001775. doi: 10.1002/14651858.CD001775.pub2

Freeman, L. (2009). Chiropractic. In L. Freeman (Ed.), *Mosby's complementary and alternative medicine: A research based approach* (3rd ed., pp. 283–309). St. Louis, MO: Mosby Elsevier.

Garcia, M. K., McQuade, J., Haddad, R., Patel, S., Lee, R., Yang, P., Palmer, J. L., & Cohen, L. (2013). Systematic review of acupuncture in cancer care: A synthesis of the evidence. *Journal of Clinical Oncology*, 31(7), 952–960. doi: 10.1200/JCO.2012.43.5818

Goertz, C., Marriott, B. P., Finch, M. D., Bray, R.M., Williams, T.V., Hourani, L.L., ……. Jonas, W.B. (2013). Military report more complementary and alternative medicine use than civilians. *Journal of Alternative and Complementary Medicine*, 19(6), 509–517.

Goldenberg, J. Z., Ma, S. S. Y., Saxton, J. D., Martzen, M. R., Vandvik, J. D., Thorlund, K., … Johnston, B. C. (2013). Probiotics for the prevention of *Clostridium difficile*–associated diarrhea in adults and children (Review). *Cochrane Database of Systematic Reviews 2013*, 5, CD006095. doi: 10.1002/14651858.CD006095.pub3

Hempel, S., Newberry, S., Ruelaz, A., Wang, Z., Miles, J. N. V., Suttorp, M. J., … Shekelle, P. G. (2011).

Safety of probiotics to reduce risk and prevent or treat disease. Evidence Report/Technology Assessment No. 200. (Prepared by the Southern California Evidence-based Practice Center under Contract No. 290-2007-10062-I.) AHRQ Publication No. 11-E007. Rockville, MD: Agency for Healthcare Research and Quality.

Hilton, M. P., Zimmermann, E. F., & Hunt, W. T. (2013). *Ginkgo biloba* for tinnitus (Review). *Cochrane Database of Systematic Reviews 2013, 3,* CD003852. doi: 10.1002/14651858.CD003852.pub3

Hunter, J., Corcoran, K., Phelps, K., & Leeder, S. (2012). The integrative medicine team: Is biomedical dominance inevitable? *Journal of Alternative and Complementary Medicine, 18*(12), 1127–1132.

Jain, S., & Mills, P. J. (2010). Biofield therapies: Helpful or full of hype? A best evidence synthesis. *International Journal of Behavioral Medicine, 17,* 1–16.

Jawad, M., Schoop, R., Suter, A., Klein, P., & Eccles, R. (2012). Safety and efficacy profile of *Echinacea purpurea* to prevent common cold episodes: A randomized, double-blind, placebo-controlled trial. *Evidence-Based Complementary and Alternative Medicine, 2012,* 841315. doi: 10.1155/2012/841315

Johnson, P. M., Ward, A., Knutson, L., & Sendelbach, S. (2012). Personal use of complementary and alternative medicine (CAM) by U.S. health care workers. *Health Services Research, 47*(1), 221–227. doi: 10.1111/j.1475-6773.2011.01304.x

Johnston, B. C., Goldenberg, J. Z., Vandvik, P. O., Sun, X., & Guyatt, G. H. (2011). Probiotics for the prevention of pediatric antibiotic-associated diarrhea (Review). *Cochrane Database of Systematic Reviews 2011, 11,* CD004827. doi: 10.1002/1465/1858.CD004827.pub3

Kim, H., Cho, S., Park, S., Sohn, I., Jung, W., Moon, S., … Cho, K. (2012). Can acupuncture affect the circadian rhythm of blood pressure? A randomized, double-blind, controlled trial. *Journal of Alternative and Complementary Medicine, 18*(10), 918–923.

Kim, L. W., & Zhu, J. (2010). Acupuncture for essential hypertension. *Alternative Therapies in Health and Medicine, 16*(2), 18–29.

Kotsirilos, V., Vitetta, L., & Sali, A. (2011). *A guide to integrative and complementary medicine.* Sydney, Australia: Elsevier.

Lau, H. L. C., Kwong, J. S. W., Yeung, F., Chau, P. H., & Woo, J. (2012). Yoga for secondary prevention of coronary heart disease (Review). *Cochrane Database of Systematic Reviews 2012, 12,* CD009506. doi: 10.1002/14651858CD009506.pub2

Linde, K., Barrett, B., Bauer, R., Melchart, D., & Woelkart, K. (2006). *Echinacea* for preventing and treating the common cold (Review). *Cochrane Database of Systematic Reviews 2006, 1,* CD000530. doi: 10.1002/14651858.CD0005350.pub2

Macpherson, H., Richmond, S., Bland, M., Brealey, S., Gabe, R., Hopton, A., … Watt, I. (2013). Acupuncture and counselling for depression in primary care: A randomized controlled trial. *PLOS Med, 10*(9), e1001518. doi: 10.1371/journal.pmed.1001581

Manheimer, E., Cheng, K., Wieland, L. S., Min, L. S., Shen, X., Berman, B. M., & Lao, L. (2012). Acupuncture for treatment of irritable bowel syndrome (Review). *Cochrane Database of Systematic Reviews 2012, 5,* CD005111. doi: 10.1002/14651858.CD005111.pub3

Nahin, R. L., Barnes, P. M., Stussman, B. J., & Bloom, B. (2009). *Costs of complementary and alternative medicine (CAM) and frequency of visits to CAM practitioners: United States, 2007.* National Health Statistics Reports, no. 18. Hyattsville, MD: National Center for Health Statistics.

National Cancer Institute. (2011). Acupuncture (health professional version). http://www.cancer.gov/cancertopics/pdq/cam/acupuncture/healthprofessional/page1

National Center for Complementary and Alternative Medicine (NCCAM). (2010a). Meditation: An introduction. http://nccam.nih..gov/health/meditation/overview.htm

National Center for Complementary and Alternative Medicine (NCCAM). (2010b). Tai chi. http://nccam.nih.gov/health/taichi/introduction.htm

National Center for Complementary and Alternative Medicine (NCCAM). (2010c). Cancer and CAM: What the science says. http://www.nccam.nih.gov/health/providers/digest/cancer_science.htm

National Center for Complementary and Alternative Medicine (NCCAM). (2012a). Facts at-a-glance and mission. http://nccam.nih.gov/about/ataglance

National Center for Complementary and Alternative Medicine (NCCAM). (2012b). Oral probiotics: An introduction. http://nccam.nih.gov/health/probiotics/introduction.htm?nav=gsa

National Center for Complementary and Alternative Medicine (NCCAM). (2012c). Acupuncture: An introduction. http://nccam.nih.gov/health/acupuncture/introduction.htm#risks

National Center for Complementary and Alternative Medicine (NCCAM). (2012d). Spotlight on modality: Yoga for health. http://nccam.nih.gov/health/providers/digest/yoga

National Center for Complementary and Alternative Medicine (NCCAM). (2012e). What is complementary and alternative medicine? http://nccam.nih.gov/sites/nccam.nih.gov/files/D347_05-25-2012.pdf

National Center for Complementary and Alternative Medicine (NCCAM). (2012f). NCCAM third strategic plan: 2011–2015: Exploring the science of complementary and alternative medicine. http://nccam.nih.gov/about/plans/2011

National Center for Complementary and Alternative Medicine (NCCAM). (2013a). What is CAM? http://www.nccam.nih.gov/health/whatiscam

National Center for Complementary and Alternative Medicine (NCCAM). (2013b). Paying for complementary health approaches. http://nccam.nih.gov/health/financial

National Center for Complementary and Alternative Medicine (NCCAM). (2013c). Using dietary supplements wisely. http://nccam.nih.gov/health/supplements/wiseuse.htm?nav=gsa#fed

National Center for Complementary and Alternative Medicine (NCCAM). (2013d). Herbs as a glance. http://nccam.nih.gov/health/herbsataglance.htm

National Center for Complementary and Alternative Medicine (NCCAM). (2013e). Spotlight on a modality: Oral probiotics: What the science says. http://nccam.nih.gov/health/providers/digest/probiotics?nav=gsa

National Center for Complementary and Alternative Medicine (NCCAM). (2013f). Ginkgo. http://nccam.nih.gov/health/ginkgo/ataglance.htm

National Center for Complementary and Alternative Medicine (NCCAM). (2013g). Traditional Chinese medicine: An introduction. http://nccam.nih.gov/sites/nccam.nih.gov/files/Backgrounder_Traditional_Chinese_Medicine_10-25-2013.pdf

National Center for Complementary and Alternative Medicine (NCCAM). (2013h). Yoga. http://nccam.nih.gov/introduction.htm#hed2

National Center for Complementary and Alternative Medicine (NCCAM). (2013i). Relaxation techniques. http://nccam.nih.gov/health/stress/relaxation.htm

National Center for Complementary and Alternative Medicine (NCCAM). (2013j). Spinal manipulation for low-back pain. http://nccam.nih.gov/heatlth/pain/spinemanipulation.htm#aboutspinal

National Center for Complementary and Alternative Medicine (NCCAM). (2013k). Five things to know about complementary health practices for cognitive function, dementia, and Alzheimer's disease. http://nccam.nih.gov/health/tips/alzheimers

National Center for Complementary and Alternative Medicine (NCCAM). (2013l). NCCAM clinical digest: Dietary supplements and cognitive function, dementia, and Alzheimer's disease. http://nccam.nih.gov/health/providers/digest/alzheimers-science

National Center for Complementary and Alternative Medicine (NCCAM). (2013m). Homeopathy. http://nccam.nih.gov/health/homeopathy#hed1

National Center for Complementary and Alternative Medicine (NCCAM). (2013n). Safe use of complementary health products and practices. http://nccam.nih.gov/health/safety.

National Center for Complementary and Alternative Medicine (NCCAM). (2013o). 6 things to know when selecting a complementary health provider. http://nccam.nih.gov/health/tips/selecting

National Center for Complementary and Alternative Medicine (NCCAM). (2014a). Massage. http://nccam.nih.gov/health/massage

National Center for Complementary and Alternative Medicine (NCCAM). (2014b). Alerts and advisories. http://nccam.nih.gov/news/alerts

National Center for Complementary and Alternative Medicine (NCCAM). (2014c). Credentialing: Understanding the education, training, regulation and licensing of complementary health practitioners. http://nccam.nih.gov/health/decisions/credentialing.htm

National Certification Commission for Acupuncture and Oriental Medicine (NCCAOM). (2012). http://www.nccaom.org

National Institutes for Health (NIH). (2014). Research portfolio online reporting tools (RePORT). http://projectreporter.nih.gov/reporter_SearchResults.cfm?icde=18913874

Natural Standard. (2013). The authority on integrative medicine. http://www.naturalstandard.com/

Natural Medicines Comprehensive Database. (2014). http://naturaldatabase.therapeuticresearch.com/home.aspx?cs=&s=ND&AspxAutoDetectCookieSupport=1\

Nicolai, S. P. A., Krudenier, L. M., Bedermacher, B. L. W., Prins, M. H., Stokmans, R. A., Broos, P. P. H. L., & Teijink, J. A. W. (2013). *Ginkgo biloba* for intermittent claudication (Review). *Cochrane Database of Systematic Reviews 2013*, 6, CD006888. doi: 10.1002/14651858.CD006888.pub3

Oguamanam, C. (2006). Biomedical orthodoxy and complementary and alternative medicine: Ethical challenges of integrating medical cultures. *Journal of Alternative and Complementary Medicine*, 12(5), 577–581.

Owens, C., Baergen, R., & Puckett, D. (2014). Online sources of herbal product information. *American Journal of Medicine*, 127, 109–115. http://dx.doi.org10.1016.j.amjmed.2013.09.016

Patel, N. K., Newstead, A. H., & Ferrer, R. L. (2012). The effects of yoga on physical functioning and health related quality of life in older adults: A systematic review and meta-analysis. *Journal of Alternative and Complementary Medicine, 18*(10), 902–917. doi: 10.1089/acm.2011.0473

Ramaratnam, S., & Sridharan, K. (2012). Yoga for epilepsy (Review). *Cochrane Database of Systematic Reviews 2002, 1,* CD001524. doi: 10.1002/14651858. CD001524. Update of 2002 review.

Schofield, P., Diggens, J., Charleson, C., Marigliani, R., & Jefford, M. (2010). Effectively discussing complementary and alternative medicine in a conventional oncology setting: Communication recommendations for clinicians. *Patient Education and Counseling, 79,* 143–151. doi: 10.1016/j.pec.2009.07.038

Sharma, H., & Clark, C. (2012). *Ayurvedic healing: Contemporary maharishi Ayurveda medicine and science* (2nd ed.). Philadelphia, PA: Singing Dragon.

Sharma, M., Haider, T., & Knowlden, A. P. (2013). Yoga as an alternative and complementary treatment for cancer: A systematic review. *Journal of Alternative and Complementary Medicine, 19*(11), 870–875.

Sibritt, D., & Adams, J. (2012). Utilizing existing data sets to investigate complementary and alternative medicine consumption: Cohort studies and longitudinal analyses. In J. Adams, G. J. Andrews, J. Barnes, A. Broom, & P. Magin (Eds.), *Traditional complementary and integrative medicine: An international reader* (pp. 26–34). New York, NY: Palgrave Macmillan.

Tait, E. M., Laditka, J. N., Laditka, S. B., Nies, M. A., Racine, E. F., & Tsulukidze, M. M. (2013). Reasons why older Americans use complementary and alternative medicine: Costly or ineffective conventional medicine and recommendations from health care providers, family and friends. *Educational Gerontology, 39*(9), 684–700. doi 10.1080/03601277.2012.734160

Tiralongo, E., Lea, E. A., Wee, S. S., Hanna, M. M., & Griffiths, L. R. (2012). Randomised, double blind, placebo-controlled trial of *Echinacea* supplementation in air travelers. *Evidence-Based Complementary and Alternative Medicine, 2012,* 417267. doi: 10.1155/2012/417267

Ulbricht, C. (2011). *Davis's pocket guide to herbs and supplements.* Philadelphia, PA: F. A. Davis.

Villemure, C., Ceko, M., Cotton, V. A., & Bushnell, C. (2013). Insular cortex mediates increased pain tolerance in yoga practitioners. *Cerebral Cortex.* PMID 23696275. doi: 10.1093/cercor/bht124

Walker, B. F., French, S. D., Grant, W., & Green, S. (2010). Combined chiropractic interventions for low back pain (Review). *Cochrane Database of Systematic Reviews 2010, 4,* CD005427. doi: 10.1002/14651858. CD005427.pub2

Wardle, J., & Adams, J. (2012). Indirect risks of complementary and alternative medicine. In J. Adams, G. J. Andrews, J. Barnes, A. Broom, & P. Magin (Eds.), *Traditional complementary and integrative medicine: An international reader* (pp. 212–219). New York, NY: Palgrave Macmillan.

Witt, C. M. (2011). Acupuncture. In G. T. Lewith, W. B. Jonas, & H. Walach (Eds.), *Clinical research in complementary therapies: Principles, problems and solutions* (2nd ed., pp. 217–234) Toronto, ON: Elsevier.

Wu, T., Munro, A. J., Guanjian, L., & Liu, G. J. (2005). Chinese medical herbs for chemotherapy side effects in colorectal cancer patients (Review). *Cochrane Database of Systematic Reviews 2005, 1,* CD004540. doi: 10.1002/14651858.CD004540. pub2

Wyatt, G., Sikorskii, A., Wills, C. E., & An, H. S. (2010). Complementary and alternative medicine use, spending, and quality of life in early stage breast cancer. *Nursing Research, 59*(1), 58–65.

Zhang, F., Kong, L., Zhang, Y., & Li, S. (2012). Evaluation of impact on health-related quality of life and cost effectiveness of traditional Chinese medicine: A systematic review of randomized clinical trials. *Journal of Alternative and Complementary Medicine, 18*(12), 1108–1120.

Zhang, J., Yang, K., Tian, J., & Wang, C. (2012). Effects of yoga on psychologic function and quality of life in women with breast cancer: A meta-analysis of randomized controlled trials. *Journal of Alternative and Complementary Medicine, 18*(110), 994–1002. doi: 10.1089/acm/2011.0514

Chapter 19

Models of Care

Barbara J. Lutz and Pamala D. Larsen

Introduction

As the population aged 65 and older increases and the healthcare system sees more individuals with chronic illness, healthcare professionals and third-party payers are considering how best to care for individuals with chronic disease on a long-term basis. Increasingly we hear about disease management models that have demonstrated better patient outcomes than "usual care." Less well publicized, however, is nursing's role in caring for individuals with chronic disease. For some nurses, it has always made sense that chronic care should be part of nursing's domain, particularly given that the nursing profession tends to look at care as opposed to cure.

The United States continues to outspend similar nations in health care. However, more money does not translate into better patient outcomes or better value for the consumer. Phrases heard today emphasize the "value-based" and "value-added" nature of products and services—whether in manufacturing, architecture, engineering, or now health care. What is the value of the health care that the patient is receiving? Robinson (2008) defines value in health care as being measured in terms of contributions of health care minus the attendant costs, with costs and contributions conceptualized broadly (p. 11).

In 2010, the United States passed healthcare reform legislation, the Patient Protection and Affordable Care Act (ACA). The provisions

of this bill are continuing to be implemented. Will they be successful in improving health outcomes? Do they address the "real" issues of our healthcare system? There have been several attempts to repeal the bill since it became law, but as of 2014 it remained in effect, and it is expected that many of its cost-saving provisions will continue to be implemented. Will provisions in this bill help us to more effectively provide quality care to those with chronic conditions?

This chapter provides an overview of models and frameworks designed to improve care for individuals with chronic illness and their families.

Historical Perspectives

Over the past several decades, in an effort to control the burgeoning costs of health care, the Centers for Medicare and Medicaid Services (CMS), formerly known as the Health Care Financing Agency (HCFA), implemented prospective payment systems for Medicare beneficiaries. One of the most well known is diagnosis-related groups (DRGs), which were first implemented in 1983. The DRG system was the direct result of trying to find a better way to pay care providers than the retrospective payment system that was in place from 1965 to 1983. It seemed that paying care providers prospectively, per diagnosis group, would decrease costs. DRGs were implemented using the International Classification of Diseases, Ninth Revision, Clinical Modifications (ICD-9-CM) (now in its 10th revision, with plans for an 11th version to appear in 2015). ICD-9-CM coding assigned individual codes to diseases, symptoms, and procedures. Although DRGs were used initially only for Medicare patients, third-party payers frequently adopted similar payment structures using the same ICD-9-CM (and now ICD-10-CM) coding.

With the advent of DRGs, acute care facilities soon developed clinical pathways or care algorithms for patients with a diagnosis that matched a specific DRG. Patients with heart failure, myocardial infarction, appendectomy, cholecystectomy, stroke, diabetes, and so forth were placed within standard care plans, care maps, clinical pathways, or algorithms (the name varied across institutions) as a way to monitor these patients and make sure they were "on track" for discharge. Because the hospital was to be paid a certain amount of money for each individual with a specific condition, it was critical that patients received accurate diagnoses, were treated swiftly and effectively, and were discharged in a timely manner. This led to more patients with chronic illnesses being discharged "sicker and quicker," in turn requiring an increase in post-acute care including home health, skilled nursing, and rehabilitation. As costs for care shifted to post-acute care settings, so did similar policies regarding prospective payment across the continuum of care. Although one would not consider prospective payment policies, such as DRGs, a disease or illness management model, these changes to Medicare in the 1980s have influenced how we manage care today. This has led to multiple different models for dealing with chronic illness in efforts to better manage patient care, improve outcomes, and reduce costs.

Impact

The direct and indirect costs associated with providing appropriate care for someone with multiple chronic conditions cannot be overstated. In 2010, Medicare beneficiaries with two or more chronic conditions accounted for 93% of the program's spending (CMS, 2012). From a cost perspective alone, the need to provide high-quality care efficiently drove the development of both formal and informal disease and care management programs. These programs originated from federal and state agencies as well as from for-profit and not-for-profit companies.

Disease Management Versus Illness Management

While there is wide variation in disease management programs, these programs typically focus on the management of one disease, such as diabetes, congestive heart failure, or coronary artery disease, and often exclude patients with complex conditions. According to the Congressional Budget Office (CBO), disease management programs should have several components. Specifically, they should educate patients about the disease and self-management strategies. They should use evidence-based guidelines and monitor clinical status and physiologic markers of disease, such as the measurement of one's glycosylated hemoglobin ($HgbA_{1c}$), the forced expiratory volume (FEV) of a patient with chronic obstructive pulmonary disease (COPD), the number of medications prescribed to a patient, the number of visits to a healthcare professional, and so forth. These programs should also coordinate disease-related care among providers (Holtz-Eakin, 2004).

Interventions

The early approach to disease management was marked by the formation of disease management companies during the mid-to-late 1990s. The primary goal of these companies was to reduce the costs of health care for those with chronic diseases. By 1999, there were 200 companies nationwide offering disease management services for such conditions as diabetes, asthma, and heart failure (Bodenheimer, 2003). Most of these programs did not originate within healthcare institutions but rather were outsourced to outside companies. Today, few of those companies exist or are profitable, primarily because their focus was on one specific disease. They did not take into consideration the impact of multiple comorbidities and the other determinants that lead to poor health outcomes.

Chronic illness management is much more complex than simply focusing on one disease. For example, factors such as income, health literacy, social support, transportation, and access to care can all affect chronic disease management. Additionally, older adults typically have multiple chronic conditions. As an example, in 2010, 98% of all 30-day hospital readmissions involved individuals with more than one chronic condition and 80% were attributed to individuals with four or more conditions (CMS, 2012). The early disease management companies offered programs that were just that—programs—with neither a systems approach nor an integration of these programs into a healthcare system or institution. In addition, a number of those disease management programs were based on physician specialty practice and not primary care. Older adults, however, may have several chronic conditions that necessitate them seeing several different specialty physicians. Therefore, programs based on specialty practice typically did not work.

The effectiveness of such programs has also proved difficult to establish through research. In meta-analyses or systematic reviews of disease management programs, it becomes difficult to figure out inclusion criteria for studies, because each program is different. Furthermore, when looking at outcomes, determining whether a specific component of the program or a combination of components acting interdependently makes a difference in the health outcome is difficult to discern.

Mattke, Seid, and Ma (2007), in their analysis of disease management programs, suggest in broad terms that disease management refers to a system of coordinated healthcare interventions and communications to help patients address chronic disease and other health conditions. Disease management programs are "big business," with 96% of the top 150 U.S. payers offering some form of disease management service and 83% of more than 500 major U.S. employers using programs to help individuals manage their health (as cited in Mattke et al., 2007, p. 670). Revenues associated with these programs grew significantly from $78 million in 1997 to nearly $1.2 billion in 2005 and were projected to top $1.8 billion by the end of 2008 (Mattke et al., 2007). What are the health outcomes that emerge from these expenditures of $1 billion to $2 billion per year? Are these programs making a difference in health outcomes, and, if so, are they reducing costs in other areas?

In their review of 3 evaluations of large-scale, population-based programs, 10 meta-analyses, and 16 systematic reviews covering 317 studies, Mattke and colleagues (2007) found consistent evidence of improved processes of care and disease control, but no conclusive support of improved health outcomes. In addition, when the costs of the programs and/or interventions were accounted for and then cost savings subtracted, there was no evidence of a net reduction in medical costs (pp. 675–676).

Tricare Management Activity, which administers healthcare benefits for U.S. military service personnel, retirees, and their dependents, developed a disease management program for beneficiaries with diabetes. A quasi-experimental approach assessed the program's impact on 37,370 beneficiaries ages 18 to 64 living in the United States. Beneficiaries were categorized as having "uncontrolled" or "controlled" diabetes based on past medical claims. The study compared observed outcomes to predicted outcomes in the absence of diabetes management. Results indicated that total annual medical savings per participant averaged $783. More active participation in the program was associated with lower medical costs (Dall et al., 2010).

Buntin, Jain, Mattke, and Lurie (2009) suggest that results from disease management programs may be skewed because of selection bias. Selection bias includes patients being recruited into programs because they are likely to realize quality and cost benefits from such participation (typically the more engaged patient is more interested in self-management). The conundrum is whether the disease management program itself produces the results or whether it is the selection of the appropriate patients that make the difference (Buntin et al., 2009).

In a 2012 report from the Congressional Budget Office, outcomes from 6 disease management and care coordination demonstration projects involving 34 programs for Medicare beneficiaries were evaluated. These programs used nurse care managers who contacted patients primarily by phone. The nurses educated patients, encouraged self-care, monitored health status, and tracked healthcare use related to the specific chronic disease. Most of the demonstration projects excluded high-use Medicare beneficiaries, persons with dementia, individuals with recent hospital stays, or those who were receiving hospice or care for complex conditions. Overall, the 34 programs "had little or no effect on hospital admissions or *regular* Medicare spending ... although the estimated effects varied considerably from one program to another" (CBO, 2012, pp. 2–3). Those programs that were able to demonstrate reductions in hospitalizations included "significant in-person interactions between care managers and patients" and those with "substantial direct interactions" with the patients' physicians (p. 4).

When considering any disease, the pathophysiology, required medications, and education are only some of the components of caring for the patient and, quite frankly, represent the easier part—the measurable part. The illness experience of an individual patient and the impact on the family; the uniqueness of the patient; and the patient's living situation, social support, and coping mechanisms—whether effective or ineffective—are other components of the patient's life that disease management programs do not address.

Additionally, it is important to consider the impact of the multiple determinants of health—such as economic, geographic, educational, cultural, political, and environmental factors—on individuals with chronic illness. When we think about chronic illness, each condition needs to be put within the larger context of "health." From a public health perspective, medical or disease management at the individual level is just one small component of managing the overall impact of chronic illness and improving the health of those persons diagnosed with chronic disease.

Several theoretical models for understanding health have been proposed. One of the most widely embraced is the social–ecological model (SEM). Several versions of the SEM exist, but all consider the influence of factors at different levels on individual health. McLeroy's version of the SEM has five levels—intrapersonal (individual), interpersonal, institutional (organizational), community, and public policy (McLeroy, Bibeau, Steckler, & Glanz, 1988). Individuals (intrapersonal) with chronic illness are considered within the larger context of interpersonal factors (e.g., family, friends, peers), organizations (e.g., church, school, work, health care), community (e.g., local government, networks, norms), and public policy factors. Within the SEM, an individual's health is influenced by factors at all of these levels, and all levels need to be considered when determining which interventions may be most effective for a particular group or individual. Early models of chronic disease management often did not consider factors outside of the intrapersonal/individual level. More recently, as a result of policy changes, newer models are beginning to include factors at the other levels.

Chronic Care Model

The best-known model for providing care to individuals with chronic disease is the chronic care model (CCM). The CCM is a comprehensive team-based model that aims to redesign primary and specialty practice. It includes six "essential factors in chronic care management: community resources, health care organization, self-management support, decision support, delivery system redesign, and clinical information systems" (Bodenheimer, 2003, p. 65).

Work on this model began in the early 1990s with the efforts of Edward Wagner, an internist and director of the Seattle-based MacColl Institute for Healthcare Innovation at the Center for Health Studies, Group Health Cooperative. Wagner identified three issues in providing care to those with chronic illness through primary care (Wielawski, 2006, p. 5):

1. Primary care offices are set up to respond to acute illnesses rather than anticipate and respond proactively to patients' needs (which is what individuals with chronic illness need).
2. Patients with chronic illness are not adequately informed about their conditions and are not supported in the self-care of their conditions beyond the physician's office.
3. Physicians are too busy to educate and support patients with chronic illness to the degree needed for them to stay healthy.

Wagner's (1998) solution was to replace the physician-centered office with a structure that supported a team of professionals who collaborated with the patient in his or her care, and considered factors beyond medical management and clinical markers.

Early implementation of the CCM model took place with 15,000 patients with diabetes at the Group Health Cooperative, a 590,000-member health maintenance organization in Seattle. Over the course of 5 years, the percentage of patients with up-to-date screening improved; blood sugar levels and the regularity of monitoring improved; patients reported higher satisfaction with their care; and admission to acute care facilities decreased.

During this period of time in the mid-to-late 1990s, Wagner and associates partnered with the Robert Wood Johnson Foundation (RWJF) to further develop the model. The model was refined and published in its current form in 1998. Improving Chronic Illness Care (2006–2014), a national program through RWJF, was launched in 1998 with the CCM as its core (**Figure 19-1**). The CCM is not a model for individual care, but rather addresses care of large populations of individuals. It does not redesign patient care, but rather redesigns clinical practices that are delivering care by implementing system and process changes.

A 2009 Intervention Review of an earlier Cochrane Review supported the use of the CCM with clients with both type 1 and type 2 diabetes. Forty-one studies with a total of 48,000 clients were involved in the review. Renders and colleagues (2000) concluded that multifaceted professional interventions can enhance the performance of healthcare professionals in managing clients with diabetes. Although using the model enhanced process outcomes, the effect on client health outcomes was less clear.

Studies from 2000 through 2009 were reviewed to determine the impact of the CCM in redesigning care. For this review, a CCM-based intervention was defined as an intervention that integrated changes that involved most or all of the six areas of the model: self-management support, decision support, delivery system design, clinical information systems, healthcare organization, and community resources (Coleman, Austin, Brach, & Wagner, 2009). Eighty-two studies were retained for analysis as part of the final study. The published evidence suggested that practices redesigned in accord with the CCM generally improve the quality of care and

Figure 19-1 The Chronic Care Model

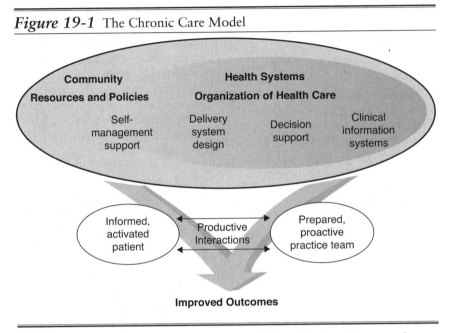

Source: Wagner, E. H. (1998). Chronic disease management: What will it take to improve care for chronic illness? *Effective Clinical Practice, 1,* 2–4.

the outcomes for patients with various chronic illnesses (p. 81).

Although the CCM is a model for primary medical care, Jacelon, Furman, Rea, Macdonald, and Donaghue (2011) have adapted it for long-term care. In their version, the six constructs of the CCM were implemented to create a model for high-quality chronic disease care.

Guided Care

Using the CCM as a basis, researchers at Johns Hopkins University developed the Guided Care model in 2006, as a means to improve the quality of life and efficiency of resource utilization for older adults with multiple chronic conditions. Guided Care enhances the use of primary care (versus specialty care) and utilizes seven principles of chronic care: disease management, self-management, case management, lifestyle modification, transitional care, caregiver education and support, and geriatric evaluation

and management (Boyd et al., 2007, p. 697). What is unique about this model is the use of registered nurses specifically trained in Guided Care concepts, who in turn use a computerized electronic health record (EHR) in working with two to five primary care physicians to meet the needs of 50–60 older adults with multiple comorbidities. The Guided Care nurse (GCN) is based in the primary care physician's office, and performs eight clinical activities, guided by scientific evidence and the patients' priorities (p. 698). Pilot versions of the Guided Care model included several of the eight core activities. The first major application of this model occurred in a cluster-randomized controlled trial (RCT) through Johns Hopkins University. The study utilized 8 sites (49 physicians) in the Baltimore–Washington, D.C., area, with 904 patients in either the experimental group (who received Guided Care) or the control group (who received usual care) (Boult et al., 2008).

Patients eligible for the study were those 65 years or older and ranking in the upper quartile of risk for using health services during the coming year. The GCN performed eight clinical activities:

1. *Assessment.* Initial assessments include medical, functional, cognitive, affective, psychosocial, nutritional, and environmental evaluations. Other tools used may include the Geriatric Depression Scale and the CAGE alcoholism scale. The client is also asked what his or her priorities are for improved quality of life.

2. *Planning.* The EHR merges the assessment data with evidence-based practice guidelines to create a preliminary care guide that manages and monitors patients' health conditions. The GCN and the primary care physician then personalize the care guide with input from the patient and family. The end result is a patient-friendly version of the plan called "My Action Plan," which is written in lay language and given to the patient.

3. *Chronic disease self-management (CDSM).* The GCN encourages the patient's self-efficacy in the management of his or her chronic conditions. The patient is referred to a free, local 15-hour CDSM course led by trained lay people and supported by the GCN. In this program—developed by Kate Lorig and associates at Stanford University (1999)—the patient learns how to operationalize the action plan.

4. *Monitoring.* The GCN monitors each patient at least monthly by telephone to address issues promptly. The EHR plays an important role in the monitoring by providing reminders about each patient (Boyd et al., 2007).

5. *Coaching.* Motivational interviewing is used to facilitate the patient's participation in care and to reinforce adherence to the action plan (Boyd et al., 2007). The GCNs are trained in motivational interviewing principles and strategies to assist in this process.

6. *Coordinating transitions between sites and providers of care.* The GCN is the primary coordinator of care for patients in this program and, therefore, is responsible for the care transitions that occur between home, the emergency room, hospitals, long-term care facilities, and other care settings.

7. *Educating and supporting caregivers.* The GCN works with family or other unpaid caregivers of the patients to educate and support them. This may include individual or group assistance, support group meetings, or ad hoc telephone consultation (Boyd et al., 2007).

8. *Accessing community resources.* Determining which community resources are appropriate for the patient, such as Meals on Wheels, transportation assistance, and so forth, are key functions of the GCN. The idea is not to duplicate services, but rather to utilize the services already available in the community.

In April 2008, 6 months into the RCT, data suggested that the Guided Care model provided improved quality of care, reduced medical care costs, and resulted in high satisfaction among both the primary care physicians and the GCNs (Boult et al., 2008). Based on these early results, two of the managed care partners in the trial, Kaiser Permanente and Johns Hopkins HealthCare, agreed to continue to pay the costs of the GCNs for an additional year. However, 18-month outcomes demonstrated few positive results. The study looked at the use of health services and included 850 older patients at high risk for using health care in the future. The only statistically significant overall effect of Guided Care was a reduction in episodes of home health care (Boult et al., 2011). The latest research findings about Guided Care appear in the Evidence-Based Practice Box.

Geriatric Resources of Assessment and Care

Geriatric Resources of Assessment and Care (GRACE) was established in 2002 as a comprehensive integrated, home-based geriatric care model for low-income elders (age 65 and older) with chronic conditions. The GRACE interprofessional team consists of a geriatrician, pharmacist, physical therapist, mental health social worker, community-based resource support person, and direct care support team that includes a geriatric nurse practitioner (GNP) and a licensed social worker (SW). The support team conducts a comprehensive medical, psychosocial, and functional assessment in the patient's home. Findings from this assessment are presented to the rest of the GRACE team and a comprehensive plan of care is developed. The support team (GNP and SW) discusses the plan of care with the patient's primary care provider and seeks additional input and suggestions from that physician. Then, the support team works with the patient to implement the plan based on the patient's goals. They conduct face-to-face visits and phone calls based on the GRACE protocols and patient need. They also coordinate care and assist the patient in securing community-based resources (e.g., transportation, medication assistance). Patient outcomes are tracked over the length of the intervention using an electronic health record system. The GNP and SW meet with the rest of the team at regular intervals to discuss ongoing care and progress of the patients enrolled in the program. The services are not covered by Medicare fee-for-service reimbursement, but are included in some Medicare Advantage Plans, large employers' healthcare programs, and Veterans Administration (VA) care. The cost of GRACE model was estimated to be $1,000 per patient per year (Counsell, Callahan, Buttar, Clark, & Frank, 2006).

A randomized controlled trial of more than 900 low-income elders demonstrated that participants enrolled in the GRACE program had fewer emergency department visits, better quality of care, and improved health-related quality of life. In a subgroup of participants at high risk for rehospitalization, GRACE participants had fewer hospital admissions during year 2 of the study (Counsell et al., 2007). Participants enrolled in the GRACE program (i.e., the intervention arm of the study) also were more likely to receive a flu shot, see their primary care provider within 6 weeks of hospital discharge, and receive information about geriatric conditions, (e.g., fall prevention, incontinence, depression, and hearing impairment) (Boult & Wieland, 2010).

Program of All-Inclusive Care for the Elderly

Although the Program of All-Inclusive Care for the Elderly (PACE) was not specifically developed for individuals with chronic illness, it is obvious that the majority of older adults accessing this program could have at least one chronic condition. PACE was developed in 1990 and is a capitated benefit authorized by the Balanced Budget Act (BBA) of 1997 that offers comprehensive health care to older adults. PACE is modeled after the successful On Lok Senior Health Services program in San Francisco. The On Lok model showed successful outcomes in a number of demonstration projects funded through the CMS (then known as HCFA) in the 1980s and 1990s. PACE is a permanent entity within the Medicare program, which enables states to provide PACE services to Medicaid beneficiaries as a state option.

Participants in PACE must be 55 years of age, live in a PACE service area, have a low income, and be certified as eligible for nursing home care. The program allows most of its participants to receive services while they continue to live at home. Capitated financing allows care providers to deliver all services that the participants need, rather than those that are limited under Medicare and Medicaid fee-for-service systems (http://www.cms.hhs.gov/pace/). PACE becomes the sole source of services for the Medicare- and Medicaid-eligible enrollees. As of 2013, there were 99 PACE providers located in 31 states (National PACE Association, 2013).

Mukamel and colleagues (2007) attempted to determine which program characteristics of PACE were associated with the risk-adjusted health outcomes of mortality, functional status, and self-assessed health. Their research examined 3,042 persons who were newly enrolled in 23 PACE programs over a 4-year period (1997 to 2001). A number of program characteristics were significantly associated with better functional outcomes: a medical director who was a trained geriatrician, medical directors who spent time providing direct patient care, programs with effective interprofessional teams, teams composed of more aides than professionals, the same ethnicity of participant and team member, and larger and older PACE programs (Mukamel et al., 2007).

A few program characteristics were associated with improved participant self-assessed health outcomes. Specifically, higher staffing levels, having more diverse services, and having a match between the ethnicity of the participant and the staff member were associated with higher self-assessed health outcomes (Mukamel et al., 2007, p. 524).

All three of these models—Guided Care, GRACE, and PACE—provide a comprehensive approach to chronic illness management. In addition to ongoing monitoring of clinical status, these models include important components for addressing the multiple determinants of health. Boult and Wieland (2010) conducted a comparative review of the evidence for these three models of care. They found that the programs offered similar approaches to providing health services to older adults with complex health issues. All three programs include an interprofessional team, a comprehensive

assessment, implementation of and adherence to an evidence-based comprehensive plan of care, ongoing monitoring of the patient's clinical status, coordination of care across sites and specialties, and enhanced access to community-based support services (e.g., transportation, adult day services, exercise programs) (p. 1939).

The GRACE and Guided Care models are not currently covered by state Medicaid, fee-for-service Medicare, or most insurance plans. The costs of these programs are relatively reasonable, with Guided Care costing approximately $1,800 per person per year and GRACE costing approximately $1,000 per person per year. In contrast, PACE is a Medicare- and Medicaid-covered managed care program available in selected states. PACE participants are required to use a primary care provider who is enrolled in the local PACE program. Only low-income elders qualify for both PACE (age 55 and older) and GRACE (age 65 and older). Availability of all of these programs is quite limited. PACE is available in just 31 states and not in all areas of those states where it is provided. Furthermore, those who have chronic illnesses but are not considered low income would not qualify for PACE or GRACE as they are currently designed. The ACA provides incentives for broader testing and implementation of models like these comprehensive care management programs for persons with chronic illnesses (Boult & Weiland, 2010).

Evidence-Based Practice Box

Boult and colleagues (2013) designed a matched-pair cluster-randomized trial of Guided Care versus usual care for high-risk older adults. It was hypothesized that Guided Care would produce better function and higher quality of life, while reducing health costs. The study was 32 months in length and involved eight community-based primary clinics. Using a predictive model, high-risk older adults were identified through fee-for-service

(continues)

Medicare, a Medicare Advantage plan, or Tricare. A registered nurse (RN) collaborated with two to five primary care physicians in providing eight services to participants: comprehensive assessment, evidence-based care planning, proactive monitoring, care coordination, transitional care, coaching for self-management, caregiver support, and access to community-based services.

Functional health was measured using the SF-36, quality of life was measured using the Patient Assessment of Chronic Illness Care tool, and health services utilization was measured by health insurance claims. The authors concluded that Guided Care increased the quality of life in high-risk older adults while reducing the adults' use of home care, but did not appear to improve functional health.

Source: Boult, C., Leff, B., Boyd, C. M., Wolff, J. L., Marsteller, J. A., Frick, K. D., ... Scharfstein, D. O. (2013). A matched-pair cluster randomized trial of Guided Care for high-risk older patients. *Journal of General Internal Medicine, 28*(5), 612–621.

Centers for Medicare and Medicaid Services

Since 1999, several disease management demonstration and pilot programs have been conducted by the CMS for the traditional fee-for-service Medicare program. These programs have included 300,000 beneficiaries in 35 programs (Bott, Kapp, Johnson, & Magno, 2009). Programs ranged in size from 257 in a case management demonstration to 200,000 in Medicare Health Support Organizations. Some programs targeted beneficiaries with specific chronic illnesses, while others focused on high-cost or high-risk beneficiaries regardless of diagnosis, and still others involved a combination of beneficiaries. These disease management programs have been defined as a system of coordinated healthcare interventions and communications for populations with conditions in which patient self-care efforts are significant components of care. Their goal is to improve the health status

of the population, improve satisfaction with the care, and reduce total healthcare costs—net of fees and the programs' implementation costs. A disease management intervention that is effective but increases spending would not be an option to add to traditional Medicare.

Results from the CMS demonstration projects have not shown widespread evidence of improvement in compliance with evidence-based care, satisfaction for providers or beneficiaries, or broad behavior change (Bott et al., 2009, p. 92). Only a few programs have produced financial savings net of fees. Foote (2009) suggests that the CMS needs to develop a new strategy with its demonstration projects. In 2007, CMS healthcare expenditures totaled $418 billion. Given this massive level of spending, the need for CMS to "get it right" cannot be overstated.

While most of the recent discussions about the ACA (passed in 2010) have focused on providing health insurance options for all Americans, the ACA also includes several provisions aimed at reducing costs while improving the quality of health care and, in particular, care for individuals with chronic illnesses. These provisions include an enhanced focus on how care is delivered across the continuum, better access to primary care and community-based services, an increased focus on prevention, better medication management, and improved patient outcomes. Goals of these provisions are to improve care coordination and transitions throughout the continuum and to implement patient- and family-centered models that promote shared decision making among providers, patients, and family caregivers.

To meet the primary aims of the ACA, a Center for Medicare and Medicaid Innovation (the Innovation Center) was established. The Innovation Center's mission is to help transform the Medicare, Medicaid, and Children's Health Insurance Programs (CHIP) to deliver better health care, better health, and reduced costs through improved services for CMS beneficiaries, and in so doing, help to transform the healthcare system for all Americans (Centers for Medicare & Medicaid Innovation, n.d., para 1). The Innovation Center was given flexibility and resources to rapidly test innovative care and payment models and scale up successful models. Innovation models are funded under the following broad categories: (1) accountable care, (2) bundled payment for care improvement, (3) innovations for Medicaid and CHIP, (4) improved care for dually eligible Medicare–Medicaid enrollees, (5) incentives to accelerate the development and testing of new payment and service delivery models, (6) initiatives to speed the adoption of best practices, and (7) primary care transformation. More information about all of these CMS Innovation Center initiatives can be found at http://innovation. cms.gov; they are profiled briefly here.

- Accountable care focuses on improving care through better coordination and transitional care while reducing costs. In this voluntary program, groups of providers, hospitals, and other healthcare organizations (e.g., home health agencies, rehabilitation providers, and nursing homes) join together to form accountable care organizations (ACOs) that accept responsibility for the cost and quality of care delivered to a specific population of patients cared for by the groups' clinicians (Shortell, Casalino, & Fisher, 2010, p. 1293).
- Bundled payment is a model that is designed to cover the costs per episode of care across the continuum. Models are being tested for several illnesses including stroke, chronic obstructive pulmonary disease, congestive heart failure, renal failure, and multiple conditions related to arthritis.
- The innovations focused on the Medicaid and CHIP populations include two areas specifically related to chronic disease. One seeks to provide incentives for Medicaid beneficiaries who participate in prevention programs and demonstrate reductions in health risk behaviors. The other area

focuses on improving psychiatric services for Medicaid beneficiaries with mental illness.
- Initiatives to improve care for recipients of both Medicare and Medicaid (dual eligibles) include better financial alignment of the two programs to improve care coordination and an initiative to reduce avoidable hospitalizations for dual-eligible nursing home residents.
- Across the United States, new service delivery and payment models to improve care coordination and service delivery while reducing costs are being tested. In 2013, 25 states were receiving funding to test improved models of care.
- The Innovation Center is also funding initiatives to improve the implementation of best practices in healthcare delivery. These include community-based care transitions programs for people with chronic illnesses who are at high risk for rehospitalization. As of 2013, there were more than 100 programs funded by this initiative.
- Comprehensive primary care transformation initiatives are aimed at fostering collaboration between public and private healthcare payers to improve primary care. Primary care providers who choose to participate in such an initiative receive incentives for outcomes reflecting better care coordination. In particular, this initiative includes the patient-centered medical home (PCMH) that is being widely implemented across the United States.

Patient-Centered Medical Homes

The patient-centered medical home model builds on the chronic care model by providing a more comprehensive approach to primary care. The PMCH emphasizes a team approach to care that is patient centered with a focus on care coordination, communication, and improved patient outcomes (National Committee for Quality Assurance [NCQA], n.d.; Williams et al., 2012). This model has also been referred to as a patient-centered healthcare home in an effort to expand the focus beyond medical care to a broader definition of health with a focus on the multiple determinants of health. While most of the research uses the term PCMH, implementation of the PCMH in many cases includes components focusing on other determinants of health.

The American Academy of Pediatrics (AAP) first used the term *medical home* in 1967 to refer to "single centralized source of care and medical record" for children with special needs (Williams et al., 2012, p. 1). Over the past several decades, the AAP, along with the American Academy of Family Physicians, the American College of Physicians, and the American Osteopathic Association, have refined the concept and expanded it to the care of all patients. There is widespread agreement that primary care is in crisis. Patients are not satisfied with their care, and purchasers and insurers are disappointed with its cost and quality. There are many highly effective primary care practices, but many others are poorly organized and not able to provide timely, quality care (Cassidy, 2010; Williams et al., 2012). Fifty percent of all patients do not understand what their primary care physician is telling them because visits are too short and do not allow patients any time to ask questions. Coordination among primary care physicians, specialists, and hospitals is often lacking, and each may be unaware of the others' treatment plans (Cassidy, 2010). Many believe that the PCMH can address these issues. Although initially focused on the physician–patient relationship, this concept has evolved to emphasize team-based care.

As defined by the four medical societies, the PCMH includes four cornerstones: primary care, patient-centered care, new-model practice, and payment reform. In the PCMH model, *primary care* is "comprehensive, first-contact, acute, chronic, and preventive care across the life span, delivered by a team led by the patient's primary care provider" (Rittenhouse & Shortell, 2009, p. 2038). It also includes care coordination across the continuum of care. Care in the PCMH is *patient centered*, with care being tailored to the preferences and goals of patients and their families. In a PCMH, communication between providers and patients should facilitate patients' engagement in decisions about all aspects of their care and access to information should be readily available. The implementation of electronic health records with patient portals is a key component in meeting this standard. The PCMH focuses on a *new model of practice* where evidence should drive care decisions and patient safety, transparency, and accountability are paramount (p. 2039). Finally, the *payment structure* in a PCMH combines fee-for-service with payment for high-quality performance. PCMHs also receive additional funds for care coordination activities (Rittenhouse & Shortell, 2009).

While no one set of specific criteria exists to identify medical homes, many states have developed their criteria based on the joint principles and cornerstones agreed to by the four medical societies. The National Committee for Quality Assurance (http://www.ncqa.org) developed the standards for PCMHs in parallel with the four medical societies' efforts. The NCQA sees the medical home concept as strengthening the provider–patient relationship and replacing episodic care with coordinated care. It has developed standards in six areas for evaluating PCMHs:

1. Access and continuity of care
2. Managing patient populations
3. Planning and managing care
4. Enhancing self-management and linking to community resources
5. Coordinating care
6. Measuring and improving performance (NCQA, 2012)

The NCQA's standards and corresponding measures generally focus on assessment of clinical status and infrastructure. According to Rittenhouse and Shortell (2009), other standards and measures that focus on the patient experience are still needed. Another challenge is that the term "medical home" may be confusing and create some resistance. Also, the idea of the primary care provider as a "gatekeeper" to access to specialty care is an issue. Finally, there are likely to be upfront costs to set up the appropriate infrastructures to make PCMHs successful in the long term; as a consequence, cost savings may not be immediately apparent (Rittenhouse & Shortell, 2009).

A health policy brief issued by *Health Affairs* in September 2010 identified more than 100 demonstration projects testing the effectiveness of PCMHs (Cassidy, 2010). Additionally, 31 states are planning or implementing medical home pilots within Medicaid or CHIP, and at least 12 states have developed medical home initiatives that involve multiple payers. One fifth of medical homes recognized by the NCQA are sole practices, although it is much more common for large practices to serve as medical homes (Abrams, Schor, & Schoenbaum, 2010).

TransforMed, funded by the American Academy of Family Physicians, launched a 24-month project in June 2006 through May 2008, involving 36 family medicine practices across the United States. The practices were small, independent practices that wished to become PCMHs. Practices were randomized into "facilitated intervention" and "self-directed" (Nutting, Crabtree, Miller, Stange, Stewart, & Jaen, 2011). Findings from the project revealed that practices made

> *heroic efforts and attempted to implement as many model components as possible over the two-year life of the project.... Many of the chronic care and health IT components may be implemented by highly motivated practices. Nevertheless, even with extensive assistance from their facilitator, the availability of expert consultation, and the incentive of being in a national spotlight, two years was not long enough to implement the entire model and to transform work processes. (Nutting et al., 2011, p. 440)*

Interestingly, the article assessing this project seems to be more focused on the processes involved rather than the patients. Isn't the end result of medical homes better patient outcomes? A systematic review of 85 studies on PCMH found "moderately strong evidence that PCMH improves patient experiences and preventive care services" (Williams et al., 2012, p. 14). The evidence also "suggests benefit" for staff experiences with PCMH. In addition, the research indicates the use of PCMHs may reduce patients' use of inpatient hospital and emergency department services, although it does not affect total costs. Overall, Williams et al. concluded that many of the studies addressing PCMHs were under-powered and more research is needed on the impact of PCMHs.

Self-Management Programs

The term *self-management* initially appeared in a book by Thomas Creer on the rehabilitation of children with chronic illness (Lorig & Holman, 2003). Creer and colleagues used the concept to indicate that the patient was an active participant in his or her own care. According to Creer and Holroyd (2006), self-management differs from adherence in that "self-management places greater emphasis on the patient's active role in decision-making, both inside and outside the consultation room" (p. 8). Self-management is also seen as different from disease management. Creer and Holroyd view disease management as being more focused on healthcare professionals' algorithms and interventions to standardize care as opposed to self-management, which emphasizes patients' involvement in defining the problems.

Lorig and her colleagues implemented a self-management model of care at Stanford in 1999. Lorig's early work is based on Corbin and Strauss's (1992) framework of medical management, role management, and emotional management, and more recently has integrated social learning theory and self-efficacy (Bandura, 1977). Her framework for self-management programs includes "five core self-management skills: problem solving, decision making, resource utilization, forming of a patient–healthcare provider partnership, and taking action" (Lorig & Holman, 2003, p. 2).

Empirical results of self-management programs have been mixed. What follows are examples taken from the literature in this area.

- In one of her early studies, Lorig and colleagues (1999) studied 952 patients, 40 years of age and older, with a diagnosis of heart disease, lung disease, stroke, or arthritis, in a 6-month-long RCT. The Chronic Disease Self-Management Program (CDSMP) consisted of seven weekly 2.5-hour sessions on making management choices and achieving success in reaching self-selected goals as opposed to prescribing specific behavior changes (p. 7). Outcome measures included health behaviors, health status, and health service utilization. At 6 months, the experimental group demonstrated improvements in weekly minutes of exercise, frequency of cognitive symptom management, communication with physicians, and self-reported health. Participants also had decreased fatigue and disability and fewer social/role-activity limitations with less health distress, fatigue, and disability. There were no differences between the groups in pain/physical discomfort, shortness of breath, or psychological well-being (p. 5).
- In a more recent study of the CDSMP, researchers, using data from previous CDSMPs delivered in English and Spanish, examined whether there were statistically significant interactions between baseline status and randomization in estimating 6-month changes in health status (Ritter, Lee, & Lorig, 2011). The results demonstrated no moderating factors that consistently predicted improved health outcomes.
- In 2013, Lorig and her colleagues reported on the effectiveness of the CDSMP in addressing the main aims of the ACA. This analysis included longitudinal data over 12 months from 22 organizations in 17 states with 1,170 enrolled participants; 825 patients completed the 12-month follow-up. Participants' diagnoses included diabetes, asthma, COPD, arthritis, and cancer. Almost one third of the patients had four or more chronic conditions. At 12 months, participants had better health outcomes as evidenced by reduced fatigue, pain, and depressive symptoms, and improved provider communication and health literacy. They also reported a perception of better value from their health care. Emergency department visits were reduced at 6 and 12 months. Hospital visits were less frequent at 6 months, but there were no differences at 12 months (Ory et al., 2013). The reduction in hospital use resulted in a net cost savings of "$364 per participant and a national savings of $3.3 billion if 5% of adults with one of more chronic condition" received the same intervention (Ahn et al., 2013, p. 1).

Chodosh and colleagues (2005) assessed the effectiveness of self-management programs through a meta-analysis. Of the 780 studies screened, 53 met the researchers' criteria for inclusion. Self-management interventions led to statistically and clinically significant results of decreased HgbA$_{1c}$ (a decrease of 0.81%), a decrease of 5 mm Hg in systolic blood pressure, and a decrease of 4.3 mm Hg in diastolic blood pressure. There were no significant results for participants with osteoarthritis in either pain or function. The researchers concluded that the studies had variable quality, making it difficult to analyze them, and publication bias may have been present (pp. 435–436). In addition, it was not clear what constituted a self-management program.

A Cochrane review of self-management programs, led by lay leaders, was completed in 2007 (Foster, Taylor, Eldridge, Ramsay, & Griffiths, 2007). The review included 17 studies that enrolled 7,442 individuals with chronic conditions such as arthritis, diabetes, hypertension, and chronic pain. Many of the programs were similar, but they differed in the conditions that they addressed and the outcomes that each researcher reported. Overall, the programs led to modest short-term improvements in patients' confidence in managing their condition and perceptions of their own health. Increases in the amount of aerobic exercise by participants were observed. While some improvements in pain, disability, fatigue, and depression were noted, the changes were not clinically significant. The programs did not improve quality of life for the individuals, alter the number of doctor visits for these individuals, or reduce hospitalizations.

Population- and Community-Based Models for Disease Prevention

The National Center for Chronic Disease Prevention and Health Promotion (NCCDPHP) of the Centers for Disease Control and Prevention (CDC) is designated as the United States' lead agency for preventing chronic disease and promoting health. NCCDPHP supports translation of research into practice and has ongoing programs focused on prevention of cancer, diabetes, heart disease and stroke, and other chronic diseases. Examples of two of its initiatives focusing on improving the health of the U.S. population are the Million Hearts and WISEWOMAN programs.

The goal of the Million Hearts program is to prevent 1 million heart attacks and strokes by 2017 (CDC, 2012) by building partnerships across federal agencies and with private-sector organizations such as the American Heart Association and the YMCA. The initiative aims to improve access to and quality of care, focus attention of clinical caregivers on prevention of cardiovascular disease, activate the public to adopt heart healthy lifestyles, and improve adherence to medication regimens aimed at preventing heart attacks and stroke. Clinical prevention efforts focus on the ABCS: appropriate aspirin therapy, blood pressure control, cholesterol management, and smoking cessation (CDC, 2012). While not a typical "model of care" as described elsewhere in this chapter, this approach to prevention is more broadly based and recognizes that improving population health requires a multitiered, systematic model that includes population-, community-, and individual-based approaches to prevention.

Another CDC program, WISEWOMAN, aims to prevent cardiovascular disease in low-income women across the United States through improved screening and interventions focused on behavior change. In the WISEWOMAN model, women receive blood pressure, cholesterol, and diabetes screening. They also have access to exercise and nutrition resources, such as healthy cooking classes, walking clubs, lifestyle counseling, and referrals to smoking cessation programs as needed. The CDC funded 21 of these community-based programs through state health departments and tribal organizations. To date, more than 40 research publications have focused on the WISEWOMAN project.

In a randomized controlled study of 1,093 Latina woman in California, those who were assigned to the WISEWOMAN program reported higher levels of moderate and vigorous exercise (Coleman et al., 2012). In another study of the same California program, those women who were randomly assigned to WISEWOMAN reported improved eating and exercise habits, and had significantly decreased their 10-year cardiovascular disease risk as compared to the usual-care group (Hayshi, Farrell, Chaput, Rocha, & Hernandez, 2010). In a review of five of the WISEWOMAN programs, researchers identified 87 best practices for lifestyle interventions to reduce cardiovascular disease risk factors. The authors developed an evidence-based toolkit which outlines these best practices (available online at http://www.mathematica-mpr.com/publications/PDFs/wisewomantoolkit.pdf) (Besulides, Zaveri, & Hanson, 2007).

Models like WISEWOMAN have demonstrated improved outcomes, but sustainability of such programs are often an issue. If the federal funding runs out, state and local organizations may not be able to provide ongoing support.

Transitional Care

Naylor, Aiken, Kurtzman, Olds, and Hirschman (2011) conducted a systematic review of the literature and summarized 21 randomized controlled trials of transitional care interventions targeting adults with chronic illness. Transitional care is defined as a broad range of time-limited services designed to ensure healthcare continuity, avoid preventable poor outcomes among at-risk populations, and promote the safe and timely transfer of patients from one level of care to another or from one type of setting to another (Coleman & Boult, 2003). Transitions have been associated with increased rates of potentially avoidable hospitalizations. A 2009 study reported that approximately 20% of Medicare beneficiaries discharged from hospitals were rehospitalized within 30 days and that 34% were readmitted within 90 days (Jencks, Williams, & Coleman, 2009).

A review of transitional care (Naylor et al., 2011) identified 21 studies focusing on adults with chronic illnesses transitioning from an acute care hospital to another setting. There was a mean sample size of 377 subjects among the studies. A variety of primary and secondary outcomes in five categories were reported: health outcomes, quality of life, patient satisfaction or perception of care, resource use, and costs. Among the 21 studies, all but one reported positive findings in at least one category (p. 749).

The 21 interventions discussed in these studies varied in terms of their nature, point of initiation, intensity, and duration (Naylor et al., 2011). The largest group of studies could be characterized as comprehensive discharge planning and follow-up with (4 studies) or without (3 studies) home visits. The remainder dealt with disease or case management (4 studies), education or psychoeducation (2 studies),

peer support (2 studies), telehealth facilitation (1 study), postdischarge geriatric assessment (1 study), and intensive primary care (1 study) (p. 749). Eighteen of the studies designated a nurse—most frequently an advanced practice nurse (10 studies)—as the intervention's clinical manager or leader. A variety of primary and secondary outcomes in five categories were reported. Overall, the authors concluded that a robust body of evidence supports the benefits of transitional care. Studies of 9 interventions demonstrated a positive effect on at least one measure of readmissions; 8 of the 9 interventions reduced all-cause readmission through at least 30 days after discharge (p. 751). Three studies effectively reduced readmissions for at least 6 or 12 months after discharge. Each of these three studies included a focus on patient self-management (Naylor et al., 2011).

Another systematic review of hospital-to-home transitional care programs, which included 17 published randomized controlled trials, explored whether the studies included patients who were at the highest risk for rehospitalization (Piraino, Heckman, Glenny, & Stolee, 2012). High risk was defined as having two or more chronic conditions, polypharmacy, cognitive impairment, depression, inadequate social support, or advanced nonmalignant diseases. The review included studies from the United States, Europe, Canada, and Asia. The authors found that only three of the studies targeted patients with two or more chronic conditions; two others reported the number of comorbidities for participants. Only one study targeted patients taking two or more medications, although three others reported the number of medications taken by participants. Cognitive impairment or dementia represented exclusion criteria in one of the studies. Only one study reported on both cognitive and depressive symptoms. More than half of the studies (9) included patients who lived alone. Finally, patients who had limited life expectancy (less than 6 months) or those receiving palliative or hospice care were excluded in 10 studies. The authors concluded that transitional care programs can reduce rehospitalizations in the populations studied, but that those persons who are at highest risk for rehospitalization may not be adequately represented in these studies and more research is needed on transitional care interventions for these high-risk patients.

Section 3026 of the ACA establishes the Community-Based Care Transitions Program (Naylor et al., 2011), which could help to address this issue. The program provides $500 million from 2011 to 2015 to health systems and community organizations that provide at least one transitional care intervention to high-risk Medicare beneficiaries. For more information about this program, see https://www.cms.gov/Medicare/Demonstration-Projects/DemoProjectsEvalRpts/downloads/CCTP_Solicitation.pdf (CMS, n.d.).

Home- and Community-Based Medicare–Medicaid Waiver Programs

Under federally funded home- and community-based Medicare–Medicaid Waiver initiatives, managed long-term services and support programs (MLTSS) were implemented across several states. The goal of these comprehensive managed care programs was to provide a community-based option for low-income elders and persons with disabilities, many of whom qualified for nursing home level of care. As of 2012, approximately 389,000 persons were receiving services under these waiver programs in 16 states. It was expected that 26 states would implement a MLTSS programs by 2014 (Saucier, Kasten, Burwell, & Gold, 2012). All of the programs operate as managed care organizations, receiving a fixed per-member, per-month premium from Medicaid and sometimes Medicare at a rate that is negotiated annually. These programs can be quite comprehensive in nature, usually providing an array of services including nursing, behavioral health, primary and acute care, and prescription drugs. Coverage levels vary by state and by program. All covered services, care management, and administrative costs are paid for and managed through the monthly payment. The cornerstone of these programs is a care management model that links home- and community-based services, acute care, and long-term care with the assistance of an interprofessional team (Saucier et al., 2012). The PACE program, described earlier in this chapter, is funded through this waiver. Another example of this type of program is described next.

VNSNY CHOICE PROGRAM

The Visiting Nurse Service of New York (VNSNY) CHOICE is a comprehensive Medicare–Medicaid waiver program that began in 1998 as a nursing home diversion program. It operates under a contract with the New York State Department of Health and is licensed by the state as a managed care organization. Clients enrolled in the program work with their nurse care manager to develop an individualized care plan that meets the client's goals. The average VNS CHOICE member is 81 years old, female, and lives either with a family member or alone. Most members speak English, Spanish, or Chinese. The average member has 3.6 chronic illnesses, with the most common being hypertension, diabetes, osteoarthritis and related disorders, and heart disease (Dehm & McCabe, 2007).

The VNS CHOICE program is very comprehensive and provides the following services: care coordination; nursing care; personal care; 24/7 support line; medication management; chore and housekeeping services; transportation to appointments; home-delivered meals; nutritional counseling; adult day services; medical equipment and supplies; home safety modifications; prosthetics; dental, eye, and foot care; hearing exams and aids; and nursing home care. The program contracts with area physicians to provide primary care (VNSNY, 2013).

Distance Chronic Disease Management Programs

Throughout the rural areas of the United States, access to face-to-face disease management programs is not possible. Thus, distance programs, whether by telephone or through the Internet, have been developed that better provide services to patients and families

Telehealth Disease Management

The Veterans Administration operates one of the largest integrated telehealth programs in the United States, providing case management and care coordination for more than 490,000 veterans with chronic illnesses. The goal of the VA telehealth program is to facilitate access to care and improve health outcomes through better care management. The VA uses home telehealth devices to collect data from veterans in their homes and link these data to the VA electronic medical record. VA clinicians monitor the clinical data and connect directly with the program participants to manage chronic conditions such as diabetes, congestive heart failure, depression, post-traumatic stress disorder, and chronic obstructive pulmonary disease. They also use clinic-based telehealth to connect primary care providers in rural outreach clinics to specialists in large VA system hospitals and clinics. This reduces long travel times for veterans who do not live close to a larger VA medical center (Darkins, Foster, Anderson, Goldschmidt, & Selvin, 2013).

In a study of more than 98,000 veterans enrolled in the VA's mental telehealth program, hospitalization rates decreased by 25% after the program was implemented (Godleski, Darkins, & Peters, 2012). In another descriptive study of veterans enrolled in the VA home telehealth program between 2003 and 2007, hospital utilization data were compared 1 year prior to enrollment in the program with data 6 months postenrollment. In the postenrollment period, a 19.74% reduction in hospital admissions was observed. The program costs approximately $1,600 per year per patient to administer (Darkins et al., 2008).

In a diabetes disease management program, researchers used the telephone to provide an educational intervention to a randomized sample of 1,220 Medicare+Choice recipients older than

age 65 in Ohio, Kentucky, and Indiana (Berg & Wadhwa, 2007). There were 610 intervention group members matched to a control group with the same number of members. The disease management program used a structured, evidence-based telephonic nursing intervention to provide patient education, counseling, and monitoring services. The self-management intervention plan included risk stratification, formal scheduled nurse education sessions, 24-hour access to a nurse counseling and symptom advice telephone line, printed action plans, workbooks, medication compliance and vaccination reminders, physician alerts, and signs and symptoms of complications. The participants in the study were high users of services, with hospitalization rates of 605 per 1,000 intervention group members and 612 per 1,000 control group members. Emergency room visit rates were also high, 700 per 1,000 in both groups during the baseline period (p. 230). The groups were well matched and could be assumed to consist of moderately ill to severely ill older adults with diabetes. The intervention group had significantly lower rates of acute service utilization compared with the control group: 23.8% increase in angiotensin-converting enzyme (ACE) inhibitor use, 13.3% increase in blood glucose regulator use, 11.8% increase in $HgbA_{1c}$ testing, 10.3% increase in lipid panel testing, 26% increase in eye exams, and 35.5% increase in microalbumin tests (p. 226).

Another study used the telephone for disease management directed toward patients with heart failure (Smith, Hughes-Cromwick, Forkner, & Galbreath, 2008). This study examined the cost-effectiveness of the approach versus the patient outcomes. Adult subjects with documented systolic heart failure or diastolic heart failure ($n = 1,069$) were randomized into one of three study groups: usual care, disease management, or augmented disease management. Subjects in the intervention arms were assigned a disease manager who was an RN; the disease manager performed patient education and medication management in conjunction with the patient's primary care provider for the full 18 months of the study. Subjects in the augmented disease management group also received in-home devices for enhanced self-monitoring. The data gathered via these devices were electronically transmitted to the disease manager. Although the program produced statistically significant survival advantages among all patients, analyses of direct and intervention costs showed no cost savings associated with the intervention. It also did not reduce healthcare utilization of the subjects (Smith et al., 2008).

Virtual Models of Disease Management

A retrospective, quasi-experimental cohort design evaluated program participants in an online disease management program (through Blue Cross Blue Shield) with a matched cohort of nonparticipants (Schwartz, Day, Wildenhaus, Silberman, Wang, & Silberman, 2010). The study was conducted with 413 online participants and 360 nonparticipants. The online program was a commercially available, tailored program for chronic disease self-management. Healthcare costs per person per year were $757 less than predicted for participants relative to matched nonparticipants, yielding a return on investment of $9.89 for every $1.00 spent on the program.

With the increasing use of smartphones, iPads, and other handheld mobile devices, the applications (apps) that individuals can use on their mobile phones or other devices to monitor and manage their chronic illnesses are expected to proliferate rapidly. Known as mHealth (mobile health), these interventions enable individuals with chronic illnesses to engage in self-monitoring activities and to report symptoms and clinical data directly to their healthcare providers through the electronic health record. The U.S. Department of Health and Human (DHHS) Services set up a "Text4Health Task Force" to encourage the development of mHealth technologies. Multiple funding initiatives are also available for development of mHealth programs (DHHS, n.d.). Interventions are currently being tested in the areas of obesity prevention and weight management, asthma self-management, medication adherence, diabetes, HIV/AIDS, and fibromyalgia.

In a systematic review of four randomized controlled trials including 182 participants, researchers found that "in certain cases mobile phone messaging interventions may provide benefit in supporting the self-management of long-term illnesses" (de Jongh, Gurol-Urganci, Vodopivec-Jamsek, Car, & Atun, 2012, p. 2). While the literature on these mobile interventions is limited, this will be an area of increasing focus and importance in the future.

Other Models

PATIENT ADVOCACY CASE MANAGEMENT

Service use and costs were examined in eight studies using the patient advocacy case management model of care with frail older adults or those with chronic illness. Results from the systematic review indicated that this model of care did not increase service use and costs, and was effective in decreasing service use and costs in two studies (Oeseburg, Wynia, Middel, & Reijneveld, 2009).

COLLABORATIVE CARE

A single-blind RCT involving 214 participants in 14 primary care clinics was conducted in the state of Washington. Patients were randomly assigned to the usual-care group or to the intervention group, in which a medically supervised nurse, working with each patient's primary care physician, provided guideline-based collaborative care management with the goal of controlling risk factors for chronic disease (Katon et al., 2010). The primary outcomes were lower HgbA$_{1c}$, low-density lipoprotein (LDL) cholesterol, and systolic blood pressure levels, and measurement of scores from the Symptom Checklist-20, a tool for detecting depression. Compared with the control group, patients in the intervention group had greater overall 12-month improvement across HgbA$_{1c}$, LDL cholesterol, systolic blood pressure, and the Symptom Checklist-20.

Shared Care

Smith, Allwright, and O'Dowd (2007) completed a systematic review of "shared care" for the Cochrane Database. These authors considered "shared care" to be the combined management or joint participation of primary care physicians and specialty care physicians in planning the delivery of care for a client. Twenty studies were identified for chronic disease management, with 19 of them being RCTs. The results were mixed. The authors concluded that there was insufficient evidence to demonstrate significant benefits from shared care, apart from improving prescribing medications.

Patient-Centered or Family-Centered Care

Many of the models described in this chapter include a goal of being patient-centered, which generally means that treatment plans and care decisions should be tailored to the patient's needs and preferences, and that healthcare professionals should use strategies to help patients become actively engaged in decisions about their care. This is a very important component of models of care designed to manage chronic illnesses, but it should be expanded to include a family-centered approach. In most instances, patients with chronic illnesses are living with and often receiving assistance from family members. These family members may help with basic and/or instrumental activities of daily living. They may responsible for implementing the chronic illness management strategies, but their needs and preferences often are not considered, nor are they explicitly included in the decision-making process. When we look to the future and decide which models of care are most appropriate for which groups of patients, we need to understand that patients are usually part of a larger family unit and the needs and preferences of that unit must be considered. Even the most independent patients often want and need to have family members involved in decisions regarding their care and treatments.

Outcomes

With any model of care for individuals with chronic conditions and their families, an expected outcome is that both the disease and the illness experience are managed appropriately and some cost savings are realized. Most of the models described in this chapter include some form of case management, most often led by a nurse care manager. The more comprehensive models include interprofessional teams who collaborate with patients, and sometimes their families, to identify their health-related goals and address their chronic illness needs. Research to date has demonstrated mixed results for the models currently in practice. It remains unclear how the U.S. health system should be organized to provide care for those persons with chronic illness. Because older adults are more likely to be affected by chronic illness, CMS has been at the forefront in developing programs or models of care through its demonstration projects. So far, there is not substantive evidence to definitively state which models provide the best outcomes. Are PCMHs the answer? Or should the focus be on more comprehensive care management strategies? Only time will tell if these entities make a difference.

What is not "measured" in these models is how the programs or models of care affect the illness experience of the individual and family. Can we say that because an individual with a chronic illness has a lower HgbA$_{1c}$, or has not been hospitalized within the last 6 months, or checks his blood glucose level regularly, has a better quality of life or experiences more life satisfaction, or—in the terms of Strauss and colleagues (1984)—is successful at normalizing his life?

CASE STUDY 19-1

Sam White is an 85-year-old retired farmer. He has a history of high blood pressure, mild congestive heart failure, chronic bronchitis, and diabetes. He lives with his daughter, Jean, who is 60 years old, divorced, and is caring for her two elementary school–aged grandchildren because their parents are unable to care for them. Jean works in the local fast-food restaurant. She gets off work in time to pick up her grandchildren from school.

Until recently, Sam was independent and able to help Jean care for the children after school and on weekends. Over the past several months, however, Sam's health has deteriorated. He had a stroke and spent 2 weeks in an inpatient rehabilitation hospital. He was recently discharged from the hospital and now needs assistance with dressing, meal preparation, and walking, and he seems depressed. He also has some issues with incontinence, and Jean has to help him to the bathroom.

Jean has been on family medical leave from her job, but she feels she must return to work because she needs the income. Jean has high blood pressure and was recently diagnosed with diabetes. Jean does not know how she will manage both her illnesses and her father's new limitations, but she does not want to place her father in a nursing home. The children are enrolled in the state's children's health insurance program because Jean cannot afford her company's health insurance program. She qualifies for the new government-sponsored health insurance program, but she is confused about her options. She spoke with the local Area Agency on Aging and found out that there were several programs offered in her area. The three that sounded the most helpful were Guided Care, GRACE, and PACE, but she does not know anything about them. She just knows she needs to get some help for her own health care and in caring for her father.

Discussion Questions

1. What are the things that Jean needs to think about as she explores the healthcare options in her area?
2. What are some questions Jean should ask about each of these programs?
3. Which program would best fit Jean's own healthcare needs? Which one might be best for her father?
4. What are the advantages and disadvantages of each program?
5. Which options should Jean consider if none of the three programs were available in her area?

CASE STUDY 19-2

Mary Brown is an 80-year-old widow living alone on her farm 5 miles from town in a western rural state. The town, with a population of 10,000, has a critical access hospital. Mary lives in the farmhouse to which she moved when she married 60 years ago. She would like to stay there as long as possible, but after her hip replacement surgery last fall, her mobility is not as good as it used to be. She is mildly hypertensive and is on medication. Her type 2 diabetes is under control with diet and medication. Mary has lots of friends in the community, but her grown children live several states away. Because of her isolation and age, she might be considered "at risk."

Discussion Questions

1. What are Mary's "at-risk" variables?
2. Which self-management tasks should be initiated with her?
3. What does Mary need? What are her potential needs? This is a small community with few resources available. Be creative and develop a model of care for her.

CASE STUDY 19-3

Maria Alvarez is a 55-year-old single woman, living alone in low-income housing in an impoverished area of a large city. There are 300 residents living in the housing complex; they include seniors and adults with disabilities from varied ethnic backgrounds and cultures. The only primary care clinic that serves these residents is a public health department across town. Most of the residents use public transportation to get to the clinic, which takes approximately 90 minutes travel time.

Maria was recently diagnosed with high blood pressure and type 2 diabetes. Her mobility is impaired due arthritis, and she has been treated for depression in the past. In addition to medications, Maria's primary care provider recommended several lifestyle changes for her, including changing her diet and increasing her exercise. Many of the other residents living in Maria's complex have similar chronic health concerns. Most of them are living on very low incomes and often have difficulty buying food and paying their utilities each month.

You are a public health nursing supervisor designated to provide services to Maria's neighborhood. Your director just let you know that the health department plans to apply for federal funding to implement a chronic illness management program to meet the needs of the residents in Maria's neighborhood. She has asked you to write a proposal to develop the best evidence-based program for the residents.

Discussion Questions

Considering the models discussed in this chapter:
1. Which might be the best program (or programs) for a neighborhood like Maria's?
2. What are the advantages and disadvantages of each program for the residents?
3. How might you tailor a program to best meet the residents' needs?
4. What are some things you should consider when designing the program?
5. Who are the key stakeholders you should include when designing the program?

STUDY QUESTIONS

1. What are the benefits of disease management models of care?
2. Identify the issues involved with a disease management model of care for an older adult.
3. How do we as nurses care for individuals and families and their *illness experiences* within a disease management model?
4. After reading about the different models of care in this chapter, what do you think should be included in a model of care for an older adult with multiple comorbidities?
5. Where does the family fit into these models of care?
6. How do self-management components of care fit within a disease management program?
7. Which role does (or should) the advanced practice nurse have in disease management?
8. How will technological advancements influence chronic illness management?

Internet Resources

Chronic Disease Self-Management Program, Stanford University: http://patienteducation.stanford.edu/programs/cdsmp.html

CMS Innovation Center: http://innovation.cms.gov/

Commonwealth Fund: http://www.commonwealthfund.org

GRACE: http://medicine.iupui.edu/iucar/research/grace/

Guided Care: www.guidedcare.org

Improving Chronic Illness Care: www.improvingchronic-care.org

Institute for Patient and Family-Centered Care: http://www.ipfcc.org/

NCQA Patient-Centered Medical Home: http://www.ncqa.org/Programs/Recognition/PatientCenteredMedicalHomePCMH.aspx

PACE: http://www.medicare.gov/Nursing/Alternatives/Pace.asp

References

Abrams, M., Schor, E. L., & Schoenbaum, S. (2010). How physician practices could share personnel and resources to support medical homes. *Health Affairs*, 29(6), 1194–1199.

Ahn, S., Basu, R., Smith, M. L., Jiang, L., Lorig, K., Whitelaw, N., & Ory, M. G. (2013). The impact of chronic disease self-management programs: Healthcare savings through a community-based intervention. *BMC Public Health*, 2013(13), 1–6. http://www.biomedcentral.com/content/pdf/1471-2458-13-1141.pdf

Bandura, A. (1977). Self-efficacy: Toward a unifying theory of behavioral change. *Psychological Review*, 84(2), 191–215.

Berg, G. D., & Wadhwa, S. (2007). Health services outcomes for a diabetes disease management program for the elderly. *Disease Management*, 10(4), 226–234.

Besculides, M., Zaveri, H., & Hanson, C. (2007). WISEWOMAN best practices toolkit: Lessons learned from selected projects. http://www.mathematica-mpr.com/publications/PDFs/wisewomantoolkit.pdf

Bodenheimer, T. (2003). Interventions to improve chronic care: Evaluating their effectiveness. *Disease Management*, 6(2), 63–71.

Bott, D. M., Kapp, M. C., Johnson, L. B., & Magno, L. M. (2009). Disease management for chronically ill beneficiaries in traditional Medicare. *Health Affairs*, 28(1), 86–98.

Boult, C., Leff, B., Boyd, C. M., Wolff, J. L., Marsteller, J. A., Frick, K. D., ... Scharfstein, D. O. (2013). A matched-pair cluster randomized trial of guided care for high-risk older patients. *Journal of General Internal Medicine, 28*(5), 612–621. http://link.springer.com /article/10.1007/s11606-012-2287-y#page-1

Boult, C., Reider, L., Frey, K., Leff, B., Boyd, C. M., Wolff, J. L., ... Scharfstein, D.O. (2008). Early effects of "guided care" on the quality of health care for multi-morbid older persons: A cluster-randomized controlled trial. *Journal of Gerontology: Medical Sciences, 73A*(3), 321–327.

Boult, C., Reider, L., Leff, B., Frick, K. D., Boyd, C. M., Wolff, J. L., ... Scharfstein, D.O. (2011). The effect of guided care teams on the use of health services: Results from a cluster-randomized controlled trial. *Archives of Internal Medicine, 171*(5), 460–466.

Boult, C., & Weiland, G. D. (2010). Comprehensive primary care for older patients with multiple chronic conditions: "Nobody rushes you through." *Journal of the American Medical Association, 304*(17), 1936–1943.

Boyd, C. M., Boult, C., Shadmi, E., Leff, B., Brager, R., Dunbar, L., ... Wegener, S. (2007). Guided care for multimorbid older adults. *The Gerontologist, 47*(5), 697–704.

Buntin, M. B., Jain, A. K., Mattke, S., & Lurie, N. (2009). Who gets disease management? *Journal of General Internal Medicine, 24*(5), 649–655.

Cassidy, A. (2010). Patient-centered medical homes: A new way to deliver primary care may be more affordable and improve quality—but how widely adopted will the model be? *Health Affairs.* http://healthaffairs. org/healthpolicybriefs/brief_pdfs/healthpolicybrief _25.pdf

Centers for Disease Control and Prevention (CDC). (2012). Million Hearts. http://millionhearts.hhs.gov /aboutmh/overview.html

Centers for Medicare and Medicaid Innovation. (n.d.). About the Innovation Center. http://innovations.cms.gov

Centers for Medicare and Medicaid Services (CMS). (2012). Chronic conditions among Medicare beneficiaries. *Chartbook, 2012.* Baltimore, MD: Author.

Centers for Medicare and Medicaid Services (CMS). (n.d.). Solicitation for applications: Community-based care transitions program. https://www.cms.gov/Medicare/ Demonstration-Projects/DemoProjectsEvalRpts/down-loads/CCTP_Solicitation.pdf

Chodosh, J., Morton, S. C., Mojica, W., Maglione, M., Suttorp, M. J., Hilton, L., ... Shekelle, P. (2005). Meta-analysis: Chronic disease self-management programs for older adults. *Annals of Internal Medicine, 143,* 427–438.

Coleman, E. A., & Boult, C. (2003). Improving the quality of transitional care for persons with complex care needs. *Journal of the American Geriatrics Society, 51*(4), 556–557.

Coleman, K., Austin, B. T., Brach, C., & Wagner, E. H. (2009). Evidence on the chronic care model in the new millennium. *Health Affairs, 28*(1), 75–85.

Coleman, K. J., Farrell, M. A., Rocha, D. A., Hayashi, T., Hernandez, M., Wolf, J., & Lindsay, S. (2012). Readiness to be physically active and self-reported physical activity in low-income Latinas, California: WISEWOMAN, 2006–2007. *Preventing Chronic Disease, 9,* 1–8. http://www.ncbi.nlm.nih.gov.lp.hscl. ufl.edu/pmc/articles/PMC3406743/pdf/PCD-9-E87 .pdf

Congressional Budget Office (CBO). (2012). Lessons from Medicare's demonstration projects on disease management, care coordination, and value-based payment. http://www.cbo.gov/publication/42860

Corbin, J., & Strauss, A. (1992). A nursing model for chronic illness management based upon the trajectory framework. In P. Woog (Ed.), *The chronic illness trajectory framework: The Corbin and Strauss nursing model* (pp. 9–28). New York, NY: Springer.

Counsell, S. R., Callahan, C. M., Buttar, A. B., Clark, D. O., & Frank, K. I. (2006). Geriatric Resources for Assessment of Care of Elders (GRACE): A new model of primary care of low-income seniors. *Journal of the American Geriatric Society, 54,* 1136–1141.

Counsell, S. R., Callahan, C. M., Clark, D. O., Tu, W., Buttar, A. B., Stump, T. E., & Ricketts, G. D. (2007). Geriatric care management for low-income seniors: A randomized controlled trial. *Journal of the American Medical Association, 298*(2), 2623–2633.

Creer, T., & Holroyd, K. A. (2006). Self-management of chronic conditions: The legacy of Sir William Osler. *Chronic Illness, 2,* 7–14.

Dall, T. M., Roary, M., Yanag, W., Zhanag, S., Zhang, S., Chen, Y. J., ... Zhang, Y. (2010). Health care use and costs for participants in a diabetes disease management program, United States, 2007–2008. *Preventing Chronic Disease, 8*(3). http://www.cdc.gov/pcd/issues/2011 /may/10_0163.htm

Darkins, A., Foster, L., Anderson, C., Goldschmidt, L., & Selvin, G. (2013). The design, implementation, and operational management of a comprehensive quality management program to support national telehealth networks. *Telemedicine and e-Health, 19*(7), 557–564.

Darkins, A., Ryan, P., Kobb, R., Foster, L., Edmonson, E., Wakefield, B., & Lancaster, A. E. (2008). The systematic implementation of health informatics, home telehealth, and disease management to support the care of veteran patients with chronic conditions. *Telemedicine and e-Health, 14*(10), 1119–1126.

Dehm, K., & McCabe, S. (2007). Managing care for adults with chronic conditions: The VNS CHOICE Model. *Policy & Practice,* 14–17.

de Jongh, T., Gurol-Urganci, I., Vodopivec-Jamsek, V., Car, J., & Atun, R. (2012). Mobile phone messaging for facilitating self-management of long-term illnesses (Review). *Cochrane Database of Systematic Reviews, 12*(12), CD0074559. doi: 002/14651858.CD007459.pub2

Foote, S. M. (2009). Next steps: How can Medicare accelerate the pace of improving chronic care? *Health Affairs, 28*(1), 99–102.

Foster, G., Taylor, S. J. C., Eldridge, S., Ramsay, J., & Griffiths, C. J. (2007). Self-management education programmes led by lay leaders for people with chronic health conditions. *Cochrane Database of Systematic Reviews, 17*(4), CD005108. doi: 10.1002/14651858.CD005108.pub2

Godleski, L., Darkins, A., & Peters, J. (2012). Outcomes of 98,609 U.S. Department of Veterans Affairs patients enrolled in telemental health services, 2006–2010. *Psychiatric Services, 63*(4), 383–385.

Hayashi, T., Farrell, M. A., Chaput, L. A., Rocha, D. A., & Hernandez, M. (2010). Lifestyle intervention, behavioral changes, and improvements in cardiovascular risk profiles in the California WISEWOMAN project. *Journal of Women's Health, 19*(6), 1129–1138.

Holtz-Eakin, D. (2004). *An analysis of the literature on disease management programs.* Washington, D C: Congressional Budget Office. http://www.cbo.gov/sites/default/files/cbofiles/ftpdocs/59xx/doc5909/10-13-diseasemngmnt.pdf

Improving Chronic Illness Care. (2006–2014). The chronic care model. http://www.improvingchroniccare.org/index.php?p=The_Chronic_Care_Model&s=2

Jacelon, C., Furman, E., Rea, A., Macdonald, B., & Donaghue, L. C. (2011). Creating a professional practice model for postacute care. *Journal of Gerontological Nursing, 37*(3), 53–60.

Jencks, S. F., Williams, M. V., & Coleman, E. A. (2009). Rehospitalization among patients in the Medicare fee-for-service program. *New England Journal of Medicine, 360*(14), 1418–1428.

Katon, W. J., Lin, E., Von Korff, M., Ciechanowski, P., ... McCulloch, D. (2010). Collaborative care for patients with depression and chronic illness. *New England Journal of Medicine, 363*(26), 2611.

Lorig, K., & Holman, H. R. (2003). Self-management education: History, definition, outcomes and mechanisms. *Annals of Behavioral Medicine, 26*(1), 1–7.

Lorig, K. R., Sobel, D. S., Steward, A. L., Brown, B. W., Bandura, A., Ritter, P., ... Holman, H.R. (1999). Evidence suggesting that a chronic disease self-management program can improve health status while reducing hospitalization: A randomized trial. *Medical Care, 37*(1), 5–14.

Mattke, S., Seid, M., & Ma, S. (2007). Evidence for the effect of disease management: Is $1 billion a year a good investment? *American Journal of Managed Care, 13,* 670–676.

McLeroy, K. R., Bibeau, D., Steckler, A., & Glanz, K. (1988). An ecological perspective on health promotion programs. *Health Education Quarterly, 15*(4), 351–376.

Mukamel, D. B., Peterson, D. R., Temkin-Greener, H., Delavan, R., Gross, D., Kunitz, S. J., ... Williams, T.F. (2007). Program characteristics and enrollees' outcomes in the Program of All-Inclusive Care for the Elderly (PACE). *Milbank Quarterly, 85*(3), 499–531.

National Committee for Quality Assurance (NCQA). (2012). NCQA PCMH 2011 standards, elements, and factors documentation guideline/data sources. http://www.ncqa.org/portals/0/Programs/Recognition/PCMH_2011_Data_Sources_6.6.12.pdf

National Committee for Quality Assurance (NCQA). (n.d.). Patient-centered medical home recognition. http://www.ncqa.org/Programs/Recognition/PatientCenteredMedicalHomePCMH.aspx

National PACE Association. (2013). PACE in the states. http://www.npaonline.org/website/download.asp?id=1741&title=PACE_in_the_States

Naylor, M. D., Aiken, L. H., Kurtzman, E. T., Olds, D. M., & Hirschman, K. B. (2011). The importance of transitional care in achieving health reform. *Health Affairs, 30*(4), 746–754.

Nutting, P. A., Crabtree, B. F., Miller, W. L., Stange, K. C., Stewart, E., & Jaen, C. (2011). Transforming physician practices to patient-centered medical homes: Lessons learned from the national demonstration project. *Health Affairs, 39*(3), 439–445.

Oeseburg, B., Wynia, K., Middel, B., & Reijneveld, S. A. (2009). Effects of case management for frail older people or those with chronic illness: A systematic review. *Nursing Research, 58*(3), 201–210.

Ory, M. G., Ahn, S., Jiang, L., Smith, M. L., Ritter, P. L., Whitelaw, N., & Lorig, K. (2013). Successes of a national study of the chronic disease self-management program. *Medical Care, 51*(11), 992–998.

Piraino, E., Heckman, G., Glenny, C., & Stolee, P. (2012). Transitional care programs: Who is left behind? A systematic review. *International Journal of Integrated Care, 12*(10). http://www.ijic.org/index

.php/ijic/article/view/URN%3ANBN%3ANL%3AUI
%3A10-1-113107/1774

Renders, C. M., Valk, G. D., Griffin, S. J., Wagner, E., vanEijk, J. T., & Assendelft, W. J. J. (2000). Interventions to improve the management of diabetes mellitus in primary care, outpatient and community settings. *Cochrane Database of Systematic Reviews*, *4*, CD001481. doi: 10.1002/14651858.CD001481

Rittenhouse, D. R., & Shortell, S. M. (2009). The patient-centered medical home: Will it stand the test of health reform? *Journal of the American Medical Association*, *301*(19), 2038–2040.

Ritter, P. L., Lee, J., & Lorig, K. (2011). Moderators of chronic disease self-management programs: Who benefits? *Chronic Illness*, *7*(2), 162–172.

Robinson, J. C. (2008). Slouching toward value-based health care. *Health Affairs*, *27*(1), 11–12.

Saucier, P., Kasten, J., Burwell, B., & Gold, L. (2012). The growth of managed long-term services and supports (MLTSS) programs: A 2012 update. Washington, DC: Centers for Medicare and Medicaid Services. http://www.medicaid.gov/Medicaid-CHIP-Program-Information/By-Topics/Delivery-Systems/Downloads/MLTSSP_White_paper_combined.pdf

Schwartz, S. M., Day, B., Wildenhaus, K., Silberman, A., Wang, C., & Silberman, J. (2010). The impact of an online disease management program on medical costs among health plan members. *American Journal of Health Promotion*, *25*(2), 126–133.

Shortell, S. M., Casalino, L. P., & Fisher, E. S. (2010). How the center for Medicare and Medicaid innovation should test accountable care organizations. *Health Affairs*, *29*(7), 1293–1298.

Smith, B., Hughes-Cromwick, P. F., Forkner, E., & Galbreath, A. D. (2008). Cost-effectiveness of telephonic disease management in heart failure. *American Journal of Managed Care*, *14*(2), 106–115.

Smith, S. M., Allwright, S., & O'Dowd, T. (2007). Effectiveness of shared care across the interface between primary and specialty care in chronic disease management. *Cochrane Database of Systematic Reviews*, *3*, CD004910. doi: 10.1002/14651858.CD004910.pub2

Strauss, A., Corbin, J., Fagerhaugh, S., Glaser, B., Maines, D., Suczek, B., & Wiener, C. (1984). *Chronic illness and the quality of life* (2nd ed.). St. Louis, MO: Mosby.

U.S. Department of Health and Human Services (DHHS). (n.d.). HRSA health information technology and quality improvement. http://www.hrsa.gov/healthit/mhealth.html

Visiting Nurse Service of New York (VNSNY). (2013). Choice health plans: Managed long term care (MLTC). http://www.vnsnychoice.org/long-term-care/2014-plan-features/managed-long-term-care-mltc/

Wagner, E. H. (1998). Chronic disease management: What will it take to improve care for chronic illness? *Effective Clinical Practice*, *1*, 2–4.

Wielawski, I. M. (2006). Improving chronic illness care. In S. L. Isaacs & J. R. Knickman (Eds.), *To improve health and health care, 10: The Robert Wood Johnson Foundation anthology* (pp. 1–17). Princeton, NJ: Robert Wood Johnson Foundation.

Williams, J. W., Jackson, G. L., Powers, B. J., Chatterjee, R., Prvu Bettger, J., Kemper, A. R., … Gray, R. (2012). *The patient-centered medical home: Closing the quality gap: Revisiting the state of the science.* Evidence Report/Technology Assessment Publication No. 208. (AHRQ Publication No. 12-E008-EF). Rockville, MD: Agency for Healthcare Research and Quality. http://www.effectivehealthcare.ahrq.gov/reports/final.cfm

Chapter 20

Home Health Care

Cynthia S. Jacelon

Introduction

The home healthcare industry delivers a variety of services to individuals with chronic health problems living in the communities. Services can be divided into two types: (1) skilled healthcare professionals, under the direction of a physician's order and supported by third-party reimbursement, and (2) supportive community services, including support for instrumental activities of daily living and personal care. Individuals and agencies provide these services on a fee-for-service basis. Some of these supportive community services may be supported through Medicaid Home and Community-Based Services (HCBS), as discussed in this chapter. It is common for healthcare professionals and supportive care workers to simultaneously provide their services to clients, often through the same agency, and to coordinate those services. The focus of this chapter is on the roles of nurses and other skilled healthcare providers in the home.

Home health nurses provide nursing care to clients with acute and/or chronic illnesses, as well meet the terminal care needs of clients, in their place of residence. The overall goal of care is to enhance the clients' quality of life or support clients at the end of life (American Nurses Association [ANA], 2008). Home health nurses use holistic strategies to work with clients, families, and informal caregivers to manage disease or disability. They practice independently, often being the only professional care provider in the home. The specialty of home health nursing differs from other nursing specialties in that care is provided in the client's home; the duration and frequency of care depend on the care delivery model and the holistic needs of the client, family, and caregivers; and the nurse must have advanced knowledge of healthcare payment systems and cost containment (ANA, 2008).

It is anticipated that the need for homecare services will increase as the population ages. Because of the unique characteristics required to be a successful homecare nurse, the shortage of qualified nurses in this setting may be more severe than in other areas of the healthcare system (Ellenbecker, 2004). Homecare nurses must possess a unique set of skills, including "flexibility, creativity, and innovative approaches to situations and problems in the context of individual and environmental differences and widely varying resource availability" (ANA, 2008, p. 7). According to *Home Health Nursing: Scope and Standards of Practice* (ANA, 2008), the nurse best suited to homecare practice is the baccalaureate-prepared nurse, owing to his or her broad-based education. Nevertheless, nurses prepared at the associate degree or diploma level are typically members of the homecare team. All nurses engaged in home care are expected to advance their ability to meet client needs in the homecare setting. This goal is accomplished by

Table 20-1 MINIMUM QUALIFICATIONS OF HOMECARE NURSES

A baccalaureate degree in nursing

Ability to incorporate communication and motivation skills and principles in the home health setting

Ability to apply critical thinking to physical, psychosocial, environmental, cultural, family, and safety issues

Ability to utilize clinical decision making in applying the nursing process to clients in their places of residence

Ability to practice as an effective member of an interdisciplinary team

Competency in applying care-management skills

Source: American Nurses Association. (2008). *Home health nursing: Scope and standards of practice.* Silver Springs, MD: Author.

supporting colleagues, structured preceptor programs, clinical experience, and lifelong learning (ANA, 2008). **Table 20-1** identifies the ANA's minimum qualifications for a homecare nurse.

In 1966, the U.S. federal government began providing for homecare services as a benefit of the then-new legislation known as Medicare. Medicare paid for the expansion of homecare services to many people, particularly the elderly who did not have access to such care. In 1973, the Medicare homecare benefit was expanded to include disabled Americans regardless of age. However, homecare advocates became increasingly concerned that the narrow scope of homecare-related legislation limited services as a means of avoiding the excessive costs of providing the full range of services that many clients needed.

Medicare-sponsored home care grew rapidly until the 1990s, when the government found that a program designed to meet the short-term needs of acutely ill individuals was also being used to care for persons with chronic illness, and the expansion was unsustainable (Buhler-Wilkersen. 2012). The growth of services was

a direct result of many reimbursement changes affecting hospitals. In an earlier effort to control the cost of care in acute care hospitals, Congress had passed the Social Security Amendments of 1983 to initiate the prospective payment system (PPS) for inpatient services (Stanhope & Lancaster, 2010). In this way, the federal government shifted reimbursement to a PPS based on diagnosis-related groups (DRGs). With reimbursement for hospital care now predetermined by client diagnosis, hospitals responded to the significant revenue reductions by decreasing the average length of stay for clients. The direct consequence was shorter hospital stays and increased referrals to home care (Stanhope & Lancaster, 2010).

In 1997, however, Congress targeted home health care as a place to reduce healthcare expenditures. The passage of the Balanced Budget Act of 1997 (BBA) imposed stricter limits on Medicare reimbursement for homecare services and required the Medicare administration to expand the prospective payment system to include homecare services (Murkofsky & Alston, 2009). The BBA narrowed the definition of those individuals eligible to receive homecare services to those persons who were deemed "homebound." Under these guidelines, Medicare recipients were no longer eligible for home care if they were able to leave home for any reason other than medical services (Maurer & Smith, 2005). As a consequence of the stricter rules, the number of persons eligible for Medicare homecare funding declined by 50% between 1997 and 2000 (Maurer & Smith, 2005). During this time, as many as 3,000 homecare agencies went out of business (Buhler-Wilkerson, 2012).

Today, the industry continues to provide holistic care in a fiscally restrained environment. Under the prospective payment system implemented in 2000, agencies are paid a set amount for each 60-day episode of care regardless of the number of visits provided. These payments are adjusted based on case mix, such that the agency receives more money for clients requiring more care (Murkofsky & Alston, 2009).

Theoretical Frameworks for Management of Chronic Illness in Home Care

Homecare nurses provide intermittent care and rely heavily on clients' ability to self-manage their health problems. As such, the nurse is in a unique position to apply frameworks for practice that help the nurse work with clients to promote independence. Mid-range theories, applied in homecare settings to help promote clients' self-management of chronic health problems, conceptualize nursing care as based on relationships and provide guidelines for collaborative decision making. The mid-range theory of relationship-based care is presented here, as well as a model for community-based care of clients with chronic illness and hospice care.

Relationship-Based Care

In this model, relationship is the basis of nursing practice (Doane, 2002). Individuals are "viewed as contextual beings who exist in relation with other people and with social, cultural, political, and historical processes" (Doane & Varcoe, 2007, p. 198). Every day, nurses engage in relationships with self, clients, other nurses, and healthcare professionals. In turn, this network of relationships forms a web of mutual dependencies (Doane & Varcoe, 2007, p. 193).

Relationship-based care is a model of human relating that reflects this web of interactions within the context of humanistic values (Hartrick, 1997). In the past, models of nursing care have been based on behavioral models in which the nurse learns a set of communication skills and applies those skills when interacting with clients. This model is unique in that it is based on the recognition of the relational nature and complexity of human experience (Hartrick, 1997, p. 524). Rather than enhancing communication between nurse and client, application of communication techniques may impede communication because the nurse may be focused on

performing these techniques and is unable to be "in-caring-human-relation" (p. 525). According to this model, "health and healing are promoted through the development of an increasing openness to learning and growth, an increasing capacity to tolerate ambiguity and uncertainty, and an increasing experience of empowerment and choice" (p. 525). For clients with chronic illness, this model of human relation may provide a means for the client, family, and nurse to grow in relationships with each other as well as in the relationship with the chronic illness. In one study, homecare nurses defined their relationships with clients in terms of knowing the client and building trust with clients and their families (Stajduhar et al., 2011).

For nurses to engage in caring relationships with others, they must first have a caring relationship with self. Such a relationship with self includes both self-knowing and self-awareness (Ledesma, 2011). Self-knowing is a process of identifying your personal values and beliefs and balancing your personal needs with your professional practice. Self-knowing, in turn, leads to self-awareness. Self-awareness is being aware of your body, mind, and spirit in the context of engaging in relationships. To be present in relationships with others, you must be centered in your self.

Once centered, nurses purposefully build relationships with other staff members. A group of workers who have developed meaningful relationships with one another can work effectively together to provide relationship-based care for clients and their families. Employing relationship-based care with clients involves engaging with clients to accomplish care goals rather than focusing solely on the tasks of care. Simple things that the nurse can do to further these goals include thinking of the person who is receiving care, sitting with the client at eye level when talking with the client or providing education, and responding to the client in a manner that acknowledges and supports the significance of the chronic illness as the client experiences it.

Hartrick (1997) identified five nurse capacities upon which to base nursing action: (1) initiative, authenticity, and responsiveness; (2) mutuality and synchrony; (3) honoring complexity and ambiguity; (4) intentionality in relating; and (5) reimaging (p. 526).

Initiative, authenticity, and responsiveness address the nurse's active concern for others (Hartrick, 1997, p. 526). Within the relationship-based care model, these concepts are intertwined. The nurse takes the initiative to engage in a relationship with the client. She or he is authentic, responding to the client and the situation in a way that is consistent with her or his personality, and showing emotions as they arise. In addition, the nurse is responsive to the feelings, needs, and goals of the client. The nurse is mindful of his or her presence with the client and is attentive to the client through conscious listening.

The concepts of mutuality and synchrony explain the nature of relationships. Mutuality refers to the commonalities experienced by people in relationships. A mutual relationship is a negotiated, collaborative process in which both client and nurse participate, make choices, and act (Doane & Varcoe, 2007, p. 193). These commonalities include shared visions and goals, while acknowledging differences in perspectives. Synchrony describes the rhythms that occur naturally within the context of the relationship, including synchrony between internal and external patterns, and periods of silence (Hartrick, 1997, p. 526).

The nurse honors complexity and ambiguity by acknowledging the complexity of human experience. The nurse, in relation with the client, seeks to uncover the numerous and possibly conflicting elements of the experience. Through this process of discovery, the nurse and client begin to mutually make connections between seemingly disparate actions, feelings, and events. Through this process, the client and nurse are able to appreciate the relevance of the experience and make choices regarding the management of the disease process (Hartrick, 1997, p. 526).

Intentionality involves the nurse exploring his or her values and then maintaining consistency between personal values and values in use during professional practice. Each nursing moment is shaped by the actions and intentions of the nurse, by the actions and responses of others, and by the contexts within which those interactions occur (Doane & Varcoe, 2007, p. 202). The intent of relational practice is to help clients understand the meaning of their health and healing experiences, and to discover choice and power within the experiences (Hartrick, 1997, p. 527).

Reimaging is the process of questioning the usual ways of being in the world. Through this process, the nurse can help clients transform their health and healing experiences and enhance their relational capacity (Hartrick, 1997, p. 527).

The nurse who engages in relational nursing practice makes a conscious commitment to act using the values and goals of the nursing profession to attend to each client's unique context and situation, helping that person grow in health. Difficulty and suffering can provide a vehicle for meaningful relationships, which is the basis for ethical decision making. In these situations, responsive nursing care creates the space for mutual experience, and for nurse and client to develop clarity and courage to act in health-promoting ways (Doane & Varcoe, 2007, p. 202).

In more recent work, Weydt (2010) identifies other characteristics necessary for effective relationship-based care—namely, clinical proficiency, interdisciplinary communication and teamwork, and continuity of nurse/patient/family relationships. In home care, where use of a primary nursing care model is common, building relationships with clients to improve their self-management of chronic disease can help clients maximize their quality of life.

In another model emphasizing relationships in home care, Funk and Stajduhar (2011) describe how families of clients receiving homecare services view relationships with care providers. Their model includes relational preconditions such as interactional opportunities, effort, and skill of the homecare nurse, as well as relational demonstrations such as knowledge, understanding, responsiveness, respect, and affection or closeness; these factors lead to the perceived quality of the relationship and the perceived quality of care.

Chronic Care Model of Disease Management

Individuals with chronic disease require a new strategy for health management. The chronic care model (CCM; **Figure 20-1**) was developed through a grant from the Robert Wood Johnson Foundation to change the way health care was delivered to individuals with chronic illness (Improving Chronic Illness Care, 2007). This model is designed to support the person with the chronic illness in self-managing his or her health using appropriate community and healthcare system resources. The home health nurse is in an excellent position to assist the client in managing his or her own health and chronic illness within this model.

Traditionally, the healthcare system in the United States has focused on providing acute care for acute illness in an episodic manner. Individuals with chronic illness require a proactive approach, combining self-management with effective use of community resources and the healthcare system (Improving Chronic Illness Care, 2007). Such care is based on evidence-based protocols, which are then tailored to the needs of the individual client. Common areas of difficulty for self-management include managing multiple medications, recognizing early warning signs of condition changes, coordinating and appearing for multiple physicians' appointments, understanding the plan of treatment, and coordinating support services (Meckes, 2005).

Figure 20-1 The Chronic Care Model

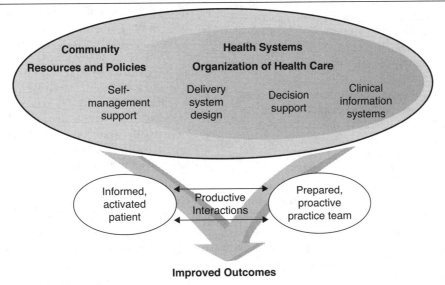

Source: Wagner, E.H. (1998). Chronic disease management: What will it take to improve care for chronic illness? *Effective Clinical Practice*, 1, 2–4.

According to the CCM, healthcare systems need to retool themselves to provide planned visits focused on maintaining wellness. In this model, clients are recognized as having the central role in managing their health. The role of healthcare professionals, by comparison, is to support clients' ability to self-manage their health (Improving Chronic Illness Care, 2007). The nurse can also affect the client's understanding of the disease process and choices for management. By being in the client's home, the homecare nurse gains a unique perspective of the client's culture and the meaning of the illness in the client's life.

Recently the CCM has been adapted to reflect care delivered by nurses in post-acute care settings such as home care (Jacelon, Furman, Rea, Macdonald, & Donoghue, 2011). In this version of the model, the nurse and the client are at the center of the model. The nurse and client form a team where the nurse coaches and advises the client in effective self-management techniques. In doing so, the home healthcare nurse may act as a case manager, helping the client navigate complicated interactions with several medical care professionals, and guiding the client to seek medical care for condition changes in a timely manner. In addition, the nurse can encourage the client to engage with community organizations to help support the client's self-management strategies; these community agencies might include food programs and disease-focused organizations (e.g., the Alzheimer's Association).

Radhakrishnan, Jacelon, Bigelow, et al. (2012) used the Jewish Geriatric Services-Chronic Care Model [JGS-CCM] (Jacelon et al., 2011) as a framework to explore how individuals with multiple chronic conditions, including heart failure, used telehealth services. These researchers conceptualized the nurse as a partner with the client to provide holistic nursing care and promote self-management. In their study, they found that individuals with heart failure and comorbidities including anemia, anxiety, musculoskeletal disorders, and depression required increased use of homecare services, whereas individuals who had heart failure and comorbidities including renal failure, cancer, and depression were more likely to discontinue telehealth services.

Home Healthcare Agencies

Home care is a unique healthcare service, in that homecare practice, by definition, takes place in the home of the care recipient. Within this context, the nurse is a guest in the client's home. Being a guest implies that an invitation must be extended from the client for the nurse to enter the home. In addition, the living arrangements of the individual receiving care are an important consideration in determining the services provided (Furaker, 2012). The home health nurse uses primary, secondary, and tertiary prevention strategies in assisting clients and families with self-management and coordination of community resources; all of these strategies are accomplished within the community, in the home of the client (ANA, 2008).

Home healthcare practitioners and standards of practice are governed by state and federal legislation. In particular, individual state regulations must be met for basic licensing of all home health agencies. If participation in the Medicare reimbursement program is desired, federal regulations that govern Medicare certification and coverage of services (Conditions of Participation and HHA-11, respectively) must also be satisfied. These federal mandates, along with individual state licensing or certification requirements, help ensure that home healthcare practitioners are qualified to provide their specialized services.

Language of Home Health Care

Several definitions are important in determining eligibility of patients for homecare services and subsequent reimbursement for the home healthcare agency. Terms are defined by federal Medicare regulations and include the following: *homebound, primary services, continuing services*, and *dependent services*.

Federal Medicare regulations include the qualifications of clients for coverage of home health services. The client must be confined to the home or to an institution that is not a hospital or skilled nursing facility (SNF). "Confined to the home" does not mean the client must be bedridden. "Homebound," or "home confined," is defined as an inability to leave the home normally, such that leaving would be taxing and require considerable effort and assistance. When the client does leave the home, the absences are infrequent and of relatively short duration, or to receive medical care.

The homebound client must be under the care of a physician and in need of skilled services on an intermittent-visit, not continuous, basis. The services must be provided in the client's home. Hospitals or nursing homes are not considered the client's home, but individuals living in assisted-living facilities or other group living situations are eligible for home care (Murkofsky & Alston, 2009).

Reimbursement is made to the homecare agency under the prospective payment system. Medicare pays the homecare agency a set amount of money for each client whose diagnosis is listed within one of 80 home health resource groups (Stanhope & Lancaster, 2010).

In addition to primary skilled services, home health aides and social work services are covered as dependent services under Medicare regulations. The client must require a skilled service to receive a home health aide or social work services, and once the skilled service is no longer required, the home health aide and social work services are not covered. These dependent services can also be continued if occupational therapy (a continuing service) is to be provided to the client.

Home Healthcare Team

The home healthcare team consists of the client, physicians, nurses, physical therapists, occupational therapists, speech therapists, medical social workers, home health aides, and informal caregivers. Each member of the team possesses a special set of skills that collectively supports a comprehensive approach to assist the client in meeting his or her care needs.

Effective home care depends on groups of independent practitioners forming teams to provide services for clients. These practitioners have different skill sets and are not always all from the same agency. The multiple practitioners on the home healthcare team have the knowledge and skills to identify clients' needs and address those needs through management of complex plans of care. Each practitioner must have a strong grasp of the rules and regulations that govern home health care, the ability to pay attention to detail, well-developed interpersonal skills, strong clinical skills, a working knowledge of the changing economics of health care, and the ability to effectively prioritize and time-manage challenging tasks and responsibilities.

Four models of team functioning have been identified: medical, multidisciplinary, interdisciplinary, and transdisciplinary (Jacelon, 2011). In a medical model team, the physician leader directs all functions of the team. Team members do not meet together, but rather communicate through the physician. This team configuration is most common in acute care settings where the physician is in daily contact with the client. Such a model is not desirable in a homecare situation, however, because the client may not be in frequent contact with the physician; the care providers are in the client's home, and independent decision making is a hallmark of this type of care.

The second type of team is the multidisciplinary team. In this model, professionals work in parallel. Each provider develops goals for his or her interaction with the client, and coordination occurs at the supervisory level. The individuals who are providing care do not usually communicate directly with one another. This model of care is common in long-term care settings in which a rigid bureaucratic structure exists. Multidisciplinary models are also observed in homecare settings.

Transdisciplinary teams are found in rehabilitation settings where team members and the client are in proximity daily. In this model, the client and primary care provider work as a team with the counsel of all other team members (Jacelon, 2011). Individual team members perform the interventions required for the client while the provider is with the client. Although this model is effective in rehabilitation settings, the nature of home care does not lend itself to this type of team function. The billing constraints in home care require that professionals perform the interventions within their scope of practice; the payment system does not reimburse for care outside of that scope. A transdisciplinary model works best in a capitated payment system, where the agency receives a predetermined amount of money for care regardless of who is providing the care.

The team configuration that is most effective in the home setting is the interdisciplinary team model. In an interdisciplinary team, professionals working with a client communicate directly with the client and with one another. In this model, the client is an integral part of the team, and professionals collaborate with the client to establish goals for care (Jacelon, 2011). Effective interdisciplinary team collaboration has been associated with benefits for both practitioner and client. For example, the registered nurse and the physical therapist may visit on different days to increase the number of days a week that a skilled provider visits the client's home. The interdisciplinary team is uniquely qualified to meet the client's psychosocial and health problems. Indeed, in chronic illness, the psychosocial and health problems are often intertwined (LoFaso, Breckman, Capello, Demopoulos, & Edelman, 2010).

Informal Caregivers

In 2009, it was estimated that 65.7 million family caregivers—nearly one-third of the U.S. population—provided care to adults who were disabled, ill, or aged (National Alliance of Caregiving [NAC], 2009). American caregivers are predominantly white, are usually female (66%), and are, on average, 48 years of age. Caregiving time averages 20.4 hours per week, and the duration of such care is, on average, 4.6 years.

In a systematic review of the literature, Roseland, Heisler, and Piette (2012), found that clients who had families that emphasized self-reliance, personal achievement, family cohesiveness, and attention to symptoms had better chronic illness outcomes than either individuals without families or individuals whose families held negative attitudes. Positive marital and family function predicted better physiologic control in chronic illness and lower mortality (p. 234).

Often both the home healthcare nurse and the care recipient rely heavily on the informal caregiver. As such, collaboration and decision making may involve a triad rather than the usual nurse–client dyad. However, the nurse must carefully negotiate the relationship to make sure that the care recipient is not silenced. Individuals with chronic illness who have families who are critical, overprotective, or controlling are at risk for poorer outcomes (Roseland et al., 2012). Homecare nurses should collaborate with both the client receiving care and informal caregivers to optimize the benefit of the available professional care. Leff (2004) found that clients demonstrated higher satisfaction with care when they were included in decision making regarding what the goals are, what the plan is, who (which disciplines and personnel) provides care, how often and which time of day visits occur, which activities occur during the visit, how care is provided, and who communicates with the physician (p. 298).

Interventions for Home Care

Coaching to Promote Self-Management

The homecare nurse is in an excellent position to coach the client and family in the management of chronic illness. Coaching is a strategy in which the nurse uses a combination of education, collaborative decision making, and empowerment to help clients manage their health needs (Butterworth, Linden, & McClay, 2007; Huffman, 2007, 2009). Health coaching has its roots in substance abuse counseling and has been found to be a relatively short-term, successful strategy. This client-centered approach to care focuses on the issues and barriers to self-management.

To employ health coaching, the home health nurse begins by asking the client what he or she is most concerned about. In this way, the nurse can capitalize on the client's interest in resolving or managing a particular problem. The next step is to validate the client's feelings about his or her capacity to manage the problem. Following this step, the nurse might help the client develop solutions to the problem by asking which strategies the client has tried in the past and which strategies he or she might like to try now (Huffman, 2007).

Recent evidence indicates that coaching is an effective intervention that improves clients' health status. Vincent and Birkhead (2013) reviewed 13 research studies that used coaching to improve clients' self-management. They found that coaching was effective in 11 of the 13 studies. Investigators in these studies used coaching to improve self-management of diseases such as type 2 diabetes and coronary heart disease as well as other long-term conditions. Coaching was an effective intervention to improve overall health in a group of older individuals with impaired activities of daily living. Other researchers used nurse coaching to promote behavior change and psychosocial health in individuals with addictions. Another group used coaching to reduce 30-day hospital readmission rates for recently hospitalized older adults. By comparison, Internet coaching was the least effective of the coaching techniques in improving overall health behaviors.

Information Technology and Telehealth

One of the fastest-growing areas of home health care is telehealth. Assistive devices in the home—such as telephones, video cameras, computers, Internet connections, and email—have the potential to improve home safety, enhance independence, and reduce the risk for injury of individuals with chronic illness. These devices provide a mechanism for clients and care providers to communicate from a distance (McLean, Nurmatov, Liu, Pagliari, Car, & Sheikh, 2011). However, Medicare does not presently reimburse for telehealth home care. In addition, some individuals—both clients and care providers—are ambivalent about the use of monitoring technology in the home because of the potential for invasion of the client's privacy (Percival & Hanson, 2006) and may lack confidence in the accuracy of the data provided by such equipment (Radhakrishnan, Jacelon, & Roche, 2012). As the home technology market has continued to explode, however, the homecare industry has embraced the use of technologies such as cellular phones, laptop computers, the Internet, and telehealth (ANA, 2008). Appropriate use of information technology and telehealth can lead to enhanced quality of care, improved client and clinician safety, and increased productivity (American Telemedicine Association [ATA], 2011).

The ATA (2011) has defined telemedicine as "the use of medical information exchanged from one site to another via electronic communications to improve clients' health status." Telemedicine may include distance monitoring of an individual's health status, routine consultations with healthcare professionals, referrals to specialists for complex problems, and consumer health information sites on the Internet. However, for reimbursement, if telemedicine is to be used for a homecare client, the plan of care and the physician's order must specify the expected number of live visits and the expected level of telehome care. Additionally, a telehealth visit may not be substituted for an in-person visit. Privacy and security risks continue to present formidable challenges in the protection of client health information (Hall & McGraw, 2014).

As the available technology expands, researchers are turning their attention to the efficacy of telemedicine and telehealth. In a study evaluating the effectiveness of a telemedicine intervention for clients with congestive heart failure (CHF) who had recently been discharged from the hospital, as opposed to a group of similar clients receiving the usual homecare services, researchers found that while the telemedicine intervention reduced the number of nursing visits, decreased home health costs, and improved clients' self-perceived quality of life, it did not affect the number of readmissions or visits to the emergency department (Myers, Grant, Lugn, Holbert, & Kvedar, 2006). Unexpected findings included a need for ongoing education and support for the clients using the telehealth equipment throughout the treatment period. In addition, several potential research participants declined or withdrew from the study because they were anxious about using the equipment (Myers et al., 2006). In a study conducted by Radhakrishnan, Jacelon, Bigelow et al. (2012), nurses also reported that some clients with CHF found the telemonitoring process a cause for anxiety. Nevertheless, in at least one study, a telehealth program was found to be efficacious for reducing rehospitalization of individuals with CHF (Smith, 2013). Telehealth has also been found to be effective in reducing emergency room visits and improving quality of life for individuals with chronic obstructive pulmonary disease (COPD) (McLean et al., 2011).

The breadth of telehealth and telemonitoring applications is expanding rapidly. Use of interactive computer video conferencing programs such as Ustream (Smith-Stoner, 2011) is becoming increasingly common. These programs provide a way for individuals to see and talk to each other across time and distance. The technology can provide an economical way to conduct consults for wound care, for example, and to hold team meetings while the team members are in different locations. This technology can also be used to include a client who would not

otherwise be available for a team meeting. In addition, interactive video can provide a way for homebound individuals to connect with family members who do not live nearby.

Other types of telehealth and telemonitoring equipment include online repositories of clients' health data, such as Microsoft Healthvault (http://www.healthvault.com/). These websites provide a place for individuals to track their progress toward health goals, store health data, and provide information to healthcare providers. Often, peripheral devices such as a blood pressure cuff, blood glucose monitoring device, or pedometer can communicate directly with the computer program, providing an easy way for individuals to monitor their health.

Preventing Rehospitalization

Homecare nurses have an important role in preventing rehospitalization. Rehospitalization is defined as a client being readmitted to an acute care facility within 30 days of the original discharge. As many as 27% of frail older adults receiving home care are readmitted to such facilities within 30 days (Delta Health Technologies, 2012). Under the Patient Protection and Affordable Care Act (ACA), hospitals are now penalized for rehospitalizations of clients with heart attack, heart failure, and pneumonia. For FY2015, rehospitalizations for three other diagnoses, COPD, elective total hip arthroplasty, and elective total knee arthroplasty, will be evaluated for potential penalties as well (Centers for Medicare and Medicaid Services [CMS], 2014). Penalties for these diagnoses will further exacerbate an already critical funding problem for healthcare facilities. The homecare agency that can effectively reduce the number of clients who return to the hospital will, therefore, become a desirable partner for acute care facilities.

Improving care transitions is one way homecare nurses can reduce the likelihood of rehospitalization. Several models have been developed to improve such transitions. Naylor (1990) developed one of the early models, called the transitional care model (TCM), to improve the quality of care transitions. This model is based on case management by an advanced practice nurse, who ensures coordination of care between the acute care and homecare settings. A key aspect of this model is the client's and family's understanding of the client's health issues, and their ability to recognize changes in the client's status.

The Care Transitions Program (Coleman, n.d.; http://www.caretransitions.org) is based on care provided by competent providers in partnership with the client. Emphasis is placed on the client's ability to manage his or her medications, a client-centered health record that is maintained by the client, the client's willingness to actively schedule and complete follow-up visits with physicians, and the client's clear understanding of events suggesting that a health condition is worsening.

All of these models rely on the client as a partner in care. In each case, the client is an informed, empowered individual who is responsible for engaging in the plan of care. The homecare nurse's use of a setting-appropriate transition of care model may well be one answer to improving the quality of care across settings, decreasing readmissions, controlling costs, and meeting the needs of patients and their families (Enderlin et al., 2013).

Outcome Assessment System and Information Set (OASIS) data are collected on all homecare clients and may potentially serve as a source for assessing risk factors for rehospitalization. Tao and Ellenbecker (2013), for example, used the OASIS database to explore which client factors increased the likelihood of an individual being rehospitalized. They found that males with a median level of cognitive ability, greater functional impairment, lack of facilitated medical care, and lack of environmental supports were more likely to be rehospitalized than other clients. In addition, being older, obese, in poorer health, requiring activities of daily living (ADL) or instrumental activities of daily living (IADL) care, and receiving less informal care were associated with higher rehospitalization rates.

Cultural Competence

As many as 40% of Americans are immigrants or the children of immigrants (Hines, 2012). As the older population grows, the diversity of those individuals with chronic illness increases. Likewise, the diversity of individuals seeking homecare services is increasing. Cultural competence is an ongoing process that involves respecting the differences among persons and planning care while keeping those differences in mind. Nurses with cultural competence apply their knowledge, skills, and understanding of diverse cultures to provide culturally competent care (Hines, 2012, p. 39). It is critical for the homecare nurse to remember that when he or she is providing care in the client's home, he or she is a guest in the client's culture. To increase the likelihood of the client adopting the self-management strategies the nurse is offering, the nurse must find a way to connect the health care that he or she is suggesting with the client's experience in the context of his or her culture.

Coordination of Care

According to the National Coalition of Care Coordination (N3C), care coordination is defined as follows:

> {A} person-centered, assessment-based, interdisciplinary approach to integrating health care and social support services in a cost-effective manner in which an individual's needs and preferences are assessed, a comprehensive care plan is developed, and services are managed and monitored by an evidence-based process which typically involves a designated lead care coordinator. (N3C, n.d., p. 1)

Homecare nurses and agencies are in an excellent position to incorporate the role of care coordinator into the role of the nurse, because homecare nurses often treat individuals who are at high risk for complications of chronic disease. Nurses are uniquely prepared to serve as the designated lead coordinator. They can coordinate the needs of the client and family with services provided by an array of care providers. In this milieu, effective care coordination often includes (1) coordination of the interdisciplinary team, (2) frequent face-to-face contact between the care coordinator and the client, (3) regular telephone contact, and (4) psychosocial services (Volland, Schraeder, Shelton, & Hess, 2013).

Home and Community Based Services

Home and Community-Based Services (HCBS) is a Medicaid program developed in 1982 to provide support for poor older adults who want to stay at home, rather than move to a nursing home, but need long-term supportive services (Kane, 2012). To be eligible for the program, older adults must be eligible for admission to a nursing home. In addition, HCBS are required to be cost neutral, meaning that the total cost of care at home cannot exceed the Medicaid cost of living in a nursing home (Ng & Harrington, 2012). HCBS can include personal care, homemaker, and nursing services, which are often provided by homecare agencies. Some HCBS programs even include medical house calls (Hayashi & Leff, 2012). HCBS are frequently coordinated by homecare agencies. Currently, most states participate in this program.

In a comparison of homecare services and nursing home services for matched clients, Marek and colleagues (2012) found that nurse-coordinated home services were less expensive than the equivalent nursing home care. Even though there is currently no mechanism for reimbursement for care coordination services, in another study Marek and colleagues (2010) calculated the costs of nurse care coordination and included the cost in their calculations—the saving to Medicare and Medicaid was more than $300 monthly.

Program of All-Inclusive Care for the Elderly

The Program of All-Inclusive Care for the Elderly (PACE) provides care for older adults with chronic illness, who are eligible for both Medicare and Medicaid, and who are living at home even though they qualify for nursing home care (Young, 2002). Through PACE, interdisciplinary teams assess individuals and provide comprehensive services across settings. By removing the financial barriers to coordination of care, the PACE concept unites the healthcare team around providing long-term care management in the least restrictive setting (National PACE Association, 2013). PACE provides comprehensive services to a group of individuals. Although these individuals usually live close together in an apartment complex or neighborhood, PACE organizations may be centered on an adult daycare site where members are bused to a central site daily. At the daycare site, the clients can receive full services including personal care, nursing and medical care, and socialization. These programs have demonstrated efficacy in controlling costs and providing comprehensive services for dual-eligible frail older adults (Hirth, Baskins, & Dever-Bumba, 2009).

Reimbursement for Home Care and Documentation of Care

Skilled services that are reimbursable by third-party payers drive the homecare industry. The majority of skilled homecare services are covered by health insurance, particularly Medicare and Medicaid. In 2000, Medicare and Medicaid paid for 72% of homecare services and 87% of hospice clients in the United States (Clark, 2008). By 2006, the percentage of homecare services reimbursed had increased to 77%, with private insurance accounting for only 12% of costs. The remaining 10% of expenditures were paid out of pocket by clients (Murkofsky & Alston, 2009). Usually, private insurance companies follow the guidelines set by Medicare. Therefore, changes in Medicare regulations and reimbursement have a major effect on the home healthcare industry.

Medicare establishes regulations that determine who is eligible to receive reimbursable homecare services. Accompanying the Medicare funding stream are strict regulations for client eligibility, homecare practice, and reimbursement mechanisms. Although the Medicare homecare benefit was designed to extend care to more people, obtaining access to this benefit was initially difficult because only certain agencies could provide care, and because restrictions limited who was eligible for care, which services clients could receive, and what the length of service could be. An additional burden on homecare agencies was a complex billing system that often resulted in extensive payment delays.

Agencies adhering to the Medicare guidelines to receive Medicare and Medicaid payment are classified as "certified." "Noncertified" home health agencies render home healthcare privately, without consideration of the Medicare guidelines, and, therefore, receive no payment from Medicare. A home health agency may choose to participate in the Medicare program and can receive payment from Medicare for those clients who meet the eligibility criteria. Agencies choosing not to participate in the Medicare program follow their respective state-established regulations that govern the provision of homecare services. However, as a quality measure, private payment agencies often follow the standards of adequate care as established by Medicare.

When a client's care can no longer be billed to Medicare, the agency is responsible for providing advanced notice to the physician and client and assisting with finding other sources of care. The client can always independently pay the agency, an arrangement that provides an alternative to third-party reimbursed care. Since the inception of the prospective payment system, many long-term care clients have paid their own bills for care. According to Medicare's definition of its payment criteria, it was never intended to pay for care other than short term, acute, intermittent, and skilled, so clients needing longer-term services require other payment sources.

If a home health agency determines that a client can no longer be served because of costs, discontinuation of care may put the agency at risk for charges of client abandonment. The definition of abandonment is cessation of services by an agency to a client who continues to require care and for whom no provision has been made, nor has the client received proper and timely notice of impending discharge from service.

In the prospective payment system, a specific dollar amount per client is given to a healthcare professional for delivery of services. The healthcare professional, in turn, becomes the coordinator of the individual's care and assumes responsibility for managing cost, risk, resources, and outcomes of care (Remington, 2000). Reimbursement amounts are determined by clinical assessment of the client's needs using the mandated assessment tool, Outcome Assessment System and Information Set. OASIS was designed to establish the national standard for collecting client outcome data that can be used to evaluate homecare services on an industry-wide basis. It is used to collect a combination of demographic, clinical, and functional client care data used in calculating Medicare payments to home health agencies.

The actual charges submitted by an agency are determined by the OASIS clinical scoring system, which assigns points to selected items in the OASIS data set as well as additional points if therapy services are needed. The OASIS scoring system is intended to calculate Medicare payments based on the severity and acuity of the client's condition; in this way, higher payments are provided for sicker clients. There are no limitations on the episodes of care that a client can receive.

The OASIS tool has been used to measure outcomes from nursing interventions. However, in their evaluation of OASIS, Schneider, Barkauskas, and Keenan (2008) did not find it to be sensitive to the effects of home healthcare nursing, as measured by intervention intensity.

The implementation of the prospective payment system in home health has led to more stringent regulations regarding which services will be reimbursed, and for how long, in some instances. This may well limit access to care for certain vulnerable groups, such as the frail elderly and individuals with chronic illness whose care is largely home based, and people who are human immunodeficiency virus (HIV) positive. Nurses and other healthcare professionals must work even more closely with families to determine the kinds of services needed to foster self-care and the optimal timing of these services (Stanhope & Lancaster, 2010).

The Future of Reimbursement

Since 2000, there has been increasing pressure by the U.S. government to slow the growth and costs of home care. Pay-for-performance demonstrations have been initiated in seven states, and Congress has instituted several caps and restrictions on reimbursement (Murkofsky & Alston, 2009). At the same time that reimbursement for skilled services through Medicare is contracting, there is an initiative to move individuals out of long-term care institutions and provide supportive services in their homes. This initiative is funded by state Medicaid budgets and represents an effort to reduce long-term care costs.

Although the ACA, signed into law in March 2010, does not specifically mention homecare services, the law will affect services. The mandate that all individuals have health insurance may not have a major effect on home care, because private insurance accounts for only 12% of homecare revenue. However, the move to expand Medicaid to include all individuals with incomes up to 133% of the poverty level could mean an increase in Medicaid-covered services.

Two provisions in the law have a direct effect on home health care. First, in January 2013, a national Medicare pilot program to develop and evaluate a bundled payment system for acute, inpatient hospital services, physician services, outpatient hospital services, and post-acute care services for an episode of care that begins 3 days prior to a hospitalization and spans 30 days following discharge

was begun. If the pilot program achieves its stated goals of improving (or not reducing) quality and reducing spending, the CMS will develop a plan for expanding the pilot program beginning in 2016. The second provision was implemented in 2012 and created the Independence at Home demonstration program to provide high-need Medicare beneficiaries with primary care services in their home and allow participating teams of health professionals to share in any savings if they reduce preventable hospitalizations, prevent hospital readmissions, improve health outcomes, improve the efficiency of care, reduce the cost of healthcare services, and achieve patient satisfaction (Kaiser Foundation, 2010).

Outcomes and Quality Management

The desired outcomes for home health care in the management of the client with chronic illness seem initially to be quite apparent. The positive effects of the health care delivered in the home to the client, as well as the positive effects of the caregiver support mechanisms that keep the client at home and do not necessitate institutionalization, are clearly important outcomes. However, establishing outcome criteria that are stable and dependable so as to measure outcome attainment is essential for determining whether positive effects are occurring to the advantage of the client and caregiver or simply because there is no alternative to providing care.

Maurer and Smith (2005) have established nine possible outcome measures for evaluating outcome attainment based on changes in the population, the healthcare system within the community, or the environment. These outcome measures include (1) knowledge; 2) behaviors and skills; (3) attitudes; (4) emotional well-being; (5) health status (epidemiology); (6) presence of healthcare system services and components; (7) satisfaction or acceptance regarding the program interventions; (8) presence of policy allowing, mandating, and funding; and (9) altered relationship with the physical environment (p. 403). Evaluating the outcomes of care rendered by any of the disciplines participating in home health care for the first five of these measures is inclusive in the care itself. The professionals and paraprofessionals who work within the homecare team function within and by delivering care using these first five principles, thereby making their use as measurement variables relatively easy and functional. The last four outcome measures, however, have been a continuous struggle for home health care throughout the 20th century and now the 21st century. These four measures are unpredictably influenced by the ups and downs of financial support, government regulations, management control in home health itself, and in the institutional care that passes clients on to in-home care.

Medicare Home Health Care Compare (HHC; http://www.medicare.gov/homehealthcompare) is a website designed to provide comparative information about the quality of homecare agencies. The information posted on HHC is obtained from OASIS data and from patient satisfaction data. HHC captures care delivery (process of care) and care outcomes data from OASIS and provides comparison information from the agency, state, and national averages for the indicator. Process of care data focus on how often home health agencies gave recommended, evidence-based care or treatments to clients. Outcome measures include client improvement measures (e.g., mobility, ADLs, and overall health) and healthcare utilization measures. HHC is an excellent tool to use as a basis for a quality improvement program. Focusing improvement efforts on processes of care and outcome measures that do not meet the average state or federal standard of care is a good way to improve care overall.

Home health nurses are in a unique position to promote clients' self-management of their chronic diseases. Such nurses can be effective in helping clients and their informal caregivers to maximize the support available to them. In addition, using strategies such as coaching and telemedicine can help clients improve their self-care abilities. OASIS is not simply a reimbursement document, but can provide a wealth of information regarding quality of care and outcomes.

Homecare Satisfaction Measures

In health care, objective measures of client satisfaction with care are often used as an indicator of positive outcomes. To report clients' experiences of care, Home Health Compare uses the Home Health Consumer Assessment of Healthcare Providers and Systems (HHCAHPS) instrument (https://homehealthcahps.org/). All Medicare-certified homecare agencies participate in the HHCAHPS. The survey data are collected by a mailed or telephone survey. The instrument includes five basic items regarding (1) professional care; (2) communication; (3) discussion of medications, pain, and home safety; (4) overall care; and (5) clients' willingness to recommend (or not) the agency to family and friends. Other items can be added as well. The publication of the HHCAHPS results, which are readily available to the public, provide a strong incentive for homecare agencies to provide high-quality care.

Ideally, outcomes and client satisfaction evaluation and analysis will demonstrate that the home healthcare process results in appropriate, adequate, and effective client care. Positive client outcomes, however, require that homecare agencies become aware of the roles that clients, family, and caregivers play before the client is admitted for service. Homecare providers, clients, families, and caregivers must enter into partnerships to provide the care needed for the client. Informal care providers need to know the significance of their roles in the plan of care, and nurses must enlist these informal caregivers to continue to provide care. In turn, the client's family must understand what can be expected from agency services.

Several forces are coming to bear on the need for homecare services. As the U.S. population ages, individuals survive longer, and chronic illnesses increase, there is a social movement to decrease institutionalization in nursing homes in favor of keeping clients in their own communities. The homecare industry is in an excellent position to create partnerships with payers, clients, and families to help clients stay in their own environments and manage their chronic illness.

CASE STUDY 20-1

John Robinson is a 73-year-old man who is preparing for discharge from the hospital following a left hip replacement. He has a history of osteoarthritis in his knees and hips, with the left hip being the worst. He has smoked 1 pack of cigarettes daily for 50 years.

Mr. Robinson lives alone in a small apartment near the center of town. The plan is for him to return home with homecare services. It is anticipated that he will meet the criteria for being home-bound and will need physical therapy for mobility, skilled nursing care for wound supervision, and respiratory assessment. He will also need a home health aide to assist with ADLs until he regains his mobility.

When the hospital case manager came to discuss Mr. Robinson's discharge plans with him, she indicated that three homecare agencies served his neighborhood. Mr. Robinson asked, "Which one is the best?" Mr. Robinson and the case manager used her laptop computer in his hospital room to look at Home Care Compare to evaluate the outcomes of the three agencies as compared to each other, state outcomes, and national outcomes. Based on the ratings, they chose Greenway Visiting Nurse Services (GVNS). From GVNS, Mr. Robinson could receive the skilled services he needs, and would also be able to obtain homemaker services to do light housekeeping and grocery shopping.

Discussion Questions

1. Which services provided to Mr. Robinson will be covered by Medicare?
2. Mr. Robinson is eligible for 3 weeks of homecare services. How would you organize care to provide the best service?
3. Which potential problems have you identified for Mr. Robinson?
4. Which other resources might be considered for Mr. Robinson?

CASE STUDY 20-2

Mrs. Chandler is an 87-year-old widow with end-stage COPD. She lives alone in subsidized senior housing. Mrs. Chandler is hospitalized three or four times each year with an exacerbation of her breathing difficulty. Currently she has just returned home from her most recent hospitalization. She is using oxygen at 2 L/min continuously, and tires extremely easily when engaging in ADLs. Currently she is relying on Meals on Wheels and friends to provide meals and groceries.

Mrs. Chandler is on Medicare and Medicaid and is nursing home eligible. She is adamant that she wants to remain in her apartment. You are the visiting nurse and are responsible for coordinating and arranging care for Mrs. Chandler. Although your agency is capable of providing skilled nursing, nurse aide, and homemaker services, Mrs. Chandler requires home oxygen services that are provided by another company.

Discussion Questions

1. What are the issues of coordinating care for Mrs. Chandler?
2. How might you incorporate telehealth into her care?
3. Which information will you need to initiate HCBS for Mrs. Chandler?
4. Which community resources might be involved in Mrs. Chandler's care?

Evidence-Based Practice Box

Parker and colleagues (2014) conducted a review of the available evidence published in English between 1990 and 2012 for several skilled homecare interventions in the United States. Four interventions had strong evidence supporting that they enhanced outcomes—namely, coordination of care, telehealth, multicomponent interventions, and data-driven quality of care monitoring. In addition, Medicaid Home and Community-Based Services hold promise for producing Medicaid savings and high consumer satisfaction.

Coordinating care among the client, informal caregivers, and healthcare providers can improve the outcomes of care. Care coordination is particularly important with respect to care transitions. It is most critical for individuals with multiple chronic conditions—these clients tend to require multiple care givers and move among healthcare settings frequently. Care coordination is challenging in part because reimbursement for these services is lacking. However, implementation of the Affordable Care Act holds promise for improving coordination of healthcare services.

Telehealth-based interventions show promise as a means to improve outcomes and reduce cost in home healthcare settings. Telehealth interventions including phone monitoring, telemonitoring, virtual visits, and email reminders have been used in this setting. Telemonitoring has the most evidence to support its efficacy.

Multicomponent interventions have been found to be effective for keeping rates of hospitalization down for individuals with chronic illness. The most successful agencies routinely used six or more evidence-based interventions to prevent hospitalizations, including fall prevention, front-loaded visits, care management, medication management, and 24-hour availability.

Recently, the OASIS database has been used to assess quality in home care. This database has provided a mechanism to evaluate the effectiveness

(continues)

of interventions across agencies. Through the online reporting system known as Home Health Compare, agencies can now compare their outcomes to the outcomes of other agencies. Public reporting of outcome measures appears to have improved the overall quality of care delivered, especially for low-performing agencies.

Medicaid Home and Community-Based Care is a Medicaid program that provides care in the community for individuals who qualify for nursing home care. Its goals are to keep the individual in his or her home and to provide services at less than the cost of nursing home care. Although to date few large research studies have evaluated the effectiveness of this program, some evidence shows that HCBS is effective in controlling the growth of Medicaid expenditures in some states.

Home health is well positioned to provide high-quality, cost-effective care for individuals with chronic illness.

Source: Parker, E., Zimmerman, S., Rodriguez, S., & Lee, T. (2014). Exploring best practices in home health care: A review of available evidence on select innovations. *Home Health Care Management Practice,* 26(1), 17–33.

STUDY QUESTIONS

1. What is the goal of home care according to the ANA?
2. Discuss the definition of *homebound*. Explain how being homebound might affect an individual's ability to go to church regularly and how it might affect the provision of health care.
3. Discuss how the homecare nurse might use the CCM to provide care to a client with chronic illness.
4. How does including telehealth in the list of interventions affect the delivery of home care?
5. Discuss strategies the homecare nurse might use to help a client and his or her family manage the chronic disease process.
6. Which skills does a nurse need to be an effective homecare nurse?
7. How can the interdisciplinary team maintain effective communication in the home?
8. Discuss how nurses might use Home Care Compare measures to improve the healthcare delivery system.

Internet Resources

Centers for Medicare and Medicaid Services: http://www.cms.gov/oasis/
Home Healthcare Nurses Association: www.hhna.org
National Association for Home Care and Hospice: www.nahc.org

Medicare Home Health Compare: http://www.medicare.gov/homehealthcompare/

References

American Nurses Association (ANA). (2008). *Home health nursing: Scope and standards of practice.* Silver Springs, MD: Author.

American Telemedicine Association (ATA). (2011). American Telemedicine Association. http://www.americantelemed.org

Buhler-Wilkersen, K. (2012). No place like home: A history of nursing and homecare in the US. *Home Healthcare Nurse, 30*(8), 446–452.

Butterworth, S. W., Linden, A., & McClay, W. (2007). Health coaching as an intervention in health management programs. *Disease Management of Health Outcomes*, 15(5), 299–307.

Clark, M. J. (2008). *Community health nursing: Advocacy for population health* (5th ed.). Upper Saddle River, NJ: Pearson.

Coleman, E. (n.d.). The Care Transitions Program. http://www.caretransitions.org

Centers for Medicare and Medicaid (2014). Readmissions reduction program. http://www.cms.gov/Medicare/Medicare-Fee-for-Service-Payment/AcuteInpatientPPS/Readmissions-Reduction-Program.html

Delta Health Technologies. (2012). The Delta study to reduce hospitalizations: A national study to reduce avoidable hospitalizations through home care. Sponsor: Delta Health Technologies. Co-sponsor: National Association for Home Care & Hospice. Affiliated sponsors: Home Health Quality Improvement (HHQI) National Campaign, NAHC Forum of State Associations, Community Health Accreditation Program, the Joint Commission, American Physical Therapy Association, and Fazzi Associates, Inc.

Doane, G. (2002). Beyond behavioral skills to human-involved processes: Relational nursing practice and interpretive pedagogy. *Journal of Nursing Education*, 41(9), 400–404.

Doane, G., & Varcoe, C. (2007). Relational practice and nursing obligations. *Advances in Nursing Science*, 30(3), 192–205.

Ellenbecker, C. (2004). A theoretical model of job retention for home health care nurses. *Journal of Advanced Nursing*, 47(3), 303–310.

Enderlin, C. A., McLeskey, N., Rooker, J. L., Steinhauser, C., D'Avolio, D., Gusewelle, R., & Ennen, K. A. (2013). Review of current conceptual models and frameworks to guide transitions of care in older adults. *Geriatric Nursing*, 34, 47–52.

Funk, L., & Stajduhar, K. (2011). Analysis and proposed model of family caregivers' relationships with home health providers and perceptions of the quality of formal services. *Journal of Applied Gerontology*, 32(2), 188–206.

Furaker, C. (2012). Registered nurses' views on competencies in home care. *Home Healthcare Management and Practice*, 24(5), 221–227.

Hall, J. L., & McGraw, D. (2014). For telehealth to succeed, privacy and security risks must be identified and addressed. *Health Affairs*, 33(2), 216–221.

Hartrick, G. (1997). Relationship capacity: The foundation for interpersonal nursing practice. *Journal of Advanced Nursing*, 26, 523–528.

Hayashi, J., & Leff, B. (2012). Medically oriented HCBS: House calls make a comeback. *Generations*, 36(1), 96–102.

Hines, D. (2012). Cultural competence: Assessment and education resources for home care and hospice clinicians. *Home Health Care Nurse*, 30(1), 39–45.

Hirth, V., Baskins, J., & Dever-Bumba, M. (2009). Program of All-Inclusive Care (PACE): Past, present, and future. *Journal of the American Medical Directors Association*, 10, 155–160.

Huffman, M. (2007). Health coaching: A new and exciting technique to enhance patient self-management and improve outcomes. *Home Healthcare Nurse*, 25(4), 271–274.

Huffman, M. (2009). Health coaching: A fresh, new approach to improve quality outcomes and compliance for patients with chronic conditions. *Home Healthcare Nurse*, 27(8), 491–496.

Improving Chronic Illness Care. (2007). The chronic care model. http://www.improvingchroniccare.org/index.php?p=The_Chronic_Care_Model&s=2

Jacelon, C. S. (2011). Health care, rehabilitation and rehabilitation nursing. In C.S. Jacelon (Ed.) *The specialty practice of rehabilitation nursing: A core curriculum* (6th ed., pp. 3-13). Glenview, IL: Association of Rehabilitation Nurses.

Jacelon, C. S., Furman, E., Rea, A., Macdonald, B., & Donoghue, L. C. (2011). Creating a professional practice model for post acute care: Adapting the chronic care model for long-term care. *Journal of Gerontological Nursing*, 37(3), 53–60.

Kaiser Foundation. (2010). Summary of new health reform law. http://www.kff.org/healthreform/8061.cfm.2/12/11

Kane, R. (2012). Thirty years of home- and community-based services: Getting closer and closer to home. *Generations*, 36(1), 6–13.

Ledesma, C. R. (2011, April). Relationship-based care: A new approach to caring. *Nursing Management*, 40–43.

Leff, E. (2004). Involving patients in care decisions improves satisfaction: An outcomes based quality improvement project. *Home Healthcare Nurse*, 22(5), 297–301.

LoFaso, V. M., Breckman, R., Capello, C. F., Demopoulos, B., & Edelman, R. D. (2010). Combining the creative arts and the house call to teach medical students about chronic illness care. *Journal of the American Geriatrics Society*, 58(2), 346–351.

Marek, K. D., Stetzer, F., Adams, S. J., Popejoy, L. L., & Rantz, M. (2010). The relationship of community-based nurse care coordination to costs in the Medicare and Medicaid programs. *Research in Nursing and Health*, 33, 235–242.

Marek, K. D., Stetzer, F., Adams, S. J., Popejoy, L. L., & Rantz, M. (2012). Aging in place versus nursing home care: Comparison costs to Medicare and Medicaid. *Research in Gerontological Nursing*, 5(2), 123–128.

Maurer, F., & Smith, C. (2005). *Community public health nursing practice*. St. Louis, MO: Elsevier Saunders.

McLean, S., Nurmatov, U., Liu, J. L. Y., Pagliari, C., Car, J., & Sheikh, A. (2011). Telehealthcare for chronic obstructive pulmonary disease. *Cochrane Database of Systematic Reviews*, 7, CD007718. doi: 10.1002/14651858.CD007718.pub2

Meckes, C. (2005). Opportunities in care coordination. *Home Healthcare Nurse*, 23(10), 663–669.

Murkofsky, R. L., & Alston, K. (2009). The past, present, and future of skilled home health agency care. *Clinical Geriatric Medicine*, 25(1), 1–17.

Myers, S., Grant, R., Lugn, N., Holbert, B., & Kvedar, J. (2006). Impact of home-based monitoring on the care of patients with congestive heart failure. *Home Health Care Management and Practice*, 18(6), 444–445.

National Alliance of Caregiving (NAC). (2009). Almost one-third of U.S. adult population plays caregiver role in households across America: 65.7 million caregivers. http://www.caregiving.org/pdf/research/CaregivinginUS09Release12309.pdf

National Coalition on Care Coordination (N3C). (n.d.). Policy brief: Implementing care coordination in the Patient Protection and Affordable Care Act. http://www.nyam.org/social-work-leadership-institute/docs/publications/N3C-Implementing-Care-Coordination.pdf

National PACE Association. (2013). PACE in the states. http://www.npaonline.org/website/download.asp?id=1741&title=PACE_in_the_States

Naylor, M. (1990). Comprehensive discharge planning for hospitalized elderly: A pilot study. *Nursing Research*, 39, 156–160.

Ng, T., & Harrington, C. (2012). The data speak: A progress report on providing Medicaid HCBS for elders. *Generations*, 36(1), 14–20.

Parker, E., Zimmerman, S., Rodriguez, S., & Lee, T. (2014). Exploring best practices in home health care: A review of available evidence on select innovations. *Home Health Care Management Practice*, 26(1), 17–33.

Percival, J., & Hanson, J. (2006). Big Brother or Brave New World? Telecare and its implications for older people's independence and social inclusions. *Critical Social Policy*, 26(4), 888–909.

Radhakrishnan, K., Jacelon, C. S., Bigelow, C., Roche, J., Marquard, J. L., & Bowles, K. H. (2012). Association of comorbidities with home care service utilization of patients with heart failure while receiving telehealth. *Journal of Cardiovascular Nursing*, 28(3), 216–227.

Radhakrishnan, K., Jacelon, C. S., & Roche, J. (2012). Perceptions on the use of telehealth for heart failure by homecare nurses and patients: A mixed method study. *Home Health Care Management & Practice*, 24(4), 175–181.

Remington, L. (2000, July/August). PPS is making people run out of excuses for a change. In: *The Remington report: Business and clinical solutions for home care and post-acute markers*. pp. 13–15.

Roseland, A. M., Heisler, M., & Piette, J. D. (2012). The impact of family behaviours and communication patterns on chronic illness outcomes: A systematic review. *Journal of Behavioral Medicine*, 35, 221–239.

Schneider, J. S., Barkauskas, V., & Keenan, G. (2008). Evaluation of home health care nursing outcomes with OASIS and NOC. *Journal of Nursing Scholarship*, 40(1), 76–82.

Smith, A. C. (2013). Effect of telemonitoring on re-admission in patients with congestive heart failure. *Medical Surgical Nursing*, 22(1), 39–44.

Smith-Stoner, M. (2011). Webcasting in home and hospice care services: Virtual communication in home care. *Home Healthcare Nurse*, 29(6), 337–341.

Stajduhar, K. I., Funk, L. M., Roberts, D., Cloutier-Fisher, D., McLeod, B., Wilkinson, C., & Purkis, M. E. (2011). Articulating the role of relationships in access to home care nursing at the end of life. *Qualitative Health Research*, 21(1), 117–131.

Stanhope, M., & Lancaster, J. (2010). *Foundations of nursing in the community: Community-oriented practice* (8th ed.). St. Louis, MO: Mosby.

Tao, H., & Ellenbecker, C.H. (2013). Is OASIS effective in predicting rehospitalization for home health care elderly patients? *Home Health Care Management & Practice*, 25(6), 250–255.

Vincent, A. E., & Birkhead, A. C. S. (2013). Evaluation of the effectiveness of nurse coaching in improving health outcomes in chronic conditions. *Holistic Nursing Practice*, 27(3), 148–161.

Volland, P. J., Schraeder, C., Shelton, P., & Hess, I. (2013). The transitional care and comprehensive care coordination debate: Which approach works best for people with chronic illness? We provide some models (and a real-life story) for study. *Generations*, 36(4), 13–19.

Wagner, E. H. (1998). Chronic disease management: What it will take to improve care for chronic illness. *Effective Clinical Practice*, 1, 2–4.

Weydt, A. (2010). Mary's story: Relationship-based care delivery. *Nursing Administration Quarterly*, 34(2), 141–146.

Young, H. M. (2002). Challenges and solutions for care of frail older adults. *The Online Journal of Issues in Nursing*, 8(2), 5.

Chapter 21

Long-Term Care

Kristen L. Mauk

Introduction

Long-term care (LTC) is an umbrella term that refers to a range of services that addresses the health, personal care, psycho-emotional, and social needs of persons with some degree of difficulty in caring for themselves (National Care Planning Council, 2014). Although family members may assist those persons with age-related functional decline or those with disabilities, LTC is often needed as time progresses to bridge the gap in care. The ideal LTC services promote independence of the person for as long as possible and allow him or her to remain at home as appropriate. LTC may be required because of disability associated with birth defects, injury, chronic illness, or the aging process. The concept of LTC may best be visualized on a continuum. Between the two ends of the spectrum—independence with minimal assistance at home versus skilled care in the nursing home—are many alternatives and options.

Care needs may be minimal or extensive (**Figure 21-1**). LTC services are offered in a variety of settings, as discussed in greater detail in this chapter. There is a growing trend toward provision of community-based services. Often, persons visualize a nursing home setting when they think of LTC, but this setting is used by only a small portion of the population at any given time.

Nurses are in an excellent position to design and implement innovative, cost-effective, and visionary care modalities to provide high-quality LTC services for patients, while preserving the individual's dignity and personhood. Because of the holistic perspective that nurses have regarding the patient, family, and community, they are in an excellent position to act as change agents in the process of healthcare reform.

In 2009, there were 39.6 million people older than age 65 in the United States. By 2030, there will be approximately 72.1 million older adults, more than twice the number in 2000 (Administration on Aging, 2011). An overview of LTC services in the United States (Harris-Kojetin, Sengupta, Park-Lee, & Valverde, 2013) provided these statistics:

In 2012, about 58,500 paid, regulated long-term care service providers served about 8 million people in the United States. Long-term care services were provided by 4,800 adult day services centers, 12,200 home health agencies, 3,700 hospices, 15,700 nursing homes, and 22,200 assisted living and similar residential care communities. Each day in 2012, there were 273,200 participants enrolled in adult day

Figure 21-1 Long-Term Care Continuum in Terms of Intensity

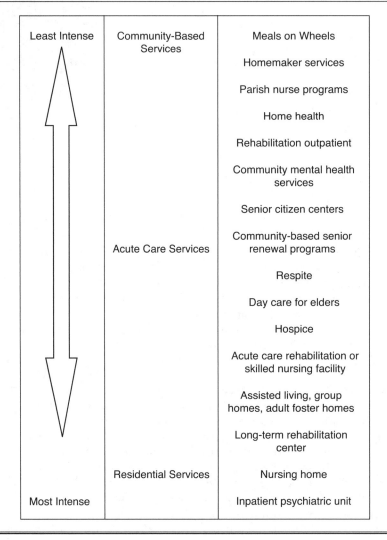

service centers, 1,383,700 residents in nursing homes, and 713,300 residents in residential care communities; in 2011, about 4,742,500 patients received services from home health agencies, and 1,244,500 patients received services from hospices. (p. viii)

For many persons, increased age is accompanied by one or more chronic illnesses. Such health conditions reported in the Health and Retirement Study (National Institute on Aging, 2007) included (in order of frequency) arthritis, hypertension, heart conditions, diabetes, psychological/emotional problems, cancer, chronic lung disease, and stroke. These chronic conditions account for many of the frequent complaints of older adults as they experience the aging process. Chronic diseases are the leading causes of death and disability in the United States and account for approximately one in seven deaths (Centers for Disease Control and Prevention [CDC], 2012). In fact, 19 million Americans reported difficulty in performing some activities of daily living due to arthritis alone (CDC, 2012). As the incidence of chronic disease grows, deficits in a person's ability to perform self-care often follow, which can eventually lead to the need for LTC services.

According to an AARP document (Houser, Fox-Grage, & Gibson, 2009), indicators of the need for LTC services include advanced age, living alone, poverty, less education, not owning a home, and not having a vehicle for transportation. There is wide variation among states as to the availability and use of LTC services (Reinhard, Kassner, Houser, & Mollica, 2011). Even though it is thought that the use of community-based services is increasing (Houser, Fox-Grage, & Ujvari, 2012), "findings from the National Study of Long-Term Care Providers (NSLTCP) suggest that in most areas of the country the supply and use of nursing homes are still greater than those of other long-term care service options" (Harris-Kojetin et al., 2013, p. 38).

Historical Perspectives

Caring for a client with complex health needs over a long period continues to be a challenge for the U.S. healthcare system. Throughout history, the consideration given to the quality of care for older adults or other vulnerable populations has been seen as a reflection of societal values (Koop & Schaeffer, 1976). In societies with more fluid resources, vulnerable populations such as the frail elderly or individuals with chronic illness are better cared for because of the availability of assistance with health care (Kalisch & Kalisch, 2004). History has demonstrated that

in societies experiencing famine, war, or social upheaval, the vulnerable may not be able to survive because of malnutrition, lack of health care, and the lack of ability of the family unit to provide support.

A review of LTC in the United States reveals several significant events that have led to the current system of providing care. Prior to the 20th century, older adults in the United States were usually cared for within extended family units (DeSpelder & Strickland, 2011). Those without family to care for them might have gone to a facility supported by a religious organization or by charitable citizens, such as a poorhouse or almshouse. Over time, changes in medical care altered hospital stays and allowed LTC to evolve, with group rest homes and private charitable homes providing care for chronically ill, dependent persons. Because life expectancies continued to increase, the demand for LTC increased. Political response to this demand came in the form of the Social Security Act in 1932, which provided services for the elderly and chronically ill.

In 1951, the first White House Conference on Aging was held. Title XVIII of the Social Security Act, which was passed in 1965 and was a part of the Great Society of President Lyndon B. Johnson, provided medical insurance for the elderly (Medicare) and further involved the federal government in health care (Centers for Medicare and Medicaid Services [CMS], 2011a). At the same time, in 1965, public policy was altered by the enactment of the Older Americans Act, which established aging networks throughout the states and funded community-based health services. Medicare opened the door for the government to dictate regulations and set the standard for care in formal caregiving settings. Evolution of this system included a restructuring of the Health Care Financing Authority into the CMS, with an emphasis on improving the overall process of coordinating care of complex illness in the context of managed care (Administration on Aging, 2008).

Part of the Social Security Amendments of 1965 was Title XIX, better known as Medicaid, to provide medical and health-related services for individuals and families with low incomes. In 1972, legislation was passed that paid for intermediate care for this population. Medicaid, a cooperative program between each state and the federal government, is the largest source of funds for services to the poor. Each state establishes its own eligibility standards, sets the rate of payment for services, and administers its own program (CMS, 2011a).

The Omnibus Reconciliation Act, passed in 1987, included the Nursing Home Reform Act, which established high quality of care as a goal, along with the preservation of residents' rights in LTC facilities. Among the changes included in this legislation was the requirement that comprehensive assessments of all nursing home residents be done to determine the functional, cognitive, and affective levels of the residents and to be used in planning care. In addition, more specific requirements for nursing, medical, and psychosocial services were designed to ensure that patients would attain and maintain the highest possible mental and physical functional statuses by focusing on patient outcomes (Harrington, Carrillo, Blank, & O'Brian, 2010).

The Patient Protection and Affordable Health Care Act (ACA) of 2010 is expected to lead to a major overhaul of the existing healthcare funding system; the ultimate goal is to provide care to all Americans. Extensions of and changes to the implementation of this legislation make it difficult to predict how the ACA will eventually impact the LTC industry.

The Continuum of Care

For the purpose of common definitions, the U.S. government recognizes five types of long-term care services: adult day service centers, nursing homes, residential care communities, home health agencies, and hospice (Harris-Kojetin et al., 2013). All will be discussed in this section, with the exception of hospice. Persons who

require long-term care services are those who need assistance with activities of daily living (ADLs) such as dressing, grooming, feeding, or bathing, and/or instrumental activities of daily living (IADLs) such as paying bills, managing money, and using the telephone (National Care Planning Association, 2014).

Long-Term Acute Care Long-term acute care hospitals (LTACHs) are units that provide extended medical and rehabilitation care to persons with complex healthcare needs. They are appropriate for persons needing hospital-level care for a longer period of time. The average length of stay at an LTACH is 25 to 30 days (Kindred Hospital, 2014). Patients requiring this level of care usually have multiple comorbidities with acute illness or disease progression that cannot be treated at a lesser level of care. Some LTACHs are free-standing, while others may occupy a floor within an acute care hospital (Amann & LeBlanc, 2014).

Community-Based Long-Term Care A variety of services are available within the LTC continuum. "Of the approximately 58,500 regulated, long-term care service providers, about two-thirds provided care in residential settings (26.8% were nursing homes and 37.9% were residential care communities), and about one-third provided care in home- and community-based settings (8.2% were adult day services centers, 20.9% were home health agencies, and 6.3% were hospices)" (Harris-Kojetin et al., 2013, p. 8). Current trends advocate using a case management approach to coordinate services and to ensure that individuals receive services in an efficient, timely fashion. Case management promotes aging in place for individuals with chronic illness, trying to keep a person in the home setting for as long as possible. The LTC system may be confusing to clients and families, but case managers can arrange and coordinate services such as Meals on Wheels, medical care, home health aides, and companion services.

The newest role is that of a geriatric care manager, a service for clients and families.

Geriatric Case Management   Professional geriatric care managers (PGCMs) help families care for their older family members while promoting independence of the older adult. The National Association of Professional Geriatric Care Managers (2011) suggests that families might expect a PGCM to provide the following services:

- Conduct care-planning assessments to identify problems and to provide solutions
- Screen, arrange, and monitor in-home help or other services, including assistance in hiring a qualified caregiver for home care
- Provide short- or long-term assistance for caregivers living near or far away
- Review financial, legal, or medical issues and offer referrals to geriatric specialists
- Provide crisis intervention
- Act as a liaison for families at a distance, overseeing care and quickly alerting families to problems
- Assist with moving an older person to or from a retirement complex, assisted care home, or nursing home
- Provide consumer education and advocacy
- Offer eldercare counseling and support

Unfortunately, neither private insurance, nor Medicare, nor Medicaid reimburses for geriatric case managers. The services are all private-pay only.

Community-Based Services   Related services for the frail elder or individual with chronic illness could also include legal services, adult protective services, area councils on aging, ombudsman programs, senior centers, and elder-advocacy groups. Older adults with chronic illnesses that are amenable to rehabilitation may receive assistance with recovery through Medicare, which pays for inpatient and limited outpatient therapies ordered by a physician. Respite care for family members who care for loved ones with chronic illness and disability is also a community-based service.

Adult Day Services   Adult day services (ADS) are an alternative for those persons wishing to remain at home but who need assisted-living services during the day (Matthiesen & Schumaker, 2010). ADS programs often provide meals, activities, some therapies, and socialization within a safe group setting for individuals when a caregiver or family member is not home during the day. These services are offered during working hours and do not include housing or overnight stays. They may be housed at organizations such as churches or community centers (Amann & LeBlanc, 2014). Use of these community services varies among ethnic groups. In a recent U.S. survey, among adult daycare participants, Latinos accounted for 20.1% and non-Hispanic blacks represented 16.7% (Harris-Kojetin et al., 2013).

PACE   The Program of All-Inclusive Care for the Elderly (PACE) is another community-based alternative that promotes aging in place (Boult & Wieland, 2010). This program comprises an evidence-based model of care whose services are often covered by Medicare and Medicaid (Medicaid.gov, 2014). According to the National PACE Association (2011), the average user is 80 years old, and preliminary studies suggest that involvement in a PACE program may slow functional decline for older adults. The PACE model combines dollars from different funding streams to deliver a comprehensive set of services focused on the health and well-being of the individual (National PACE Association, 2011). The number of states with participating organizations has increased to 30 in the last few years (the list of states with programs is found on the PACE website at http://www.npaonline.org).

Continuing evaluation of this program in terms of the cost–benefit relationship for the funding agencies may lead to it becoming available in more locations.

Retirement Communities Continuing care retirement communities (CCRCs) and naturally occurring retirement communities (NORCs) are additional options for community-based services. CCRCs may offer a range of services, from independent living to skilled nursing care. This allows for smoother care transitions, as older adults are able to age in place within the same campus community. NORCs are living communities that are designed for older adults, but do not offer medical services. NORCs generally limit residents of the property to age 55 years or older and may offer social and recreational programs, outside property maintenance, healthcare programs, meals, and transportation (Amann & LeBlanc, 2014). Both of these models are designed to help older adults age in place in a safe environment.

Residential Long-Term Care Settings

Residential LTC facilities are formal, organized agencies that provide care for persons who are unable to live alone because of physical or other problems, but who do not require hospitalization. Persons living in residential care are not called patients, but residents, because the LTC setting is their home. The three most common types of residential LTC facilities are group homes, assisted-living centers, and nursing homes. Many retirement communities combine independent-living facilities and assisted-living facilities, although they actually represent two different levels of care. Those living independently in a retirement community may do so because of declining health caused by chronic illness, safety factors, frailty, and the need for socialization. The decision to move from one's own home to a community living situation is difficult, however, and often involves the advice

of family members who are concerned about the older adult's ability to live alone safely. LTC residents are a vulnerable population who tend to have more chronic illnesses and may require advocacy from health or social professionals.

Group Homes Group homes are also referred to as personal care homes, foster homes, domiciliary care homes, board and care homes, and congregate care homes. Their philosophy embraces a home environment with a limited number of residents who share common characteristics in needing assistance with such things as activities of daily living, shopping, cleaning, and medication management. Much like a boarding house, the owner of the home provides services such as meals, laundry and cleaning, medication management, and a safe environment (Amann & LeBlanc, 2014). These homes are licensed by the state. Group-home care is most appropriate for persons with uncomplicated medical problems. Payment for group homes can be private, although in some states it may be covered by welfare programs. The Robert Wood Johnson Foundation (2014) has sponsored research in creating innovative and livable homes under the Green House Project (more information may be found in the research literature and at www.thegreenhouseproject.org).

Assisted-Living Facilities Persons in assisted-living facilities (ALFs) are those who require some type of help with activities of daily living. According to the National Center for Assisted Living (2011), more than 900,000 individuals currently reside in ALFs; of those persons, 64% require help with bathing, 39% need help with dressing, 26% need help with toileting, 19% need help with transferring, and 12% need help with eating. Of all residents, 81% need help with medication management. Because Medicare, Medicaid, and the U.S. Department of Veterans Affairs (VA) do not pay for assisted-living care (except in certain circumstances through the VA for veterans), the cost for this living arrangement and services are paid for out of pocket. Assisted-living centers may be found as free-standing facilities, as part of retirement communities, or attached to nursing homes to allow for smoother transition of care for those expected to need skilled nursing in the future.

Data from the 2010 National Survey of Residential Care Facilities survey revealed the following points about ALFs (Caffrey, Sengupta, Park-Lee, Moss, Rosenoff, & Harris-Kojetin, 2012):

- The majority of residents were non-Hispanic and female, and more than half were 85 years of age or older.
- Nearly 4 of 10 residents received assistance with at least three ADLs, typically bathing and dressing.
- More than three-fourths of the residents had at least 2 of the 10 most common chronic diseases. High blood pressure and Alzheimer's and other dementias were the most common.
- The median length of stay for all residents was 671 days, or nearly 2 years.

Although assisted-living facilities are accountable to a board of directors and may employ a registered nurse (RN) consultant, the care is generally provided by aides, with licensed practical nurses (LPNs) used regularly to supervise daily services. Such facilities provide autonomy for older adults, allowing them to live in a safe, home-like environment adapted for those with physical challenges. Assisted-living arrangements provide personal space in the form of apartments or suites, meals through community dining, and transportation and social activities.

Green House Model for Assisted Living
The Green House model supports de-institutionalization of long-term care by creating a home-like atmosphere in which high-quality skilled care is provided. This model was created by Dr. William Thomas, a geriatrician, with the hope of providing a place where older adults would get the care they need, but within a home environment. Green houses are larger than an average home and may house 10 residents, each of whom has a private bathroom, but who share a common living area and kitchen. There were 260 Green Houses in 26 states as of 2014 (Robert Wood Johnson Foundation, 2014).

All of the services provided in a long-term care facility may be present in a Green House, but the emphasis is on autonomy and choice of the residents, supporting dignity, fostering meaningful relationships, and giving comprehensive care in a more nurturing environment (Robert Wood Johnson Foundation, 2014). Nurse practitioners are mid-level providers who may help manage care in this setting.

Skilled Nursing Facilities or Nursing Homes
Nursing home is a term used to refer to a facility that has either skilled nursing services and/or intermediate care. Nursing homes are LTC facilities for individuals with chronic illness, who are medically frail, or who are disabled (Harris-Kojetin et al., 2013). The level of care may be described as residential, long-term, nonemergent, or custodial care. Some facilities may include an intermediate care or rehabilitation unit for individuals who need assistance in reestablishing self-care abilities. The larger nursing care facilities offer services such as traditional nursing care, assisted and independent living, memory care units, therapies, pharmacy services, and hospice.

The majority of such agencies are "for profit" entities. Some of the largest nursing home chains in the United States include Golden Living (Beverly), Life Care Centers of America, HCR ManorCare, Kindred, and Genesis (*Provider Magazine*, 2012). The few nonprofit agencies are generally associated with churches or other nonprofit organizations such as the VA, which refers to its nursing homes as community living centers (U.S. Department of Veterans Affairs, 2014). The Veterans Health Administration (VHA) has predicted that the number of veterans older than age 85 will double in the next decade, and that the VHA-enrolled veterans in this oldest-old age group will increase sevenfold, resulting in a 22% to 25% increase in both nursing home and community-based services.

Agencies that receive income from the CMS are required to meet minimum state and federal standards. These standards address items such as nutritional and fluid intake; provision of social interaction and activities; and support services such as physical therapy, rehabilitation therapy, housekeeping, and laundry services. There is a continued concern by those employed in LTC settings that facility structure and staffing are often based on minimal standards that place a priority on containing costs instead of first considering what is desirable or needed for the client. However, as the baby boomer generation ages, it is expected that interest in this issue will increase and creation of higher standards will occur, leading to a higher quality of care in LTC facilities.

Approximately 5% of the elderly population reside in nursing homes in the United States, and 28% pay for their own care. Care in nursing homes may be funded by the individual (self-pay), insurance, Medicare (with limits), or Medicaid. To be eligible for Medicaid payment for residential care, the client must have limited assets with which to pay for the services required. Often a LTC resident will enter a nursing home and pay for services until his or her estate is spent down, at which point Medicaid pays for care until the client's death (AARP, 2010).

Much of the care provided in the traditional nursing home setting is considered custodial care. Rehabilitative services are provided for those persons who have the capacity to regain function. Because the institutionalized individual may require a great deal of help with the physical aspects of care, such as bathing, dressing, eating, and space maintenance, his or her cognitive needs (emotional, psychological, and spiritual) may be considered less important. Activity programs are sometimes geared toward only one segment of the facility population. Care in LTC settings should include not only appropriate physical care, but also appropriate social and cognitive stimulation.

Long-Term Care Recipients: A Vulnerable Population

Vulnerable individuals are those who are at increased risk for loss of autonomy, loss of self-will, injustice, loss of privacy, and increased risk for abuse. A vulnerable adult is defined as an individual who is either being mistreated or is in danger of mistreatment and who, because of age and/or disability is unable to protect himself or herself (Teaster, 2002). Examples of vulnerable persons in LTC may include those with physical, mental, or emotional problems; the elderly; those with dementia; and those who have been in prison. In a culture that values youth, energy, strength, and the ability to work, many devalue elders or those with chronic illness. Laws and practices differ between states in the areas of abuse, neglect, and protective services. Ultimately, it is the care providers and administrators in LTC who are responsible for maintaining an environment that supports the unique personhood of the client and protects the vulnerable.

Vulnerable older adults living in long-term care facilities face special challenges. In Connecticut, for example, state data revealed a large number of nursing home residents were not receiving adequate dental care and suffered from tooth decay (Connecticut Department of Public Health, 2013). Seemingly simple problems such as these can easily lead to tooth infection, abscess, and even sepsis.

Many individuals requiring LTC have already lost some autonomy and self-will because of illnesses that affect the individual's ability to make decisions or carry out intentional behavior. Vulnerability is of special concern in these individuals. Decisions must be made for them regarding many aspects of life, such as eating, bathing, medication administration, socialization, and exercising religious practices. Some persons may benefit from the services of a guardian, discussed later in this chapter.

Abuse in the home or in a residential facility is an extreme threat to the autonomy of the client. If the nurse providing care is the first to observe signs and symptoms of mistreatment, reporting these observations to Adult Protective Services (or another public agency, as designated in the particular state) is required by law. In the home, the home healthcare nurse may be in a position to discover abuse and act as the primary advocate to prevent further abuse. The nurse may work with various agencies to ensure that appropriate intervention is made. Because elder mistreatment is often subtle, the nurse must be persistent in reporting signs until action is taken. If abuse or neglect of the community-based client is profound, a move to residential care may be indicated.

Problems and Issues in Long-Term Care

There are a number of challenges related to LTC, ranging from overall system breakdown to individual treatment issues for clients in the system. The issues mentioned in this chapter are not all-inclusive, but merely provide an introduction to current problems.

Provision of Care

Along the continuum of LTC, problems in the provision of care include organization of services care transition, assessment in long-term care, access to care, gaps in public policy, funding, staffing, and standards of care. Specific issues vary within individual states or communities. It is imperative that the professional nurse involved in LTC is cognizant of the local and state issues that affect delivery and quality of LTC services.

Being a political activist to advocate on behalf of the recipients of LTC is also important.

Organization of Services

It was not surprising that the second most important resolution that came from the White House Conference on Aging in 2005 was the need for a more comprehensive and well-coordinated LTC strategy (Lomastro, 2006). Another issue, end-of-life care, did not receive any attention. According to Moody (2008), "the whole range of end-of-life decision making was overlooked by the 2005 White House Conference on Aging" (p. 25). The next White House Conference on Aging will occur in 2015.

In community-based LTC, the array of services in a given community may not be organized according to any hierarchy. Each specialized service, such as home care, elder daycare, hospice, or nutrition programs, was most likely initiated in response to a specific need or business opportunity in the community. It is often necessary for a program of LTC to be pieced together from a number of different organizations to meet one client's needs. This is especially true for community-dwelling residents.

Partial help with this problem comes from the United Way, a nonprofit service-based agency whose mission is to help others to give, advocate, and volunteer (United Way, 2014). The United Way publishes a resource book in larger cities that describes community programs and services. (This publication can be obtained by calling the local United Way office; the list of resources is available online at http://www.unitedway.org.) This resource book assists clients, family, and care providers in identifying appropriate services, phone numbers, and eligibility requirements. Many times individuals with chronic illness and their families are not aware that when they are involved with one system (such as a nursing home), they have access to other services (such as hospice). Individuals with chronic illnesses often view access to the LTC system as complicated and overwhelming.

Those with chronic illnesses and their families may have a limited amount of energy to invest in problem solving and identifying the best options. Often, access to the LTC system is controlled by gatekeepers who have minimal training and experience with complex medical conditions. Rules may be seen as arbitrary, and appear to exclude the very individuals intended to benefit from programs. Many states partner with their long-term care ombudsmen to advocate for the needs of older adults in nursing homes.

With the increased utilization of case management for individuals with chronic illness, whether through the local or federal VA, state health and human services divisions, or private companies, some progress is being made in assisting community-dwelling individuals to more effectively access LTC services. However, for most clients and families, access to the LTC system remains confusing and complex. Ongoing issues with organization of care have led to some new initiatives aimed at smoothly transitioning patients within the system of care.

Care Transitions

Transitioning from one point of care to another is a growing problem in the U.S. healthcare system, especially for the elderly, those with disabilities, and other vulnerable populations. Key risk factors leading to poor outcomes during the transition of care include lack of education for clients and families in managing illness, poor care coordination among healthcare professionals and settings, poor communication between professionals, inadequate assessment at the point of care, medication errors, lack of follow-up, health literacy problems, poor support systems, and cultural barriers (Amann & Blanc, 2014). These factors may lead to care that is fragmented, disorganized, and inefficient (Association of Rehabilitation Nurses [ARN], 2013). Families and patients can easily become frustrated when looking at post-acute care settings. According to

CMS (2013), such system factors may also lead to increased rates of rehospitalization. The ARN suggests that rehabilitation nurses are the professionals with the most appropriate skill set to address care transitions; it encourages organizations to take advantage of the knowledge of these experts during times of change in care settings (ARN, 2013).

Admission and Assessment in the Long-Term Care Setting

Admission to a nursing home can be very distressing to anyone. From the individual's perspective, the move to a nursing home or even assisted living away from their personal home may symbolize the reality of the loss of health, autonomy, personal relationships, economic power, productivity, and independence. Adjustment to such facilities may evoke a mix of emotions. The stress of going into a facility in which one is surrounded by strangers can be difficult. In addition, the individual must adjust to schedules determined by others, instead of following routines established throughout a lifetime. In many nursing homes, eating and bathing schedules are relatively fixed. Although not ideal, the resident is often the one who must change expectations to make allowance for the workload of the nursing home staff.

The decision to move to a nursing home is usually made after much consideration by the client and family. The transition may be made more smoothly when the client retains as much participation in the process as possible. The client should be encouraged to have input into choosing the facility and planning the move. Retention of personal items gives the individual a better sense of self in the new facility.

Admission to a nursing home may be one of life's most traumatic transitions. The nurse needs to assist in making the adjustment of the client to the facility as smooth as possible. The client experiencing psychological and emotional difficulty during the admission and transition into any LTC facility needs support from the attending nursing staff. The use of therapeutic communication techniques by the staff in addition to spending adequate time with a transitioning resident can make a difference in the level of anxiety and stress experienced. If indicated, the nurse should initiate a referral for the resident to be seen by mental health services. These services are generally an underused resource for elders.

Accessing community-based LTC services may seem a natural and necessary transition for an elder needing help with either rehabilitation or assistance with other aspects of care. For others, accessing services may create significant emotional turmoil. Once a frail elder can no longer stay in the community environment, the individual and family may decide that a move to another environment that provides needed services is necessary. For those persons who can afford assisted living, this option may be less emotionally traumatic. In such a setting, individuals feel they have retained a great deal of autonomy while paying for the services that they can no longer perform, such as food preparation, laundry, housekeeping, and medication management.

An accurate assessment of the client is the critical beginning for the client's experience in the LTC system. During the admission process to a LTC facility, the care provider completes a battery of paperwork that documents the client's condition and reason for admission. In residential nursing homes, this assessment is important because it provides the basis upon which the care plan is developed and helps set the course for interventions designed to promote the highest level of functioning possible. It is imperative that the admission process not be limited to completing paperwork, but also include gaining insight into the client to provide individualized care (ARN, 2013).

The Minimum Data Set (MDS) for Resident Assessment and Care Screening was developed for use by nursing homes in response to the Nursing Home Reform Legislation of 1987. The MDS provides extensive data about individual residents, but it also makes possible the establishment of a nationwide database regarding nursing home residents. Information requested by the MDS covers the areas of the resident's functional, medical, cognitive, and affective status at the time of admission and periodically thereafter (Sehy & Williams, 1999). This type of information also helps in tracking the improvement or decline of a resident over time, and indicates whether quality indicators for care are being met. In the initial or follow-up assessment, the assessment protocol summarizes vulnerable aspects of the client's life that may require special care planning, interventions, and reporting of progress or problems in the resident's chart.

The reliability of the information obtained varies with the knowledge that evaluators are able to obtain about the client. The latest revision to the MDS system (3.0) (CMS, 2010) has the following broad goals:

- To make the MDS more clinically relevant, while still achieving the federal payment mandates and quality initiatives
- To improve ease of use and efficiency
- To integrate selected standard scales
- To elicit resident voices by introducing interview questions

Other assessment tools are available and can provide more specific or multidimensional information. Tools can help the nurse determine the client's level of functioning in the cognitive, communication, behavioral, and social support domains. Other instruments measure vision, personality, depression, affect, comorbidity, and quality of life. Examples of individual tools that are readily available in the literature include the Katz Index of Activities of Daily Living (Katz, Downs, Cash, & Grotz, 1970), Older American Resources and Services (Fillenbaum, 1988), the Beck Depression Rating Scale (Beck, Rush, Shaw, & Emery, 1979), the Mini-Cog (Borson, Scanlan, Chen, & Ganguli, 2004: Borson, Scanlan,

Hummel, Gibbs, Lessig, & Zuhr, 2007), and the Arthritis Impact Measurement Scale (Meenan, 1985).

A helpful website with a list of more than 30 assessment tools that can be downloaded for immediate use is located at http://hartfordign .org/Practice/ConsultGeriRN/. For each assessment tool in the *Try This* series from the American Association of Colleges of Nursing (AACN)/Hartford Foundation, an explanation of the tool by an expert, validity and reliability information, the tool itself, and instructions on how to use it are succinctly provided.

Gaps in Public Policy

In the United States, the primary responsibility for paying for LTC services lies with the individuals who need those services. Medicare pays for limited skilled nursing care, up to 100 days associated with an acute illness requiring at least 3 days of hospitalization (Houser et al., 2009; Medpac, 2010). Partly because of the funding sources and partly because of the method of development of services, however, gaps in LTC services persist. Much policy work needs to be done related to the transitions that individuals experience when moving from one type of service to another, because no overall umbrella of comprehensive care exists. The current healthcare reform effort is at least to some extent aimed at making such transitions more seamless. Pharmaceutical costs, extended home health care, and rehabilitative services are problematic for many in LTC. Unfortunately, some who are unable to self-pay may go without services or medications.

Funding

The gaps in both LTC-related service and public policy are related to funding issues. Devising ways to afford long-term care services is a major issue for older adults, persons with disabilities, and their families. It also poses a major challenge for state and federal governments (Commission on Long-Term Care, 2013; Reinhard et al., 2011). In 2009, $144 billion was paid by state

and federal agencies to free-standing nursing home facilities (Harrington et al., 2010). An estimated $306 billion was spent on long-term care services in 2010. Excluding home health and skilled nursing care, other long-term care services costs totaled $237.7 billion in 2010 (Hartman, Martin, Benson, & Caitlin, 2013). As previously mentioned, a significant number of residents in nursing homes and other residential care facilities pay privately for their care until their estate is spent down, at which time state and federal funding may take over payments (Houser et al., 2009). Many persons may be eligible for both Medicare and Medicaid. Although these persons do not generally report difficulty obtaining medical care, 58% of those who need LTC report their needs as being unmet.

Private insurance and nonprofit organizations also provide services for those in need of LTC. However, beyond the nursing home setting, piecing together a comprehensive LTC program for a frail elder with comorbidities who wishes to remain in the community is challenging. Certification of eligibility for certain benefits, such as extended home care, is strict and lasts for a limited amount of time only.

Resources for LTC, whether private or public, are limited. Community-dwelling elders may be eligible for Medicare benefits in regard to certain services, such as home health care, but only as long as some rehabilitation progress can be documented. Once progress stops and the condition is considered chronic, the individual may have to pay privately for rehabilitative and home services. However, a new law that revised Medicare's rule regarding therapy was passed in January 2013. The settlement in the *Jimmo v. Sebelius* court case allows Medicare beneficiaries to receive health services needed to maintain their current level of functioning (AARP, 2013). For individuals who have lived through the Great Depression, World War II, and other historical events that required genuine frugality, spending nearly $100 to pay for less than an hour of a home visit from an agency RN is not a viable option. Many older adults from working-class backgrounds do without needed care rather than pay privately for such services. This reality suggests that state policies can make a difference in the health care of their citizens.

A key issue of debate is the entitlement to care for older adults and those with chronic illness conferred by the Social Security programs. These programs were designed to provide some comfort and security to the older individual. One view is that society has an obligation to provide for those in need, particularly the elderly, because of the labor and service that they have provided (Tobin & Salisbury, 1999). Another view is that society is obligated to provide care for frail and chronically ill elders because of the sanctity of all human life, rather than simply because of work during an adult's life. These philosophical origins of social services programs play an important part not only in the establishment and continuation of programs, but also in setting standards for ongoing programs.

Alternative financing for LTC needs to be explored. Although both PACE and social managed care plans offer alternatives to nursing homes and promote aging in place, it is evident that their scope and availability are significantly limited. In addition, a few strategies to fund LTC costs have arisen from the financial sector—notably, reverse mortgages and life settlement. Both concepts focus on helping individuals liquidate assets (for example, a home or life insurance policy) to provide the cash needed to privately pay to enter or remain in a facility. Only since 2000 has use of one's life insurance been considered as a financial tool to obtain relatively quick cash. Any individual considering this option should consult with a financial adviser, however.

STAFFING

Healthcare agencies that receive Medicare and Medicaid funding are licensed by each state or are accredited by a recognized accrediting agency. Each agency must meet requirements in staffing. Two main issues in staffing are the training of the staff member and the staff-to-client ratio (Harrington et al., 2010).

Standards for required staff training are often minimal. For example, medication aides working in an assisted-living center may be required to attend a 6-week training course, yet the medication regimens for the assisted-living center clientele may be extremely complex. For proper medication management, much more time is required to educate a person on the pharmacologic effects of medications, side effects, and complications. Although assisted-living centers are required to have an RN available, that single RN may act as a consultant for multiple centers under the same ownership umbrella. The actual individual who "supervises" the medication aides may be an LPN who works a 40-hour week.

Qualifications for the director or administrator of an assisted-living center are minimal, with a 2-year degree generally required and a 4-year degree preferred. The average salary for this position in 2012 was approximately $73,000 per year (Severson, 2014). An assisted-living administrator can earn certification in as little as 40 hours of continuing education. The majority of staff working in such facilities may be minimally trained personnel, and client safety is a legitimate concern. For example, resident assistants may have no additional training beyond high school, and the median salary for this position is about $20,000 (Miller, 2014). Staffing challenges in providing home health care are also significant. State requirements vary for home health aides, but no training program is more than 8–12 weeks in length. Often, aides are trained and then expected to work independently, with little supervision.

Staffing in nursing homes is a continuing issue. Conclusive evidence shows that a positive relationship exists between nursing staffing and quality of nursing home care (Mullaney, 2014). Fewer RN and nursing assistant hours are associated with quality-of-care deficiencies (Arling,

Kane, Mueller, Bershadsky, & Degenholtz, 2007; Families for Better Care, 2013). "States whose nursing homes employed an abundance of professional nurses and frontline caregivers translated to higher marks ... and only seven states provided more than one hour of professional nursing care per resident per day while 96% of states offered residents fewer than three hours of direct resident care per day" (Families for Better Care, 2013, p. 1). The turnover rate for nursing assistants can be as high as 40% to 100% in some facilities; high turnover rates have been associated with poor-quality care (Castle, Engberg, & Men, 2007). Recruitment and retention of qualified nursing assistants is an ongoing problem. Nursing staff turnover in nursing homes has been associated with negative outcomes for residents of these facilities. Thomas, Mor, Tyler, and Hyer (2013) found that "nursing homes that experienced a 10% increase in their licensed nurse retention had a 0.2% lower rehospitalization rate, which equates to two fewer hospitalizations per nursing home (NH) annually" (p. 211). Creating an environment that promotes teamwork, addresses care-related stressors, promotes positive communication, reduces paperwork inefficiencies and staffing shortages, and has high organizational morale has been shown to increase job satisfaction and commitment to the organization, but there are many other factors to consider in the complex process of staff turnover in these settings (AACN, 2011; Arling et al., 2007; Cherry, Ashcraft, & Owen, 2007). More recently, a positive trend in staff turnover has been noted. According to the American Healthcare Association (2012), "from 2008 to 2010, turnover decreased for all nursing staff in direct care roles, as well as nurses with administrative duties and for all nursing staff" (p. 12).

To complicate this situation, there is a projected shortage of healthcare professionals. Half of the RN workforce is at least 45 years old. It is estimated that by 2025 there will be a shortage of at least 260,000 RNs because of a number of significant factors, including the population growth, retirement of nurses in the current workforce, and the lack of qualified faculty to educate willing students in nursing programs (Harrington, 2008).

STANDARDS

Residential and community-based LTC facilities that accept government payments are regulated by federal and state mandates. Agencies and institutions involved in providing LTC that receive outside funding are required to meet certain standards and undergo regular inspection (Harrington et al., 2010).

Requirements for LTC facilities change frequently. Part of the responsibility of both the facility administrator and the director of nursing in any LTC facility is to be aware of and implement changes that are made necessary as a result of changes in state and federal requirements. In home health agencies, the number and type of visits that can be reimbursed by insurance or Medicare are limited. If evidence regarding why visits were made and which health-related goal was achieved is unclear, the payer may bill the agency back for those services, which can be financially devastating to the organization.

Nursing homes undergo an initial survey to become certified and then undergo inspection no less than every 15 months, with the average frequency of inspection being every 12 months (Harrington et al., 2010). State surveyors evaluate both processes and outcomes of nursing home care in several areas. Tags are assigned depending on the severity of the violation. If deficiencies are found, follow-up surveys may be conducted. If care is so poor that residents are deemed to be in danger, facilities can be fined large amounts of money, be prohibited from admitting any residents, and even be closed for severe violations. Agencies must demonstrate that the staff meet educational requirements, that residents are receiving adequate care, and that documentation is appropriate. Requirements vary for different types of agencies, however, and are inevitably complicated. Most states post the results of surveys on a public website, where family members can access information and compare facilities when making decisions about placing loved ones into LTC. Current national survey results are available through the CMS website (http://www.cms.gov). Families for Better Care (2013) also posts a Nursing Home Report Card that presents a synthesis of data in a user-friendly format (http://nursinghomereportcards.com/). On this report card, states are given a grade of A to F based on data related to care provision and staffing.

CMS sets standards for nursing home care. Standards address issues such as nursing care hours per client, nursing assessments, care plans, accidents, fall prevention, prevention of pressure sores, use of physical restraints, nutrition, use of certain medications, and housekeeping services.

Facilities are to provide care for residents in a manner that maintains dignity and respect by providing grooming, appropriate dress, and promotion of independence in dining; allowing private space and property; and interacting respectfully. For example, nursing staff must not perform any invasive assessment or task in a public area, but should take the resident to his or her room for procedures such as listening to lung sounds or checking a glucometer reading.

Harrington and colleagues (2010) point out that the quality of care provided in nursing homes has long been a matter of great concern to consumers, healthcare professionals, and policy makers. If the regulation and inspection process is ignored, LTC residents may suffer. Examples of system failures can be found at both the local and state levels. Deficiency reports are readily available online through the CMS. The RN, at times, is required to act as an advocate for the residents and to ensure compliance with minimal standards.

Standards by which care is measured were outlined in 2002 by the CMS. These standards have since undergone major revisions, however, and the LTC (specifically nursing homes) system is currently undergoing change to incorporate the newest and most patient-oriented measurement standards (CMS, 2011b). CMS data indicate that trends are improving with regard to

nursing home deficiency citations, particularly those more serious citations that indicate harm to residents.

Ethical Issues in Long-Term Care

Individuals with chronic illness or who are frail represent a vulnerable population and are often at the mercy of the caregivers in the LTC system. Healthcare professionals in LTC should have a solid understanding of the ethics involved in this type of care. Principles upon which decisions should be made include autonomy, nonmaleficence, beneficence, and justice (Beauchamp & Childress, 2009; Jonsen, 2007). The manner in which these principles are executed in the professional nurse–client relationship can make a visible difference in the quality of life of the LTC resident. Some of the more common ethical issues are discussed next.

CLIENT AUTONOMY VERSUS DEPENDENCE

One principle of critical importance in LTC is autonomy. Healthcare professionals and caregivers should observe the essential rule of bioethics: Respect the autonomy of persons (Jonsen, 2007). The abilities to make one's own decisions and to act independently are important aspects of autonomy in a long-term care setting (Wulff, Kalinowski, & Drager, 2010). Autonomy is sometimes misapplied or ignored in long-term care. The need for help in long-term care has been associated with residents' reported feelings of being ill, dependent, inferior, and at the mercy of others (Moe, Hellzen, & Enmarker, 2013). It is possible for an individual to gradually lose increments of his or her autonomy because of limitations imposed by sensory deprivation, immobility, weakness, and cognitive impairment (Mezey, Mitty, & Ramsey, 1997). Research suggests that even frail elderly individuals who are homebound have a greater sense of personal control than those in nursing homes (Crain, 2001), making those living in facilities at greater risk for loss of decision making and independence. Loss of autonomy and development of dependence are problems for many LTC clients.

Custodial Care

When basic ethical principles are applied, an issue arises regarding whether providing minimal physical care for those with chronic illness is acceptable versus providing more comprehensive care extending beyond custodial physical care. This balancing act is particularly challenging in a residential LTC environment. As a result of regulation, funding, and staffing patterns for Medicare/Medicaid residential facilities, the goal inadvertently becomes custodial care. CMS defines custodial care as "non-skilled, personal care, such as help with activities of daily living like bathing, dressing, eating, getting in or out of a bed or chair, moving around, and using the bathroom. It may also include care that most people can do themselves, like using eye drops" (CMS, 2012a, para 1). Medicare does not pay for custodial care—a factor that poses a dilemma for persons who need some help but cannot afford assisted living in the home and must pay for it privately. New care models are needed to address these financial challenges.

Mental Health Issues

Physical issues of the LTC facility resident are important, but those issues should not be the only focus of care. Mental health needs should also be considered in the chronically ill and elderly populations. With limited attention to these needs, the client is at risk of suffering boredom, anxiety, and, consequently, depression. In 2004, persons age 65 and older accounted for 16% of suicide deaths, although they represented only 12% of the entire U.S. population at that time (National Institute of Mental Health [NIMH], 2010).

Appropriate referral for mental health services is a responsibility of the nurse who detects symptoms of emotional difficulties. Signs of depression include feeling nervous, empty, guilty, tired, restless, irritable, and unloved, and believing that life is not worth living. Physical symptoms associated with mental health problems include eating more or less than normal, sleep disturbances, headaches, stomachaches, and an increase in chronic pain (Varcarolis & Halter, 2010). The risk of depression in the elderly increases with the presence of chronic illness and a loss of physical function (NIMH, 2010). If symptoms of depression are present in an LTC client, services are available to provide assistance.

End-of-Life Decision Making

Difficult and complex decisions at the end of life are an inherent component of LTC. Many older adults lack the resources—or lack knowledge of the available resources—that could help with decision making during this stage of life. Although most older adults are approached about completing written documents to outline treatment preferences, many choose not to do so. Making one's wishes known in the event of terminal illness or incapacity is one approach to preserving autonomy for the older adult. However, family issues may impact the elder's willingness to do so.

Cultural and religious beliefs play an important part in end-of-life decision making. Some religions dictate that everything should be done to preserve life; others support allowing natural death. For example, African Americans are generally opposed to placing a loved one in a nursing home, preferring family members to die at home. Healthcare professionals should familiarize themselves with the major traditions and practices of their clients so that culturally appropriate care can be provided.

Approximately "28% of home health care patients, 65% of nursing home residents, and 88% of discharged hospice care patients had at least one advance directive (AD) on record" (Jones, Moss, & Harris-Kojetin, 2011, para 1). The use of ADs varies by age and population, with blacks using ADs less frequently than whites. Blacks, Hispanics, and Asians in long-term care facilities are also less likely to have an AD on record (Frahm, Brown, & Hyer, 2013). The most commonly used advance directives in these long-term care populations were living wills and DNR orders. Nursing home residents and hospice patients are more likely than home health patients to have an AD on record (Jones et al., 2011). These statistics underscore the need for healthcare professionals to address advance directives with persons while they are capable of expressing their end-of-life wishes.

In many states, an older person can make his or her wishes known by completing a legally recognized document. Three such documents are described here: Five Wishes, AND, and POLST.

The Five Wishes program, sponsored by Aging with Dignity, is unique relative to other living will declarations, in that it addresses all aspects of the person's life: emotional, spiritual, personal, and medical (Aging with Dignity, 2010). This document is legally recognized in 42 states and allows the person to use his or her own lay language to express end-of-life desires. Five Wishes documents the following information for the older adult's family and doctors (Aging with Dignity, 2010):

• Which person should make healthcare decisions
• The kind of medical treatment the person wants and does not want
• How comfortable the person wishes to be made
• How the person wants others to treat him or her
• What the person wants loved ones to know

The allow natural death (AND) order focuses on allowing death as the natural end of a terminal illness. AND is considered more positive in that is allows persons to describe comfort measures they would prefer that also promote a natural death (Warring & Krieger-Blake, 2014).

POLST—physician's orders for life-sustaining treatment—differs from the other AD documents in that it provides instructions for emergency personnel about treatment while the person is at home, before emergency treatment is given. "The POLST Paradigm is designed to ensure that seriously ill patients can choose the treatments they want and that their wishes are honored by medical providers" (POLST, 2012, para 1). Paramedics and other emergency responders have been trained to check the refrigerator for a copy of the person's AD. The POLST form contains items that address CPR, medications, and nutrition, and has a place where the physician signs after consultation with the patient about the AD.

Healthcare professionals play an important role in educating older adults about advance directives. Residents in long-term care especially need healthcare professionals to advocate for their wishes at end of life and to be certain that these requests are legally documented.

ABUSE AND NEGLECT OF VULNERABLE ADULTS

The incidence of abuse and neglect of vulnerable adults is difficult to estimate. The National Adult Protective Services Association (2014) estimates that anywhere between 500,000 and 5 million elders and other vulnerable adults in the United States are in some way victims of abuse each year. Other sources indicate that nearly 6 million cases of elder abuse occur every year (Elder Abuse Daily, 2010), with 1 in 10 older adults suffering some kind of abuse but fewer than half reporting it (National Center for Elder Abuse, 2014). It is believed that cases of abuse, neglect, or exploitation are grossly underreported because of fear, intimidation, lack of sound research, or other factors. Nursing home residents are particularly vulnerable to being victims of abuse, with as many as 44% to 95% of nursing home residents reporting abuse or neglect (National Center for Elder Abuse, 2014). Families for Better Care's Nursing Home Report Card, based on data analysis from several key sources, showed that "1 in 5 nursing homes abused, neglected, or mistreated residents in almost half of all states" (2013, p. 1).

Abuse can be categorized as domestic or institutional. Within these categories, physical, sexual, and emotional/psychological abuse may occur as well as neglect, self-neglect, abandonment, and financial exploitation (National Center for Elder Abuse, 2011). Because of the longer life expectancies for those with chronic illness, it is very likely that the incidence of abuse will increase in the future (Mauk & Urban, 2014). The individual with chronic illness, if cognitively competent, may be hesitant to discuss the mistreatment because he or she fears the loss of the relationship or other reprisal by the perpetrator. If the individual is not capable of expressing information regarding the abuse, identification may be by forensic evidence.

Physical abuse is the actual assault of an individual, for which evidence may include the presence of unexplained bruises, fractures, cuts, or burns in various stages of healing. Sexual abuse also falls within this category. The victim of such treatment is in danger and requires immediate advocacy. Physical abuse often escalates from neglect or other forms of abuse. Perpetrators often share similar characteristics such as lack of social support, history of being an abuse victim, and mental or emotional problems.

Neglect is defined as the lack of provision of basic necessities, such as food, water, and medical care. Neglect may be evidenced by poor hygiene, malnutrition or dehydration, pressure ulcers, and reports of being left in an unsafe condition or being left without resources to obtain necessary medications. Neglect can take place because of willful intention or because home management has become overwhelming to the client's aging spouse or family. This type of abuse may be seen more frequently in homes where the caregiver lacks the knowledge or resources to provide care. Neglect can also include self-neglect (Mauk, 2011), which is defined as an individual losing the will or the ability to properly care for himself. Abandonment is the extreme form of neglect.

Another type of elder abuse, exploitation, is defined as the use of an elder's resources without knowledge or consent for the gain of another. Signs of elder exploitation include the disappearance of monetary resources or the "taking over" of personal belongings without permission or consent (Hildreth, 2011). Financial abuse in the form of fraud or deception may also be considered exploitation and may come through family members who borrow money with no intention to repay it, or from mail fraud schemes that attempt to cheat persons out of money by promising prizes and rewards.

Each state has established an Adult Protective Services (APS) agency to protect the rights and health of older people and people with disabilities who are in danger of being mistreated or neglected, unable to protect themselves, and have no one to assist them. APS helps by "assessing each individual's unique needs, then developing a service plan to maintain his/her safety, health and independence" (National Adult Protective Services Association, 2014, para 2). APS is responsible for receiving the report of abuse, investigating the report, assessing the individual's risk, developing and implementing case plans, service monitoring, and evaluating. Some agencies may provide more in-depth services including housing, medical care, social support, and economic and legal services. Healthcare professionals and paraprofessionals such as RNs, physicians, nurse aides, and homemaker aides are mandated by law to report suspected adult or elder abuse.

Interventions

Preservation of Autonomy of the Person

Healthcare professionals dealing with clients in LTC should carefully consider their own position as a moral force. Making decisions with a moral component is a part of everyday practice for most nurses. Understanding the concepts that provide the moral foundation for human existence is important. Those concepts typically include the following: autonomy, nonmaleficence, beneficence, justice, and professional–patient relationships (Beauchamp & Childress, 2009). Autonomy is in the forefront in LTC and the concept is rooted in the idea of self-rule and independent decision making.

AUTONOMY

The role of the nurse in providing LTC along the continuum of care is to preserve the autonomy of the client. At the same time, the client must be protected from harm. Balancing these issues is not always easy. It is imperative that the care provider not assume that because an individual has lost some physical autonomy, such as requiring personal assistance with daily hygiene, that the individual has given up his or her autonomy or is incapable of making his or her own decisions. Promotion of autonomy is accomplished by allowing the individual to make as many decisions as possible. In decisions that can impact health or health care, the nurse must provide the appropriate information to enable the client to make an informed decision. To more fully understand the concept of autonomy, the caregiver is encouraged to think about autonomy from the client's perspective when making caregiving decisions. Nursing home residents "often experience greater dependency, and with it, a greater likelihood that they will have their interests and values overridden by others" (Sherwin & Winsby, 2011, p. 183). Paternalism can become more commonplace in an institutional or clinical setting.

Individual decision making is a complex and multifaceted issue (Wulff et al., 2010). Loss of decision-making capacity in one area does not indicate loss of *all* decision-making capacity. Decision-making capacity may fluctuate through the course of an illness, and determining the best approach to preserving safety and autonomy concurrently is at times challenging. At some point after decision-making capacity comes into question, it will be appropriate to consider legal guidelines set in place by the state in which the patient resides. The law in some states defines the line of authority for decision making when competence is in question. In cases where the person has been legally deemed unable to make his or her own decisions, the designated family member or legal guardian must be informed of all important aspects of the person's life and is responsible for making decisions that are in the person's best interest—that is, on his or her behalf or at his or her behest. When a person has lost some degree of autonomy, the nurse must also act in a judicious way that protects the individual from harm or exploitation.

It is also possible for someone who has legally lost autonomy (been declared incompetent) to continue to participate in the decision-making process (Mauk, 2011). For example, a person with early-stage dementia may have a legal guardian who is ultimately responsible for decision making in the person's best interest. However, as much as the person is able, the guardian would involve the person in the decision-making process, seeking input and finding out the wishes of the person prior to taking any action. This kind of consideration can make a significant positive contribution to quality of life for the LTC resident.

Decision making or autonomy can be viewed on a continuum. An example might be when a person with advanced dementia decides to walk the halls. Autonomous decision making in a small way is appropriate as long as other principles, such as the client's safety and the safety of others, are considered. It is the nurse's responsibility to recognize an individual's capacity for autonomy and preserve that capacity as much as possible (Casada da Rocha, 2009). Sometimes, the nurse must compromise what he or she perceives to be the best treatment so as to incorporate client preferences. An example would be a client's bathing twice a week as opposed to more frequent bathing. In that case, the nurse might alter other interactions, such as frequency of spot baths or application of lotion to ensure skin integrity, while respecting the autonomy of the client.

GUARDIANSHIP

One of the ways in which the healthcare system provides for those who are unable to make informed decisions for themselves because of a cognitive or other health problem is to appoint a legal guardian. The responsibility of the guardian is to ensure the safety of and quality care for the person and to make decisions in the person's best interest. The guardian may be a family member, a friend, or a healthcare professional appointed by the court. In complex cases involving large estates, difficult family relationships, or divorce, the court may choose to appoint a professional guardian or person who will assist in making legal decisions for the incompetent person (Mauk, 2011). The appointment of a guardian by the court usually follows a legal determination of the individual's incapacity. The person who has been declared by the court to be an incapacitated person is then no longer able to make any type of contractual decision independently. The guardian of the person is responsible to the court for getting to know the person sufficiently to be able to make decisions in his or her best interest and to provide documentation to the court as needed on the status of the person. The guardian may also be responsible for a variety of tasks related to the individual, ranging from healthcare advocacy to managing finances to ensuring that daily care needs are being met.

Guardianship guidelines vary from state to state and even from county to county within states. There is no established fee for these services, and guardians may be paid a small fee monthly or a significant hourly fee as a consultant if additional services such as case management are being provided—if there are funds from the estate to cover such costs. These arrangements are generally agreed upon through the court as part of the legal guardian's acceptance of this responsibility.

Some controversy exists regarding the methods and process used for assigning guardianship and assessment of a person's capacity. A tri-state study (Moye, Butz, Marson, & Wood, 2007) found that the quality of written clinical evidence to establish the need for guardianship was significantly lacking and that key information about the individual's values, preferences, and wishes was rarely documented. The persons for whom guardianship was sought were rarely present at the hearing. Functional assessments of persons should be routinely used during the evaluation of the need for guardianship. An assessment template that incorporates six assessment domains of interest to the court is recommended; the areas that should be addressed, according to one such model, include medical condition, cognition, functional abilities, values, risk for injury and supervision needed, and ways to enhance capacity (Moye et al., 2007). Ongoing communication between clinical and legal team members is needed to protect the rights of vulnerable persons.

Nurses and social workers often make excellent guardians, because they are able to professionally address these areas and provide a holistic approach to care for the incapacitated person. Some court systems develop a rapport with certain professionals who act as guardians and will request their appointment in cases such as for older adults with dementia who reside in LTC facilities. To preserve the autonomy of persons as long as possible, guardians should encourage as much participation of the individual as possible in decision making, while keeping in mind the goal of safety and quality care for the incapacitated person.

Advocacy: The Role of the Ombudsman

The LTC ombudsman is an advocate charged with the protection of the rights of all residents in LTC. The purpose of this role is to enhance quality of life for LTC residents and do the following:

- Advocate for residents' rights and quality care
- Educate consumers and providers
- Resolve residents' complaints
- Provide information to the public (National Long-Term Care Ombudsman Resource Center, 2014, p. 1)

The ombudsman program is administered by the Administration on Aging (AoA). The network has 8,813 volunteers certified to handle complaints and 1,167 paid staff. Most state ombudsman programs are housed in their State Unit on Aging. Nationally, in 2011 the ombudsman program investigated over 200,463 complaints on behalf of 131,078 individuals and provided information on long-term care to another 288,698 people. (National Long-Term Care Ombudsman Resource Center, 2014, para 2)

The LTC ombudsman is a person hired by a state LTC service agency under the auspices of the state or local health department or the statewide aging services. Volunteers who report to the ombudsman supervisor may perform many of the actual investigations. The contact information for the ombudsman should be posted conspicuously in each LTC facility. Complaints may come from the LTC resident, concerned family, or caregivers. Findings must be reported to the client and/or family, and the ombudsman is responsible for achieving an equitable settlement between the resident and the LTC facility. The role of the ombudsman is founded in ethical principles and is implemented on behalf of the vulnerable client. (Updates on the organizational activities contacts can be found at http://www.ltcombudsman.org.)

Nursing Care

Nursing care is the primary service provided by residential LTC facilities. The further one progresses along the LTC continuum, the more intense are the nursing care needs. Nursing care in LTC settings is much more complex than it has been in the past and requires greater knowledge and expertise on the part of the nursing staff to manage comorbidities and provide high-quality care to all residents.

Care that nurses provide in LTC facilities should be holistic and multidimensional. Because most persons in LTC settings are older,

nurses would benefit from education in gerontology. The AACN, with funding from the Hartford Foundation, has released a set of standards outlining geriatric content for inclusion in the baccalaureate educational process for nurses; each program should periodically review and update the curriculum to stay current and prepare expert nurses for practice (AACN & Hartford Institute for Geriatric Nursing, 2010). More nursing curricula are adding stand-alone courses in gerontological nursing and/or integrating these concepts into the BSN curricula.

PAIN MANAGEMENT

It is important for the nurse in LTC to adequately assess pain and to provide adequate treatment of that pain (Fink & Gates, 2010). Of particular importance is assessing clients' suffering from the pain associated with arthritis, osteoporosis, or neuralgia. A great deal of information is available on appropriate pain management strategies, and the nurse dealing with such clients should access this body of literature. When implementing pain management strategies in the LTC setting, follow-up is critical. Pain relief varies for many reasons, and current pain might not be relieved by a method that had previously been successful for the client. When pain is chronic and affects the ability of the client to function, treatment strategies may include routine regular administration of medication to manage the pain. Breakthrough pain—that is, pain experienced intermittently when a client is on routine pain medication—is then treated with "as-needed" medication. Addiction is not generally considered to be a major problem for elders suffering from chronic pain, but tolerance can become problematic.

For individuals unable to verbally express pain, its presence is noted in other ways. Evidence of pain may include facial expression (grimacing), groaning, body position, bracing, guarding, and rubbing of the painful body part. Alternative methods of dealing with pain should be considered. Massage, heat, cold, and support mechanisms such as knee or back braces may be helpful. The quality of life of the LTC client can be greatly affected by pain. With current advances in pharmacology and treatment, however, most pain can be managed effectively.

End-of-life care requires an intense management of comfort levels. If the individual is suffering intractable pain, use of palliative sedation may be necessary. Guidelines for such aggressive symptom management must be accessed through a process of evidence-based practice to ensure the most appropriate approach is used (Melnyk & Fineout-Overholt, 2010).

DISEASE PREVENTION/HEALTH PROMOTION

Although it may be impossible to prevent some of the chronic diseases seen in the LTC population, others are certainly preventable. An important preventive health measure is the provision of flu and pneumonia vaccines to LTC residents. A vaccination program in residential facilities is essential and usually mandated by public health guidelines; in such settings, infections such as influenza can spread rapidly and cause deaths among the frail elderly (American Lung Association, 2014). These types of infections may affect a number of residents at one time, creating a difficult burden for staff as they struggle to deal with a number of acutely ill clients. Admission of clients to acute care settings in such circumstances is not unreasonable to ensure that all clients receive adequate nursing care during an outbreak of illness.

Certain screenings are recommended for older adults and can be helpful with early identification and treatment initiation. The following screenings are recommended by the U.S. Preventive Services Task Force and *Healthy People 2020* for older adults with chronic illness: nutrition, tobacco, safety, immunizations, depression, alcohol abuse, lipids, hypertension, osteoporosis, vision and hearing, breast cancer, and colorectal cancer. Each of these screenings is rated as beneficial and supported by at least fair evidence that health outcomes and benefits outweigh the screening risk (Nelson, 2014).

Several key areas are considered standard for health promotion in older adults—namely, exercise, not smoking, maintaining a healthy weight, social support, medication adherence, a safe environment, and activities that strengthen cognition and memory (Hardin, 2010). Social support is an important factor is maintaining good health (Haber, 2014). Thus health promotion, even for those with existing chronic illness, emphasizes the same important strategies that healthcare professionals should encourage in LTC residents.

DELIRIUM

Individuals in LTC who have cognitive impairment caused by an acute condition (delirium) need to receive immediate intervention to reverse the cause of the impairment before permanent disability or death results. Delirium is an acute condition brought on by one or more conditions that have altered brain functioning. The chief symptoms include sudden disturbance in consciousness and/or cognition. The underlying condition can be a single factor or a combination of conditions, which include but are not limited to fever, infection, allergic reaction, malnutrition, vitamin deficiency, drug toxicity (over-the-counter or prescription medications), drug interactions, food supplement toxicity, hyperglycemia or hypoglycemia, and hypoxia (Tullman, Mion, Fletcher, & Foreman, 2008). The underlying condition can be life threatening and must be corrected to prevent the incident from leading to the client's death. If the nurse providing care in the LTC setting determines that a client is suffering from delirium, it may be necessary to arrange transportation to an acute care facility where appropriate emergent care can be provided.

In addition to these physiologic processes, cognitive impairment can be brought about by psychosocial factors such as depression, change in health brought on by aging or disease, or change in location such as a move from a long-time home to live with another family member or a move to an institutionalized setting.

The nurse assessing the patient should consider these possibilities when selecting the appropriate interventions.

Because of the physiologic changes that occur with aging, the signs of delirium in a frail elder may develop over a period of days as a subclinical condition worsens to a crisis point. In addition, in a patient who has a complicated medication regimen, symptoms of increased confusion may initially be mild. The astute nurse will make the appropriate observations to detect delirium even when the symptoms are subtle. In a client population with fluctuating cognition, such as the individuals found at many residential facilities, detection of delirium becomes more challenging.

Delirium is treated by addressing the cause. Some causes of delirium in the LTC population include urinary tract infections, pneumonia, electrolyte imbalance, dehydration, polypharmacy or medication side effects, fever, or untreated pain (Rose, 2014). Nursing interventions should be focused at the diagnosis and the appropriate treatment of the underlying condition.

DEMENTIA

Individuals in LTC may suffer cognitive impairment from a variety of pathologic processes. These processes may be either acute or chronic. Individuals with cognitive impairment caused by irreversible causes such as closed head injuries; stroke; or dementia from a number of pathologic processes, such as Alzheimer's disease, multi-infarct dementia, or Lewy body disease, often need special assistance to manage activities of daily living. Dementia differs from delirium in that the condition is chronic and the underlying pathologic process is progressive and irreversible. An estimated 5.2 million individuals had Alzheimer's disease in 2013; of those persons, 5 million were older than age 65, whereas 200,000 had younger-onset disease (Alzheimer's Association, 2014). In addition, between 40% and 80% of those persons living in nursing homes are believed to have a cognitive impairment (CDC, 2009a), with nearly half of all nursing home residents in the United States having a diagnosis of Alzheimer's disease (Harris-Kojetin et al., 2013). Dementia is defined as the development of multiple cognitive deficits manifested by memory impairment and other problems, such as aphasia (inability to speak), apraxia (loss of ability to use familiar objects or carry out purposeful movements not caused by loss of sensory ability), and agnosia (loss of ability to determine the significance of sensory input, such as recognition of a familiar face or voice) (American Psychological Association, 2000).

In the United States, as much as 80% of dementia care is delivered in the home by unpaid caregivers (Alzheimer's Association, 2014). In the community LTC setting, the role of the nurse is to support the family caregiver with problem solving or identifying resources such as respite care, adult daycare, or the local chapter of the Alzheimer's Association. The nurse may play a key role in the decision making that takes place when caregiving for a demented loved one is negatively affecting the health of the spousal caregiver (Maas et al., 2004). When caregiving becomes overwhelming at home, the decision to place the individual with dementia in a residential facility is appropriate.

Nursing interventions that deal with dementia generally address one or more of three symptom domains: cognitive, functional, and behavioral. All clients with dementia demonstrate functional difficulties, whereas only some demonstrate behavioral problems. Dealing with individuals suffering from permanent cognitive impairment takes patience and understanding. It is important that the caregiver not lose sight of the client's perspective. It is more important to validate the client's personhood rather than to insist that he or she achieve "reality orientation." The client may find comfort in some behavior, such as carrying a doll; this behavior, although not grounded in immediate reality, reflects the reality of a universal human behavior regarding caring for others, specifically infants.

An evidence-based practice approach should be used in structuring care and the environment in LTC facilities responsible for patients with dementia. This ensures that the patient will benefit from the latest research findings regarding best practice in dementia care.

Many nursing homes and even some assisted-living centers have special care units for dementia clients. The environment in such settings allows for safe wandering. Ideally, the staff has received training specific to caring for clients with dementia. The units are generally set up with consideration given to lighting, color, noise levels, congregate areas, and room setups. Such considerations are used to make the environment more pleasant for the residents. Those with mild dementia may still enjoy activities requiring personal interaction and following rules such as games or group singing. Those with more advanced dementia may enjoy more isolated activities such as the opportunity to fold laundry or a task related to food preparation. Again, an evidence-based practice approach will ensure that the latest research findings are incorporated into the caring regimen.

DEPRESSION AND ANXIETY

Approximately 20% of the older population has some type of mental health disorder, with depression and anxiety being the most common diagnoses (Touhy & Jett, 2010). Depression and anxiety often are seen together as geriatric syndromes in older adults, but may go unrecognized and untreated. This combination of diagnoses can lead to a decline in health and even death in older adults (Vink, Aartsen, & Schovevers, 2008). The prevalence of depression in LTC facilities has been estimated to be as high as 29% (Seitz, Purandare, & Conn, 2010). Depression is a leading cause of disability (World Health Organization [WHO], 2012). Anxiety tends to occur more in females, in persons with increased frailty and chronic illness, and after a recent traumatic event (Lochner &

Byrd, 2014). Mixed anxiety and depression may produce the following symptoms:

- Irritability
- Problems concentrating
- Hopelessness
- Insomnia or hypersomnia
- Eating disturbances
- Fear of dying
- Physical symptoms: dizziness, sweating, feelings of choking, shortness of breath, muscle tension (Lochner & Byrd, 2014)

Managing these syndromes usually involves an interprofessional team approach that includes a combination of medication and therapeutic interventions. Some common treatment strategies include counseling, establishing a daily routine, cognitive therapy, medication, stress management, sleep promotion, increased physical activity, avoiding triggers, and group therapy support. Appropriate assessment and early diagnosis and treatment are key in managing these mental health issues and promoting quality of life in long-term care.

SUBSTANCE ABUSE

Substance abuse is considered a growing problem among older adults. Because illicit drug use declines with advancing age, this problem in long-term care is presently less than in the broader community population. However, it is expected that there will be a growing number of substance abusers in the future because of baby boomers who have a history of marijuana use and other substances (Elioupoulos, 2014).

The most commonly abused substance in older adults is alcohol. The U.S. Preventive Services Task Force (USPSTF, 2012) recommends screening for alcoholism, but no connection between screening and positive outcomes has been made. Healthcare professionals should recognize the following signs and symptoms of alcohol abuse: drinking a fifth of whiskey or the equivalent daily; having blood alcohol levels greater than 150 mg/100 mL; reports of blackouts, convulsions, tremors, or delirium tremens when abstaining from drinking; negative effects on family, job, and social functioning; negative health effects such as gastritis or cirrhosis of the liver; and inability or refusal to stop drinking even when advised to do so by a physician (Elioupoulos, 2014). Counseling has been shown to reduce the amount of drinking and help maintain it (Tran & Karlamangla, 2014). One study showed that an integrated care approach that incorporated a harm-reduction program within the treatment regimen and an enhanced referral system resulted in a significant decrease in number of drinks and number of binge drinking episodes over a 3-month period (Lee, Mericle, Ayalon, & Arean, 2009). Groups such as Alcoholics Anonymous or Seniors in Sobriety have experienced success through a 12-step accountability recovery program.

The three other most commonly used illicit drugs among the elderly are cocaine, heroin, and marijuana. As far as percentage of use per ethnicity, blacks are first, followed by whites and Latinos. Most illicit drug abusers older than age 50 admitted to the emergency room are males between the ages of 50 and 54. Risk of abuse of these substances is higher among members of the over-55 age group who are in prison, with more than 30% of them reporting drug usage (Taylor & Grossberg, 2012). Unfortunately, few treatment programs are specifically geared toward the elderly population, who in this regard represent a doubly vulnerable population. Early identification and treatment in an inpatient facility are recommended (Taylor & Grossberg, 2012). More research is needed on strategies for effective substance abuse recovery in the older adult population.

FALL RISK REDUCTION AND SAFETY

One of the most important functions of the nurse in an LTC setting is to reduce risk and ensure client safety. In a community setting, part of the home assessment includes a thorough examination of the environment to detect possible hazards and correct them.

The most obvious hazards include throw rugs, electrical cords strung across traffic areas, stairs (especially those without handrails), loose tiles in the shower, slick flooring, small pets, and similar environmental conditions. In residential settings, the nurse has similar responsibilities to ensure client safety. Facilities should provide a safe environment with adaptations for those with chronic health problems that would place them at higher risk for injuries or falls.

Safe patient handling has become an important issue in best nursing practice. Organized safety programs have been linked to positive outcomes for both patients and staff (Nelson, 2006; Nelson, Collins, Siddharthan, Matz, & Waters, 2008). For example, researchers found that implementing a safe patient-handling program in an LTC through the VA system resulted in better quality of patient care for residents. Safe-handling programs include four key interventions: appropriate patient-handling equipment and devices, assessment protocols, safe lifting policies, and patient lift teams. Key areas of change for residents after implementation of the program included improved physical functioning, decreased sedentary states of residents, less deterioration in activities of daily living, decreased fall rate, and increased wakeful states in the mornings (Nelson et al., 2008).

Falls are a significant problem in LTC. In 2009, 2.2 million emergency room visits were as a result of falls and almost 600,000 resulted in hospitalizations (CDC, 2012). The cost of medical care related to falls was approximately $19 billion in 2000 (Dean, Harrison, & Zwicker, 2014).

Originally, restraints were thought to prevent injury to clients and were applied to ensure patient safety through limiting movement. Research has demonstrated, however, that restraints do the opposite and are likely to cause injury (Mion, Halliday, & Sandhu, 2008; Oliver, Healey, & Haines, 2010). Both physical and chemical restraints in LTC facilities are now strictly regulated. The most current reports regarding restraint use are available online (Agency for Healthcare Research and Quality, 2009; CMS, 2011c).

In 2010, the American Geriatrics Society (AGS) and British Geriatrics Society (BGS) convened the Panel on Prevention of Falls in Older Person, which recommended comprehensive fall risk assessment and intervention strategies. The preferred approach to decreasing falls is a multifactorial intervention tailored to each individual with a plan for follow-up on fall prevention strategies (AGS/BGS, 2010; Wallis & Campbell, 2011). All LTC facilities should have an exercise plan and program available to residents. The ideal environment for LTC residents is restraint free, with environmental and staffing accommodations made to meet the needs of each resident and promote optimal physical functioning through exercise, adequate nutrition, and safety.

PALLIATIVE AND HOSPICE CARE

Palliative care is defined as follows:

> {A}n approach that improves the quality of life of patients and their families facing the problem associated with life-threatening illness, through the prevention and relief of suffering by means of early identification and impeccable assessment and treatment of pain and other problems, physical, psychosocial and spiritual. (WHO, 2008, para 1)

The goal of this care is not curative, but rather centers on comfort. Palliative care is both a philosophy of care and a treatment system, and is not necessarily just for those considered terminally ill. In palliation, physiologic needs are met and aggressive measures are taken for pain relief. A holistic view of the client should be maintained, and the personhood of the client is of primary consideration in this type of nursing care. Palliative care may be used in conjunction with life-prolonging care. For adults, WHO (2008,

para 2) identified that palliative care has the following characteristics:

- Provides relief from pain and other distressing symptoms
- Affirms life and regards dying as a normal process
- Intends neither to hasten nor to postpone death
- Integrates the psychological and spiritual aspects of patient care
- Offers a support system to help patients live as actively as possible until death
- Offers a support system to help the family cope during the patient's illness and in their own bereavement
- Uses a team approach to address the needs of patients and their families, including bereavement counseling, if indicated
- Enhances quality of life and may also positively influence the course of illness
- Is applicable early in the course of illness, in conjunction with other therapies that are intended to prolong life, such as chemotherapy or radiation therapy, and includes those investigations needed to better understand and manage distressing clinical complications

A person with chronic illness may benefit from palliative care services and yet not qualify for hospice. Hospice is a type of palliative care that is usually delivered in the home by a team of trained professionals who address the needs of the patient and the entire family. Hospice teams may also come into nursing homes to augment and oversee comfort care. Hospice is covered under Medicare Part A, which pays for most of the needed services for the terminally ill. However, Medicare will not pay for curative treatment in hospice. The general requirement for Medicare reimbursement for hospice service is that a physician must certify that the patient probably has 6 months or less to live (CMS, 2007). Determination of the terminal phase of an illness is sometimes difficult, and patients may improve during that 6-month period of time. Patients must be recertified by their physician as having a terminal condition to continue receiving hospice services. Once hospice services are begun for community-dwelling elders, other LTC services may not be allowed by reimbursement policy.

In the terminal phase of life, appropriate care includes pain relief, comfort, and emotional and spiritual support for the client and family. The client and family can be referred for grief counseling related to the experience of incurable illness (Ferrell & Coyle, 2010). Death is a natural part of life, and the nurse should be prepared to facilitate the client's end-of-life transition and provide support to the family survivors (DeSpelder & Strickland, 2011).

Research in Long-Term Care

The science of caring for those with chronic illness is changing rapidly. Approximately 133 million Americans have at least one chronic illness, with 25% of those individuals reporting some type of difficulty with ADLs (CDC, 2009b). This growing burden of care for long-term health problems accounts for 78% of the United States' total healthcare spending. Research often begins with clinical observations of problems or recurring events that require solutions. A number of nurse researchers have undertaken focused research programs dealing with chronic illness and issues related to the nursing home experience (e.g., Cornelia Beck, Kathleen Buckwalter, Jeanne Kaiser-Jones, Meridian Maas, Matty Mezey, and Terri Fulmer). Nurses in a clinical role should take the opportunity to define a problem and propose a solution. A novice researcher may partner with a more experienced researcher to develop an idea into a researchable question. Regional research organizations such as the Southern Nursing Research Society, the Midwest Nursing Research Society, and local chapters of Sigma Theta Tau are available to provide assistance.

As the body of literature grows, more opportunities for implementation of evidence-based practice and translational research will emerge (Capezuti, Zwicker, Mezey, & Fulmer, 2008). One model of evidence-based practice known for its ease of use at the bedside is the PICO method—patient, intervention, compared to, and outcomes. Using the PICO model, questions can be formulated and the literature searched quickly to find studies that can bring insight into specific problem solving for those in LTC (see http://pubmedhh.nlm.nih.gov/nlm/picostudy/pico3.html for a search engine designed for the PICO question).

Outcomes

Simple medical models are rarely sufficient to address desired outcomes for those persons with complicated chronic medical conditions. It is not enough to consider the quality of life based on absence of sickness; rather, one must consider the overall well-being of the client. Outcomes will vary along the LTC continuum. For community-based clients, the overall outcome may be to remain in their homes as long as possible. Interventions to support that outcome may include client and family teaching on medication management, safety issues, or wound care. Rehabilitation may be a desired outcome for a community-based client following hospitalization (Mauk, 2012; Mauk & Patel, 2011).

For the resident in an LTC facility, outcomes are different and may include a reduction in the exacerbations of a chronic illness such as congestive heart failure. A client in the rehabilitative area of the facility may determine living independently again to be an outcome. Desired outcomes for other individuals may be to function at the highest potential within the limitations imposed by the chronic illness. A decrease in pain and/or nausea might be an appropriate outcome for an individual in palliative care. Living each day with optimal quality of life is an outcome for most clients in LTC. Nurses can empower frail older persons to obtain better outcomes by using good listening skills, working with them to identify the meaning of frailty to each person, and identifying positive coping and self-care solutions (Dean et al., 2014).

Evidence-Based Practice Box

The purpose of this systematic review was to examine the effectiveness of advanced practice nurses in long-term care. The authors searched 12 electronic databases, contacted leading experts, and used other reference lists, journals, and websites. Four studies and 15 papers were included in the review. The results showed that long-term settings that had advanced practice nurses working in them had decreased rates of the following conditions: depression, urinary incontinence, pressure ulcers, restraint use, and aggressive behaviors. In addition, family members expressed greater satisfaction with care, and residents felt they met more of their personal goals. The authors concluded that having advanced practice nurses in long-term facilities resulted in positive outcomes for residents and families.

Source: Donald, F., Martin-Misener, R., Carter, N., Donald, E. E., Kaasalainen, S., Wickson-Griffiths, A., Lloyd, D….& DiCenso, A. (2013). A systematic review of the effectiveness of advanced practice nurses in long-term care. *Journal of Advanced Nursing, 69*(10), 2148–2161.

CASE STUDY 21-1

Mrs. Sanchez is an 86-year-old widow who has lived in her family home for her entire life. Her husband died from lung cancer 10 years ago. Mrs. Sanchez has a large extended family of five sons and two daughters, all of whom live within an hour's drive of her house. Over their traditional holiday family gathering, Mrs. Sanchez's adult children and grandchildren noticed a change in her memory and behavior. After being diagnosed with Alzheimer's disease, already in the middle stages, her daughters suggest that Mrs. Sanchez consider an assisted-living facility within a continuing care retirement community where a memory care unit would be available later when needed. Mrs. Sanchez is very resistant to this suggestion and feels that her children are trying to force her out of her home so they can steal her money. After an unfortunate incident in which Mrs. Sanchez experienced a fall and hip fracture with bruising and lacerations to her face, the adult children got together to discuss options for new living arrangements for their mother.

Discussion Questions

1. Which factors prompted Mrs. Sanchez's children to encourage her to consider another living arrangement?
2. Based on the information in this chapter, what are some viable options for care for Mrs. Sanchez? Justify your response.
3. Which problems and issues with adaptation to her living situation is Mrs. Sanchez likely to face?
4. Which family and nursing interventions might be helpful to assist with her adjustment?

CASE STUDY 21-2

Mr. Hendricks is a 92-year-old man who resides in an Alzheimer's disease special care unit that is part of a nursing home. Mr. Hendricks has never been married and has no children. All of his brothers and sisters are deceased. He had been living alone in his own home until neighbors noticed that he was not keeping up with the yard work, and he seemed increasingly confused and disoriented when they talked to him. One of the neighbors called APS after Mr. Hendricks fell in his yard and refused to go to the hospital. Eventually, the Area Council on Aging was called in and appointed by the court as Mr. Hendricks's guardian because of lack of available family members willing to assume this job.

Mr. Hendricks spends much of his time wandering the halls on the Alzheimer's unit and sometimes displays combative, aggressive behavior. The nursing staff members try to get him more involved in group activities such as playing games and doing art projects, but his behavior becomes agitated at these attempts. He has scratched or bitten some of the nursing assistants when they try to engage him in activities.

Discussion Questions

1. Is it necessary for Mr. Hendricks to be involved in group activities such as games and music therapy? What are the benefits or drawbacks to insisting on his involvement in these types of activities?
2. Is Mr. Hendricks's wandering a common problem for persons with dementia? How is this best handled by the nursing staff?
3. Which interventions can address Mr. Hendricks's behaviors that have injured staff members?
4. What are the chances that Mr. Hendricks has a problem with substance abuse?

STUDY QUESTIONS

1. There are a number of issues in LTC today. What are the most essential issues for the federal government to address first?
2. Discuss the ethical principle of autonomy when constructing an appropriate plan of care for a recipient of long-term care.
3. Discuss the principle of autonomy in relation to the community-dwelling client versus the person in a residential facility.
4. Analyze nursing interventions that would most likely support the goals of an ideal LTC system.
5. How is LTC defined?
6. What is the difference between an LTACH, a CCRC, and an NORC?
7. Describe the major settings in which LTC is provided, giving a specific example of each in your local community.
8. What are some of the precipitating factors for an individual to access the long-term care system?
9. What are the major problems facing both caregivers and clients in today's long-term care continuum?
10. What are the most commonly abused illicit substances among older adults?
11. Which individuals are considered vulnerable populations?

Internet Resources

Across the States 2006: Profiles of Long-Term Care and Independent Living: http://assets.aarp.org/rgcenter/health/d18763_2006_ats.pdf

Geriatric Nursing Education Project: http://www.aacn.nche.edu/gnec.htm

Hartford Institute for Geriatric Nursing: http://hartfordign.org

Leading Age (formerly American Association of Homes and Services for the Aging): http://www.leadingage.org

Long-term care planning tool from CMS: http://www.medicare.gov/LTCPlanning/Include/DataSection/Questions/SearchCriteria.asp?version=default&browser=IE%7C6%7CWinXP&language=English&defaultstatus=0&pagelist=Home

Medicare and You, 2012 (Centers for Medicare and Medicaid Services publication): http://www.medicare.gov/Publications/Pubs/pdf/10050.pdf

Long-Term Care Ombudsman: http://www.ltcombudsman.org

Medicare Hospice Benefits: http://www.medicare.gov/publications/pubs/pdf/02154.pdf

National Gerontological Nursing Association: http://www.ngna.org

National Association of Professional Geriatric Care Managers: http://www.caremanager.org

National Center for Assisted Living: http://www.ahcancal.org/ncal/Pages/default.aspx

National Hospice and Palliative Care Organization: http://www.nhpco.org

Practicing physician education in geriatrics: http://www.gericareonline.net

Senior Care Central: http://www.seniorcarecentral.net

Scope and Standards of Assisted Living Practice: http://www.alnursing.org/alnursecert/SCOPE_AND_STANDARDS_FINAL2_09-19-06.pdf

References

AARP. (2010). Prepare to care: A planning guide for families. http://www.aarp.org/relationships/caregiving/info-04-2010/prepare-to-care.html

AARP. (2013). Medicare ruling means no more "improve or you're out." http://blog.aarp.org/2013/02/06/amy-goyer-medicare-pays-for-skilled-therapy-for-maintenance-with-chronic-illness/

Administration on Aging. (2008). The 2005 White House Conference on Aging. http://www.whoa.gov/

Administration on Aging. (2011). A profile of older Americans: 2010. http://www.aoa.gov/AoARoot/Aging_Statistics/Profile/2010/2.aspx

Agency for Healthcare Research and Quality (AHRQ). (2009). Elderly long-term care: Use of physical restraints in nursing homes creates substantial adverse consequences for residents. http://www.ahrq.gov/research/mar09/0309RA9htm

Aging with Dignity. (2010). Five Wishes 2010 edition. http://www.agingwithdignity.org/five-wishes.php

Alzheimer's Association. (2014). Alzheimer's facts and figures. http://www.alz.org/alzheimers_disease_facts_and_figures.asp#quickFacts

Amann, C. A., & LeBlanc, R. G. (2014). Caring across the continuum. In K. L. Mauk (Ed.), *Gerontological nursing: Competencies for care* (3rd ed., pp. 857–878). Burlington, MA: Jones & Bartlett Learning.

American Association of Colleges of Nursing (AACN). (2011). Nursing shortage. http://www.aacn.nche.edu/media-relations/fact-sheets/nursing-shortage

American Association of Colleges of Nursing (AACN) & Hartford Institute for Geriatric Nursing. (2010). *Recommended baccalaureate competencies and curricular guidelines for the nursing care of older adults.* New York, NY: Author.

American Geriatrics Society (AGS) & British Geriatrics Society (BGS). (2010). Clinical practice guideline: Prevention of falls in older adults. http://www.medcats.com/FALLS/frameset.htm

American Healthcare Association. (2012). Quality report. http://www.ahcancal.org/quality_improvement/Documents/AHCA%20Quality%20Report%20FINAL.pdf

American Lung Association. (2014). Pneumonia fact sheet. http://www.lung.org/lung-disease/influenza/in-depth-resources/pneumonia-fact-sheet.html

American Psychological Association. (2000). *Diagnostic and statistical manual*, 4th ed., text revision. Arlington, VA: Author.

Arling, G., Kane, R., L., Mueller, C., Bershadsky, J., & Degenholtz, H. B. (2007). Nursing effort and quality of care for nursing home residents. *The Gerontologist*, 47(1), 672–682.

Association of Rehabilitation Nurses (ARN). (2013). *The essential role of the rehabilitation nurse in facilitating care transitions: A white paper by the Association of Rehabilitation Nurses.* Glenview, IL: Author.

Beauchamp, T. L., & Childress, J. F. (2009). *Principles of biomedical ethics* (6th ed.). New York, NY: Oxford University Press.

Beck, A. T., Rush, A. J., Shaw, B. F., & Emery, G. (1979). *Cognitive therapy of depression.* New York, NY: Guilford.

Borson, S., Scanlan, J. M., Chen, P., & Ganguli, M. (2003). The Mini-Cog as a screen for dementia: Validation in a population-based sample. *Journal of the American Geriatrics Society, 51*(10), 1451–1454.

Borson, S., Scanlan, J., Hummel, J., Gibbs, K., Lessig, M., & Zuhr, E. (2007). Implementing routine cognitive screening of older adults in primary care: Process and impact on physician behavior. *Journal of General Internal Medicine, 22*(6), 811–817.

Boult, C., & Wieland, G. D. (2010). Comprehensive primary care for older patients with multiple chronic conditions. *Journal of the American Medical Association, 304*(17), 1936–1943.

Caffrey, C., Sengupta, M., Park-Lee, E., Moss, A., Rosenoff, E., & Harris-Kojetin, L. (2012). Residents living in residential care facilities: United States 2010. NCHS Data Brief, April (91), 1–8.

Capezuti, E., Zwicker, D., Mezey, M., & Fulmer, T. (2008). *Evidence-based geriatric nursing protocols for best practice.* New York, NY: Springer.

Casada da Rocha, A. (2009). Towards a comprehensive concept of patient autonomy. *American Journal of Bioethics, 9*(2), 37–38.

Castle, N. G., Engberg, J., & Men, A. (2007). Nursing home staff turnover: Impact on nursing home compare quality measures. *The Gerontologist, 47*(1), 650–661.

Centers for Disease Control and Prevention (CDC). (2009a). National nursing home survey: 2004 overview. http://www.cdc.gov/nchs/data/series/sr_13/sr13_167.pdf

Centers for Disease Control and Prevention (CDC). (2009b). Chronic disease and health promotion. http://www.cdc.gov/chronicdisease/overview/index/htm

Centers for Disease Control and Prevention (CDC). (2012). Chronic diseases and health promotion. http://www.cdc.gov/chronicdisease/overview/index.htm

Centers for Medicare and Medicaid Services (CMS). (2007). Medicare hospice benefits. http://www.medicare.gov/publications/pubs/pdf/02154.pdf

Centers for Medicare and Medicaid Services (CMS). (2010). State operations manual. http://www.cms.gov/manuals/downloads/som107c01.pdf

Centers for Medicare and Medicaid Services (CMS). (2011a). Overview. http://www.cms.gov/history

Centers for Medicare and Medicaid Services (CMS). (2011b). Nursing home quality indicators. http://www.cms.gov/NursingHomeQualityInits/01_Overview.asp#TopOfPage

Centers for Medicare and Medicaid Services (CMS). (2011c). 482.13(e) Standard: Restraint or seclusion. http://www/cms.gov/manual/downloads/som107ap_a_hospitals.pdf

Centers for Medicare and Medicaid Services (CMS). (2012a). A glossary of terms for caregivers. http://www.medicare.gov/files/ask-medicare-types-of-care.pdf

Centers for Medicare and Medicaid Services (CMS). (2012b). Nursing home data compendium 2012. http://www.cms.gov/Medicare/Provider-Enrollment-and-Certification/CertificationandComplianc/Downloads/nursinghomedatacompendium_508.pdf

Centers for Medicare and Medicaid Services (CMS). (2013). Transitional care management services fact sheet. http://www.cms.gov/Outreach-and-Education/Medicare-Learning-Network-MLN/MLNProducts/Downloads/Transitional-Care-Management-Services-Fact-Sheet-ICN908628.pdf

Cherry, B., Ashcraft, A., & Owen, D. (2007). Perceptions of job satisfaction and the regulatory environment among nurse aides and charge nurses in long-term care. *Geriatric Nursing, 28*(3), 183–192.

Commission on Long-Term Care. (2013). http://ltccommission.org/

Connecticut Department of Public Health. (2013). DPH study finds dental care lacking among long-term care residents and vulnerable older adults. http://www.ct.gov/dph/cwp/view.asp?A=4386&Q=531622

Crain, M. (2001). Control beliefs of the frail elderly. *Case Management Journal, 3*(1), 42–46.

Dean, M., Harrison, B., & Zwicker, D. (2014). Falls in older adults. In K. L. Mauk (Ed.) *Gerontological nursing: Competencies for care* (pp. 457–480). Burlington, MA: Jones & Bartlett Learning.

DeSpelder, L. A., & Strickland, A.L. (2011). *The last dance: Encountering death and dying* (2nd ed.). New York, NY: McGraw-Hill.

Donald, F., Martin-Misener, R., Carter, N., Donald, E. E., Kaasalainen, S., Wickson-Griffiths, A., … DiCenso, A. (2013). A systematic review of the effectiveness of advanced practice nurses in long-term care. *Journal of Advanced Nursing, 69*(10), 2148–2161.

Elder Abuse Daily. (2010). Elder abuse data and statistics. http://www.eadaily.com/15/elder-abuse-statistics/

Elioupoulos, C. (2014). *Fast facts for the gerontology nurse.* New York, NY: Springer.

Families for Better Care. (2013). Top 10 Key findings from Nursing Home Report Card. http://nursinghomereportcards.com/key-findings/

Ferrell, B., & Coyle, N. (2010). *Textbook of palliative nursing.* New York, NY: Oxford University Press.

Fillenbaum, G. G. (1988). *Multidimensional functional assessment of older adults: The Duke older americans resources and services procedures.* Hillsdale, NJ: Lawrence Erlbaum Associates.

Fink, R. M., & Gates, R. A. (2010). Pain assessment. In B. Ferrell & N. Coyle (Eds.), *Oxford textbook of palliative nursing* (3rd ed., pp. 137–160). New York, NY: Oxford University Press.

Frahm, K. A., Brown, L. M., & Hyer, K. (2013). Racial disparities in end-of-life planning and services for deceased nursing home residents. *Journal of the American Medical Directors Association, 13*(9), 819. e7–11. doi: 10.1016/j.jamda.2012.07.021

Haber, D. (2014). Promoting healthy aging. In K. L. Mauk (Ed.), *Gerontological nursing: Competencies for care* (3rd ed. pp. 187–222). Burlington, MA: Jones & Bartlett Learning.

Hardin, S. (2010). Promoting quality of life. In K. L. Mauk (Ed.), *Gerontological nursing: Competencies for care* (2nd ed., pp. 618-630). Sudbury, MA: Jones and Bartlett.

Harrington, C., Carrillo, H., Blank, B. W., & O'Brian, T. (2010). Nursing facilities, staffing, residents and facility deficiencies, 2004 through 2009. http://www .pascenter.org/nursing_homes/nursing_trends_2009.php

Harrington, L. (2008). Interview with a quality leader: Peter Buerhaus on workforce issues. *Journal for Healthcare Quality, 30*(6), 31–36.

Harris-Kojetin, L., Sengupta, M., Park-Lee, E., & Valverde, R. (2013). *Long-term care services in the United States: 2013 overview.* Hyattsville, MD: National Center for Health Statistics.

Hartman, M., Martin, A. B., Benson, J., & Catlin, A. (2013). National Health Expenditure Accounts Team. National health spending in 2011: Overall growth remains low, but some payers and services show signs of acceleration. *Health Affairs, 32*(1), 87–99.

Healthy People 2020. (2011). http://www.healthypeople .gov/hp2020

Hildreth, C. J. (2011). Elder abuse. *Journal of the American Medical Association, 306*(5), 568.

Houser, A., Fox-Grage, W., & Gibson, M. J. (2009). Across the states: Profiles of long-term care and independent living (8th ed.). http://assets.aarp.org/ rgcenter/health/d18763_2006_ats.pdf

Houser, A., Fox-Grage, W., & Ujvari, K. (2012). *Across the states: Profiles of long-term services and supports* (9th ed.). Washington, DC: AARP Public Policy Institute. http://www.aarp.org/content/dam/aarp /research/public_policy_institute/ltc/2012/across-the- states-2012-full-report-AARP-ppi-ltc.pdf

Jones, A. L., Moss, A. J., & Harris-Kojetin, L. D. (2011). Use of advance directives in long-term care populations. NCHS Data Brief Number 54. Hyattsville, MD: National Center for Health Statistics.

Jonsen, A. R. (2007). A history of bioethics as discipline and discourse. In N. S. Jecker, A. R. Jonsen, & R. A. Pearlman (Eds.), *Bioethics: An introduction to the history, methods, and practice* (pp. 3–16). Sudbury, MA: Jones and Bartlett.

Kalisch, P. A., & Kalisch, B. J. (2004). *American nursing: A history* (4th ed.). Philadelphia, PA: Lippincott Williams & Wilkins.

Katz, S., Downs, T. D., Cash, H. R., & Grotz, R. C. (1970). Progress in development of the index of ADL. *The Gerontologist, 10,* 20–30.

Kindred Hospital. (2014). What is long-term acute care? http://www.khchicagonorth.com/about-us/what-is-ltac/

Koop, C. E., & Schaeffer, F. (1976). *Whatever happened to the human race?* Old Tappan, NJ: Fleming H. Revell.

Lee, H. S., Mericle, A. A., Ayalon, L., & Arean, P.A. (2009). Harm reduction among at-risk elderly drinkers: A site-specific analysis from the multi-site Primary Care Research in Substance Abuse and Mental Health for Elderly (PRISM-E) study. *Geriatric Psychiatry, 24*(1), 54–60.

Lochner, L., & Byrd, M. (2014). Anxiety and depression in the older adult. In K. L. Mauk (Ed.), *Gerontological nursing: Competencies for care* (3rd ed., pp. 513–544). Burlington, MA: Jones & Bartlett Learning.

Lomastro, J. A. (2006). The White House Conference on Aging: A positive view. *Nursing Homes: Long-Term Care Management, 55*(1), 14–16, 18.

Maas, M. L., Reed, D., Park, M., Specht, J. P., Schutte, D., Kelley, L. S., ... Buckwalter, K.C. (2004). Outcomes of family involvement in care interventions for caregivers of individuals with dementia. *Nursing Research, 53*(2), 76–86.

Matthiesen, S., & Schumaker, C. (2010). *Adult day services: Providing support and care for seniors and families.* CARF International. http://www.carf.org/WorkArea /DownloadAsset.aspx?id=23809

Mauk, K. L. (2011). Ethical perspectives on self-neglect among older adults. *Rehabilitation Nursing, 36*(2), 60–65.

Mauk, K. L. (2012). *Rehabilitation nursing: A contemporary approach to practice.* Sudbury, MA: Jones and Bartlett.

Mauk, K. L., & Patel, U. (2011). Geriatric rehabilitation. In C. Jacelon (Ed.), *The specialty practice of rehabilitation nursing: A core curriculum* (pp. 475–504). Glenview, IL: Association of Rehabilitation Nurses.

Mauk, K. L., & Urban, K. (2014). Abuse and mistreatment of older adults. In K. L. Mauk (Ed.), *Gerontological nursing: Competencies for care* (3rd ed., pp. 810–829). Burlington, MA: Jones & Bartlett Learning.

Medicaid.gov. (2014). Program of All-Inclusive Care for the Elderly (PACE). http://www.medicaid.gov /Medicaid-CHIP-Program-Information/By-Topics /Long-Term-Services-and-Support/Integrating-Care /Program-of-All-Inclusive-Care-for-the-Elderly-PACE /Program-of-All-Inclusive-Care-for-the-Elderly-PACE .html

Medpac. (2010). Report to the Congress: Medicare payment policy. www.medpac.gov/documents/Mar10 _EntireReport.pdf

Meenan, R. F. (1985). New approaches to outcome assessment: The AIMS questionnaire for arthritis. *Advances in Internal Medicine, 31*, 167–185.

Melnyk, B. M., & Fineout-Overholt, E. (2010). *Evidence based practice in nursing and healthcare: A guide to best practice* (2nd ed.). Philadelphia, PA: Lippincott Williams & Wilkins.

Mezey, M., Mitty, I., & Ramsey, G. (1997). Assessment of decision making capacity: Nursing's role. *Journal of Gerontological Nursing, 23*(3), 28–34.

Miller, A. (2014). Job description for resident assistant at assisted living. http://work.chron.com/job-description-resident-assistant-assisted-living-18081.html

Mion, L. C., Halliday, B. L., & Sandhu, S. K. (2008). Physical restraints and side rails in acute and critical care settings: Legal, ethical, and practice issues. In E. Capezuti, D. Zwicker, M. Mezey, & T. Fulmer. (2008). *Evidence-based geriatric nursing protocols for best practice* (3rd ed., pp. 503–520). New York, NY: Springer.

Moe, A., Hellzen, O., & Enmarker, I. (2013). The meaning of receiving help from home nursing care. *Nursing Ethics, 20*(7), 737–747.

Moody, H. R. (2008). The White House Conference on Aging in 2015: The shape of things to come. *Public Policy and Aging Report, 16*(1), 24–26. http://assets. aarp.org/www.aarp.org_/articles/research/oaa /whconf_2015.pdf

Moye, J., Butz, S. W., Marson, D. C., & Wood, E. (2007). A conceptual model and assessment template for capacity evaluation in adult guardianship. *The Gerontologist, 47*(5), 591–603.

Mullaney, T. (2014). Better staffing means better care, new nursing home rankings suggest. http://www. mcknights.com/better-staffing-means-better-care-new-nursing-home-state-rankings-suggest /article/307083/

National Adult Protective Services Association. (2014). Get help. http://www.napsa-now.org/get-help /how-aps-helps/

National Association of Professional Geriatric Care Managers. (2011). What can a PGCM do for me?

http://www.caremanager.org/displaycommon .cfm?an=1&subarticlenbr=87

National Care Planning Council. (2014). About long-term care. http://www.longtermcarelink.net/eldercare /long_term_care.htm

National Center for Assisted Living. (2011). Resident profile. www.ahcancal.org/ncal/resources/Pages /ResidentProfile.aspx

National Center for Elder Abuse. (2011). Definitions of elder abuse. http://www.ncea.aoa.gov/NCEAroot /Main_Site/FAQ/Basics/Definition.aspx

National Center for Elder Abuse. (2014). Statistics/data. http://www.ncea.aoa.gov/Library/Data/index.aspx#problem

National Institute on Aging. (2007). Growing older in America: The health and retirement study. http://www .nia.nih.gov/ResearchInformation/ExtramuralPrograms /BehavioralAndSocialResearch/HRS.htm

National Institute of Mental Health (NIMH). (2010). Older adults: Depression and suicide facts. http://www .nimh.nih.gov/health/publications/older-adults-depression-and-suicide-facts.shtml#how-common

National Long-Term Care Ombudsman Resource Center. (2014). About ombudsman. http://www .ltcombudsman.org/about-ombudsmen

National PACE Association. (2011). About NPA. http:// www.npaonline.org/website/article.asp?id=5

Nelson, A. (Ed.). (2006). *Safe patient handling and movement: A practical guide for health care professionals.* New York, NY: Springer.

Nelson, A., Collins, J., Siddharthan, K., Matz, M., & Waters, T. (2008). Link between safe patient handling and patient outcomes in long-term care. *Rehabilitation Nursing, 33*(1), 33–43.

Nelson, J. M. (2014). Identifying and preventing common risk factors in the elderly. In K. L. Mauk (Ed.), *Gerontological nursing: Competencies for care* (3rd ed., pp. 223–266). Burlington, MA: Jones & Bartlett Learning.

Oliver, D., Healey, F., & Haines, T. P. (2010). Preventing falls and fall-related injuries in hospitals. *Clinics in Geriatric Medicine, 26*, 645–692.

POLST. (2012). What is POLST? http://www.polst.org/

Provider Magazine. (2012). 2012 top 50 nursing facility companies. http://www.providermagazine.com /reports/Pages/0612/2012-Top-50-Largest-Nursing-Facility-Companies.aspx

Reinhard, S. C., Kassner, E., Houser, A., & Mollica, R. L. (2011). Raising expectations: A state scorecard on long-term services and supports for older adults, people with physical disabilities, and family caregivers. http:// www.longtermscorecard.org/~/media/Microsite/Files /Reinhard_raising_expectations_LTSS_scorecard _REPORT_WEB_v5.pdf

Robert Wood Johnson Foundation. (2014). The Green House Project. http://www.rwjf.org/en/grants/grantees/the-green-house-project.html

Rose, S. S. (2014). Delirium. In K. L. Mauk (Ed.), *Gerontological nursing: Competencies for care* (3rd ed., pp. 483–512). Burlington, MA: Jones & Bartlett Learning.

Sehy, Y. B., & Williams, M. P. (1999). Functional assessment. In W. C. Chenitz, J. Takano Smith, & S. A. Salisbury (Eds.), *Clinical gerontological nursing: A guide to advanced practice* (2nd ed., pp. 175–199). Philadelphia, PA: Saunders.

Seitz, D., Purandare, N., & Conn, D. (2010). Prevalence of psychiatric disorders among older adults in long-term care homes: A systematic review. *International Psychogeriatrics*, 22(7), 1025–1039.

Severson, D. (2014). Assisted living facility administrator salaries. http://work.chron.com/assisted-living-facility-administrator-salaries-27818.html

Sherwin, S., & Winsby, M. (2011). A relational perspective on autonomy for older adults residing in nursing homes. *Health Expectations*, 14(2): 182–190.

Taylor, M. H., & Grossberg, G. T. (2012, July 12). The growing problem of illicit substance abuse in the elderly: A review. *Primary Care Companion of CNS Disorders*, 14(4). http://www.ncbi.nlm.nih.gov/pmc/articles/PMC3505129/

Teaster, P. B. (2002). *A response to the abuse of vulnerable adults: The 2000 survey of state adult protective services.* Washington, DC: National Center on Elder Abuse.

Thomas, K. L, Mor, V., Tyler, D. A., & Hyer, K. (2013). The relationships among licensed nurse turnover, retention, and rehospitalization of nursing home residents. *The Gerontologist*, 53(2), 211–221. doi: 10.1093/geront/gns082

Tobin, P., & Salisbury, S. (1999). Legal planning issues. In J. T. Stone, J. F. Wyman, & S. A. Salisbury (Eds.), *Clinical gerontological nursing: A guide to advanced practice* (2nd ed., pp. 31–44). Philadelphia, PA: Saunders.

Touhy, T., & Jett, K. (2010). Mental health and wellness in late life. In *Ebersole and Hess' Gerontological nursing and healthy aging* (3rd ed., pp. 406–434). St. Louis, MO: Mosby.

Tran, H. T., & Karlamangla, A. S. (2014). Health promotion screening. In E. A. Capezuti, M. L. Malone, P. R. Katz, & M. D. Mezey (Eds.), *The encyclopedia of elder care* (3rd ed., pp. 358–362). New York, NY: Springer.

Tullman, D. F., Mion, L. C., Fletcher, K., & Foreman, M. D. (2008). Delirium. http://consultgerirn.org/topics/delirium/want_to_know_more

United Way. (2014). About United Way worldwide. http://www.unitedway.org/pages/about-united-way-worldwide/

U.S. Department of Veterans Affairs. (2014). http://www.va.gov

U.S. Preventive Services Task Force (USPSTF). (2012). Screening and behavioral counseling intervention in primary care to reduce alcohol misuse. http://www.uspreventiveservicestaskforce.org/uspstf12/alcmisuse/alcmisusefinalrs.htm#summary

Varcarolis, E. M., & Halter, M. J. (2010). *Foundation of psychiatric mental health nursing: A clinical approach.* Philadelphia, PA: Saunders.

Vink, D., Aartsen, J. J., & Schovevers, R. A. (2008). Risk factors for anxiety and depression in the elderly: A review. *Journal of Affective Disorders*, 106, 29–44.

Wallis, S. J., & Campbell, G. A. (2011). Preventing falls and fractures in long-term care. *Reviews in Clinical Gerontology*, 21(4), 346–360.

Warring, P., & Krieger-Blake, L. (2014). End of life care. In K. L. Mauk (Ed.), *Gerontological nursing: Competencies for care* (3rd ed., pp. 880–928). Burlington, MA: Jones & Bartlett Learning.

World Health Organization (WHO). (2008). WHO definition of palliative care. http://www.who.int/cancer/palliative/definition/en/

World Health Organization (WHO). (2012). Depression. Fact Sheet No. 369. http://www.who.int/mediacentre/factsheets/fs369/en/index.html

Wulff, I., Kalinowski, S., & Drager, D. (2010). Autonomy in the nursing home: Conceptual considerations regarding self-determination and capacity to act on the basis of a model. *Pflege*, 23(4), 240–248.

Chapter 22

Palliative Care

Barbara M. Raudonis
and Pamala D. Larsen

Introduction

The aging American population—the so-called silver tsunami—is one of the critical public health challenges of the 21st century (Morrison, 2013). The number of aging adults experiencing multiple chronic health problems continues to rise as well (Ritchie & Zulman, 2013). Four chronic diseases—heart disease, cancer, cerebrovascular disease, and chronic respiratory disease—remain the leading causes of death for older adults (Centers for Disease Control and Prevention [CDC], 2013). Chronic diseases share protracted illness trajectories that include phases of decline resulting in progressively advanced disease and disability. Individuals who have illness trajectories, such as those in chronic disease, can benefit from palliative care.

In examining palliative care from a worldwide perspective, data from the World Health Organization (WHO, 2014a) suggest that only 1 in 10 people who need palliative care currently receive it. This unmet need was described for the first time in the *Global Atlas of Palliative Care at the End of Life*, published jointly by WHO and the Worldwide Palliative Care Alliance. The greatest need is in low- and middle-income countries and for noncommunicable diseases (Worldwide Palliative Care Alliance, 2014). The *Global Atlas* calls on all countries to include palliative care as an essential component in every modern healthcare system as countries move toward more universal health care. The Sixty-Seventh World Health Assembly met in May of 2014 and passed a resolution that emphasized the need to strengthen palliative care services in all countries (WHO, 2014b). Currently, only 20 countries worldwide have palliative care well integrated into their healthcare systems (WHO, 2014a).

Historical Perspectives

Palliative care grew out of the hospice movement. Hospice is both a philosophy of care and an organized form of healthcare delivery. Dame Cicely Saunders, considered the founder of the modern hospice movement, was educated as a nurse, social worker, and physician, and founded St. Christopher's Hospice in Sydenham, England, in 1967. St. Christopher's Hospice was the first research and teaching hospice and is known for innovations in pain and symptom management, providing a holistic approach to care, home care, family support throughout the illness, and bereavement follow-up (Meier, 2010). Based on Saunders's work, palliative care services have spread throughout the United Kingdom and the world (Hansford, 2010). The first hospice in the United States was founded in New Haven, Connecticut, in 1971.

In the 1990s, two reports—*Study to Understand Prognosis and Preferences for Outcomes and Risks of Treatments* (SUPPORT, 1995) and an Institute of Medicine (IOM) report, *Approaching Death: Improving Care at the End of Life* (Field & Cassel, 1997)—set off a wave of concern regarding the status of end-of-life care in the United States. As a result of the attention, improving end-of-life care was placed on the national healthcare agenda. Palliative care, however, may or may not be end-of-life care.

The SUPPORT study (1995) findings identified several problems related to palliative care. Patient suffering included dying in pain with a severe symptom burden. Poor communication among patients, families, and their physicians led to undesired resuscitation efforts and extensive use of hospital resources.

The IOM study, *Approaching Death: Improving Care at the End of Life* (Field & Cassel, 1997), revealed a critical need for improvement in the education and training of healthcare professionals in palliative and end-of-life care. Healthcare professionals have traditionally received inadequate education and training in the safe and effective management of pain and other symptoms. They also lack the skills and confidence to address the psychological, social, and spiritual aspects of care (Sullivan, Lakoma, & Block, 2003).

In August 2011, the National Institute of Nursing Research (NINR) sponsored a summit, titled "The Science of Compassion: Future Directions in End-of-Life and Palliative Care." Presenters at the summit examined the state of research and clinical practice in end-of-life and palliative care. The Executive Summary is available online (https://www.ninr.nih.gov/sites/www.ninr.nih.gov/files/science-of-compassion-executive-summary.pdf). Dr. June Lunney closed the third plenary session of the NINR summit with the following words:

Palliative care is a field that encompasses the paradox of living and dying at the same time. Compassion involves understanding the unique and complex aspects of family dynamics during the dying process. The goal of the science of compassion

is to ensure that the appropriate support teams are with patients as they journey through life's health stages, including the time as they are approaching EOL. (NINR, 2011, p. 15)

Future directions in research based on themes discussed during the summit were also recommended:

- Multiple comorbidities, which influence both Medicare spending and the care at end of life
- Use of technology to improve health outcomes of individuals and their families
- A focus on the quality of the science of palliative care
- Development and nurturing of the next generation of practitioners and researchers in the field

Oftentimes the terms *hospice* and *palliative care* are used interchangeably, even in medical and nursing textbooks. Talk of symptom management and palliative care quickly moves to end-of-life care issues—not using the term *hospice*, but rather *end-of-life*. Receiving palliative care does *not* mean that clients are receiving end-of-life care. The differences are clear: Patients may receive curative treatment during palliative care, but not during hospice or end-of-life care. All hospice care is palliative care—that is, symptom management and comfort care—but not all palliative care is hospice or end-of-life care.

The hospice nurse has come to do her "intake" interview and paperwork for Randy's admission to outpatient hospice care. I have two questions. Will he be allowed to have an esophageal dilation during hospice care? Thankfully, he will, because it is a comfort measure, receiving nourishment. However, his radiation treatment that he is receiving tonight to hopefully lessen the pain from the cancer growing in his chest is not "covered" ... even though it is only symptom management. So Randy will have his radiation treatment tonight at the hospital before going home in the morning.

I think back on all of the questions I had about hospice and what was possible and what wasn't. Little did either of us know that he would die within 6 weeks of leaving the hospital. So much for the prognosis of 3 to 6 months after discharge from the hospital.

—Jenny

Defining Palliative Care

The definition of palliative care that characterizes such care in the United States, and one supported by both the U.S. Department of Health and Human Services' (HHS) Centers for Medicare and Medicaid Services (CMS) and the National Quality Forum (NQF), is as follows:

Palliative care means patient- and family-centered care that optimizes quality of life by anticipating, preventing, and treating suffering. Palliative care throughout the continuum of illness involves addressing physical, intellectual, emotional, social, and spiritual needs and to facilitate patient autonomy, access to information, and choice (Dahlin, 2013).

A more thorough description of palliative care includes these characteristics:

- Provides relief from pain and other distressing symptoms
- Affirms life and regards dying as a normal process
- Intends neither to hasten nor to postpone death
- Integrates the psychological and spiritual aspects of patient care
- Offers a support system to help patients live as actively as possible near death
- Uses a team approach to address the needs of patients and their families, including bereavement counseling, if indicated
- Enhances quality of life, and may also positively influence the course of illness
- Is applicable early in the course of illness, in conjunction with other therapies that are intended to prolong life,

such as chemotherapy or radiation therapy, and includes those investigations needed to better understand and manage distressing clinical complications (Clark, 2010, p. 10).

Clinical Practice Guidelines for Palliative Care

Landmark studies, such as the SUPPORT study and the IOM report, recognized the need for integration of palliative care into health care for all individuals with chronic, debilitating, and life-limiting illnesses. The National Consensus Project, supported by the American Academy of Hospice and Palliative Medicine (AAHPM), the Center to Advance Palliative Care (CAPC), the Hospice and Palliative Nurses Association (HPNA), the National Association of Social Workers (NASW), the National Hospice and Palliative Care Organization (NHPCO), and the National Palliative Care Research Center, established the first *Clinical Practice Guidelines for Quality Palliative Care* (NCPQPC) in 2004; it was followed by the second edition in 2009 and the third edition in March 2013.

A number of specific events necessitated development of the 2013 guidelines: an increase in the number of hospice and palliative care programs since the second-edition guidelines were published in 2009; a growing integration of palliative care throughout healthcare settings; major developments in the evidence base for palliative care; passage of the Patient Protection and Affordable Care Act (ACA), which included aspects of palliative care; advanced palliative certification by The Joint Commission in 2011; and new quality measures (Dahlin, 2013). Given that responsibility for palliative care is shared across a variety of healthcare settings, the emphasis of this document is on collaborative partnerships within and between hospitals, community centers, hospices, and home health agencies to ensure quality, continuity, and access to palliative care.

There are eight domains of care in the 2013 guidelines:

- Domain 1: Structure and Processes of Care
- Domain 2: Physical Aspects of Care
- Domain 3: Psychological and Psychiatric Aspects
- Domain 4: Social Aspects of Care
- Domain 5: Spiritual, Religious, and Existential Aspects of Care
- Domain 6: Cultural Aspects of Care
- Domain 7: Care of the Patient at the End of Life
- Domain 8: Ethical and Legal Aspects of Care

Source: Dahlin, C. (2013), *The Clinical Practice Guidelines for Palliative Care, 3e, p. 10-11. Reprinted with permission of Hospice and Palliative Nurses Foundation (HPNF)*

These areas are delineated and elements of best practice are described in the 2013 document.

The *Clinical Practice Guidelines* serve as a manual or blueprint to create new programs and guide developing programs. In each edition, the *Clinical Practice Guidelines* are revised to reflect current practice. Except for Domain 7, for which the title has been changed from "Care of the Imminently Dying Patient" to "Care of the Patient at the End of Life," the domains have remained consistent in each of the three editions (Dahlin, 2013). The underlying tenets of palliative care in this document continue to be patient- and family-centered palliative care; comprehensive palliative care with continuity across health settings; early introduction of palliative care at diagnosis of a serious disease or life-threatening condition; interdisciplinary collaborative palliative care; clinical and communication expertise within palliative care team members; relief of physical, psychological, emotional, and spiritual suffering and distress of patients and families; a focus on quality; and equitable access (http://www.nationalconsensusproject.org/GuidelinesTOC.pdf).

A summary of the revisions made to each domain in the third edition follows (Dahlin, 2013, pp. 10–11):

- Domain 1: The Structure and Process Domain was enhanced to describe and accentuate the current state of the field, with emphasis on interdisciplinary team (IDT) engagement and collaboration with patients and families. Clarity and specificity of interdisciplinary team composition, team member qualifications, necessary education, training, and support are more thoroughly described. Finally, the quality assessment process and improvement section incorporates the new mandates for quality under the ACA.
- Domain 2: The Physical Domain continues to emphasize the assessment and treatment of physical symptoms with appropriate, validated tools. Management of symptoms is multidimensional, involving pharmacologic, interventional, behavioral, and complementary interventions.
- Domain 3: The Psychological and Psychiatric Domain was revised and expanded to focus on the collaborative assessment process of psychological concerns and psychiatric diagnoses. Essential elements are described and include patient–family communication on assessment, diagnosis, and treatment options for common conditions in the context of respect for goals of care of the patient and family. New to the domain are the description and required elements of a bereavement program.
- Domain 4: The Social Domain has a greater emphasis on interdisciplinary engagement and collaboration with patients and families. Elements of a palliative care social assessment are defined. The role of the professional social worker with a bachelor's or master's degree in social work is described.
- Domain 5: The Spiritual Domain includes a definition of spirituality, stressing

assessment, access, and staff collaboration in attending to spiritual concerns throughout the illness trajectory. Requirements for staff training and education in provision of spiritual care are offered. There is stronger emphasis on the responsibility of the interdisciplinary team, inclusive of an appropriately trained chaplain, to explore, assess, and attend to spiritual issues of the patient and family. The domain promotes spiritual and religious rituals and practices for comfort and relief.

- Domain 6: Revised definitions of culture and cultural competence for the interdisciplinary team underscore culture as a source of resilience and strength for the patient and family. New content accentuates cultural and linguistic competence, including plain language, literacy, and linguistically appropriate service delivery.

- Domain 7: This domain highlights communication and documentation of signs and symptoms of the dying process in the circle of care—that is, among the patient, the family, and all other involved health providers. The importance of meticulous assessment and management of pain and other symptoms is underscored. The essential attention to family guidance as to what to expect in the dying process and the post-death period is emphasized. Bereavement support, beginning with anticipatory grief in the period before the actual death and continuing through the actual death, is stressed. Social, spiritual, and cultural aspects of care are of utmost concern throughout the process.

- Domain 8: The Ethical and Legal Domain is now restructured into three sections—advance care planning, ethics, and the legal aspects of care. The responsibility of the palliative care team to promote ongoing discussion about goals of care, along with completion and documentation of advance care planning documents, is emphasized. There is acknowledgment and affirmation

of the frequency and complexity of ethical issues in palliative care. Team competencies in the identification and resolution of commonly encountered ethical issues are described, with emphasis on the importance of seeking advice and counsel from ethics committees. There is acknowledgment of the complex legal and regulatory issues that arise in palliative care that require team members to understand their respective scope of practice within the provision of palliative care. Finally, there is new emphasis on the necessity of and access to expert legal counsel, which is essential for navigating the intricate and sensitive legal and regulatory issues in palliative care.

Palliative Care Medicine

Palliative medicine asserts boldly and optimistically that even in the face of overwhelming illness, suffering can and must be relieved.... there may be pragmatic, economic, geopolitical, or social reasons that make it difficult to provide palliative care, but these do not diminish from duty of care to seek the adequate relief of suffering of persons with incurable illness. (Hanks, Cherny, Portenoy, Kaasa, Fallon, & Christakis, 2010, p. 1)

The path to recognition of a subspecialty in palliative medicine began in 1988 with the creation of the Academy of Hospice Physicians, later renamed the American Academy of Hospice and Palliative Medicine (AAHPM). In 2006, the Accreditation Council for Graduate Medical Education and the American Board of Medical Specialties approved and recognized a new specialty in hospice and palliative medicine (Clark, 2010).

Palliative Care Nursing

The theoretical foundation for palliative care nursing continues to develop. Historically, it emerged from a philosophy of care, practice models, and guiding principles rather than a consistent application of theory. Wu and Volker (2012) applied Paterson and Zderad's (1976) humanistic theory to hospice and palliative care. Based on theoretical publications and research findings, humanistic theory is an appropriate framework for hospice and palliative nursing practice and research. The goal of person-centered comfort care is synergistic with the theory's emphasis on nurse–patient interactions promoting well-being and existential growth (Wu & Volker, 2012).

Coyle (2010) describes a distinct feature of palliative care nursing as "a whole person" philosophy of care: "Palliative nursing care is a combination of state-of-the-art clinical competence with fidelity to the patient, the ability to listen and to remain present in the face of much suffering and distress, and communication at a deeply personal level with the patient and family" (p. 3). This care is provided across the lifespan, in different care settings throughout the illness trajectory, the patient's death, and the family's bereavement. A nurse's individual relationship with the patient and family is a critical part of the healing relationship. This healing relationship, together with scientific knowledge (effective pain and symptom management) and clinical skills (addressing the emotional, psychosocial, and spiritual needs, and cultural values), is the essence of palliative care nursing, setting this specialty apart from other nursing specialty areas (pp. 5–6). As a philosophy of care and therapeutic approach, palliative care can be practiced by all nurses (Coyle, 2010).

Palliative Care and Hospice Data

The Center to Advance Palliative Care (CAPC) provides the most current data regarding palliative care. However, what is lacking are the "numbers" that document individuals receiving palliative care. Certainly, one can extrapolate that patients in hospice are receiving palliative care, but data demonstrating that persons are receiving such care outside of hospice are lacking.

CAPC (2014) provides some broad statements about palliative care:

- Palliative care is appropriate at any age and at any stage in a serious illness, and may be provided with curative treatment.
- According to a 2010 study in the *New England Journal of Medicine*, patients receiving early palliative care experienced less depression, had improved quality of life, and survived 2.7 months longer.
- Illnesses most commonly treated by palliative care are heart disease, cancer, stroke, diabetes, renal disease, Parkinson's disease, and Alzheimer's disease.
- Approximately 68% of Medicare costs are related to people with four or more chronic conditions—the typical palliative care patient.
- If palliative care fully penetrated into U.S. hospitals, the total savings could amount to $6 billion per year.
- Palliative care growth in hospitals has been exponential. The number of teams has doubled over the last 6 years. Currently, there are more than 1,500 hospitals with a palliative care team.
- Approximately 63% of all hospitals with more than 50 beds have a palliative care team today.

The National Hospice and Palliative Care Organization (2013) estimated there were 5,500 operational hospice programs throughout the United States in 2012, with an estimated 1.6 million patients served by these programs. These figures illustrate the enormous growth and progress in hospice care in the United States since 1974. The majority of hospice patients (68.6%) die at their place of residence. This could be their private residence, nursing home, or residential facility (NHPCO, 2013). In 2012, the median length of stay in hospice care was 18.7 days, while the average length of stay was 71.8 days (NHPCO, 2013). These numbers suggest that late referrals remain a problem. Non-cancer primary diagnoses accounted for 63.9% of hospice admissions in 2012, compared to 39.6% for cancer diagnoses. As evidence of the aging population, 83.4% of hospice patients were 65 years or older and one-third of those were 85 years or older (NHPCO, 2013).

Although these numbers portray tremendous growth in the use of hospice services, the patients admitted to such programs were 81.5% white/Caucasian. This is not a new finding, but rather continuing evidence that not all those in need of hospice services receive such care.

Professional Associations Related to Hospice and Palliative Care Nursing

The Hospice and Palliative Nurses Association (HPNA) was founded in 1986 and is the largest and oldest professional nursing organization dedicated to promoting excellence in palliative nursing care. The organization's foundation was incorporated in 1998 for two purposes: (1) to support research and education in end-of-life care and 2) to strive to meet the strategic goals of the HPNA. The foundation believes that evidence-based practice is the key to quality care for people with life-limiting and terminal illness. HPNF is a funding source for research, and it supports education related to hospice and palliative care to both individuals and groups. The 2012–2015 HPNA Research Agenda builds on the organization's first agenda (2009–2013) by identifying gaps in the knowledge that are barriers to quality palliative care.

In the past, the Alliance for Excellence in Hospice and Palliative Nursing (AEHPN, 2011) had a mission to "be the unified voice of professional membership, certification, research and education to advance quality palliative care for the benefit of the public at large." However, on December 1, 2013, the individual boards of its founding organizations—Hospice and Palliative Nurses Association (HPNA), the Hospice and Palliative Nurses Foundation (HPNF), and the National Board of Certification for Hospice and Palliative Nurses (NBCHPN)—decided to dissolve the Alliance.

The Center to Advance Palliative Care (CAPC) is the leading resource for palliative care program development and growth. CAPC provides access to essential palliative care tools, education, resources, and training for healthcare professionals.

The National Board for Certification of Hospice and Palliative Care Nurses is the only organization that offers specialty certification for all levels of the hospice and palliative nursing care team and administrators. Each certification is valid for a 4-year period, at which time the professional may renew his or her credential. To date, NBCHPN has certified more than 17,000 healthcare professionals in this subspecialty. Certification exams include those for the advanced certified hospice and palliative nurse (ACHPN), certified hospice and palliative nurse (CHPN), certified hospice and palliative pediatric nurse (CHPPN), certified hospice and palliative licensed nurse (CHPLN), certified hospice and palliative nursing assistant (CHPNA), certified hospice and palliative care administrator (CHPCA), and certified in perinatal loss (CPLC) professional (NBCHPN, 2014).

Problems and Barriers Related to Palliative Care

Barriers to palliative care exist for numerous reasons. The major underlying resistance to palliative care stems from a medical philosophy that emphasizes cure and prolongation of life over quality of life and relief of suffering (Morrison & Meier, 2003). Insurance reimbursement also forces consumer choice between cure and comfort care. Regular Medicare reimburses for curative treatment only, leaving the Medicare hospice benefit to cover comfort care (Fisher, Wennberg, Stukel, Gottlieb, Lucas, & Pinder, 2003).

Ohlen, Gustafsson, and Friberg (2013) suggest a combination of cancer therapy and palliative care coupled with greater awareness of the rehabilitative and palliative purposes of care is firmly in line with current descriptions of palliative care. However, this approach deviates from the image held by most healthcare professionals, who support that palliative care is exclusively for dying patients. In another arm of their study, these authors suggest that "making sense" of receiving palliative treatment is important to patients with advanced gastrointestinal cancer.

Late Identification of Palliative Care Needs

It is often difficult to determine when treatment of chronic disease should move from therapeutic interventions to palliative care strategies. Although diagnostic criteria for the need for palliative care may be clearer in patients with cancer, patients with heart failure (HF) and end-stage respiratory disease may be representative of a group of patients for whom there are no specific criteria. Fitzsimons and colleagues' (2007) study points to the fact that patients with HF and end-stage respiratory disease (and their caregivers) may have unmet clinical needs. The authors suggest earlier acknowledgment of symptoms and implementation of palliative care precepts.

Howlett (2011) concurs, noting that in comparison to patients with cancer, patients with HF are less likely to access palliative care resources and more likely to access inpatient care and cardiovascular procedures. What makes providing palliative care to HF patients and their families difficult is that for a majority of patients with advanced HF, symptoms are typically ones not readily associated with end-stage cardiac disease, but rather may include anxiety, anorexia, mood and sleep disturbances, personality change, and cognitive disturbance. Many of these symptoms are not addressed in a cardiovascular care setting (p. 145).

Lack of Knowledge About Palliative Care

The public's lack of understanding of the options available to dying patients and their families may result in delayed access to hospice and palliative care services (Field & Cassel, 1997). Surveys consistently indicate patients prefer to die at home. In 2009, 68.6% of all hospice patients died at a place they called "home"—40.1% died in their private residence, 18.9% died in nursing homes, 9.6% died in residential facilities, and 21.2% died in hospice inpatient units (NHPCO, 2013). Consumers' and communities' lack of understanding of what comprehensive palliative care programs offer, poor communication about patient and family preferences, and denial of death all impede timely referrals to palliative care services (End-of-Life Nursing Education Consortium [ELNEC], 2009).

Unfortunately, because palliative care is so closely associated with hospice care (in organizations, in medical and nursing textbooks, and in the community), most of the public believe that palliative care is the same as hospice care. Although the first part of this chapter clearly defined the differences between the two, it can be difficult to explain the distinction to the public and other caregivers.

Hospice is a specific type of palliative care, and in the United States it is generally considered a philosophy or program of care rather than a building of bricks and mortar. Hospice programs provide state-of-the-art palliative care and supportive services to dying persons and their families. This comprehensive care is available 24 hours a day, every day of the year, in community-based settings, patients' homes, and facility-based care settings. A medically directed interdisciplinary team (patients, family members, professionals, and volunteers) provides physical, psychosocial, and spiritual care during the final phase of an illness, the process of imminently dying, and the period of bereavement (NCPQPC, 2009). In hospice care, the dying person and the family are the unit of care. Patient and family values direct the care. However, the current Medicare hospice benefit eligibility criteria for hospice services include a terminal diagnosis and a 6-month prognosis. In addition, patients must discontinue curative or life-prolonging treatments to access comprehensive hospice care.

Identification of Patients Needing Palliative Care

One barrier to patients receiving needed palliative care is the lack of criteria in some communities and facilities for identifying appropriate candidates for care. This lack of criteria, combined with professional caregivers who struggle to communicate with patients about the option of palliative care, makes it hard to discern if patients are being treated appropriately.

Both criteria and tools are available to appropriately assess patients. However, use of these criteria and tools is inconsistent across the United States. Moreover, their use may be more common in teaching hospitals in urban areas compared with community hospitals and facilities in rural areas.

The Center to Advance Palliative Care website has resources for identifying appropriate patients in the community, pediatrics, long-term care, the intensive care unit (ICU), and others for a palliative care consultation. A consensus panel from CAPC reviewed existing palliative care literature as well as a number of well-known palliative care services in the United States to create relevant criteria (Weissman & Meier, 2011). For patients being admitted to a hospital, criteria for a palliative care consultation includes a potentially life-limiting or life-threatening condition *and*

- Primary criteria (the following are examples)
  - The "surprise question": You would not be surprised if the patient died within 12 months or before adulthood

- Frequent admissions (e.g., more than one admission for the same condition within several months)
- Admission prompted by difficult-to-control physical or psychological symptoms that are moderate to severe for more than 24 to 48 hours
- Complex care requirements (e.g., functional dependency, complex home support for ventilator/antibiotics/feedings)
- Decline in function, feeding intolerance, or unintended decline in weight
- Secondary criteria
  - Admission from long-term care facility or medical foster home
  - Elderly patient, cognitively impaired and with an acute hip fracture
  - Metastatic or locally advanced incurable cancer
  - Chronic home oxygen use
  - Out-of-hospital cardiac arrest
  - Current or past hospice program patient
  - Limited social support
  - No history of completing an advance care planning document (Weissman & Meier, 2011, p. 3)

Nelson and colleagues (2013) developed screening criteria for a palliative care consultation in the ICU. These authors performed a literature review from the inception of MEDLINE to December 2012 for English-language articles. A number of studies were reviewed, and although there were similarities between studies, each had its own criteria for a palliative care consultation. To summarize Nelson et al.'s findings, criteria for primary palliative assessment and consultation have been developed within one or more of the following domains: symptom distress, family distress, poor prognosis for survival or acceptable recover, and intensive utilization of healthcare resources (p. 2322). These authors also suggest that all stakeholders be involved in developing screening criteria for ICU palliative care consultation—for example, physician and nurse ICU leaders, the palliative care clinical team, the hospital administration, primary attending physician staff, nursing staff, patients, families, social work, case management, ethics consultation service, risk management, and patient relations.

Communication

In Fitzsimons and colleagues' (2007) study of unmet palliative care needs in the final stages of patients' illnesses, perhaps the most illuminating finding was the "expressed reluctance of some specialist clinicians to face the palliative care needs of their patients" (p. 321). These clinicians had known their patients for many years, but because they were unable to offer therapeutic/curative options to patients, palliative care and/or end-of-life care options were difficult for clinicians to communicate with their patients.

Interventions

Nursing Assessment

Effective symptom management begins with a thorough assessment. Research findings support the practice of routine and standardized symptom assessment with validated instruments (Morrison & Meier, 2003). Benefits attributed to routine assessments include identification of overlooked or unreported symptoms, particularly in older adults (Morrison, 2013). Dissemination and increased use of the same validated instruments facilitate the comparison of findings across practice settings and research studies. The Center to Advance Palliative Care (http://www.capc.org) and Brown University's Center for Gerontology and Health Care Research provide access to clinically useful instruments through their respective websites. Brown's website features a tool kit of instruments to measure end-of-life care (http://www. chcr.brown.edu/pcoc/toolkit.htm).

The initial nursing assessment may vary little from a standard nursing assessment. However, the framework for organization of the assessment utilizes Ferrell's (1995) quality of life framework, which includes four domains: physical, psychological, social, and spiritual well-being (Glass, Cluxton, & Rancour, 2010). It is recommended that because of changing needs of the patient and family across the illness trajectory, a comprehensive assessment should occur at four different intervals: (1) at the time of diagnosis, (2) during treatments, (3) after treatments (long-term survival or terminal phase), and (4) during active dying (Glass et al., 2010, p. 87). Glass and colleagues provide a detailed outline of such an assessment in their chapter in the *Oxford Textbook of Palliative Nursing*, edited by Betty Ferrell and Nessa Coyle (2010).

Other assessment tools are also available. McIlfatrick and Hasson (2013) offer the following domains in their brief holistic assessment and referral screening tool: physical health, social and occupational well-being, mental health and emotional well-being, family and close relationships, spiritual well-being, and awareness and decision making.

Before beginning any assessment interview and physical examination, it is important that the nurse establish a relationship with the patient. These beginning steps of developing a relationship with the patient and family are critical. What follows are suggestions for developing such a relationship:

- Introduce yourself to the patient and family.
- Verify that this is the correct patient.
- Determine how the patient would like to be addressed.
- Explain the purpose of the interaction and approximately how long you intend to spend with the patient.
- Ask the patient's permission to proceed with the assessment. Be mindful of the fact that some patients want their significant others present, whereas others do not.
- Take a seat near the patient, being respectful of closeness as an issue in some cultures.

- Invite the patient to tell about his or her illness, from how the patient learned about it until the present day.
- Take care not to interrupt the patient. Use communication techniques such as probing, reflecting, clarifying, responding empathetically, and asking open-ended questions to encourage detail (Glass et al., 2010, p. 88).

Palliative care patients are often very ill and do not have the energy, patience, or interest in answering a myriad of questions that they have answered many times in the past. Therefore, use individualized assessments based on prioritized symptoms. One issue that frequently arises in an assessment is the discussion and decision making about code status. This is a difficult subject to bring up. It is suggested that one way to introduce the topic to the patient and family is this: "We hope for the best, but try to prepare for the worst. If despite our best efforts, your breathing and/or heart stopped, would you want us to try to revive you?" (Glass et al., 2010, pp. 88–89).

When Randy entered hospice care in March 2012, he was asked to sign a form saying he was a "no code." Even though he was very aware of the purpose of hospice care, he told me he just couldn't sign it yet. We were both hanging onto that little bit of hope that maybe we would get the 3–6 months of time we wanted or that somehow the cancer that had metastasized to his lung would disappear. I didn't fight Randy about not signing it. It was his decision. However, it soon became apparent that he would lose his battle with cancer. Approximately 2 weeks before he died, and in a coherent moment for him, I asked him to sign the form. He didn't say a word, but signed his name on the form.

—Jenny

When performing a psychosocial assessment, the framework includes the following elements:

- Determining the types of losses (physical, psychosocial, and spiritual)
- Observing emotional responses
- Assessing the need for information
- Identifying coping styles
- Assessing the need for control

Additionally, the assessment would include differentiating between normal grief and depression and a general mental health assessment (Glass et al., 2010, p. 90).

The spiritual well-being assessment is an important part of the comprehensive assessment of the patient. Spiritual issues that arise after a diagnosis of a serious or life-threatening illness are abundant and varied. Additionally, as the patient progresses along the illness trajectory, more questions arise. Patients may begin asking questions such as "Why me?", "Why now?", "What does this all mean?", and "Is there life after death?" Maslow's (1987) theory places human needs on a hierarchy from the most basic physical and survival needs to the more transcendent needs. Thus a patient's willingness to discuss such questions may occur only after more fundamental issues of care are addressed.

In a classic article about palliative care, Colleen Scanlon (1989) suggests that the two most important assessment questions that nurses or other professional caregivers can ask are "What is your greatest concern?" and "How can I help you?"

Determining the Goals of Care

Palliative care interventions logically flow from the goals of care. Therefore, the first step in palliative care is to establish these goals (Morrison & Meier, 2003). In the context of chronic, debilitating, and life-threatening illness, realistic and attainable goals of care that relieve pain and other symptoms, improve quality of life, limit the burden of care, enhance personal relationships, and provide a sense of control are crucial to individuals and their families.

Healthcare professionals must work with patients and families to establish appropriate goals of care (Vollrath & von Gunten, 2011). All too frequently, the goals of care become the professional caregivers' goals of care and not the patient's or family's goals. Caregivers need to *listen more* and *talk less* with patients and families. Using open-ended and probing questions may be helpful when interviewing the patient and family.

Goals of care are dynamic across the trajectory of a disease. Several trigger situations invite the patient and healthcare professional to discuss new goals: general advance care planning, a new diagnosis, a change in therapy, the transfer to a new healthcare professional or facility, and—probably most commonly—when interventions to cure or control the disease are no longer effective or desired (Vollrath & von Gunten, 2011, p. 57).

Early Use of Palliative Care Strategies

The American College of Cardiology Foundation/American Heart Association's (ACC/AHA) Guidelines for the Management of Heart Failure recommend palliative care in the context of Stage D heart failure or at the end of life. However, in a qualitative study that interviewed 33 adult outpatients with symptomatic HF and 20 of their family caregivers, the participants wanted palliative care early in their illness, prior to Stage D HF or at end of life. That is, they wanted palliative care *concurrent with their disease-specific care.* Themes from the interviews included the following points: early support adjusting to the limitations and future course of the illness, relief of symptoms, and the involvement of family caregivers using a team approach (Bekelman et al., 2011). In another study, Howlett (2011) concurs that there is a large care gap in the provision of palliative care at all stages of heart failure, from initial presentation to end-stage care.

Communication

Communication is a core skill of palliative care, so it is important that professional caregivers understand how to appropriately communicate with the patient and family. The definition of communication, however, may vary. Many consider that communication is the transmission of information. Wittenberg-Lyles, Goldsmith, Ferrell, and Ragan (2013, p. 1) suggest that communication is, instead, the mutual creation of meaning by both communicators.

There are two central laws of communication (as cited in Wittenberg-Lyles et al., 2013). First, one cannot *not* communicate. Although that point sounds quite simple, it should remind professional caregivers that all of their words, gestures, facial expressions, gaze, touch, and tone of voice communicate loudly. Even silence "says something" to the patient and family. Second, every message has two levels of meaning: the content level and the relationship level. The content could be instructing, diagnosing, encouraging, or supportive. In contrast, the relationship level of meaning is determined by how words are spoken—for example, is the nurse glancing at the chart while asking the patient a question, is the nurse making eye contact with the patient, is the nurse standing at the door of the patient's room instead of the bedside, or does the tone of the nurse's voice denote a rote greeting or a genuine inquiry of the patient. The patient will likely interpret the questions asked by the nurse according to the relationship level of meaning (Wittenberg-Lyles et al., 2013, pp. 3–4).

Communication can be affected by a variety of factors. These factors include, but are not limited to, education level of the patient and family; health literacy; cultural issues; families where English is a second language; stress, coping, and anxiety; use of medical jargon and acronyms; and assumed understanding of the topic.

Listening is one of the most important ways that healthcare professionals can understand and communicate with patients and families. Many clinicians do not "hear" or "listen" to the patient or family, but rather have their own litany of topics to discuss. Generally, caregivers talk too much and listen too little. Some caregivers are afraid of silence and feel as if someone needs to be talking—usually them. However, silence is a powerful tool of communication: It allows both the patient and the caregiver time to reflect, gather their thoughts, or develop questions.

An issue with communication is often that there is a need for clinicians to share bad news and/or a poor prognosis. This discussion is often postponed due to the discomfort of the clinician with the topic; alternatively, in efforts to protect patients, censored comments may be provided by the professional caregiver. Such misguided attempts are made at all levels of the illness trajectory. Economy with the truth often leads to conspiracies of silence that result in fear, anxiety, and confusion (Fallowfield, 2010). Although ambiguous statements provide patients and families with short-term benefits, in the long term the trust and the relationship between the patient and caregiver are eroded. Realistic hopes and aspirations can be generated only from honest disclosure.

Dahlin (2010, p. 122) suggests the following guidelines when delivering bad news:

- Create a physical setting that is quiet and comfortable, and one in which all participants can be seated and free of distractions.
- Determine who should be present.
- Clarify and clearly state your own and the patient's goals throughout the meeting.
- Determine what the patient and family know about the patient's condition and what they have been told.
- Provide an overview of the patient's illness.
- Give a warning—"Unfortunately, I have some bad news to share with you" or "I wish things were different"—and then pause.
- Sit quietly and allow the patient and family to absorb the information. Wait for the patient to respond. After being silent, ask the patient, "I have just told you some serious news. Do you feel comfortable sharing your thoughts with me?"

- Listen carefully and acknowledge the patient's and family's emotions. Give them an opportunity for questions.

Howlett (2011) suggests that all cardiovascular care practitioners have a basic knowledge of palliative care principles, and be able to integrate such principles into the day-to-day care of their patients with advanced cardiovascular disease. Some clinicians are simply unable to bring up the subject of palliative care and/or end-of-life care with patients and families. Howlett suggests that those clinicians consider consultation with others in how to initiate these sensitive discussions. Current evidence suggests that patients, particularly those who are acutely ill or hospitalized, actually desire that such discussions take place (p. 145).

The use of the Internet has supported certain aspects of care of individuals and families with chronic illness, with this venue typically used for sharing information and/or blogs and formal support groups. A systematic review of the literature on the effectiveness of eHealth interventions and information needs in palliative care offers clear suggestions on the power of the Internet for such patients and families (Capurro, Ganzinger, Perez-Lu, & Knaup, 2014). The authors asked two broad questions to guide their research:

- Which eHealth interventions with proven efficacy exist for use in palliative care?
- What is known about the information needs of the participants in the palliative care process?

Seventeen articles were included in the review. All of these studies were conducted in high-income countries, except for one study that was conducted in Africa. Unfortunately, none of the studies involved randomized controlled trials, nor did any of the included studies describe patient-relevant clinical outcomes.

The most commonly used intervention was the implementation of telephone-based support infrastructures. Other interventions aimed to simplify various aspects of documentation. Eight studies described their eHealth interventions as being effective with regard to the following aspects of palliative care: better-quality care, improved communication, reduction of documentation effect, and reduction of costs (Capurro et al., 2014). The most prevalent information need that was identified was information related to pain management, such as recommended drug combinations and dosages. Informal caregivers are important participants of palliative care; however, they were not included in any study reviewed in this meta-analysis.

Attributes of Professional Caregivers Providing Palliative Care

Most professional caregivers are aware of their preferences for acute care nursing in the moment (ER and ICU) versus longer-term care of patients. Pavlish and Ceronsky (2009) surveyed oncology nurses to see what they believed were important attributes to provide palliative care. The oncology nurses emphasized the importance of *perceptive attentiveness,* meaning that nurses were tuned in to the patient and saw the patient behind the equipment. Another attribute was being *deliberate,* in that nurses heard what the patient and family had to say and allowed the patients and families to consider their options before proceeding. Simon, Ramsenthaler, Bausewein, Krischkie, and Geiss (2009) identified *authenticity*—which they described as being present, being open, and having unconditional regard for the patient and family—as another important attribute of professional caregivers in regard to palliative care.

Advance Directives

Discussions among families, patients, and healthcare professionals related to prognosis, preferences, and the establishment of the goals of care are recommended prior to making treatment decisions (Hanson & Winzelberg, 2013). Goals of care reflect the values, beliefs, and culture of the person with a serious, life-threatening illness. Following such discussions, the next logical step is the completion of advance directives.

Shared decision making is critical when serious illness is confronted and the treatment outcomes are uncertain (Hanson & Winzelberg, 2013). Serious illness without a cure results in a priority shift that focuses on the goals of function and comfort in the context of family support. The literature suggests that the focus of advance care planning should shift to determine an acceptable quality of life and goals of care (Fried, Bradley, Towle, & Allore, 2002; Meier & Morrison, 2002). This type of discussion is the crucial element, not the mere completion of the forms.

Consumers and healthcare professionals can use a variety of resources when pondering these issues, such as the *Caring Conversations Program* developed through the Center for Practical Bioethics (2011). Workbooks can be purchased that help families discuss their values and wishes regarding medical treatment if they cannot speak for themselves.

It is also important to be aware of each state's required documents and process for the completion of advance directives. The process and forms vary from state to state. The names of the documents may also vary. The basic two forms are (1) power of attorney for health care (this document appoints an agent or proxy who becomes the decision maker when the client can no longer do so) and (2) directive to physician (living will; this document gives direction to a physician regarding which type of care/procedures are wanted or not wanted—for example, artificial nutrition, hydration, or mechanical ventilation—if the individual cannot speak for himself or herself).

Psychosocial, Spiritual, and Bereavement Needs

Psychosocial, spiritual, and bereavement care are key components of palliative care. Professional and accrediting bodies such as The Joint

Commission require documentation of spiritual assessments of patients. Members of interprofessional palliative care teams assess and intervene to meet the spiritual and psychosocial needs of patients and their families. Bereavement support is part of the follow-up after an individual dies. Research demonstrates that family members with spiritual and psychological distress are more likely to experience an extended or complicated grief and bereavement process (McClain, Rosenfield, & Breitbart, 2003).

The act of acknowledging spiritual distress can be an intervention. However, a common language and mutual comfort must be present for a meaningful exchange to occur (Chochinov, 2004). Helping patients die with dignity is a basic tenet of palliative care. Empirical work with dying patients found that the paradigm of dignity, which includes matters of spirituality, meaning, purpose, and other psychosocial issues related to dying, includes acceptable language and topics for discussion (Chochinov, Hack, Hassard, Kristjanson, McClement, & Harlos, 2004). This work is adding to the growing body of empirical evidence that palliative care is more than symptom management and must include spiritual, psychosocial, and existential concerns. Such care must be person centered and maintain a person's dignity through his or her last breath of life.

Chochinov and associates developed a dignity-conserving model and interventions based on the analysis of 50 qualitative interviews of patients with advanced cancer. The interviews were conducted in an attempt to understand the patients' perceptions of dignity. The dignity-conserving model of care encompasses three areas of influence on a person's perception of dignity: (1) influences stemming directly from the illness, (2) influences from the person's psychological and spiritual resources or self (dignity-conserving repertoire), and (3) environmental influences (social dignity inventory) (Chochinov, 2011, p. 354). This model serves as the basis for the psychotherapeutic intervention known as

dignity therapy. In dignity therapy, dying patients are interviewed about aspects of their life that they would like recorded and remembered. The interviews are transcribed and edited to read "like well-honed narratives." The narratives are returned to the patient and ultimately given to the patient's loved ones. Chochinov reported that 76% of the 100 patients in a clinical trial of the dignity therapy intervention reported a sense of heightened dignity, and 91% were satisfied with the intervention (Chochinov, Hack, Hassard, Kristjanson, McClement, & Harlos, 2005). Ninety-five percent of the family members of the dignity therapy participants reported that they would recommend dignity therapy for other patients and families faced with a terminal illness; 77% would continue to use the recorded narratives as a source of remembrance and comfort (McClement, Chochinov, Hack, Hassard, Kristjanson, & HarlosarlosH, 2007). These researchers acknowledge that dignity-conserving care must be validated in diverse populations. However, they urge that the concept of "conserving dignity in end-of-life care should become part of the palliative care lexicon and the overarching standard of care for all patients nearing death" (Chochinov, 2011, p. 359).

Education for Healthcare Professionals

The American Association of Colleges of Nursing (AACN) and City of Hope National Medical Center received major funding from the Robert Wood Johnson Foundation for the development and dissemination of the End-of-Life Nursing Education Consortium in February 2000 (ELNEC, 2014). Versions for baccalaureate, graduate, continuing education/in-service, pediatric, oncology, and geriatric nurses and nurse educators have been developed, with train-the-trainer methodology being utilized. A quarterly newsletter, *ELNEC Connections*, is sent to all ELNEC trainers. It provides updates, ongoing resources, and project ideas from the ELNEC staff as well as a list of the trainers throughout the United States. Collegial sharing is in the spirit of improving and disseminating the science and art of palliative care nursing. Nurses and healthcare professionals from all 50 states as well as individuals from 78 international countries have participated in ELNEC.

Physicians have a parallel program to ELNEC, called Education on Palliative and End-of-Life Care (EPEC). The mission of EPEC (2014) is to educate *all* healthcare professionals on the essential clinical competencies in palliative care. Conferences using the train-the-trainer methodology are also held. In addition, the entire curriculum is available online (http://www.epec.net).

Another useful resource for healthcare professionals is the End of Life/Palliative Education Resource Center (EPERC, n.d.). Its purpose is advancing end-of-life care through an online community of educational scholars. Case studies, presentations, and articles are a few of the resources available. The website offers access to a palliative care blog, *Pallimed*. The site has a main page for discussion and posts, an arts page (i.e., book reviews related to hospice and palliative medicine topics), and a page of case studies for discussion (EPERC, n.d.).

Research in Palliative Care

A variety of tools may be used for measurement of palliative care outcomes; however, each has its own conceptual framework, whether it be clinical outcomes, quality of life, well-being, and so forth. These tools include the Edmonton Symptom Assessment Scale (ESAS), the Center for Epidemiological Studies—Depression Scale (CES-D), and the Karnofsky Performance Scale (KPS). Another tool with well-supported reliability and validity is the Functional Assessment of Chronic Illness Therapy—Palliative Care (FACIT-Pal) Scale. This multidimensional measure of self-reported health-related quality of life (FACT-G) can be used with disease and symptom-specific subscales (Lyons, Bakitas, Hegel, Hanscom, Hull, & Ahles, 2009). FACT-G has

27 items; FACIT-Pal adds 19 items and is the palliative care subscale.

A major focus of palliative care is nursing research (Payne & Turner, 2008). Unfortunately, the palliative care research agenda has lagged behind the research agenda for clinical practice. Development of a solid nursing research agenda in palliative care is needed and will be essential in moving the science forward. However, research in palliative care requires diversity in research methods (Ferrell, 2010). Researchers must carefully weigh subject burden. "Time" for the palliative care and/or end-of-life patient is precious; thus time for research must be dedicated to meaningful research. Qualitative methods are especially needed in describing the *lived experience* of patients.

Leaders in the specialties of geriatric and palliative medicine are making the case for integrated geriatric and palliative medicine to meet the care needs of older adults while improving the quality and cost-effectiveness of that care. Although the need for such integration is recognized, the evidence-based knowledge to support palliative care in older adults is sparse and must be expanded (Kelley, 2013).

On January 31, 2013, a groundbreaking meeting of researchers in aging and palliative care was sponsored by the National Palliative Care Research Center, the National Institute on Aging (NIA), and the Icahn School of Medicine at Mount Sinai Claude D. Pepper Older Adult Independence Center. This meeting had a threefold purpose: (1) examine the state of the science in geriatric palliative care; (2) identify research priorities that could, if identified, lead to improved palliative care in older adults; and (3) identify studies needed to fill the gaps. The proceedings were published as a series of NIA White Papers by the *Journal of Palliative Medicine* from July 2013 through December 2013. The topics covered included epidemiology of serious illness; research methods; multimorbidity; nonpain symptoms; informal caregiving; establishing goals, values, and preferences; long-term care; disparities; and policy initiatives.

In parallel to the publication of the NIA White Papers, the NIA released a program announcement describing funding opportunities at the R01, R03, and R21 levels. These funding opportunities specifically target geriatric palliative care with the intention of moving the care earlier in the illness trajectory. Hospice and end-of-life research are not part of this call because the National Institute of Nursing Research already addresses that area of science.

As yet, few studies have been published that have tested the effectiveness of interventions with patients diagnosed with advanced cancer. Bakitas and colleagues (2009) conducted a randomized controlled trial (RCT) to determine the effectiveness of a nursing-led intervention on quality of life, symptom intensity, mood, and resource use in patients with advanced cancer. The RCT involved 322 patients from November 2003 through May 2008. Advanced practice nurses led Project ENABLE (Educate, Nurture, Advise, Before Life Ends), a multicomponent, psycho-educational intervention for four weekly sessions and a monthly follow-up session until death or completion of the study (*n* = 161); the group that received this intervention was compared with a group that received the usual care (*n* = 161). The intervention group had higher scores for quality of life and mood, as well as improvements in symptom intensity scores or reduced days in the hospital, ICU, or ER visits, as measured by the Functional Assessment of Chronic Illness Therapy for Palliative Care instrument.

In a follow-up to the Bakitas et al. (2009) article, researchers examined the patient perspectives of participation in the ENABLE study. Benefits, from the patients' perspectives, included enhanced problem-solving skills, better coping, feeling empowered, and feeling supported or reassured. Three other themes related to participation in the clinical trial were also identified: helping future patients and contributing to science, gaining insight through completion of questionnaires, and trial/intervention aspects to improve (Maloney, Lyons, Zhongze, Hegel, Ahles, & Bakitas, 2013).

Temel and colleagues' (2010) randomized controlled trial of early palliative care for patients with metastatic non-small-cell lung cancer demonstrated significant improvements in both quality of life and mood. Those patients who received early palliative care were provided with less aggressive care but experienced longer survival. This RCT was a landmark study in palliative care that demonstrated outcomes of early initiation of palliative care. The Bakitas and Temel studies demonstrate the feasibility and outcomes of rigorous palliative care research.

Zimmerman and colleagues (2008) conducted a systematic review of the effectiveness of specialized palliative care. What was clear in the studies reviewed was that "evidence" for benefits of specialized palliative care was sparse and mostly limited by methodological shortcomings. The authors advocated for carefully planned trials, using a standardized palliative care intervention and measures constructed specifically for this population (p. 1698).

Palliative Care and Genomics

The sequencing of the human genome was completed in April 2003 by the Human Genome Project. Advances in technology now allow the exploration of genetic material ranging from genetic screening to genomic-based therapies (Conley & Tinkle, 2007). The genetic risk for many diseases, such as Huntington's disease, can now be determined, but as yet there is no cure available for these diseases (Heitkemper & Bond, 2003). How does this technological advance apply to hospice and palliative care? This discussion focuses on three connections between palliative care and genomics: pharmacogenomics, family history, and nurse competencies in genetics and genomics. **Table 22-1** defines the key terms used in this section.

Table 22-1 KEY TERMS RELATED TO GENETICS AND GENOMICS

Allele: An alternative form of a gene.

Genetics: The study of individual genes and their impact on relatively rare single-gene disorders (Guttmacher & Collins, 2002).

Genomics: The study of the functions and interactions of all the genes in the genome, including their interactions with environmental factors (Guttmacher & Collins, 2002).

Genotype: A person's genetic makeup as reflected by his or her DNA sequence.

Pharmacogenetics: The study of genetic factors that influence an organism's reaction to a drug (Howe & Eggert, 2007).

Pharmacogenomics: The study of how an individual's genetic inheritance affects the body's response to drugs (Howe & Eggert, 2007).

Phenotype: The clinical presentation or expression of a specific gene or genes, environmental factors, or both (Guttmacher & Collins, 2002).

Pharmacogenetics (the study of the role of inheritance in individual variations in drug response) has converged with knowledge from the sequencing of the human genome, resulting in pharmacogenomics (the study of the effect of DNA sequencing on the effect of a drug; science combining pharmacology and genomics) (Weinshilboum, 2003). Medications are a major intervention for symptom management in palliative care. It is important that physicians and nurses, including those in palliative care, understand the impact of genotypic variation on the therapeutic effect and adverse effects of medications. Two examples are presented here to illustrate the impact of pharmacogenomics in providing safe and effective care regardless of the trajectory of illness.

First, the cytochrome P450 system offers an example of how these factors are intertwined. A specific cytochrome enzyme, CYP2D6, converts codeine to morphine. Genotypic variants of the CYP2D6 enzyme in 5% to 10% of the population results in too little or no CYP2D6 enzyme produced. Therefore, individuals with such variants cannot change codeine into morphine and thus obtain little or no analgesic relief from codeine or codeine-derivative medications (e.g., hydrocodone, oxycodone, ethylmorphine, and dihydrocodeine) (Howe & Eggert, 2007; Meyer, 2000; Prows, 2004).

Second, scientists have discovered genetic variations in the gene that plays a major role in an individual's initial sensitivity to warfarin treatment (Schwarz et al., 2008). Members of the National Institutes of Health (NIH) Pharmacogenetics Research Network found that these variations explain why some patients require a higher or lower dose to realize the therapeutic benefit of this drug. The U.S. Food and Drug Administration (FDA) now recommends genetic testing to assist in the quick and precise determination of optimal warfarin doses.

In palliative care, the patient and the family are the unit of care. But what is the impact of a family's health history? Is the patient who is receiving palliative care worried about an illness that may be transmitted to other family members? Are family members concerned that they may be carriers of an incurable disease? The U.S. Surgeon General spearheaded the Family History Initiative. Family history is the best, most inexpensive, noninvasive genetic test available (http://familyhistory.hhs.gov). Many diseases "run in families." Detailed family histories allow individuals at risk to be identified and to implement disease-prevention strategies. Caregivers must realize that patterns of inheritance may be sources of guilt in persons with advanced disease or concerns of bereaved individuals. Nevertheless, the current palliative literature has yet to discuss these types of concerns.

What is the role of palliative care for individuals diagnosed with genetic diseases? How can palliative care providers help those diagnosed with the genotype for a terminal disease that is not yet expressed? Huntington's disease is such an example: Individuals may know that they will develop this disease years before symptoms become evident. These individuals would benefit from the support of palliative care.

The HPNA, along with 48 other professional nursing organizations, has endorsed the Genetic and Genomic Nursing Competencies (http://www.genome.gov/pages/careers/healthprofessionaleducation/geneticscompetency.pdf). Regardless of their specialty and setting, all nurses need to understand that all diseases have genetic and genomic components. Patients and their families may turn to the nurse seeking genetic and genomic information related to prevention, screening, diagnostics, prognostics, and selection of and effectiveness of treatment. Within the context of hospice and palliative care, requests for this information may occur during bereavement, thereby adding another layer of complexity to the grief process. The following are two examples of the competencies relevant to the preceding discussion (Consensus Panel, 2006):

- *Domain: Professional Responsibility.* Incorporate genetic and genomic technologies and information into RN practice.
- *Domain: Professional Practice.* Demonstrate an understanding of genetics/genomics to health, prevention, selection of treatment, monitoring of treatment effectiveness.

It might seem strange to some readers to find a section of this chapter dealing with genomics and palliative care, but palliative care is not practiced in a vacuum. Nurses must be aware of the advances in science that impact the health of patients and their families prior to interacting with them. The advances in the science of comfort and the art of caring must converge to improve the quality of life for those with life-limiting or terminal illness.

Outcomes

Outcomes research in palliative care continues to develop. There is consensus about the broad domains related to the end of life: physical or psychosocial symptoms, social relationships, spiritual or philosophical beliefs, hopes, expectation and meaning, satisfaction, economic considerations, and caregiver and family experiences. Quality of life is also considered an outcome, but quality of life needs a clearer definition and consistent measurement to strengthen the relationship.

The CAPC (2014) has identified four major outcomes of palliative care: (1) relief of pain and other distressing symptoms; (2) clear communication and decision making regarding goals of care and development of treatment plans; (3) completion of life-prolonging or curative treatments; and (4) increased patient and family satisfaction. The next steps in palliative care are to develop the science, the care delivery systems, and the instruments to deliver and evaluate the outcomes of quality palliative care.

The Center to Advance Palliative Care convened a consensus panel to develop recommendations for specific clinical and customer metrics that palliative care programs should track. The panel agreed on four key domains of clinical metrics and two domains of customer metrics. Clinical metrics include daily assessment of physician-identified, psychological, and spiritual symptoms by a symptom assessment tool; establishment of patient-centered goals of care; support to patient and family caregivers; and management of transitions across care sites. Customer metrics include patient/family satisfaction and referring clinical satisfaction (Weissman, Morrison, & Meier, 2010).

As the science and practice of palliative care continue to mature, the following description will become reality: "Coordinated palliative care matched to patient needs improves quality of care for vulnerable patients with serious illness and reduces costly use of hospitals and emergency rooms" (Unroe & Meier, 2013, p. 1503).

Evidence-Based Practice Box

Metastatic non-small-cell lung cancer is a debilitating disease with a high symptom burden, poor quality of life, and a prognosis of death within a year of diagnosis. The purpose of this study was to examine the effect of early palliative care given simultaneously with standard oncologic care on patient-reported outcomes among patients with metastatic non-small-cell lung cancer in an ambulatory care setting. A randomly assigned sample of 151 patients (a power of 80% and an effect size of 0.5 SD) required 120 patients. To account for the loss of any participants, an additional 30 patients were enrolled in the study. Patient-reported measures included health-related quality of life as measured by the Functional Assessment of Cancer Therapy—Lung (FACT-L) scale. This scale assesses multiple dimensions of quality of life, including physical, functional, emotional, and social well-being. Mood was measured with the Hospital Anxiety and Depression Scale (HADS) and the Patient Health Questionnaire 9 (PHQ-9). Data on the patients' use of health services and end-of-life care were collected from the electronic medical record.

The patients receiving early palliative care met with a member of the palliative care team within 3 weeks of enrollment in the study and at least monthly in the outpatient setting until death. Guidelines for the palliative care visits were adopted from the NCPQPC and were part of the study protocol. The patients who received standard care did not meet with members of the palliative care team unless specifically requested by the patient, family, or oncologist. All participants in the study continued to receive routine oncologic care.

These two groups were well matched, and there were no significant differences in their demographic characteristics. Participants receiving early palliative care had an average of four visits within the first 12 weeks of the study. When they compared the quality of life scores at 12 weeks, the researchers found that the patients assigned to early palliative care had significantly higher scores than the standard-care group. Depression scores in the palliative-care group were also significantly lower at 12 weeks. Patients assigned to the standard-care-only group received more aggressive end-of-life care and had less documentation regarding their resuscitation preferences in their electronic medical records.

This study clearly demonstrated the effect of palliative care when provided from the time of diagnosis through death for advanced lung cancer—namely, prolonged survival by 2 months and improved quality of life and mood. The authors of the study hypothesized that improvements in quality of life and mood might account for the increased survival, a benefit of early palliative care.

Source: Temel, J. S., Greer, J. A., Muzikansky, A., Gallaher, E. R., Admane, S., Jackson, V. A., et al. (2010). Early palliative care for patients with metastatic non-small cell lung cancer. *New England Journal of Medicine, 363*, 733–742.

CASE STUDY 22-1

Mrs. Chase is an 88-year-old widow with a history of hypertension, coronary heart disease, osteoporosis, and a recent hospitalization for pneumonia. Her surgical history includes a partial colectomy secondary to a cancerous polyp. Her follow-up colonoscopies have been negative for the past 10 years.

Mrs. Chase's chief complaint over the past 2 years has been fatigue—so debilitating that it limits her functioning. She describes it as "exhaustion and sleepiness." Although she lives alone, her apartment is connected to her son's apartment in the same house. She has an advance directive and requested a do not resuscitate order during her recent hospitalization for pneumonia. Her son is her designated healthcare power of attorney.

Mrs. Chase's goals of care focus on comfort. During the hospitalization, the hospitalist reported that her chest X-rays appear to show signs of pulmonary disease. Mrs. Chase has a long history of smoking, albeit not in the past 20 years. Upon discharge, an appointment was made for pulmonary function tests. Several weeks after the pneumonia, the tests revealed that Mrs. Chase has severe restrictive lung disease, with a forced vital capacity of 34%. Since her episode of pneumonia, Mrs. Chase has been more dependent on oxygen for her daily activities. She does not like the oxygen, and it makes her anxious and self-conscious. Her pulmonologist warned that every time she gets a cold or other respiratory illness, she is at risk for a major respiratory event and hospitalization. Mrs. Chase has repeatedly stated that she does not want to be placed on a breathing machine, but still wants to be taken to the hospital.

Discussion Questions

1. What is the next step in planning care for Mrs. Chase?
2. How might Mrs. Chase benefit from an out-of-hospital DNR?
3. Identify some examples of when Mrs. Chase might be transitioning from palliative care to hospice care.
4. Why is it important that Mrs. Chase's son, her designated healthcare power of attorney, be involved in the discussion regarding her future healthcare goals of care?
5. How would you respond to Mrs. Chase when she says, "I want to go to the hospital if I have trouble breathing, but do not put me on any machine!"

STUDY QUESTIONS

1. Describe how the goals of care might differ for an 85-year-old man diagnosed with heart failure at the time of diagnosis and in an advanced stage of the illness.
2. Explain the following statement: Hospice care is palliative care, but not all palliative care is hospice care.
3. List the domains of end-of-life care as identified by the NCPQPC.
4. Identify barriers to palliative care for an individual with a serious, life-limiting illness.
5. Identify the components of Ferrell's framework/model for quality of life.
6. What is your vision of palliative care?
7. List three online resources for use in continuing your education in palliative care.
8. Go online and find support information appropriate for the family caregiver of a palliative care patient.
9. Identify two nurse competencies in genetics and genomics.
10. Discuss how pharmacogenomics can help relieve the pain for future patients receiving hospice care.
11. How would palliative care assist a man diagnosed with Huntington's disease?
12. Discuss your vision for integrating genomics into palliative care.

Internet Resources

American Association of Colleges of Nursing, End-of-Life Care: http://www.aacn.nche.edu/elnec

American Pain Society: http://www.ampainsoc.org

Edmonton Regional Palliative Care Program: http://www.palliative.org

Education in Palliative and End-of-Life Care: http://www.epec.net

Hospice and Palliative Nurses Association: http://www.hpna.org

HPNA Research Agenda: http://www.hpna.org/PicView.aspx?ID=828

National Consensus Project: http://www.nationalconsensusproject.org

National Consensus Project for Quality Palliative Care: http://www.nationalconsensusproject.org

National Guideline Clearinghouse: http://www.guideline.gov

National Hospice and Palliative Care Organization: http://www.nhpco.org

National Palliative Care Research Center: http://www.npcrc.org

Oncology Nursing Society: https://www.ons.org

Pain Resource Center: http://prc.coh.org

Palliative Care: http://www.getpalliativecare.org

Palliative Care Framework: http://www.nhpco.org/i4a/pages/index.cfm?pageID=5122

Toolkit of Instruments to Measure End of Life Care (TIME): http://www.chcr.brown.edu/pcoc/-toolkit.htm

---

References

Alliance for Excellence in Hospice and Palliative Nursing. (2011). Mission statement. http://www.hpna.org/DisplayPage.aspx?Title=Mission%20of%20HPNA

Bakitas, M., Lyons, K. D., Hegel, M. T., Brokaw, F. C., Seville, J., Hull, J. G., ... Ahles, T. A. (2009). Effects of a palliative care intervention on clinical outcomes in patients with advanced cancer. *Journal of the American Medical Association, 302*(7), 741–749.

Bekelman, D. B., Nowels, C. T., Retrum, J. H., Allen, L. A., Shakar, S., Hutt, E., ... Kutner, J. S. (2011). Giving voice to patients' and family caregivers' needs in chronic heart failure: Implications for palliative care programs. *Journal of Palliative Medicine, 14*(12), 1317–1324.

Capurro, D., Ganzinger, M., Perez-Lu, J., & Knaup, P. (2014). Effectiveness of eHealth interventions and information needs in palliative care: A systematic literature review. *Journal of Medical Internet Research, 16*(3), 372. doi: 10.2196/jmir.2812

Center for Practical Bioethics. (2011). Caring conversations. http://practicalbioethics.org/about /model-and-methodology/making-your-wishes-known-for-end-of-life-care/

Center to Advance Palliative Care (CAPC). (2014). Palliative care facts and stats. http://www.capc.org /news-and-events/press-kit/press-kit-palliative-care-facts.pdf

Centers for Disease Control and Prevention (CDC), National Center for Health Statistics. (2013). Deaths: Final data for 2010. *National Vital Statistics Report, 61*(4).

Chochinov, H. M. (2004). Interventions to enhance the spiritual aspects of dying. In *National Institutes of Health state-of-the science conference on improving end-of-life care program & abstracts.* Bethesda, MD: U.S. Department of Health and Human Services, National Institutes of Health.

Chochinov, H. M. (2011). Dignity-conserving care: A new model for palliative care: Helping the patient feel valued. In S. J. McPhee, M. A. Winker, M. W. Rabow, S. Z. Pantilat, & A. J. Markowitz (Eds.), *Care at the close of life: Evidence and experience* (pp. 353–362). New York, NY: McGraw-Hill.

Chochinov, H. M., Hack, T., Hassard, T., Kristjanson, L. J., McClement, S., & Harlos, M. (2004). Dignity and psychotherapeutic considerations in end-of-life care. *Journal of Palliative Care, 20*(3), 134–142.

Chochinov, H. M., Hack, T., Hassard, T., Kristjanson, L. J., McClement, S., & Harlos, M. (2005). Dignity therapy: A novel psychotherapeutic intervention for patients near the end of life. *Journal of Clinical Oncology, 23*(24), 5520–5525.

Clark, D. (2010). International progress in creating palliative medicine as a specialized discipline. In G. Hanks, N. I. Cherny, N. A. Christakis, M. Fallon, S. Kaasa, & R. K. Portenoy (Eds.), *Oxford textbook of palliative medicine* (4th ed., pp. 9–16). Oxford, UK: Oxford University Press.

Conley, Y. P., & Tinkle, M. B. (2007). The future of genomic nursing research. *Journal of Nursing Scholarship, 39*(2), 17–24.

Consensus Panel. (2006). *Essential nursing competencies and curricula guidelines for genetics and genomics.* Washington, DC: American Nurses Association.

Coyle, N. (2010). Introduction to palliative nursing care. In B. R. Ferrell & N. Coyle (Eds.), *Oxford textbook of palliative nursing* (3rd ed., pp. 3–11). Oxford, UK: Oxford University Press.

Dahlin, C. (2010). Communication in palliative care. In B. R. Ferrell & N. Coyle (Eds.), *Oxford textbook of palliative nursing* (3rd ed., pp. 107–133). Oxford, UK: Oxford University Press.

Dahlin, C. (Ed.). (2013). National Consensus Project for Quality Palliative Care. Clinical practice guidelines for quality palliative care (3rd ed.). http://www.national-consensusproject.org/

End of Life Nursing Education Consortium (ELNEC). (2009). *Module 1: Nursing at the end of life.* American Association of Colleges of Nursing and City of Hope National Medical Center. Washington, DC: Author.

End of Life Nursing Education Consortium (ELNEC). (2014). ELNEC fact sheet. http://www.aacn.nche.edu /elnec/factsheet.htm

End of Life/Palliative Education and Resource Center (EPERC) (n.d.). Home page. http://www.eperc.mcw .edu/EPERC.htm

EPEC Project. (2014). Education on palliative and end-of-life care. http://www.epec.net

Fallowfield, L. (2010). Communication with the patient and family in palliative medicine. In G. Hanks, N. I. Cherny, N. A. Christakis, M. Fallon, S. Kaasa, & R. K. Portenoy (Eds.), *Oxford textbook of palliative medicine* (4th ed., pp. 333–341). Oxford UK: Oxford University Press.

Ferrell, B. R. (1995). The impact of pain on quality of life: A decade of research. *Nursing Clinics of North America, 30,* 609–624.

Ferrell, B. R. (2010). Palliative care research: Nursing response to emergent society needs. *Nursing Science Quarterly, 23*(3), 221–225.

Ferrell, B. R., & Coyle, N. (Eds.). (2010). *Oxford textbook of palliative nursing* (3rd ed.). New York, NY: Oxford University Press.

Field, M. J., & Cassel, C. K. (Eds.). (1997). *Approaching death: Improving care at the end of life.* Committee on Care at the End of Life, Division of Health Care Services, Institute of Medicine. Washington, DC: National Academies Press.

Fisher, E. S., Wennberg, D. E., Stukel, T. A., Gottlieb, D. J., Lucas, F. L., & Pinder, E. L. (2003). The implications of regional variations in Medicare spending: Health outcomes and satisfaction with care. *Annals of Internal Medicine, 138,* 288–298.

Fitzsimons, D., Mullan, D., Wilson, J. S., Bonway, B., Corcoran, B., Dempster, M., ... Fogarty, D. (2007). The challenges of patients' unmet palliative care needs in the final stages of chronic illness. *Palliative Medicine, 23*, 313–322.

Fried, T. R., Bradley, E. H., Towle, V. R., & Allore, H. (2002). Understanding the treatment preferences of seriously ill patients. *New England Journal of Medicine, 346*, 1061–1066.

Glass, E., Cluxton, D., & Rancour, P. (2010). Principles of patient and family assessment. In B. R. Ferrell & N. Coyle (Eds.), *Textbook of palliative nursing* (3rd ed., pp. 87–105). New York, NY: Oxford University Press.

Guttmacher, A., & Collins, F. (2002). Genomic medicine: A primer. *New England Journal of Medicine, 347*, 1512–1520.

Hanks, G., Cherny, N. I., Portenoy, R. K., Kaasa, S., Fallon, M., & Christakis, N. (2010). Introduction to the fourth edition: Facing the challenges of continuity and change. In G. Hanks, N. I. Cherny, N. A. Christakis, M. Fallon, S. Kaasa, & R. K. Portenoy (Eds.), *Oxford textbook of palliative medicine* (4th ed., pp. 1–5). Oxford, UK: Oxford University Press.

Hansford, P. (2010). Palliative care in the United Kingdom. In B. R. Ferrell & N. Coyle (Eds.), *Oxford textbook of palliative nursing* (3rd ed., pp. 1265–1274). Oxford, UK: Oxford University Press.

Hanson, L. C., & Winzelberg, G. (2013). Research priorities for geriatric palliative care: Goals, values and preferences. *Journal of Palliative Medicine, 16*(10), 1174–1179. doi: 1089/jpm.2013.9475

Heitkemper, M. M., & Bond, E. F. (2003). State of nursing science: On the edge. *Biological Research for Nursing, 4*(3), 151–162; discussion 163–164, 170.

Howe, L. A., & Eggert, J. (2007). Influence of pharmacogenomics on disease and symptom management. *International Journal of Nursing Intel Dev Dis, 3*(2), 2. http://journal.ddna.org

Howlett, J. G. (2011). Palliative care in heart failure: Addressing the largest care gap. *Current Opinion in Cardiology, 26*, 144–148.

Kelley, A. (2013). Epidemiology of care for patients with serious illness. *Journal of Palliative Medicine, 16*(7), 730–733. doi: 10.1089/jpm.2013.9498

Lyons, K. D., Bakitas, M., Hegel, M. T., Hanscom, B., Hull, J., & Ahles, T. A. (2009). Reliability and validity of the Functional Assessment of Chronic Illness Therapy—Palliative Care (FACIT-Pal) Scale. *Journal of Pain and Symptom Management, 37*(1), 23–32. doi: 10.1016/j.jpainsymman.2007.12.015

Maloney, C., Lyons, K. D., Zhongze, L., Hegel, M., Ahles, T. A., & Bakitas, M. (2013). Patient perspectives on participation in the ENABLE II randomized controlled trial of a concurrent oncology palliative care intervention: Benefits and burdens. *Palliative Medicine, 27*(4), 365–383.

Maslow, A. H. (1987). *Motivation and personality* (3rd ed.). Hummelston, PA: Scott-Foreman Wesley.

McClain, C. S., Rosenfield, B., & Breitbart, W. (2003). Effect of spiritual well-being on end-of-life despair in terminally ill cancer patients. *Lancet, 361*, 1603–1607.

McClement, S., Chochinov, H. M., Hack, T., Hassard, T., Kristjanson, L. J., & Harlos, M. (2007). Dignity therapy: Family member perspectives. *Journal of Palliative Medicine, 10*(5), 1076–1082.

McIlfatrick, S., & Hasson, F. (2013). Evaluating a holistic assessment tool for palliative care practice. *Journal of Clinical Nursing, 23*, 1064–1075. doi: 10.111/jocn.12320

Meier, D. E. (2010). The development, status, and future of palliative care. In D. E. Meier, S. L. Isaacs, & R. G. Hughes (Eds.), *Palliative care: Transforming the care of serious illness* (pp. 4–76). San Francisco, CA: Jossey-Bass.

Meier, D. E., & Morrison, R. S. (2002). Autonomy reconsidered. *New England Journal of Medicine, 346*, 1087–1089.

Meyer, U. A. (2000). Pharmacogenetics and adverse drug reaction. *Lancet, 356*(b), 1667–1671.

Morrison, R. S. (2013). Research priorities in geriatric palliative care: An introduction to a new series. *Journal of Palliative Medicine, 16*(7), 726–729. doi: 10.1089/jpm.2013.9499

Morrison, R. S., & Meier, D. E. (Eds.). (2003). *Geriatric palliative care.* New York, NY: Oxford University Press.

National Board for Certification of Hospice and Palliative Nurses (NBCHPN). (2014). Home page. https://www.nbchpn.org/

National Consensus Project for Quality Palliative Care (NCPQPC). (2009). Clinical practice guidelines for quality palliative care (2nd ed.). http://www.nationalconsensusproject.org/guideline.pdf

National Hospice and Palliative Care Organization (NHPCO). (2013). NHPCO facts & figures: Hospice care in America. http://www.nhpco.org/sites/default/files/public/Statistics_Research/2013_Facts_Figures.pdf

National Institute of Nursing Research (NINR). (2011). The science of compassion: Future directions in end-of-life and palliative care: Executive summary. https://www.ninr.nih.gov/sites/www.ninr.nih.gov/files/science-of-compassion-executive-summary.pdf

Nelson, J. E., Curtis, J. R., Mulkerin, C., Campbell, M., Lustbader, D. R., Mosenthal, A. C., ... Weissman, D. E. (2013). Choosing and using screening criteria for palliative care consultation in the ICU: A report from the Improving Palliative Care in the ICU (IPAL-ICU) Advisory Board. *Critical Care Medicine, 41*(10), 2318–2327.

Ohlen, J., Gustafsson, C. W., & Friberg, F. (2013). Making sense of receiving palliative treatment. *Cancer Nursing, 36*(4), 265–273. doi: 10.1097 /NCC.0b013e31826e96d9

Paterson, J. G., & Zderad, L. (1976). *Humanistic nursing.* New York, NY: John Wiley & Sons.

Pavlish, C., & Ceronsky, L. (2009). Oncology nurses' perceptions of nursing roles and professional attributes in palliative care. *Clinical Journal of Oncology Nursing, 13*(4), 404–412.

Payne, S. A., & Turner, J. M. (2008). Research methodologies in palliative care: A bibliometric analysis. *Palliative Medicine, 22,* 336–342.

Prows, C. A. (2004). Medication selection by genotype. *American Journal of Nursing, 104*(5), 60–70.

Ritchie, C. S., & Zulman, S. M. (2013). Research priorities in geriatric palliative care: Multimorbidity. *Journal of Palliative Medicine, 16*(8), 843–847. doi: 10.1090 /jpm.2013.9491

Scanlon, C. (1989). Creating a vision for hope: The challenge of palliative care. *Oncology Nursing Forum, 16,* 491–496.

Schwarz, U. I., Ritchie, M. D., Bradford, Y., Li, C., Dudek, S. M., Fry-Anderson, A., ... Stein, C.M.. (2008). Genetic determinants of response to warfarin during initial anticoagulation. *New England Journal of Medicine, 358,* 999–1008.

Simon, S., Ramsenthaler, C., Bausewein, C., Krischkie, N., & Geiss, G. (2009). Core attitudes of professionals in palliative care: A qualitative study. *International Journal of Palliative Care, 15*(8), 405–411.

Sullivan, A. M., Lakoma, M. D., & Block, S. D. (2003). The status of medical education in end-of-life care: A national report. *Journal of General Internal Medicine, 18,* 685–695.

SUPPORT Principal Investigators. (1995). A controlled trial to improve care for seriously ill, hospitalized patients: The study to understand prognoses and preferences for outcomes and risks of treatments (SUPPORT). *Journal of the American Medical Association, 274,* 1591–1598.

Temel, J. S., Greer, J. A., Muzikansky, A., Gallaher, E. R., Admane, S., Jackson, V. A., ... Lynch, T.J.. (2010). Early palliative care for patients with metastatic non-small cell lung cancer. *New England Journal of Medicine, 363,* 733–742. doi: 10.1056/ NEJMoa1000678

Unroe, K. T., & Meier, D. E. (2013). Research priorities in geriatric palliative care: Policy initiatives. *Journal of Palliative Medicine 16*(12), 1503–1508. doi: 10.1089 /jpm.2013.9464

Vollrath, A. M., & von Gunten, C. F. (2011). Negotiating goals of care: Changing goals along the trajectory of illness. In L. L. Emanuel & S. L. Librach (Eds.), *Palliative care: Core skills and clinical competencies* (2nd ed., pp. 56–68). Philadelphia, PA: Saunders/Elsevier.

Weinshilboum, R. (2003). Inheritance and drug response. *New England Journal of Medicine, 348*(5), 529–537.

Weissman, D. E., & Meier, D. E. (2011). Identifying patients in need of a palliative care assessment in the hospital setting. *Journal of Palliative Medicine, 14*(1), 1–7. doi: 10:1089/jpm.2010.0347

Weissman, D. E., Morrison, R. S., & Meier, D. E. (2010). Center to Advance Palliative Care clinical care and customer satisfaction metrics consensus recommendations. *Journal of Palliative Medicine, 13,* 179–184. doi: 10.1089.jpm.2009.0270

Wittenberg-Lyles, E., Goldsmith, J., Ferrell, B., & Ragan, S. L. (2013). *Communication in palliative nursing.* Oxford, UK: Oxford University Press.

World Health Organization (WHO). (2014a). First ever global atlas identifies unmet need for palliative care. http://www.who.int/mediacentre/news/releases/2014 /palliative-care-20140128/en/

World Health Organization (WHO). (2014b). World health assembly progress on noncommunicable disease and traditional medicine. http://www.who.int /mediacentre/news/releases/2014/WHA-20140523/en/

Worldwide Palliative Care Alliance. (2014). Global atlas of palliative care at the end of life. http://www.thewpca .org/resources/global-atlas-of-palliative-care/

Wu, H-L., & Volker, D. L. (2012). Humanistic nursing theory: Application to hospice and palliative care. *Journal of Advanced Nursing, 68*(2), 471–479.

Zimmermann, C., Riechelmann, R., Krzyzanowska, M., Rodin, G., & Tannock, I. (2008). Effectiveness of specialized palliative care: A systematic review. *Journal of the American Medical Association, 299*(14), 1698–1709.

Chapter 23

Health Policy

Anne Deutsch

Introduction

For individuals with a chronic illness, access to high-quality healthcare services that are safe, effective, patient centered, timely, affordable, and equitable is critical. Although many Americans receive high-quality healthcare services, care is not high quality for every patient during every episode of care (Institute of Medicine [IOM], 2001; Kohn, Corrigan, & Donaldson, 2000). Quality problems include underuse of needed services, overuse of unnecessary services, and an unacceptable level of errors (IOM, 2001; Kohn et al., 2000). Much of the work that healthcare professionals perform and experience as they deliver care to patients is influenced by laws, regulations, and other policies. For example, policy affects the availability of affordable health insurance for individuals and families, as well as coverage of home healthcare services, outpatient therapy, and durable medical equipment. Further, changes in health policies can positively or negatively affect utilization of the healthcare delivery system and the quality of care delivered. For example, policies can identify and incentivize opportunities for quality improvement when performance gaps exist.

Increasingly, nurses are expected to have knowledge of key health policy issues and to contribute to policy development and refinement. Understanding health policy is fundamental for nurses who want to improve the healthcare delivery system by influencing the policy-making process. To have an impact on patient care and nursing practice, nurses should be able to: (1) assess and understand current health policies, (2) identify the strengths and limitations of these healthcare policies, and then (3) act to influence changes in health policy to improve care for patients with chronic illnesses and their caregivers.

Health Policy Defined

Policy can be defined as the decisions made based on "choices that a society, segment of society, or organization makes regarding its goals and priorities and the ways to allocate its resources to attain those goals" (Mason, Leavitt, & Chafee, 2007, p. 8). *Health policy* refers to the decisions intended to influence health or health care (Chaffee, Mason & Leavitt, 2014).

The U.S. healthcare delivery system is a complex mix of private- and public-sector policies. Private-sector policies are decisions made by executives at private entities, such as private insurance companies and pharmaceutical companies, whereas public health policy decisions are made within any of the three branches of government (executive, legislative, or judicial) and at any level of government (federal, state, or local) (Longest, 2010). Examples of federal legislation include the Patient Protection and Affordable Care Act of 2010 (ACA), Medicare's prescription drug program, and funding of the National Institutes of Health to support research related to chronic diseases such as stroke, arthritis, Alzheimer's disease, and diabetes. Local government examples include city or county governments restricting smoking in public buildings. State and local boards of health have policies that monitor water quality and provide minimum safety requirements for nursing homes and daycare centers.

Because health is determined by many factors, including behaviors, physical and social environments, and access to and delivery of healthcare services, discussions of health policy can be either broad or more focused. This chapter primarily addresses health policy related to the access to and delivery of healthcare services.

Major Stakeholders in the U.S. Healthcare Industry

An important feature of the U.S. healthcare delivery system is its diverse and large number of stakeholders (Kovner & Knickman, 2011; Sultz & Young, 2013), which can make the process of developing and modifying policies challenging. Health policies can affect individuals with a common characteristic (e.g., nurses, the elderly, the disabled, the poor) or certain types of organizations (e.g., hospitals, skilled nursing facilities [SNFs], health plans, biotechnology companies, or employers). A stakeholder group's interest level and its support for or opposition to health policy changes vary by issue, and it is not uncommon for some stakeholder groups to agree on one issue, but disagree on another issue (Kovner & Knickman, 2011; Sultz & Young, 2013). For most stakeholder groups, their perspective on key issues can be anticipated. For example, a key stakeholder group is *consumers*, who tend to favor comprehensive insurance coverage, high-quality healthcare delivery, and low out-of-pocket expenses, and who tend to oppose limited access to care and increased patient payments.

A second key stakeholder group is *providers*, including both individuals (e.g., nurses) and entities (e.g., hospitals), which tend to favor maintaining income, autonomy, and comprehensive coverage, and tend to oppose limits on provider payments. Another key stakeholder group is *taxpayers*, who tend to favor limits on provider payments and oppose higher taxes. *Regulators* (government) are also a stakeholder group; they tend to favor disclosure and reporting by providers, cost containment, access to care, and high-quality health care, and tend to oppose provider autonomy. *Employers* tend to favor cost containment, administrative simplification, and the elimination of cost shifting, and tend to oppose government regulation. *Pharmaceutical manufacturers, biotechnology companies, assistive technology vendors,* and *suppliers* tend to favor comprehensive coverage and oppose limits on provider payments, whereas *private insurance companies* tend to favor business autonomy. *Consumer organizations*, such as the American Stroke Association and the Paralyzed Veterans Association, focus on securing money for research and public education.

Key Issues

U.S. Health Care: A Fragmented System of Healthcare Delivery

The United States does not have a national healthcare delivery system or health insurance system. Nevertheless, policy makers have implemented policies that support health insurance coverage for certain segments of the population, such as the elderly and the disabled, the poor, and children. This has led to separate insurance coverage programs for the elderly and disabled (Medicare), the poor (Medicaid), and uninsured children (Children's Health Insurance Program [CHIP]). Policy makers also provide healthcare insurance coverage to those who have provided service to the nation (military veterans) through the Veterans Affairs organization. More recently, the ACA established health insurance exchanges and expanded the Medicaid program. The existence of privately funded healthcare coverage, in addition to these publicly funded programs, has resulted in a fragmented and complex healthcare delivery system. To better understand this system, an overview of health insurance, including privately and publicly funded options, is provided here.

Health Insurance

Most Americans younger than the age of 65 have private health insurance coverage through an employer, and almost all individuals 65 years and older receive coverage through Medicare. Medicaid and CHIP provide insurance for millions of non-elderly individuals who have low incomes and children (Kaiser Commission on Medicaid and the Uninsured [KCMU], 2012). However, program limits and gaps in employer coverage have resulted in many people not having health insurance. In 2012, 18% of individuals younger than age 65 (47 million people) were uninsured (Kaiser Family Foundation, Health Research and Education Trust [KFF, HRET], 2013). The ACA sought to increase the number of people with health insurance by making affordable coverage more accessible through health insurance exchanges, expanding the Medicaid program, and requiring that individuals obtain health insurance. Importantly for individuals with a chronic illness, the ACA also mandated that no one could be denied health insurance coverage because of a preexisting health condition.

Health insurance coverage, however, does not always ensure access to care. There are often limitations on coverage for special services, such as behavioral health care, preventive care, post-acute care, long-term care, catastrophic illnesses or accidents, and psychiatric care. Most health insurance plans include copayments or deductibles to discourage overuse of services and to reduce premium costs. Copayments and high deductibles can discourage some patients from seeking essential care for the management of a chronic condition. This is particularly a problem for low-income populations. Rising costs have become a major problem for insured people with chronic conditions. In 2012, 26.8% of families in the United States had problems paying medical bills, with higher rates of difficulty reported among families below the poverty level, families with children, and families with a member who is uninsured (Cohen & Kirzinger, 2014).

TRADITIONAL OR CONVENTIONAL HEALTH INSURANCE

In the 1970s, the most common type of health insurance was the traditional fee-for-service (FFS) plan. Traditional health insurance plans generally allowed the insured person to choose a healthcare provider, and the healthcare provider made most healthcare decisions with minimal oversight by the insurance company. The covered services included acute care services, such as hospitalization, medication, and medical equipment, with little or no emphasis on prevention, health maintenance, or supportive healthcare services. This type of coverage limited the services needed to prevent chronic conditions and long-term care services. The number of traditional or conventional plans has declined dramatically, however, such that they accounted for fewer than 1% of all covered individuals in 2013 (KFF, HRET, 2013).

A major problem with the traditional FFS plans has been the lack of control on healthcare service use that led to high costs. In such plans, healthcare providers and consumers have few incentives to control costs. Therefore, insurance premiums must increase to cover the rising costs of services. Rising insurance costs have become a major issue for employers, which pay for some of the insurance premiums for their employees.

MANAGED CARE ORGANIZATIONS AND HIGH-DEDUCTIBLE HEALTH PLANS

As the cost of providing insurance continued to rise, employers often looked for less costly options to provide coverage for their employees.

One solution for employers has been to select managed care organizations (MCOs) and high-deductible plans (HDP) for health insurance. MCOs generally refer to health insurance plans that attempt to contain costs and manage the delivery of care (Sultz & Young, 2013). MCOs can be classified as health maintenance organizations (HMOs), preferred provider organizations (PPOs), and point-of-service (POS) plans. With the increase of MCOs in the 1990s, many became hopeful that this system would promote health and assist in preventing disease, thereby reducing costs. MCOs, it was thought, could help eliminate inappropriate overutilization of services and offer advantages by utilizing standard protocols to provide preventive healthcare services. Most experts agree that the main system change MCOs, especially HMOs, have emphasized is that of controlling costs.

Consumer-directed health plans or high-deductible health plans with savings options (HDHP/SO) are health insurance plans that have lower premiums, but higher deductibles and out-of-pocket spending limits. Under these plans, then, there are financial disincentives to seek healthcare services.

In 2013, employees selected PPO plans 57% of the time, HMO plans 14% of the time, POS plans 9% of the time, and HDHP/SO 20% of the time (KFF, HRET, 2013). Average family annual premiums in 2013 were as follows: HMO—$5,124 per employee and $11,419 per employer; PPO—$4,587 per employee and $12,084 per employer; POS—$5,590 per employee and $10,840 per employer; and HDHP/SO—$3,649 per employee and $11,578 per employer (KFF, HRET, 2013).

MEDICARE

Medicare was implemented in 1965 through Title XVIII of the Social Security Act—Health Insurance for the Aged and Disabled (Pulcine & Hart, 2014). In 2013, Medicare provided health insurance coverage to 52.3 million people, of whom 43.5 million were age 65 or older and 8.8 million people had permanent disabilities and were younger than 65 (U.S. Department of Health and Human Services [HHS], 2013). Medicare expenditures in 2012 were approximately $553.9 billion (HHS, 2013); they accounted for 16% of the federal budget and 21% of the national health expenditures (KFF, 2013a).

Medicare includes four components:

- *Part A: Hospital Insurance.* The hospital insurance component includes coverage for inpatient hospital stays, home health-care visits (skilled care only), hospice care, and skilled nursing facility (SNF) stays. Most Medicare beneficiaries do not pay a monthly premium for the hospital insurance plan, but are responsible for a deductible ($1,216 in 2014) for a hospital stay and coinsurance for an extended hospital stay ($304 per day for days 61–90 and $608 for each "lifetime reserve day" after day 90 for each benefit period in 2014). For qualified SNF stays, there is a coinsurance requirement for extended stays ($152 per day for days 21–100 and all costs after 100 days in 2014) (KFF, 2013a). Medicare Part A is financed through the Hospital Insurance Trust Fund by taxes paid by employers and their employees.

- *Part B: Supplemental Medical Insurance.* The supplementary medical insurance program covers physician, outpatient, home health, and preventive services. It is financed through the Supplementary Medical Insurance Trust Fund by federal taxes and premiums paid by beneficiaries (most people paid $104.90 per month in 2014) (KFF, 2013a). A majority of individuals who are covered under Part A of Medicare purchase Part B.

- *Part C: Medicare Advantage.* The Medicare Advantage program allows beneficiaries to enroll in a private health plan as an alternative to Medicare Part A and Part B coverage. Medicare Advantage covers hospital and physician care, and often (87% in 2014) includes prescription drug coverage (KFF, 2013b). Plans include PPOs, provider-sponsored organization (PSOs), private FFS plans, high-deductible plans linked to medical savings accounts, and special needs programs (SNPs) for individuals who are dually eligible for Medicare and Medicaid. The plans receive payments from Medicare to provide Medicare-covered benefits; Part C is not separately financed from Parts A, B, and D. Medicare Advantage enrollees generally pay the monthly Part B premium and often pay an additional premium directly to their plan (the average premium was $39 per month in 2014) (KFF, 2013b). Approximately 28% (14.4 million people) of Medicare beneficiaries were enrolled in Medicare Advantage in 2013 (KFF, 2013b).

• *Part D: Prescription Drug Benefit.* The prescription drug benefit is a voluntary program that provides coverage for outpatient prescription drugs offered through private companies that contract with Medicare. Coverage varies depending on the plan chosen. The prescription drug benefit is financed through taxes, beneficiary premiums, and state payments for individuals with both Medicare and Medicaid coverage. In 2013, an estimated 67% (35 million people) of Medicare enrollees had Part D drug coverage (Hoadley, Summer, Hargrave, & Cubanski, 2013).

Medicare services may seem comprehensive and clearly defined, yet—as with all health insurance programs—when assessing how a policy is implemented, either through specific laws or administrative regulations, services are often found to be neither comprehensive nor clearly defined. For example, to receive home health care through Medicare, an individual must meet each of the following requirements: (1) the person must be generally restricted to his or her home; (2) a physician (or certain other healthcare providers) must see the person face-to-face before a doctor can certify that there is a need for home health services; (3) a physician must prescribe the treatment; (4) the person must need skilled nursing care, physical therapy, or speech therapy; and (5) the services must be provided by a certified home health agency participating in the Medicare program (HHS, Centers for Medicare and Medicaid Services [CMS], 2012). Therefore, if a nurse practitioner's patient with diabetes and congestive heart failure needed skilled nursing care for leg ulcers, the person would first have to be referred by a physician. In addition, if the patient leaves his or her home regularly, the person would not be eligible to receive home health services through Medicare. It is also important to note, especially for those with chronic illness and disabilities, that Medicare does not cover long-term (i.e., nursing facility) care.

MEDICAID

Medicaid was an amendment to Title XIX of the Social Security Act in 1965 and was implemented in 1966 (Pulcine & Hart, 2014). Medicaid was established to provide health insurance to people who have a low income. In 2013, the average number of Medicaid monthly enrollees was 62 million people, and Medicaid spending was approximately $428.5 billion in 2012 (HHS, 2013). Individual states define the program, and it is jointly funded by federal and state governments. Medicaid covers a wide range of health and long-term care services (institutional and community-based care), but because this coverage is administered at the state level, it varies from state to state, and there are differences in who is eligible for coverage (KCMU, 2013). Medicaid managed care and nonmanaged care options are available, although some states require enrollment in a managed care plan.

To receive matching federal dollars, the state Medicaid program must offer certain basic medical services, such as inpatient and outpatient hospital care and physician and family nurse practitioner services. Covered services include long-term care, mental health care, and services and supports needed by individuals with disabilities. Medicaid covers comprehensive services for eligible children. It is the largest funding source of institutional long-term care, providing benefits to approximately 63% of all nursing facility residents (KFF, 2013c). Medicaid also covers services such as prescription drugs, eyeglasses, and hearing aids. It covers those persons with disabilities and the elderly who are enrolled in Medicare (known as "dual eligibles") but have incomes below a certain level. This coverage for low-income Medicare beneficiaries assists these individuals with premiums, deductibles, and coinsurance.

Children's Health Insurance Program

The Balanced Budget Act of 1997 expanded health insurance coverage to children through CHIP by helping states cover uninsured children who do not meet Medicaid eligibility requirements (KCMU, 2012). In 2013, more than 5.7 million children were enrolled in CHIP (KCMU, 2012). Similar to Medicaid, CHIP is administered through states, and the type of program offered varies by state. As employer insurance coverage has declined, the rate of children who are uninsured has risen. When their families lack health insurance, children often do not receive care to prevent chronic conditions or illnesses such as complications from diseases that could have been prevented by immunizations or disabilities created because of lack of treatment (e.g., hearing loss from otitis media).

Costs, Access, and Quality

Costs

The increasing cost of delivering health care has been a challenge for policy makers for several decades. In 2010, the United States spent approximately $2.6 trillion on health care, which is an average of $8,402 per person (KFF, 2012). The national health expenditures represented 7.2% of U.S. gross domestic product (GDP) in 1970—a share that increased to 17.9% of the GDP in 2010

(KFF, 2012), and is expected to reach 20% by 2021 (Wayne, 2012).

The rising costs can be attributed to many factors, including the growth of the older population, advances in healthcare technology, increased utilization of services, increasing labor costs, and increases in the costs of pharmaceuticals and malpractice insurance. While almost everyone agrees that rising healthcare costs are a problem, development of policies aimed at controlling costs has been a challenge, because one or more stakeholder groups may receive less money, or access to care may become more limited. Solutions that have been proposed to control costs include managed care, use of information technology, evidence-based care, management initiatives, controlling prescription drug costs, Medicare and Medicaid payment reform, using competition, fraud prevention and detection, and price controls.

In the 1980s, in an effort to reduce institutional costs, Medicare began a shift away from a retrospective cost-based payment system for acute care hospitals and toward a prospective payment system. The implementation of the acute care Inpatient Prospective Payment System in 1983 resulted in shorter acute care stays and higher utilization of care delivered in post-acute care settings, including SNFs, inpatient rehabilitation facilities, home health agencies, and long-term care hospitals. The implementation of post-acute care prospective payment systems beginning in 1998 decreased Medicare post-acute care expenditures for a few years, but then overall post-acute care expenditures increased as patients began increasingly receiving care in multiple post-acute care settings during an episode of care.

Concerns about the increasingly fragmented U.S. healthcare system has led to several initiatives that would move away from the current siloed provider-centric healthcare delivery system that rewards volume (i.e., acute care stay followed by multiple post-acute care stays, each paid separately) and toward a more patient-centered episode-based system that rewards efficient, high-quality, and safe care.

ACCESS TO CARE

There are many reasons why individuals do not have equal access to healthcare services. The most common reason for reduced access to necessary health services is the inability to pay for such care (Sultz & Young, 2013). When individuals and families are either uninsured or underinsured, they are less likely to have a usual source of care outside of the emergency room, often go without screenings and preventive care, often delay or forgo needed medical care, are sicker and die earlier than those who have insurance, and pay more for their care. This lack of access places a higher burden on those with chronic illness. In the United Kingdom, Canada, and the Netherlands, individuals state they rarely forgo needed medical care because of cost; yet in the United States, 54% of those with chronic diseases "had skipped medications, not seen a doctor when sick, or foregone recommended care in the past year because of costs" (Schoen, Osborn, How, Doty, & Peugh, 2009). More than 84% of individuals who are considered high users of the emergency room have chronic conditions (Peppe, Mays, Chang, Becker, & DiJulio, 2007). The ACA seeks to address the issues of lack of insurance and under-insurance, with some provisions already implemented and more significant ones due for implementation in 2014 and beyond.

Individuals can also have limited access to care, particularly specialty care, because healthcare personnel and facilities are not close to where they live (e.g., rural locations), culturally acceptable, or capable of providing the type of care needed (Sultz & Young, 2013).

QUALITY

Quality can be defined as the "degree to which health services for individuals and populations increase the likelihood of desired health outcomes and are consistent with current professional knowledge" (IOM, 2006, p. 468). The IOM (2006) noted that the only way to know if healthcare quality is improving is to document performance using standardized measures of quality. The term *quality measure* has been defined as the "quantification of the degree to which a desired health care process or outcome is achieved or the extent that a desirable structure to support health care delivery is in place" (IOM, 2006, p. 42).

Quality measures (also known as quality indicators, performance measures, and performance indicators) evaluate healthcare performance in a manner that permits comparisons across facilities and across time. Quality measures may improve care through public reporting, quality improvement, and performance-based payment (i.e., pay-for-performance) activities (IOM, 2006). The Centers for Medicare and Medicaid Services and private-sector payers have been leaders in using quality measures for public reporting and performance-based payment, with hundreds of quality measures used across 20 quality reporting programs for clinicians, acute care hospitals, and post-acute care providers. Proponents of public reporting of quality information argue that it helps patients, referring physicians, and purchasers of health care make better, more informed choices by identifying those providers that offer the best care. Another use of quality measures is rewarding providers that demonstrate better quality of care based on performance data (i.e., pay-for-performance programs).

Several classification systems for quality methods have been proposed. Donabedian (2005) classified quality measures as structure measures, process measures, or outcome measures. *Structure measures* document whether a particular mechanism or system is in place, *process measures* track performance of a particular action, and *outcome measures* document the end results of care, such as functional status, morbidity, and mortality resulting from a disease.

The IOM (2001) offers another classification system for quality measures based on the six aims of healthcare delivery: safety, effectiveness, patient centered, timeliness, efficiency, and equity. *Safety* refers to care that avoids injuries to patients as a result of care. *Effectiveness* means that services are based on scientific knowledge and provided to all who could benefit and not provided to those who would not likely benefit from those services. *Patient-centered care* refers to care that is respectful of and responsive to individual patient preferences, needs, and values. *Timeliness* refers to care that reduces wait times. *Efficient care* avoids waste, including waste of equipment, supplies, ideas, and energy. *Equity* refers to care that does not vary in quality because of personal characteristics (e.g., gender, ethnicity, geographic location, and socioeconomic status).

In the report *Crossing the Quality Chasm*, the IOM (2001) proposed 10 rules for redesigning healthcare processes to improve care:

1. *Care based on continuous healing relationships.* Care should be available 24 hours a day, 7 days a week, and access to care should occur over the Internet, by telephone, and by other means as well as in face-to-face encounters.
2. *Customization based on patient needs and values.* The system should meet the most common types of patient needs and have the ability to respond to patient choices and preferences.
3. *The patient as the source of control.* Patients should be given the necessary information and the opportunity to be involved in shared decision making.
4. *Shared knowledge and the free flow of information.* Patients should have access to their own medical information and clinical knowledge.
5. *Evidence-based decision making.* Patients should receive care based on the best scientific knowledge.
6. *Safety.* Patients should be safe from injury that is caused by the healthcare delivery system.
7. *Transparency.* The system should make information available to patients and their families that allows them to make informed decisions when selecting a health plan, hospital, or clinician.

8. *Anticipation of needs.* The system should anticipate patients' needs.
9. *Continuous decrease in waste.* The health system should not waste resources, including patients' time.
10. *Cooperation among clinicians.* Clinicians and institutions should actively collaborate and communicate to foster greater coordination of care and integration.

Two themes that emerge from these recommendations—patient engagement and care coordination—are critical components of high-quality care for individuals with chronic illness, who may be seeing more than one healthcare professional. Patient engagement refers to a patient's knowledge, skills, ability, and willingness to manage his or her own health and care, as well as the interventions that increase these factors in a way that promotes positive behavior (James, 2014). Patients who are actively involved in their health and health care tend to have better outcomes and lower costs compared to individuals who are not actively involved in their own care (James, 2014).

There is also a need for care coordination between healthcare providers, including acute care hospitals, post-acute care providers, and outpatient providers. The ACA includes several initiatives that focus on improving the coordination of healthcare services. One initiative, known as medical homes, involves healthcare settings that offer comprehensive primary care services, as well as nonemergent primary, secondary, and tertiary care. The medical home primary care provider directs and coordinates care for patients. The CMS Innovation Center also has several initiatives under way, including the Accountable Care Organizations and the Bundled Payments for Care Improvement project (http://www.innovations.cms.gov/initiatives/index.html). Evaluation of these new models of care is beginning to provide insights about the effectiveness of these approaches, but it is unclear which models of care might continue beyond the initial testing or how any model might evolve.

Opportunities to improve care of patients clearly exist. Nevertheless, designing a delivery system that aligns incentives for key stakeholders, including patients, providers, payers, and policy makers, remains challenging.

Interventions: Engaging in Policy Discussions

Public policy has greatly influenced the U.S. healthcare delivery system. Basic health services are available to many Americans, but the system remains fragmented and complex, making it difficult to navigate. Policy reforms have the potential to benefit individuals with chronic illness, but to do so requires participation in policy discussions. Being engaged in policy discussions provides nurses with the opportunity to shape policy that influences the care individuals with chronic illness receive and gives nurses an opportunity to partner with clients to meet common goals. Helping individuals with chronic conditions and their families understand the political process and the power of politics can empower them to work to improve the healthcare system.

Many policy issues affect individuals with chronic illness, including affordable health insurance, essential benefits of health insurance plans, costs of care, quality of care, and research funding. In turn, there are many opportunities to intervene to influence policy. There is also growing recognition that the healthcare delivery system is likely responsible for only a modest proportion of what makes and keeps Americans healthy, and that healthcare providers, individuals, and organizations should also work with public health agencies, community-based organizations, schools, businesses, and others to identify and solve the problems that contribute to poor health.

Stages of Influencing Policy

Public policy may be influenced at several key stages: (1) policy formulation (agenda setting and legislation), (2) policy implementation, and (3) policy modification (Longest, 2010). At each phase, individuals and organizations can take on an important role in the development of policy, which can have a significant impact on healthcare delivery.

The first stage, policy formulation, begins with agenda setting, which refers to the identification of problems and possible solutions. As conditions in society change or there is a shift in values and beliefs, new agenda items can take on more importance. Issues found on recent agendas have included affordable health insurance, patient safety, quality, healthcare fraud, and gun control. Once an agenda becomes recognized, governmental officials can legislate programs and develop or change policies to address problems identified during agenda setting (Longest, 2010). However, only a small number of issues reach policy formulation or legislation.

For those issues that do become part of a law, policy implementation provides another opportunity for input. Policy implementation, which includes rule making and policy operation, is the responsibility of the executive branch of the government. Cabinet departments such as the Department of Health and Human Services and its agencies, such as the Centers for Disease Control and Prevention (CDC) and the CMS, oversee the implementation of these laws.

The last stage, policy modification, occurs when decisions and policies made in the past are reviewed, and the outcomes, perceptions, and consequences of existing policies are evaluated.

Nursing Interventions: Action Steps

To affect public policy, nurses need to learn the skills necessary to influence policy makers at all stages of policy development. Knowledge about a key issue, communication, and collaboration are key components of political influence.

Knowing when a bill is in committee and knowing the chairperson and committee members are important information that can help one attempt to apply influence. In addition to directly trying to influence public policy makers, indirect influence can be a strategy. Communicating with Congressional/executive staff members, the media, and constituents can influence policy makers. Skillful communication, including listening skills, can be influential in the political process. Knowing who one is trying to influence and how one wants to influence their actions are key factors.

Once these details are determined, there are several communication approaches that one can use. For example, a nurse might send a message and/or position statement by email, fax, or letter. In small states, it may be possible to contact legislators directly; in larger states or at the national level, the nurse can either talk with a staff person or leave a short message. Email, fax, or phone calls are typically the best ways to communicate with legislators. In addition, many elected or policy leaders have their own websites where there is usually a mechanism to send a message (**Table 23-1**). Nurses advocating a particular policy might also write letters to newspaper editors or seek out opportunities to talk on the radio/television. Other communication options are to visit legislators and/or their staff (**Table 23-2**) and testify at public hearings. Finally, it is important to vote and to get others to vote.

Working to change policy at any level of government requires group action and collaboration. National and state professional and community organizations also work for policy initiatives that impact their organizations or members of their organizations. For example, the American Nurses Association has testified on many key issues relevant to nursing and the patients whom nurses serve, including healthcare reform, Medicare funding, and funding for nursing education programs. The American Heart Association has specific legislative goals related to heart disease and stroke. It works with individuals and groups in policy initiatives, including keeping the public informed about policy issues that impact the organization's stated goals. Professional and community organizations, especially at the local

Table 23-1 Guidelines for Writing an Email, Letter, or Fax to Policy Makers and Their Staff

Writing to a policy maker is one of the easiest and most effective ways for individuals and groups to correspond with policy makers.

1. Be professional. Use the proper forms of address when writing to any policy maker. Use a polite tone and present your message clearly, concisely, and with respect.
2. State who you are and why you are writing.
3. Be concise and informed.
4. Personalize your letter by including a description of a personal experience or patient story.
5. Be accurate and clear.
6. Be modest with the request.
7. Offer your assistance as a resource.
8. Express thanks for the policy maker's time and consideration.
9. Ask for a response.
10. If you do not get a response in about 1 month, follow up with the policy maker.

Source: Data from Association of Rehabilitation Nurses. (2014). Health policy toolkit. Retrieved from http://www.rehabnurse.org/advocacy/content/Advocacy-Toolkit.html.

level, can provide great mentoring opportunities. These organizations are often looking for individuals to help with their advocacy strategies and may often help in the development of those skills. Advocacy groups such as the American Association of People with Disabilities (2007) can help professionals or families of individuals with disabilities provide testimony at public hearings.

Sometimes diverse groups (i.e., stakeholders) can work together on a mutual issue, even if they disagree on other issues. Influencing policy changes requires patience, perseverance, and compromise. Working with those who share similar values, beliefs, and convictions will be of great assistance when working for change.

Table 23-2 Guidelines for Meeting with Policy Makers and Their Staff

1. Be prepared and be on time for your appointment. Always introduce yourself, even if this is your third or fourth meeting. State that you are a registered nurse, or if a client is speaking, have that person share the nature of the chronic condition he or she or the family member has.
2. Thank the legislator for seeing you and then briefly and clearly identify the issue you want to discuss. If it is a specific bill, state its number, its title, your position, and what you want the legislator to do.
3. Provide a real-life example or personal story to illustrate your position.
4. Listen to the policy maker's/staffer's comments and respond to any questions.
5. Ask the policy maker's/staffer's position on the issue.
6. Bring written materials on the issue that can be left with policy makers.
7. Leave your contact information, such as a business card.
8. Summarize your requests of the policy maker.
9. Follow up your visit with a thank-you note.
10. Summarize your meeting in writing and share this information with the organization(s) with which you are working.

Source: Data from Association of Rehabilitation Nurses. (2014). Health policy toolkit. Retrieved from http://www.rehabnurse.org /advocacy/content/Advocacy-Toolkit.html.

The strategies discussed in this section emphasize influencing policy at the national level. The same strategies can also be used to influence local and state policy, as well as policy makers in work and community organizations.

It is important for nurses to be involved in policy discussions, or they risk being excluded from important decisions that affect nursing practice or the care provided to their patients with chronic illness. Becoming involved in policy discussions can be an overwhelming experience. As a beginner, you can start by voting. Next, choose an issue about which you feel passionate (e.g., the inability of your clients with chronic illness to get home care). Educate yourself on the issue, and communicate with others who are interested in the issue. Communicate your position and rationale and present any research or data that support your position to the key players. Know that your cause is just, and be proud of the political influence you, your clients, and your colleagues can accomplish.

Evidence-Based Practice Box

The evidence demonstrates that health policy impacts the health of individuals.

- Medicare beneficiaries who qualify for Medicare as a result of disabilities, when compared with the beneficiaries who qualify because of age, report more problems with accessing care and finding affordable care. Beneficiaries who are disabled report a higher rate of health consequences as a result of delayed or missed care because of cost concerns, including a worsening in the primary disability or existing medical condition; more problems that require medical attention; a higher level of a significant amount of stress or anxiety; and a higher level of a significant amount of physical pain (Cubanski & Neuman, 2010).
- Using data from the 2002–2004 Medical Expenditure Panel Survey, researchers found that among 92 million adults with chronic conditions, 21% experienced at least 1 month uninsured during the average year. The gaps in health insurance coverage were associated with significantly higher levels of access problems, fewer ambulatory visits, and higher out-of-pocket costs (Gulley, Rasch, & Chan, 2010).

Outcomes

The National Strategy for Quality Improvement, which was initially released in 2011, set priorities for improving the delivery of healthcare services, patient health outcomes, and population health (HHS, 2011). It identifies three primary aims—better care, healthy people/healthy communities, and affordable care—and six priorities:

1. Making care safer by reducing harm caused in the delivery of care
2. Ensuring that each person and family are engaged as partners in their care
3. Promoting effective communication and coordination of care
4. Promoting the most effective prevention and treatment practices for the leading causes of mortality
5. Working with communities to promote wide use of best practices to enable healthy living
6. Making quality care more affordable for individuals, families, employers, and governments (HHS, 2011)

The National Quality Strategy does not include metrics for these aims and priorities, but rather serves as a framework for the development and selection of specific metrics for the different sectors of the healthcare delivery system.

The Department of Health and Human Services releases a set of goals and objectives each decade through the Healthy People initiative (www.HealthyPeople.gov). *Healthy People 2020* is the current version, which builds on the three previous versions. It specifies key health indicators that monitor progress toward the promotion of health, prevention of disease and disability, elimination of disparities, and improvement in quality of life. The 26 leading health indicators include metrics that target the healthcare delivery system (e.g., persons with medical insurance, persons with a usual primary care provider, adults who receive a colorectal cancer screening, adults with hypertension whose blood pressure is under control) as well as broader public health topics (Air Quality Index exceeding 100, children aged 3 to 11 years exposed to secondhand smoke, adults who are obese, total vegetable intake for persons aged 2 years and older).

CASE STUDY 23-1

As a nurse who works in home care with patients who have experienced a stroke, you recognize the importance of care coordination as your patients transition from the hospital setting to home, including the role of communication among the hospital staff, the patient and family, and the patient's primary care physician and home care services.

Discussion Questions

1. Which national and state advocacy organization might be able to mentor/assist you in advocacy efforts to improve care coordination?
2. If your state had a bill pending that required each patient to receive a reconciled medication list and a transition record with specified elements at hospital discharge, how would you learn more about the bill to decide whether you do or do not support passage of the bill?
3. Who are the potential stakeholders interested in care coordination issues, and how might you work with these individuals or entities?

STUDY QUESTIONS

1. Describe how trends of chronic illness are significant in relation to health policy.
2. Differentiate between Medicare and Medicaid.
3. Describe how the current U.S. healthcare system affects persons with chronic illness.
4. Identify key skills necessary for political influence, and explain how each is important.

Internet Resources
How to Find and Communicate with Legislators and Stakeholders

House of Representatives: http://www.house.gov
/representatives
Senators: http://www.senate.gov/general/contact
_information/senators_cfm.cfm

Policy/Political Resources

Federal Legislative link site: http://thomas.loc.gov
Health System Change policy analysis site: http://www
.hschange.com
Summary of national political news: http://www
.politicalwire.com
State policy and politics: http://www.stateline.org/live

Government Websites

Centers for Medicare and Medicaid Services: http://
www.cms.gov
Department of Veterans Affairs: http://www.va.gov
U.S. House of Representatives and U.S. Senate: http://
www.house.gov

Advocacy or Other Relevant Websites

Leading Age (formerly AAHSA): http://www
.leadingage.org

American Association of People with Disabilities: http://
www.aapd.com
American Heart Association: http://www.heart.org
/HEARTORG/Advocate/Advocate_UCM_001133
_SubHomePage.jsp
American Nurses Association-government affairs:
http://www.nursingworld.org/MainMenuCategories
/ANAPoliticalPower.aspx
Consortium for Citizens with Disabilities: http://www
.c-c-d.org
Families USA: http://www.familiesusa.org
National Alliance for Caregiving: http://www
.caregiving.org
National Citizen's Coalition for Nursing Home Reform:
http://www.nccnhr.org
National Respite Coalition: http://www.archrespite.org
Partnership to Fight Chronic Disease: http://www
.fightchronicdisease.org
Preventing Chronic Disease journal: http://www.cdc
.gov/pcd
United Cerebral Palsy: http://www.ucp.org
World Health Organization, Chronic Disease and Health
Promotion: http://www.who.int/chp/en

References

American Association of People with Disabilities. (2007).
AAPD policy positions and activities. http://www
.aapd.com/site/c.pvI1IkNWJqE/b.5606943/k.669B
/AAPD_Policy_Positions.htm
Association of Rehabilitation Nurses. (2014). Health
policy toolkit. http://www.rehabnurse.org/advocacy
/content/Advocacy-Toolkit.html

Chaffee, M. W., Mason, D. J., & Leavitt, J. K. (2014). A
framework for action in policy and politics. In D. J.
Mason, J. K. Leavitt, & M. W. Chaffee (Eds.), *Policy
and politics in nursing and health care* (revised reprint,
6th ed.). St. Louis, MO: Elsevier Saunders.
Cohen, R. A., & Kirzinger, W. K. (2014). *Financial
burden of medical care: a family perspective.* National

Center for Health Statistics Data Brief, No. 142. U.S. Department of Health and Human Services. Centers for Disease Control and Prevention. http://www.cdc.gov/nchs/data/databriefs/db142.pdf

Cubanski, J., & Neuman, P. (2010). Medicare doesn't work as well for younger, disabled beneficiaries as it does for older enrollees. *Health Affairs, 29*(9), 1–9.

Donabedian, A. (2005). Evaluating the quality of medical care. *Milbank Quarterly, 83*(4), 691–729.

Gulley, S. P., Rasch, E. K., & Chan, L. (2010). Ongoing coverage for ongoing care: Access, utilization, and out-of-pocket spending among uninsured working-aged adults with chronic health care needs. *American Journal of Public Health, 101*(2), 368–375.

Hoadley, J., Summer, L., Hargrave, E., & Cubanski, J. (2013). *Medicare Part D prescription drug plans: The marketplace in 2013 and key trends, 2006–2013.* Menlo Park, CA: Kaiser Family Foundation. http://kff.org/medicare/issue-brief/medicare-part-d-prescription-drug-plans-the-marketplace-in-2013-and-key-trends-2006-2013/

Institute of Medicine (IOM). (2001). *Crossing the quality chasm: A new health system for the 21st century.* Washington, DC: National Academies Press.

Institute of Medicine (IOM). (2006). *Performance measurement: Accelerating improvement.* Washington, DC: National Academies Press.

James, J. (2014, February 14). Health policy brief: Patient engagement. *Health Affairs.* http://www.healthaffairs.org/healthpolicybriefs/brief.php?brief_id=86

Kaiser Commission on Medicaid and the Uninsured (KCMU). (2012). Health coverage of children: The role of Medicaid and SCHIP. http://www.kff.org/uninsured/upload/7698.pdf

Kaiser Commission on Medicaid and the Uninsured (KCMU). (2013). *Medicaid: A primer.* Menlo Park, CA: Kaiser Family Foundation. http://www.kff.org/medicaid/7334.cfm

Kaiser Family Foundation (KFF). (2012). *Health care costs: A primer.* Menlo Park, CA: Author. http://kff.org/health-costs/report/health-care-costs-a-primer/

Kaiser Family Foundation (KFF). (2013a). *Medicare: A primer.* Menlo Park, CA: Author. http://www.kff.org/medicare/7615.cfm

Kaiser Family Foundation (KFF). (2013b). *Medicare Advantage: A primer.* Menlo Park, CA: Author. http://kff.org/medicare/fact-sheet/medicare-advantage-fact-sheet/

Kaiser Family Foundation (KFF). (2013c). *Overview of nursing facility capacity, financing, and ownership in the United States in 2011.* Menlo Park, CA: Author.

Kaiser Family Foundation (KFF), Health Research and Education Trust (HRET). (2013). *Employer health benefits 2013 annual survey.* Menlo Park, CA: Author. http://kaiserfamilyfoundation.files.wordpress.com/2013/08/8466-employer-health-benefits-2013_summary-of-findings2.pdf

Kohn, L. T., Corrigan, J. M., & Donaldson, M. S. (2000). *To err is human: Building a safer health system.* Washington, DC: National Academies Press.

Kovner, A. R., & Knickman, J. R. (Eds.). (2011). *Jonas and Kovner's health care delivery in the United States* (10th ed.). New York, NY: Springer.

Longest, B. B. (2010). *Health policymaking in the United States* (5th ed.). Chicago, IL: Health Administration Press.

Mason, D. J., Leavitt, J. K., & Chaffee, M. W. (2007). Policy and politics: A framework for action. In D. J. Mason, J. K. Leavitt, & M. W. Chaffee (Eds.), *Policy and politics in nursing and health care* (5th ed.). St. Louis, MO: Saunders Elsevier.

Peppe, E. M., Mays, J. W., Chang, H. C., Becker, E., & DiJulio, B. (2007). Characteristics of frequent emergency department users. http://www.kff.org/insurance/7696.cfm

Pulcine, J. A., & Hart, M. A. (2014). Financing health care in the United States. In D. J. Mason, J. K., Leavitt, & M. W. Chaffee (Eds.), *Policy and politics in nursing and health care* (revised reprint, 6th ed., pp. 135–146). St. Louis, MO: Elsevier Saunders.

Schoen, C., Osborn, R., How, S. K. H., Doty, M. M., & Peugh, J. (2009). In chronic condition: Experiences of patients with complex health care needs, in eight countries, 2008. *Health Affairs, 28*, w1–w16.

Sultz, H. A., & Young, K. M. (2013). *Health care USA: Understanding its organization and delivery* (8th ed.). Burlington, MA: Jones & Bartlett Learning.

U.S. Department of Health and Human Services (HHS). (2011). *Report to Congress: National Strategy for Quality Improvement in Health Care.* Washington, DC: Author. http://www.ahrq.gov/workingforquality/nqs/nqs2011annlrpt.htm

U.S. Department of Health and Human Services (HHS). (2013). *2013 CMS statistics.* Baltimore, MD: Author. http://www.cms.gov/ResearchGenInfo/02_CMSStatistics.asp#TopOfPage

U.S. Department of Health and Human Services (HHS), Centers for Medicare and Medicaid Services (CMS). (2012). *Documentation of requirements for home health prospective payment system (HH PPS) face-to-face encounter.* Medicare Learning Network MSE1405. Baltimore, MD: Author. http://www.cms.gov/Outreach-and-Education/Medicare-Learning-Network-MLN/MLNMattersArticles/downloads/SE1405.pdf

Wayne, A. (2012, June 12). Health-care spending to reach 20% of U.S. economy by 2021. *Bloomberg News.* http://www.bloomberg.com/news/2012-06-13/health-care-spending-to-reach-20-of-u-s-economy-by-2021.html

Chapter 24

Rehabilitation

Kristen L. Mauk

Introduction

Rehabilitation is both a philosophy and a process through which persons with physical challenges or disabling conditions learn to regain maximal function, independence, and/or restoration (Mauk, 2012). Rehabilitation assists individuals with long-term health alterations to adapt to changes that have occurred as a result of deviations in their health status. A popular rehabilitation saying is that "rehabilitation begins day one" and, therefore, should be considered as part of the overall plan of care for most episodes of acute illness and throughout the duration of most chronic illnesses.

Rehabilitation is commonly associated with certain disorders or illnesses in which therapeutic interventions have been shown to be effective. These include health alterations such as stroke, spinal cord injury, and traumatic or other brain injury; neurologic diseases such as Parkinson's disease, multiple sclerosis (MS), and Guillain-Barré syndrome; orthopedic problems such as arthritis, fractures, and joint replacements; and, less commonly, burns, cancer, and respiratory disorders. In each of these conditions, persons can be assisted to regain maximal functioning that may have been altered because of a disease process, injury, or congenital defect.

The primary goal of rehabilitation is to achieve the highest level of independence possible for the client. This goal is highly individualized. For example, a person with a mild stroke may have the goal to walk again and resume gainful employment at the same job he held previously. Another person with a high-level spinal injury may realistically have a goal of being able to be mobile independently with the use of a mechanically adapted wheelchair such as a Sip-N-Puff chair. Both persons have achievable goals that are based on their capacity and functional limitations that have resulted from illness or injury.

The objectives of rehabilitation may be summarized with a few concepts: restoring or maximizing the level of function, facilitating independence, preventing complications, and promoting quality of life. Rehabilitation typically involves a team of professionals working toward a common goal. The client and family are considered the most important team members. Professional team members may include physicians, nurses, therapists, social workers, vocational counselors, nutritionists, orthotists, prosthetists, and chaplains. Additional professionals may be consulted as necessary to help meet the unique needs of the individual.

One of the foci of the rehabilitation process is community reintegration or reentry, sometimes referred to as resocialization. Through this process, individuals are reintegrated into society after a life-altering health condition or situation changes their previous roles and abilities. Within a rehabilitation setting, reintegration is an ongoing goal. Rehabilitation professionals work with disabled clients or individuals with chronic illness and their families to help them reenter their communities; they may have to accomplish significant adjustments to adapt to changes that have occurred in each area of their lives. Often this process involves the client relearning self-care with activities of daily living (ADLs) such as bathing, grooming, toileting, eating, and dressing. Rehabilitation is a hopeful process that encourages individuals to maximize their strengths while making positive adaptations to their limitations.

Definitions

REHABILITATION

Rehabilitation refers to services and programs designed to assist individuals who have experienced a trauma or illness that results in impairment that creates a loss of function (physical, psychological, social, or vocational). Common themes among the various definitions of rehabilitation should be considered. Concepts include the complex, dynamic interactions among the individual, the disease or health condition, and the environment. Most definitions of rehabilitation include assisting an individual with a limitation to attain his or her maximal independence and function. The Institute of Medicine (IOM) has defined rehabilitation as "the process by which physical, sensory or mental capacities are restored or developed.... Rehabilitation strives to reverse what has been called the disabling process, and may therefore be called the enabling process" (Brandt & Pope, 1997, pp. 12–13).

PHYSICAL MEDICINE AND REHABILITATION

Also called physiatry, physical medicine and rehabilitation (PM&R) is one of 24 recognized medical specialties. Physiatrists specialize in preventing, diagnosing, and treating disorders that may result in temporary or permanent impairment. Usually these health problems are related to the brain, nervous system, spine, bones, or muscles (American Academy of Physical Medicine and Rehabilitation, 2014).

REHABILITATION NURSING

Rehabilitation is a continuous process, and clients rehabilitate themselves through a comprehensive approach to care provided by the rehabilitation nurse. Rehabilitation nurses "help individuals across the lifespan who are affected by chronic illness or physical disability to achieve their greatest potential, adapt to their disabilities, and work toward productive, independent lives" (Association of Rehabilitation Nurses [ARN], 2012, para 2). The ARN (2008) defines rehabilitation nursing as "the diagnosis and treatment of human responses of individuals and groups to actual or potential health problems related to altered functional ability and lifestyle" (p. 13).

General information for rehabilitation nurses and advanced rehabilitation nurses is included in the *Standards and Scope of Rehabilitation Nursing Practice* (ARN, 2008). Because of the growth of the specialty of rehabilitation nursing, many subspecialties are associated with this field. The ARN has developed role descriptions for each of the emerging areas where rehabilitation nurses work.

RESTORATIVE CARE

"Restorative care nursing, more recently referred to as function-focused care, is a philosophy of care that enables caregivers to actively help older adults achieve and maintain their highest level of function" (Resnick, Galik, Bolz, & Pretzer-Aboff, 2012, p. xiii). Restorative care differs from rehabilitation in that it does not include activities directed by therapists, but rather emphasizes nursing interventions that promote adaptation, comfort, and safety within a long-term care setting. Restorative care focuses on maximizing an individual's abilities, helping to rebuild self-esteem and to achieve appropriate goals (Resnick et al., 2012). Such care often focuses on assisting individuals with ADLs as well as walking and mobility exercises, transferring, amputation/prosthesis care, and communication. Self-care skills, such as management of one's diabetes, ostomy care, or medication setup and administration, are also emphasized. Restorative care, although conceptually similar to rehabilitation, is most appropriate for those individuals who have already reached their maximal functional level and need to maintain that function, and for those who are not appropriate candidates for intensive rehabilitation services.

VOCATIONAL REHABILITATION

Vocational rehabilitation assists the disabled individual to return to gainful employment and focus on financial independence through programs specifically designed for this purpose. The federal government requires each state to have an office of vocational rehabilitation to provide services for people with disabilities, and it provides funding and support to integrate clients into the work community (Parker & Neal-Boylan, 2007; Rehabilitation Services Administration, 2014). The Rehabilitation Services Administration (2014), through the U.S. Department of Education, provides leadership and resources to help states and agencies develop vocational rehabilitation so that persons with disabilities can maximize their employment potential and independence.

Rehabilitation Models and Classification Systems

Despite 50 years of research into rehabilitation, this specialty still lacks a grand theory or model to guide practice (Dijkers, Hart, Tsauosides, Whyte, & Zanca, 2014). Models are used to help explain, guide, or direct practice or processes. Rehabilitation models can aid

in understanding how chronic conditions and disability develop and progress, or how they can be managed. Several major classification systems are used to document rehabilitation processes and outcomes (Brandt & Pope, 1997; World Health Organization [WHO], 1980, 2002), including the Functional Limitations System (FLS), the Enabling–Disabling Model, and the WHO International Classification of Functioning, Disability, and Health (ICF). In addition, the American Congress of Rehabilitation Medicine (ACRM) has proposed a taxonomy of rehabilitation treatments that is described in this section (Fasoli & Chen, 2014).

The IOM recommends the use of the Enabling–Disabling Process Model, whereas the WHO recommends the use of the ICF to help standardize and effectively communicate information about diagnoses, care, and treatment. The ACRM has proposed an alternative approach to standardization in rehabilitation by describing the treatment versus the process. The model used may depend largely on the facility and its preferences. The use of standard terminology within these models can help facilitate communication, but rehabilitation professionals must be thoroughly familiar with the chosen model and understand the terminology within it.

THE ENABLING–DISABLING PROCESS

The Enabling–Disabling Process was developed at the IOM in 1997 as a framework for professional rehabilitation practice. It emphasizes the uniqueness of each individual client by revising the original Disability in America model generated by the IOM (Pope & Tarlov, 1991). A committee of professionals enhanced the 1991 IOM model "to show more clearly how biological, environmental (physical and social), and lifestyle/behavioral factors are involved in reversing the disabling process, i.e., rehabilitation, or the enabling process" (Brandt & Pope, 1997, p. 13). In the Enabling–Disabling

Process, "disability does not appear in the model since it is not inherent in the individual but [rather is] a function of the interaction of the individual and the environment" (Brandt & Pope, 1997, p. 11). Disability is seen as a product of the interaction of an individual with the environment. The model posits that rehabilitation depends largely upon the individual and his or her unique characteristics, and that the disabling process may even be reversed with appropriate rehabilitation interventions (Lutz & Bowers, 2003; Whyte, 2014). The basic concepts of this model include pathology, impairment, functional limitation, disability, and society limitation (Brandt & Pope, 1997). **Table 24-1** summarizes the concepts of the Enabling–Disabling Process.

The IOM report entitled *Enabling America* (Brandt & Pope, 1997) urged rehabilitation professionals to adopt a framework that better described the rehabilitation process. Since its introduction, however, the Enabling–Disabling Model has not received the recognition or use within healthcare professions that was probably hoped for by the IOM. A search of several notable scholarly databases over a number of years revealed few articles written by rehabilitation professionals in healthcare professions that mentioned this process or used it as a framework for research.

INTERNATIONAL CLASSIFICATION OF FUNCTIONING, DISABILITY, AND HEALTH

In 1980, WHO developed a classification system that was widely used for years internationally. WHO originally defined impairment as a loss related to structure and function; a disability was related to a loss of ability to perform an activity, and a handicap was a disadvantage for a person related to the environment.

The ICF is WHO's framework for measuring health and disability at both individual and population levels: "ICF is a classification of health and health related domains that describe body functions and structures, activities and

participation. The domains are classified from body, individual and societal perspectives" (WHO, 2007, p. 1). The ICF provides a shift in viewing disability as gradually becoming a part of the majority of the person's life over time. It provides a holistic look at the process of disability related to health, considering all aspects of the condition, not just the medical or physical characteristics (WHO, 2007). The four major sections of the classification document are body functions (by system and including mental health), body structures (by system), activities and participation (such as learning, communication, self-care, and community involvement), and environmental factors (such as products, technology, attitudes, service, and policy) (WHO, 2007). **Table 24-2** provides an overview of the ICF.

REHABILITATION TREATMENT TAXONOMY

In a document newly published in 2014, the ACRM proposed a framework for creating a rehabilitation treatment taxonomy (RTT), stating that there is a lack of universally accepted terms and concepts about rehabilitation treatment. This inconsistency makes education and training of new clinicians difficult, so a cross-disciplinary conceptual framework is needed. Such a framework would be the beginning of a new classification system (Dijkers, 2014) **(Figure 24-1)**. The proposed conceptual framework differs from the ICF model in that only what the clinician actually does for the patient is included in the scope of classification. It also "places the therapeutic hour in the context of the entire rehabilitation enterprise" (Dijkers, 2014, p. S2). Formal assessments are not considered treatment, so they are excluded from the classification system. According to proponents of the RTT, "ICF provides a useful overarching theory to help organize the RTT by characterizing enablement and disablement at several conceptual levels ... and proposing that all of these are affected by both Personal Factors and Environmental Factors" (Dijkers, Hart,

Table 24-1 CONCEPTS OF THE ENABLING–DISABLING PROCESS

Pathophysiology	Impairment	Functional Limitation	Disability	Societal Limitation
Interruption of or interference with normal physiologic and developmental processes or structures	Loss and/or abnormality of cognition, and emotional, physiologic, or anatomic structure or function, including all losses or abnormalities, not just those attributable to the initial pathophysiology	Restriction or lack of ability to perform an action in the manner or within a range consistent with the purpose of an organ or organ system	Inability or limitation in performing tasks, activities, and roles to levels expected within physical and social contexts	Restriction, attributable to social policy or barriers (structural or attitudinal), that limits fulfillment of roles or denies access to services and opportunities that are associated with full participation in society
Level of Impact				
Cells and Tissues	Organs and Organ Systems	Function of the Organ and Organ System	Individual	Society
Structural or functional	Structural or functional	Action or activity performance or organ or organ system	Task performance by person in physical, social contexts	Societal attributes relevant to individuals with disabilities
Patient Examples				
Lacunar infarct of the cerebellum (right hemisphere) related to microvascular changes associated with chronic hypertension	Neuromotor function of the brain	Left hemiparesis or difficulty with spatial–perceptual tasks, difficulty sequencing, memory deficits	Deficits in ambulation, self-care, shopping, work	Lack of adaptations in the work environment that would enable the person to continue employment

Source: Reprinted from *Archives of Physical Medicine and Rehabilitation*, 79(11), Whyte, J., Enabling America: A report from the Institute of Medicine 1998, with permission from Elsevier

Table 24-2 CONCEPTS OF THE INTERNATIONAL CLASSIFICATION OF FUNCTIONING, DISABILITY, AND HEALTH

Health Condition	Impairment	Activity Limitation	Participation Restriction
Diseases, disorders, and injuries (e.g., leprosy, diabetes, spinal cord injury)	Problems in body function or structure such as a significant deviation or loss (e.g., anxiety, paralysis, loss of sensation of extremities)	Problems in body function or structure such as a significant deviation or loss (e.g., anxiety, paralysis, loss of sensation of extremities)	Problems an individual may experience in involvement in life situations (e.g., unable to attend social events, unable to use public transportation to get to church, unable to perform job functions)
Example			
Spinal cord injury	Paralysis	Incapable of using public transportation	Unable to attend religious activities

Source: Data from World Health Organization. (2002). Towards a common language for functioning, disability and health ICF. Retrieved from www.who.int/classifications/icf/training/icfbeginnersguide.pdf.

Figure 24-1 Focus of the RTT within the Larger Care System

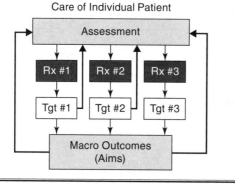

Reprinted from Hart, T., Tsaousides, T., Zanca, J. M., Whyte, J., Packel, A., Ferraro, M., & Dijkers, M. P. (2014). Toward a theory-driven classification of rehabilitation treatment. *Archives of Physical Medicine and Rehabilitation*, 95(1 suppl 1), S33–S44. Copyright (2014), with permission from Elsevier.

Tsauosides, et al., 2014, p. S12). The purpose of the RTT is to provide a way of identifying and describing treatments that result from the rehabilitation process so as to better understand the work and interventions of clinicians within the interprofessional team and to suggest a terminology and taxonomy that captures this process. The group working on the RTT describes it as a work in progress (Hart et al., 2014).

The work done thus far on the RTT presents treatment groupings by target domains. The treatment groupings include structural tissue properties, organ functions, skilled performances, and cognitive/affective representatives (**Table 24-3**). Structural tissue properties target size, shape, and flexibility; a clinical example would be wound healing. Organ functions target capacity such as change in functional output of an organ; examples would be prosthetic limbs or aerobic exercise to improve cardiovascular endurance. Skilled performances include speed and quality that require learning, such as gait training or ADLs. Cognitive/affective representations target the amount and completeness of knowledge as well as changes in attitudes or beliefs (emotions). Examples would include patient/caregiver education or referrals to community services (Hart et al., 2014).

Table 24-3 TREATMENT GROUPINGS BY TARGET DOMAINS IN A PRELIMINARY TAXONOMY OF REHABILITATION TREATMENTS

Attributes of Groupings	Structural Tissue Properties	Organ Functions	Skilled Performances	Cognitive/ Affective Representations
Typical targets	Size (Length) Shape Flexibility	Output Efficiency Capacity (of normative function) Response dynamics of system	Speed/efficiency of performance Quality (compared with standard of completeness, independence, appropriateness to context, etc.) Automaticity	Amount, completeness, accuracy of knowledge Changes in emotional reactions, emotional nuances of cognition (attitudes, beliefs, etc.)
Mechanisms of action	Tissue remodeling processes (or microscopic)	Up- or down-regulation Nonvolitional learning mechanisms (habituation, classical conditioning) Substitution of function	Learning: mix of implicit and explicit mechanisms	Semantic/affective information processing Semantic memory
Essential ingredient	Application of energy to tissues	Change in functional output of organ (system)	Facilitation of performance on part of recipient	Facilitation of acquisition of information on part of the recipient
Active ingredients (examples)	Type(s) of energy applied (thermal, mechanical, electromagnetic, etc)	Methods to enhance effort on part of recipient (eg, motivational interventions)	Set manipulations (instructions, rationales, motivational aids) Coaching guidance/cues during performance Feedback, reinforcement, response to error Provision of strategies Methods to promote generalization	Attributes of information presented (modality, organization, complexity, etc) Methods of facilitating acquisition (didactic, socratic, prompting, modeling, persuasion, etc) Methods to enhance comprehension/retention/ use

(*Continues*)

Table 24-3 TREATMENT GROUPINGS BY TARGET DOMAINS IN A PRELIMINARY TAXONOMY OF REHABILITATION TREATMENTS (CONTINUED)

Attributes of Groupings	Structural Tissue Properties	Organ Functions	Skilled Performances	Cognitive/ Affective Representations
Typical dosing parameters	Amount, intensity, schedule of energy applied Progression in Physical demands on tissue to maximize change	Progression in demand on system to maintain optimal challenge level	Progression in demands on performance to maintain optimal challenge level Schedules of practice (intensity, number/duration, patterning)	Amount of information per unit time Amount/ spacing of repetition and rehearsal
Clinical examples	Tendon lengthening (ranging, casting) Wound healing	Muscle strengthening Cardiovascular endurance exercise Deep brain stimulation Tilt table (up-regulate baroreceptor system) Transcranial direct current stimulation Prosthetic Limbs	Training in gait, activities of daily living, use of memory orthotics, alternative responses to anger triggers, etc. Dexterity/motor control exercises Mental rehearsal of physical movements	Patient/ caregiver education Adjustment counseling/ psychotherapy Referrals to community services How to (without practice)

Source: Reprinted from *Archives of Physical Medicine and Rehabilitation*, 95(1 Supplement 1), Hart, T., Tsaousides, T., Zanca, J. M., Whyte, J., Packel, A., Ferraro, M. & Dijkers, M. P., Toward a theory-driven classification of rehabilitation treatment, Pages S33–44, Copyright 2014, with permission from Elsevier.

The RTT is still in its infancy, and the creators of this taxonomy acknowledge that there is much work to be done to develop, refine, and test the framework (Dijkers, Hart, Whyte, Zanca, Packel, & Tsaousides, 2014). "Any taxonomy must be put to work in the real world to demonstrate that it can be applied to empirical data and to show that it is fruitful in research that assesses whether the outcomes of treatment support theory-driven hypotheses" (Dijkers, Hart, Tsaousides, et al., 2014, p. S10).

Historical Perspectives

Rehabilitation as a specialty within medicine, and later within nursing, was slow to develop. A general apathy toward the poor, disabled, disenfranchised, and elderly prevailed in European countries and the United States. England was the first developed country to pass legislation, in the form of the Poor Relief Act of 1662, to provide assistance to the poor and disabled (Jacelon, 2011a; Williams, 2011).

Some interest in rehabilitation emerged in the 1800s, mainly with regard to helping "crippled" children. In the first half of the 1900s, society began to focus more on the needs of persons with physical limitations. Susan Tracy, a nurse and teacher, helped to develop the discipline of occupational therapy. The first medical social service department was established at Bellevue Hospital in New York City, and Lillian Wald began the first visiting nursing service (Williams, 2011).

World War I and II provided an impetus for the growth of rehabilitation. The large number of American soldiers wounded in World War I led to the establishment of a national rehabilitation program for veterans. It is interesting to note that rehabilitation services at this time were not generally available to the public. With the discovery of sulfa drugs and antibiotics, those injured in World War II had a much greater chance of survival. In turn, the numerous veterans of World War II who came home with multiple trauma, amputations, traumatic brain injuries, and spinal cord injuries necessitated a more comprehensive rehabilitation program. During this time, Dr. Howard Rusk (1965) emerged as both a pioneer and a champion for rehabilitation, believing that these therapeutic services should be available not just to veterans, but to the entire world population. He demonstrated to military leaders through his personal assistance with the rehabilitation of those persons whom other medical professionals deemed a lost cause, that rather than convalescence, rehabilitation could promote recovery (Kottke, Stillwell, & Lehmann, 1982). Rusk showed that disabled persons could still be productive members of society and enjoy a good quality of life. As technology advances continued to expand in the 1940s, the number of civilians with industry and motor vehicle injuries increased, leading to a need for rehabilitation to address continuing disability. In 1947, Rusk established the first hospital-based medical rehabilitation services for civilians (Edwards, 2007).

The American Academy of Physical Medicine and Rehabilitation was established in 1938, and rehabilitation medicine was recognized as a board-certified medical specialty in 1947. In 1974, the Association of Rehabilitation Nurses (ARN) was created, recognizing rehabilitation as a nursing specialty.

Legislation has affected rehabilitation services in many ways. In 1954, the Hill-Burton Act (PL 83-565) provided greater financial support, research and demonstration grants, state agency expansion, and grants to expand rehabilitation facilities. The Vocational Rehabilitation Act (PL 89-333) expanded and improved vocational rehabilitation services, and the Rehabilitation Act of 1973 (PL 93-112) expanded services to more severely disabled individuals by giving them priority. It also provided affirmative action in employment and nondiscrimination in facilities. Additional laws passed in the mid-1970s provided free appropriate education for handicapped children in the least restrictive setting, and the National Housing Act Amendments of

1975 mandated removal of barriers in federally supported housing.

In the 1980s, freestanding rehabilitation hospitals were reimbursed based on reasonable costs with limits through the Tax Equity and Fiscal Responsibility Act (TEFRA). Diagnosis-related groupings (DRGs) were established in 1984 to decrease Medicare payments through a prospective payment system for acute care, and in 1989 the Omnibus Budget Reconciliation Act (OBRA) raised the standards for nursing care in nursing homes and contained significant legislation related to nursing home reform.

In 1990, the Americans with Disabilities Act (ADA; PL 101-336) established the concept of "reasonable accommodation" to avoid discrimination on the basis of disability. In 2001, the prospective payment system (PPS) was mandated for inpatient rehabilitation facilities, with the phase-in being completed in 2003 and case-mix groups (CMGs) then used as the basis for reimbursement. In 2004, the Centers for Medicare and Medicaid Services (CMS) modified the criteria used to classify inpatient rehabilitation facilities by phasing in the 75% rule; it said that by 2007, 75% of the population treated in a rehabilitation facility must match one or more specified medical conditions. In 2013–2014, a 60% rule was in effect, but return to the 75% rule is under discussion with CMS and its stakeholders (Jacelon, 2011a). The Patient Protection and Affordable Care Act (ACA) has proposed bundled payments for selected diagnoses. The ACA is still in the process of being implemented, however, and there are many unknowns related to its impact on rehabilitation services and reimbursement (Scott, 2010). Organizations such as the American Medical Rehabilitation Providers Association (AMRPA) continue to lobby and advocate for rehabilitation services and funding across settings.

As societies continue to pursue medical and technological advances that would allow persons with extreme levels of physical disability to live longer, rehabilitation has become a specialty in high demand. In the civilian population, more persons are living with disabilities, as first responders are now better equipped to aid them in surviving serious injury. However, the need to address continuing adjustment to disability remains. In addition, as life expectancy in developed countries has increased, chronic illness rates have also risen, providing additional opportunities for rehabilitation professionals to enhance quality of life for those aging with disability or acquiring it with age.

For soldiers, the types of weapons used in the wars in Iraq and Afghanistan have resulted in polytraumatic injuries never seen before. Rehabilitation professionals are being called upon to address multiple injuries in these individuals that may include a combination of multiple traumatic amputations, burns, internal organ and soft-tissue damage from explosive forces, brain and spinal injuries, as well as posttraumatic stress.

Public Policy and Rehabilitation

There are several ways in which rehabilitation services may be paid for, including Medicare, Medicaid, worker's compensation, private insurance, and Social Security disability benefits. Rehabilitation professionals should be familiar with these types of reimbursement and understand what is covered by the client's insurance provider. Case managers and social workers are team members who are excellent resources regarding payment for rehabilitation.

MEDICARE

Medicare is a federal social insurance program that provides care for persons older than the age of 65 and for certain younger persons with disabilities. The coverage and costs for Medicare change each year, so clients need to be alert to the potential for changes on an annual basis. Medicare Part A consists of the hospital insurance portion of the Medicare program, providing funds for hospital care, skilled nursing, hospice, and home health care. Medicare Part B covers medically necessary services as well as some preventive services. After a client's deductible is met, Part B covers 80% of the costs of Medicare-approved physician services, and other services including physical and occupational therapy, durable medical equipment, cardiac rehabilitation, pulmonary rehabilitation (for those persons with moderate to severe chronic obstructive pulmonary disease [COPD] within certain parameters), and prosthetics and orthotics (CMS, 2014). However, many services that a rehabilitation client may need are not covered under Medicare. For example, Medicare has limited coverage for eye or hearing exams in special cases, but it does not cover routine foot care or nursing home care. Medicare Part C, referred to as the Medicare Advantage Plan, is a combination of Parts A and B, and functions much like a preferred provider organization or health maintenance organization using managed care. Medicare Part D (CMS, 2014) is a prescription drug plan in which private companies issue plans through Medicare. Part D is available for anyone with Medicare regardless of income. Costs vary greatly within this plan, and clients would be wise to compare and review various plans each year prior to re-enrollment or plan changes.

Rehabilitation facilities and hospitals, collectively called inpatient rehabilitation facilities (IRFs), currently receive reimbursement using a PPS through the Social Security Act (CMS, 2011). The IRF PPS uses information from the Uniform Data System for Medical Rehabilitation (UDSMR), better known as the Functional Independence Measure (FIM) tool, "to classify patients into distinct groups based on clinical characteristics and expected resource needs. Separate payments are calculated for each group, including the application of case and facility level adjustments" (CMS, 2011, para 2). Codes are assigned to case-mix groups (CMGs), and Medicare pays a specific amount per discharge.

Since 2004, Medicare has been phasing in new rules for IRFs. The case-mix classifications for 2013 used the same criteria as those for 2007. The 13 medical diagnoses that are covered under the 60% IRF rule are stroke, brain injury, spinal cord injury, congenital deformity, amputation, multiple major trauma, neurologic disorders, hip fracture, burns, systemic vasculitides with joint inflammation, severe advanced osteoarthritis, rheumatoid arthritis, and certain joint replacements (CMS, 2013). Under the Affordable Care Act, more changes to rehabilitation services will likely be seen.

Medicare limits the amount it pays for physical, occupational, and speech therapy services. There is a deductible for Part B Medicare, after which Medicare pays 80% and the individual pays 20% up to the set limits for medically necessary therapies. There are some allowable exceptions to this rule, and appropriate documentation by the provider is essential.

Medicaid

Medicaid is a state-run program that is funded by both the state and the federal government; it is the largest source of medical care payments for persons with low income and limited resources. In 2007, President George W. Bush introduced a plan to place new restrictions on the rehabilitative services (called the rehab option) allowed through Medicaid, with the goal of saving the federal government $2.29 billion over 5 years. Nearly 75% of persons receiving rehab services under Medicaid were persons with mental health needs, and they were responsible for 79% of the rehab option spending (Kaiser Commission, 2007). The vast majority of states provide some type of mental or physical health services under the rehab option.

Establishing Medicaid is a complex process that varies among states. Although each state sets standards for its own programs, the federal government provides broad guidelines for those who may qualify under categorically needy, medically needy, and special groups (such as some persons with disabilities). However, therapy caps are determined on a calendar-year basis and have been in effect since 2011 (CMS, 2011). The current and predicted implementation of the Affordable Care Act suggests that definitions of who qualifies for Medicaid may change and become broader. States must provide long-term care for persons who are Medicaid eligible. State Medicaid programs offer a variety of services within a variety of settings. Services that are provided relative to rehabilitation for the categorically needy include hospitalization, lab tests and X-rays, nursing facilities for those age 21 and older, physician and some nurse practitioner services, medical–surgical dental needs, and home health (CMS, 2011).

WORKER'S COMPENSATION

Worker's compensation is a state income-supported program. For a person to be eligible for this benefit, the injury or condition must be work related. Four major disability compensation programs exist: wage replacement benefits, medical treatment, vocational rehabilitation, and other benefits (U.S. Department of Labor, 2014). Benefits are usually calculated as a percentage of the employee's weekly earnings at the time the injury occurred. Each state places restrictions on the maximum amount of benefits, which is often set at two-thirds of the employee's gross salary (Deutsch & Dean-Baar, 2007). The types of benefits may range from temporary partial or total disability, to permanent partial or total disability, to death. Some states have a maximum benefit period, and some may require a waiting period. Disabled workers may be compensated through spousal benefits (in case of death), medical and rehabilitation expense coverage, and lost wages. The current set of worker's compensation programs are more restrictive than they once were; they limit physician choice and eligibility, provide lower benefits, and use managed care for cost containment (U.S. Department of Labor, 2014).

PRIVATE INSURANCE

Most private insurance pays for at least some rehabilitative services. There is generally a deductible and often a copayment, which may be higher if the provider is not a member of the network of providers contracted by the insurance company. In the case where the person has private insurance and Medicare as a secondary payer, much of the therapy services may be covered, provided there is sufficient and ongoing documentation of medical necessity and progress toward goals. Private insurance may also provide disability income insurance, accidental death and dismemberment insurance, or other benefits.

SOCIAL SECURITY DISABILITY INCOME

Social Security Disability Income (SSDI) was established in 1956 as part of the Social Security Disability Act of 1954. This federally administered disability insurance program covers those persons who meet the strict definition of disability under Social Security. The criteria for disability are threefold: (1) the person cannot do the same work he or she did before; (2) it is determined that the person cannot adapt to other work because of the existing medical condition; and (3) the disability has lasted for at least 1 year, or is expected to result in death (Social Security Administration, 2014). The person must also have worked and paid into the Social Security program before the disability. SSDI is paid as a monthly benefit.

Supplemental Security Income (SSI) may provide disability benefits for persons who have not worked long enough to receive SSDI. The SSI program pays benefits to disabled adults and children with limited income and resources, and to certain older persons with severely limited income. Persons may receive a monthly check. The SSI program also helps individuals to access Medicare benefits and take advantage of other possible assistance through the federal government. Eligibility for the program is based on income and resources (Social Security Administration, 2014).

DISABILITY BENEFITS FOR VETERANS

The Department of Veterans Affairs (VA) provides a number of benefits for veterans: "Disability compensation is a benefit paid to a veteran because of injuries or diseases that happened while on active duty, or were made worse by active military service. It is also paid to certain veterans disabled from VA health care" (U.S. Department of Veterans Affairs, 2011). These benefits are tax free and may include a monthly stipend (ranging from $123 to $2,673), priority medical care through the VA, clothing and housing allowances (to make accommodations), adaptive equipment, and various grants as needed (U.S. Department of Veterans Affairs, 2010). The VA also provides vocational rehabilitation by maintaining working relationships with many businesses that employ veterans with physical, mental, or emotional disabilities. Consultation is available in many areas including employment, assistive technology, case management, work-site and job analysis, and help in addressing ADA compliance issues (U.S. Department of Veterans Affairs, 2014).

VOCATIONAL REHABILITATION

Vocational rehabilitation is an important part of the rehabilitation process, carrying heavier weight for those of working age and certain racial/ethnic groups for whom work is part of personal identity and reputation. In 1918, Congress passed the Smith-Sears Act to assist with national vocational rehabilitation services to veterans who served in World War I. In 1920, the Smith-Fess Act made vocational rehabilitation services available for all persons with disabilities, not just those with war-related injuries (Buchanan, 1996). More significant legislation was enacted when the Rehabilitation Act of 1973 provided funds to support state vocational rehabilitation programs.

The Rehabilitation Services Administration (RSA) of the U.S. Department of Education coordinates vocational rehabilitation services. The RSA "oversees grant programs that help individuals with physical or mental disabilities to obtain employment and live more independently through the provision of such supports as counseling, medical and psychological services, job training and other individualized services" (U.S. Department of Education, 2014, p. 1). This is accomplished through dispensing funds to state grant programs to assist them with finding work-related services or programs for persons with disabilities, particularly the severely disabled. The RSA is the Congressionally appointed federal agency charged with implementing the various titles associated with the Rehabilitation Act of 1973. This agency acts as a resource for information and a leader in advocating at all levels for national programs that help to remove barriers for persons with disabilities (U.S. Department of Education, 2014).

The services provided in vocational rehabilitation are many, but generally include personal counseling, mental and physical health services, and assistance with vocational placement and job training (U.S. Department of Education, 2014). In addition, the RSA helps administer projects among specific groups of persons such as migrant and seasonal farm workers, American Indians, older adults, and the visually impaired.

One principle of vocational rehabilitation is that informed consumer choice promotes enhanced employment outcomes. For vocational rehabilitation to be effective and enhance quality of life for the person with mental disabilities, the agency and counselors must work closely with the employer and the client to find the working environment best suited to that individual (Inman, McGurk, & Chadwick, 2007; Morgan, 2007). Employment outcomes are most frequently used as the measure of the success (Kosciulek, 2007).

Vocational rehabilitation may not be a goal for all rehabilitation clients. Many older adults requiring rehabilitation services are retired, for example, so employment is not a goal. However, for those younger persons with functional limitations or mental health impairments, work may be directly related to their sense of self and identity within their culture. For these persons, vocational rehabilitation plays an important role in the comprehensive rehabilitation process, and the vocational rehabilitation counselor is an essential team member.

AMERICANS WITH DISABILITIES ACT

The ADA, which was enacted in 1990, guarantees individuals with physical disabilities equal access to public accommodations related to transportation, education, and employment. Employment discrimination of qualified applicants because of disabilities is prohibited by this law (U.S. Equal Employment Opportunity Commission, 2008). Although the Rehabilitation Act of 1973 and its amendments covered accessibility to buildings of organizations that received federal financial assistance, the ADA requires private organizations to comply with accessibility and employment laws. The concept of reasonable accommodation was introduced with the ADA, requiring employers to make those accommodations within reason that may be necessary for a person with disability. The ADA addresses four major areas: employment, public services, public accommodations services by practice entities, and telecommunications relay.

Rehabilitation Issues and Challenges

Rehabilitation services provided by an interprofessional team within a variety of settings suggest several possible challenges for providers. In particular, problematic issues include the rising costs of care, caregiver burden, inequities among those with disabilities, the negative image of disability, the changing composition of

the disabled population, ethical issues, providing culturally competent care, and professional and informal caregiver issues.

Rising Care Costs

An estimated 133 million Americans have at least one chronic illness, with 25% of those individuals having one or more daily activity limitations (Centers for Disease Control and Prevention [CDC], 2009). Forty-two million persons (17% of the U.S. population) were uninsured in 2012 (although with implementation of the ACA, those numbers may decrease) and 32 million (13%) received Medicaid assistance. Of those uninsured, the major reason cited was cost.

Approximately 10.7 million (5%) adults are unable to work because of health-related problems. Some 39.7 million persons (12%) are limited in their usual activities due to a chronic health problem (U.S. Department of Health and Human Services, 2013). Persons with less education and low incomes are less likely to be able to work because of health problems (Adams, Kirzinger, & Martinez, 2011). The U.S. government spends about $260 billion per year on assistance for persons with disabilities (Hall, 2013).

Given these statistics, major challenges for rehabilitation professionals are to assist persons to attain and regain their health and become productive, working members of society, and to explore other means of providing access to health care.

Caregiver Burden

Because an event requiring rehabilitation happens to the entire family and community, not just the client, it is important to address the needs of caregivers throughout the rehabilitation process and/or chronic illness trajectory. Approximately 52 million persons in the United States serve as caregivers to adults (aged 18 or older) with a disability or illness. The typical caregiver is a 48-year-old female providing care to a family member for an average of 4.6 years (National Alliance for Caregiving & AARP, 2009).

> *The Home Alone study—a study of family caregivers who provide complex chronic care—found that nearly half of the caregivers surveyed (46% or 777) performed medical and nursing tasks. More than 96% (747) also provided activities of daily living (ADLs) supports (e.g., personal hygiene, dressing/undressing, or getting in and out of bed) or instrumental activities of daily living (IADLs) (e.g., taking prescribed medications, shopping for groceries, transportation, or using technology) supports, or both. Of these caregivers, nearly two-thirds (501) did all three types of tasks. Of the non-medical family caregivers, two-thirds (605) provided IADL assistance only. (Family Caregiver Alliance, 2012)*

Minority caregivers also experience disparities in this role. For example, minority caregivers providing care for seniors in urban areas have been found to be poorer, have Medicaid coverage, and have higher rates of disability. Hispanics have more unmet hours of care, and caregiver services appear "less likely to help African Americans remain at home" (Herrera, George, Angel, Markides, & Torres-Gil, 2013, p. 35).

The caregiver's ability to cope with the family member's care demands is influenced by a variety of factors, including the type and severity of illness, the length of quality of recovery, social support, inherent caregiver factors, and coping ability. This may hold true for both formal and informal caregivers (Bushnik, Wright, & Burdsall, 2007). For example, the caregiver spouse of a person with uncomplicated coronary bypass surgery may be able to meet care demands over a limited period of rehabilitation. By comparison, the older spouse caregiver of a stroke survivor with severe aphasia and functional deficits may be facing years of caregiving—a burden that is often overwhelming.

Caregiver burden—referring to the effects of caregiving-related stress on family members or other care providers—has been associated with a number of health problems in caregivers. These problems, which are well documented in research originating in many countries, suggest that caregiver burden or caregiver strain is a universally experienced phenomenon. Emotional distress, anxiety, depression, decreased quality of life, hypertension, lowered immune function, decreased marital quality, impaired family functioning, and increased mortality are among the concerns noted by researchers of caregivers (Al-Krenawi, Graham, & Gharaibeh, 2011; Bayen et al., 2013; Cecil, Thompson, Parahoo, & McCaughen, 2013; De Souza Olivereira, Cordeiro Rodrigues, Carvalho De Sousa, De Sousa Costa, De Oli7vereira Lopes, & De Araujo, 2013; Grunfeld et al., 2004; King, Hartke, & Denby, 2007; Rattanasuk, Nantachaipan, Sucamvang, & Moongtui, 2013; Ski & O'Connell, 2007). There is sufficient research to demonstrate that the burden of caregiving over time can have deleterious effects on the health of the family caregiver.

Caregiver burden is thought to be greater when more care is required. Research suggests that although education and training programs have some effect on caregiver stress levels, the benefit is short term and caregivers are likely to need ongoing involvement from care professionals to help maintain their own health (Draper, Bowring, Thompson, Van Heyst, Conroy, & Thompson, 2007; Halm, Treat-Jacobson, Lindquist, & Savik, 2007; King et al., 2007). The perceived rewards of caregiving, however, may have an effect on the well-being of caregivers (Rattanasuk et al., 2013).

Assessment of caregiver burden should be included in the rehabilitation plan of care. Early identification and interventions related to managing caregiver stress may result in better outcomes for the entire family, and appropriate discharge planning and follow-up are an important part of the process.

Inequities Among Disabled Americans

The Office of Minority Health and Health Equity "aims to accelerate CDC's health impact in the U.S. population and to eliminate health disparities for vulnerable populations as defined by race/ethnicity, socio-economic status, geography, gender, age, disability status, risk status related to sex and gender, and among other populations identified as at-risk for health disparities" (CDC, Office of Minority Health and Health Equity, 2013, para 1). Those racial and ethnic populations considered minorities include Asian Americans, blacks or African Americans, Hispanics or Latinos, and Native Hawaiians and Other Pacific Islanders.

According to the National Health Interview Survey (NHIS) on disability (CDC, 2014), there are 34 million to 43 million people in the United States with physical and mental disabilities. In 2006, 5.9% of the working-age population in the United States received disability benefits. The Disability Statistics Compendium (2013) indicates that persons with disabilities account for more than 12% of the U.S. population.

Although the 2013 CDC Health Disparities and Inequalities Report showed an improvement in morbidity and mortality among minority groups as a result of the *Healthy People 2010* and *Healthy People 2020* initiatives, non-Hispanic black adults were still at least 50% more likely to die of heart disease or stroke prematurely (i.e., before age 75 years) than non-Hispanic whites in the same cohort. Diabetes prevalence among adults is higher among Hispanics, non-Hispanic blacks, and those of other or mixed races than among Asians and non-Hispanic whites; it is also higher among persons without a college degree and members of lower socioeconomic groups (CDC, Office of Minority Health and Health Equity, 2013).

In the United States, the groups considered vulnerable populations (in which disparities in access to health care and transportation are often most prominent) include some minority groups, children, the elderly, the poor, those living in rural areas, those with intellectual and developmental disabilities, and those with mental illness (CDC, 2014; President's Committee for People with Intellectual Disabilities, 2009). The nearly 8 million persons with intellectual and developmental disabilities make up approximately 3% of the population (President's Committee for People with Intellectual Disabilities, 2009; Ward, Nichols, & Freedman, 2010). Individuals in this subgroup often have challenges with language, self-care, and mobility.

Both older age and poverty are factors that are associated with poorer health status and increased disability. The poor elderly population is three to four times more likely to need assistance with ADLs and IADLs than those who are not poor (Adams, Dey, & Vickerie, 2007).

Many persons in minority groups experience a double jeopardy or double minority status when they acquire disability. Caucasians and Asians, for example, are more likely to report excellent health than African Americans. Hispanic persons younger than age 65 (34%) are more than 2.5 times as likely as non-Hispanics (14%) in the same age cohort to be uninsured.

Studies suggest that there is also disparity between ethnic groups with regard to stroke rehabilitation. African Americans may have less positive outcomes from stroke rehabilitation than Caucasian Americans. "In addition to health status, the rehabilitation care of [African Americans with stroke] may be influenced by cultural and or racial similarities or differences that exist between themselves and their physical therapists" (Greene, 2013, p. 1). Additional research is needed in many areas of rehabilitation related to ethnic and racial diversity.

An example of the importance of cultural sensitivity and knowledge is the practice of pain management among different ethnic or cultural groups. Clients might not take their pain medications because of fear of addiction or out of a belief that pain is a punishment they deserve for some wrongdoing (Monisvais, 2011). Chronic pain rehabilitation and functional outcomes are poorer among African Americans than Caucasians (Hooten, Knight-Brown, Townsend, & Laures, 2012). Persons with chronic pain may also constitute a subgroup whose members share similar behaviors such as overdramatizing, underusing the healthcare system, and not fully disclosing information to providers (Monisvais & Engebretson, 2011).

Stigma of Disability

Stigma is defined as "the application of set attitudes about and stereotypes of people with disabilities" (Jacelon, 2011b). The Framework Integrating Normative Influences of Stigma (FINIS) provides a means of better understanding of the effects of stigma on the lives of persons with disabilities (Pescosolido, Martin, Lang, & Olafsdottir, 2008).

Although much progress has been made on a national policy level toward dispelling the negative image and stigma associated with disability through modifying rehabilitation models (Brandt & Pope, 1997; WHO, 2002), many persons with disabilities still report feelings of negative reactions from others regarding their differences. The impact of the disability could range from something as relatively invisible as a hearing aid worn by an adolescent (Kent & Smith, 2006) to obvious employment discrimination for a person with mental illness (Lloyd & Waghorn, 2007; Stuart, 2006). One study found that a positive factor, such as exercise done by a person with a physical disability, may undermine the negative impressions that some persons have and fight the stigma of disability (Arbour, Latimer, Ginis, & Jung, 2007).

Ethical and Legal Issues

Rehabilitation professionals are often in positions that require difficult decision making. Ethics refers to the reasons or beliefs that guide thinking and behavior (Bratcher, Farrell, Stevens, & Vanderground, 2012). Beauchamp and Childress (2008), in their classic text on principles of biomedical ethics, emphasize the four cornerstone principles: respect for person, nonmaleficence, beneficence, and justice. These principles play into many aspects of rehabilitation practice and programming. Common ethical (and often legal) issues that pertain particularly to rehabilitation clients have been identified by a variety of authors (Bratcher et al., 2012; Hackman, 2011; Kothe, 2014; Tapper, Vercler, Cruze, & Sexson, 2010).

Ethical dilemmas arise when there is conflict between such principles (**Table 24-4**). As an example, consider the situation of a nonterminal rehabilitation client who has just told his nurse that he does not wish to be resuscitated if he should "code." However, the paperwork for advance directives has yet to be completed, signed, or placed on the chart. Minutes after having the conversion with the client, the nurse finds the client without a pulse or respirations. Although she must call the code team in this situation, the nurse is in conflict because she has intimate knowledge that this was action was contrary to the client's wishes. The nurse experiences an ethical dilemma because on the one hand she wants to support the patient's autonomy and right to choose, but on the other hand she must follow the law and the policies of her facility.

Rehabilitation professionals are advocates for the patient, but they must also follow the dictates of ethical and moral principles as well as the laws of the state. Hospital or organization ethics boards can help sort out matters when difficult decisions must be made or there is a lack of agreement among patients, family, and staff members.

Ethics committees are established in acute care hospitals and even retirement communities to assist in difficult decision making (Tapper et al., 2010). An ethics committee is a team of healthcare professionals that is established specifically to address ethical dilemmas that occur in a particular setting. Persons serving on this committee may include physicians, nurses, advanced practice nurses, physician assistants,

Table 24-4 POTENTIAL ETHICAL CONFLICTS

Withholding or withdrawing treatment	Determining competence in decision making
Do not resuscitate (DNR) orders	Use of physical or chemical restraints
Genetic screening	Organ donation
Guardianship	Research on human subjects
Use of stem cells and stem cell research	Disagreement between family members about treatment options
Use of complementary or alternative medicine	
Advance directives	Life-prolonging declarations, living wills
Informed consent	HIV/AIDS rehabilitation
Medical futility	Estate planning
Determining legal death or brain death	Substance abuse
Rehab of a person with terminal disease	Confidentiality
Defining quality of life	Self-termination or assisted suicide
Euthanasia	Abuse of the vulnerable
Allocation of resources	Long-term care placement

social workers, therapists, pastoral care personnel, members of the community, and ethicists. The benefits of an ethics committee include allowing many perspectives to be discussed, providing a forum for communication, fostering development of related policies, promoting awareness of existing and potential issues, and focusing on the patient (Masters-Farrell, 2007). Some disadvantages include the potential for inefficiency and political influence, and lack of time for participation. Common topics that ethics committees discuss or provide consultation on may include confidentiality, medical futility, brain death, or staff errors. At large medical centers, ethical consults are more common in the areas of obstetrics, general medicine, surgery, and pregnancy, than in rehabilitation (Tapper et al., 2010).

Cultural Competency

Cultural sensitivity involves an awareness and consideration of a group's beliefs, values, communication styles, language, and behavior. Providing culturally sensitive rehabilitation care will be an even greater challenge in the United States in the future, given the country's changing demographics and increasing minority elderly population (Cot, 2013). How clients and families perceive disability and participate in rehabilitation is heavily influenced by cultural norms and expectations (Buse, Burker, & Bernacchio, 2013; Campinha-Bacote, 2001). For example, cultural variations in resilience after a trauma have been examined, with the research suggesting that individuals who were raised in a collectivist society may not benefit from the normal emphasis that Western rehabilitation therapists place on individual goals and recovery (Buse et al., 2013). The first step in becoming culturally sensitive is to know one's own self.

Although some generalizations will be discussed here related to the major ethnic–racial groups, professionals should avoid stereotyping and seek individual information from each client. Because of the vast differences between and within the many cultural groups that rehabilitation professionals serve, it is wise to ask clients about their particular beliefs and practices. If needed, the services of a translator (not a family member) should be used.

African Americans are a group at high risk for many disabilities and chronic illnesses that warrant rehabilitative care, including hypertension, stroke, diabetes, and heart disease. African Americans typically have a close family structure, maintain deep religious affiliations, and share a strong belief against placing older parents in long-term care facilities. They are generally open to rehabilitation programs and tend to experience disabling conditions at a younger age than do Caucasians. Career counseling for African Americans with disabilities should take into account the effects of double minority status: disability and racial. Rehabilitation professionals should realize that prejudice, oppression, and stigma are often attached to both of these factors, and a multidimensional, multicultural approach to care should be used (Mpofu & Harley, 2006; Shannon & Hassler, 2014).

Hispanic and Latino Americans also enjoy strong family bonds. There is generally good family involvement for clients experiencing rehabilitation. However, severe disability may be seen as a punishment from God for some evil or wrongdoing and, therefore, may stigmatize a person or family. Latinos tend to continue to work with a disability, but in some instances may show poorer outcomes, such as difficulty adjusting to life after stroke (Cook, Stickley, Ramey, & Knotts, 2005). In addition, Latino Americans may experience more difficulty with vocational rehabilitation if they are less enculturated in the U.S. health system and have limited English language skills. There may be a mistrust of vocational rehabilitation services as well (Velcoff, Hernandez, & Keys, 2010).

Among Asian cultures, there is a diversity of beliefs. However, a respect for healthcare professionals as well as Eastern healers often means that Asians will seek treatment for rehabilitative conditions. In Chinese and Japanese cultures, there is belief in the need for balance between positive and negative forces, between the hot and cold, between the male and female. These opposing and related forces are referred to as the yin and the yang. When the body is out of harmony, or lacks balance, illness may occur; emotional problems are believed to be linked to a weak character. There may be feelings of guilt and shame in having a disability, because it could indicate punishment for wrongdoing. Work is seen as fundamental to a successful and honorable life, but in Hong Kong, only 2.5% of Chinese males with psychiatric disabilities are permitted to seek employment (Shannon & Hassler, 2014).

According to the 2012 census, there were approximately 5.2 million American Indians and Alaskan Natives in the United States. There are 565 recognized populations, each with its own customs and beliefs (CDC, 2013a). These groups, in general, embrace the interrelatedness of the earth with the body and spirit, but tribes often have their own culturally distinct practices. They rely on a relatively private extended community and kinship ties. Most traditional American Indians value folk medicine over Westernized medical treatments and facilities. There is an innate distrust of persons outside their community, given these minorities' history of oppression. Mortality has been drastically higher for American Indians when compared to the general U.S. population related to the following conditions: chronic liver disease/cirrhosis, 368%; diabetes mellitus, 177%; unintentional injuries, 138% ; assault/homicide, 82%; and intentional harm/suicide, 65% (Indian Health Services [IHS], 2014). In 2009, the leading causes of death in the American Indian population were heart disease, cancer, unintentional injuries, diabetes, chronic liver disease and cirrhosis, chronic lower respiratory disease, stroke, and suicide (CDC, 2013a).

Rehabilitation professionals must be aware that today's American Indians may come from a mixed background of tribal customs, and that many still believe in folk healers.

Professional Caregiver Issues

As the U.S. population increases and the oldest of the old become the fastest-growing age group, there will be a lack of physicians and nurses who are prepared to meet the demand for care of the many persons with chronic illness and disability. Currently, there are 10,000 board-certified physiatrists in the United States (Association of Academic Physiatrists, 2014) and more than 10,000 nurses who hold the certified rehabilitation registered nurse (CRRN) credential. The ARN has strongly advocated for certification in rehabilitation. However, few nursing programs provide rehabilitation education as a separate course or have dedicated content to this specialty area. Getting healthcare professionals such as physicians and nurses interested in the specialty has been difficult because of its limited visibility in traditional educational programs (Thompson, Emrich, & Moore, 2003). However, part of the ARN's (2013) strategic plan is to integrate rehabilitation nursing concepts into all aspects of health care. Initiatives are currently under way toward meeting that objective.

With more than 40.4 million people in America older than 65 years of age as of 2010 (Lehman & Wirt, 2014), there is an increased need for professionals trained to provide quality care to older adults. Older adults with one chronic condition number account for nearly 80% of the elderly population, and 50% have at least two chronic conditions. Heart disease, cancer, and stroke remain the leading causes of death among those aged 65 and older (National Center for Chronic Disease Prevention and Health Promotion, 2009). Yet, most nursing schools in the United States have no full-time faculty certified in geriatric nursing and only a few of the nation's medical schools have a geriatric department. Fewer than 1% of RNs and

fewer than 3% of advanced practice nurses are certified in geriatrics. As of 2005, fewer than one-third of nursing programs required a course in geriatrics (Robert Wood Johnson Foundation, 2012).

Despite concerted efforts to change this perception, care of older adults continues to have a negative stigma among nursing students. Without education in gerontology, healthcare professionals may not realize the rehabilitation potential of many of these older adults. The common rehabilitative disorders are often seen in the older age group, and even small improvements in function and independence can allow older adults to age in place and remain at home. Even those persons who make long-term care or retirement communities their home can improve their strength and function with small lifestyle changes and exercise.

There is also a growing number of persons whose caregiving needs go unmet.

The Affordable Care Act (ACA) appropriately recognized the need to increase the number of highly skilled nurses available to care for an aging population and created a number of important tools to better ensure that all Americans can have access to quality health care when and where they need it. Through its funding for the new Centers for Medicare and Medicaid Services Innovation Center and funding for nurse-managed clinics, the ACA also provides important opportunities to promote and highlight nursing leadership. (Winnifred Quinn, as quoted in Robert Wood Johnson Foundation, 2012, p. 1)

More than 34 million persons are limited in some way from usual activities because of chronic illness. In the United States, an estimated 3.8 million adults with disabilities require assistance with ADLs and 7.8 million need help with IADLs (Adams et al., 2007). Persons who need assistance are more likely to be poor, older, and less educated. Persons whose needs are not met are more likely to experience discomfort, weight loss, dehydration, falls, and burns (LaPlante, Kaye, Kang, & Harrington, 2004). Further research is needed to help identify the consequences of their unmet caregiving needs as well as strategies to address this growing problem.

Interventions

The Rehabilitation Process

Rehabilitation is both a philosophy and a discipline (Jacelon, 2011a). It is based on the premise that all individuals have self-worth and are deserving of dignity, respect, and quality health care regardless of their limitations. Many concepts are embedded in the field of rehabilitation and are reflected through such common sayings as the following:

- Rehabilitation begins day one.
- What you do not use, you lose.
- Progress is measured in small gains.
- Independence is better than dependence.
- Motivation is a key to success.
- All care should include rehabilitation principles.
- Activity strengthens and inactivity wastes.
- If it can be corrected, it probably could have been prevented.

Rehabilitation should begin from the first day the person is in the hospital. When healthcare professionals forget the basic principles of rehabilitation, complications such as contractures, pressure sores, and incontinence ensue. Rehabilitation includes nursing, medical therapies, and social services. It is an interprofessional team process focused on maintaining or restoring function, preventing complications, promoting independence and self-care, and enhancing quality of life.

Team Approach

The team approach is most effective when working with clients with complex needs such as those requiring rehabilitative services. Although several models are used with this approach, the common threads are that the team members work toward goals that are mutually established with the client.

Prevailing models are either multidisciplinary, interdisciplinary, or transdisciplinary. Multidisciplinary teams involve professionals from different disciplines, each treating the client within his or her particular area; however, these professionals may not coordinate their efforts in the care of a client (Jacelon, 2011a). The advantage of this type of model is that all professionals bring their education and expertise to promote the best outcomes for the client. The major weakness is that communication between and across the disciplines may be lacking.

In the transdisciplinary model, each client has a primary therapist from the team, who may be a nurse, physical therapist, or occupational therapist. One therapist is cross-trained to provide comprehensive care to the client (Behm & Gray, 2012). Although this model may provide for continuity of care, issues surrounding licensure, scope of practice, and accountability abound. In addition, team members are often out of their comfort zone in providing services that they were not specifically trained for. Turf issues may complicate this type of care as well. Lastly, some organizations that have tried this model have given it up for a different approach because the team was not motivated to embrace it.

The most preferred rehabilitation team model is the interdisciplinary team (**Table 24-5**). This approach involves each team member communicating on a regular basis with each other team member and establishing common goals for clients (Behm & Gray, 2012; Jacelon, 2011a; Williams & Doeschot, 2011). This is often accomplished through weekly team meetings in which the entire team reviews the progress of each client and mutual goals are discussed and updated. The client and family are an important part of the team as well. Nontraditional team

---

Table 24-5 MEMBERS OF THE
REHABILITATION TEAM

Physiatrist

Certified rehabilitation registered nurse

Certified nursing assistant

Physical therapist

Physical therapist assistant

Occupational therapist

Certified occupational therapy assistant

Speech therapist/speech-language pathologist

Audiologist

Dietitian/nutritionist

Social worker

Psychologist

Therapeutic recreation specialist

Pastoral counselor

Prosthetist/orthotist

Case manager

---

members may be added to the team based on the client's specific needs.

EVALUATION OF THE CLIENT

An important element in considering rehabilitation as an option for any client is proper evaluation of rehabilitation potential. Many factors may be considered as part of such an evaluation, but several forces play a major role. These include the severity of the illness, injury, or defect; the client's functional level and cognitive status; physical indicators such as range of motion and muscle strength; and socioeconomic factors (Koenig, Teixeira, & Yetzer, 2014).

Rehabilitation Potential   For purposes of insurance coverage (i.e., the healthcare payers), clients receiving inpatient rehabilitation need to meet the minimum requirements of being

able to tolerate at least 3 hours of therapy per day (Jacelon, 2011a). Generally, a professional is assigned to do an evaluation of rehabilitation potential before the client is admitted to a program. This professional may be a social worker, nurse, case manager, clinical nurse specialist, or other clinician with appropriate education and evaluation skills. No one type of client provides a perfect profile of the usual patient. Rather, the evaluator uses his or her assessment skills to consider all the aspects of the person's life that could contribute to success in an intensive therapeutic program, such as the likelihood of functional improvement given the person's illness or injury, internal motivation, and available support.

Although general criteria are followed for admission to a rehabilitation program, the uniqueness of each individual is considered by the evaluator. Over time, healthcare professionals develop an intuition that aids them in selecting clients who are appropriate rehabilitation candidates. There may be occasions when, for example, a person who has a low level of functioning as a result of traumatic brain injury but is highly motivated and has strong family support achieves a better rehabilitation outcome than a stroke patient with minimal functional deficits but whose negative attitude is a deterrent to readiness for intensive therapy. Sometimes clients will be referred to a transitional care unit or post-acute care prior to rehabilitation admission, and then days or weeks later they may feel the motivation to enter acute rehabilitation.

Strengths of the Client, Family, and Environment   Another important factor in the evaluation process is the identification of the client's and family's strengths. Questions to ask during this assessment include the following: What can the client do for himself or herself? What does the client see as his or her own strengths and weaknesses? What are the family's strengths and weaknesses? Which coping mechanisms does the client typically use, and will they be sufficient for the current crisis? Which community resources are available to the family and client? What are the client's personal goals? A highly motivated client and supportive family are important to the success of the rehabilitation process.

Functional Assessment   Although functional assessment is important, the evaluator should not forget that a true evaluation of rehabilitation potential must consider all factors, not just physical or function related. Functional assessment includes an evaluation that identifies one's ability to perform self-care and physical activities. The two approaches generally used to perform this assessment are asking questions and observation (Guse, 2014).

A number of tools are available to assess function, although they are mainly aimed at screening for disability. Functional assessment tools include "(1) the development of a client problem list, (2) goal setting based on identified strengths and weaknesses of the client, (3) evaluation of the client's progress and outcomes, (4) measurement of treatment interventions, (5) cost–benefit effectiveness of care, (6) assistance in the rehabilitation program's evaluation and audit, and (7) research" (Remsburg & Carson, 2006, p. 601). Some commonly used assessment tools are discussed later in this section.

Evaluators may use a variety of methods to complete a functional assessment. Generally, a combination of self-report, in the form of a questionnaire completed by either the person or the interviewer, and observation are used. An example of an easy-to-use tool to assess general geriatric health is the Timed Up and Go (TUG) test. In this test, the person is asked to rise up from a chair, walk 10 feet, turn around, walk back to their chair and sit back down. Increased TUG times have been associated with falls in the elderly (Podsiadlo & Richardson, 1991).

The FIM (Uniform Data System for Medical Rehabilitation, 1997) is the most widely accepted and used performance-based measure of ADLs (**Figure 24-2**). A revised version of the FIM (called the Wee-FIM) is available for pediatric patients. The FIM instrument is completed by a trained evaluator, who assesses the client on 18 performance items using a 7-level scale. The tool is completed upon admission, at discharge, and often several times in between to monitor progress. The total score of all categories can help to show improvement over time. The evaluator may be one person, or different team members may complete various parts of the FIM tool based on their expertise. For example, the nurse may complete the sphincter control item and the speech therapist may complete the communication section. Team members base their evaluation on direct observation of the subject. The items assessed include self-care, sphincter control, transfers, locomotion, communication, and social cognition. The evaluator quantifies each category by determining how much assistance is required in each category. A score of 1 means total assistance was needed and the subject provided less than 25% of the effort. A score of 7 signifies complete independence in a timely and safe manner (i.e., the subject is completely independent in that activity).

The usefulness or accuracy of some of these tools has been called into question by some critics. It is wise to investigate the development path of the instrument and to determine which patient groups were used during its development. In addition, the outcomes of a tool are generally somewhat dependent upon the person using it, so it is essential that evaluators are properly educated in the use of the instrument. Many tools have questionable generalizability to older adults and may not take into consideration the normal effects of aging.

Rehabilitation Nursing

Rehabilitation is a growing specialty, and nursing is an emerging leader in this field.

Figure 24-2 FIM Instrument.

LEVELS	7 Complete Independence (Timely, Safely) 6 Modified Independence (Device)	NO HELPER
	Modified Dependence 5 Supervision (Subject = 100%+) 4 Minimal Assist (Subject = 75%+) 3 Moderate Assist (Subject = 50%+) **Complete Dependence** 2 Maximal Assist (Subject = 25%+) 1 Total Assist (Subject = less than 25%)	HELPER

	ADMISSION	DISCHARGE	FOLLOW-UP
Self-Care A. Eating B. Grooming C. Bathing D. Dressing - Upper Body E. Dressing - Lower Body F. Toileting			
Sphincter Control G. Bladder Management H. Bowel Management			
Transfers I. Bed, Chair, Wheelchair J. Toilet K. Tub, shower			
Locomotion L. Walk/Wheelchair M. Stairs	W Walk C Wheelchair B Both	W Walk C Wheelchair B Both	W Walk C Wheelchair B Both
Motor Subtotal Score			
Communication N. Comprehension O. Expression	A Auditory V Visual B Both V Vocal N Nonvocal B Both	A Auditory V Visual B Both V Vocal N Nonvocal B Both	A Auditory V Visual B Both V Vocal N Nonvocal B Both
Social Cognition P. Social Interaction Q. Problem Solving R. Memory			
Cognitive Subtotal Score			
TOTAL FIM Score			

NOTE: Leave no blanks. Enter 1 if patient not testable due to risk.

Specialties such as rehabilitation nursing are often impacted by the wars that create larger numbers of veterans with multiple traumatic injuries that require rehabilitation. Rehabilitation nurses are finding themselves working in a wider variety of settings and subspecialties to meet the growing demand for their services.

In 1984, the ARN offered the first certification for registered nurses (RNs) working with rehabilitation clients. This credential, the CRRN, is the basic designation for this nursing specialty. There are more than 10,000 CRRNs today (ARN, 2010). In 1997, an advanced practice certification, the certified rehabilitation registered nurse—advanced (CRRN-A) was offered, but because of the smaller number of nurses sitting for the exam and changes in certification methods, it was phased out in 2009. The ARN (2010) also supports a variety of specialized practice roles for rehabilitation nurses. Role descriptions that have been developed by the ARN for rehabilitation nurses for the subspecialties are listed in (**Table 24-6**).

Table 24-6 Rehabilitation Nursing Roles

Gerontologic rehabilitation nurse
Homecare rehabilitation nurse
Pain management rehabilitation nurse
Pediatric rehabilitation nurse
Rehabilitation nurse manager
Rehabilitation admissions liaison nurse
Advanced practice rehabilitation nurse
Rehabilitation nurse case manager
Rehabilitation nurse educator
Rehabilitation staff nurse
Rehabilitation nurse researcher

Source: Data from Association of Rehabilitation Nurses. (2010). Role description brochures. Retrieved from http://www .rehabnurse.org/pubs/role/index.html.

Rehabilitation Settings

Rehabilitation services are offered in a wide variety of settings and are considered a philosophy of care, rather than being defined by the setting. Settings in which such care is delivered may include freestanding rehabilitation facilities, acute rehabilitation units within hospitals, long-term care facilities, or the home. Regardless of the setting for care, services should be provided by an interdisciplinary team of trained professionals. In the past, rehabilitation units, especially those within hospitals, served patients with diverse diagnoses. However, as the specialty has grown and the body of research and evidence-based practice has expanded, it is becoming more common for larger rehabilitation facilities to target services for groups of clients with specific diagnoses, such as multiple trauma, traumatic brain injury, stroke syndromes, spinal cord injury, cancer, burns, or human immunodeficiency virus (HIV), or at least provide dedicated units for persons with similar diagnoses.

Subacute Care Units

Subacute care units, which may also be called transitional or progressive care units, are intended for patients who require more intensive nursing care than the traditional long-term care facility or nursing home can provide, but less than the care provided by the acute care hospital or skilled care unit (Amann & LeBlanc, 2014). Clients seen in subacute care are typically those who need additional time to transition to the community. Clients may stay in such a unit for periods of time ranging from days to several weeks. Persons who need rehabilitation services but would be unable to tolerate the intensive therapy of acute rehabilitation may be candidates for this level of care. Persons receiving subacute rehabilitation services still demonstrate measurable functional improvements (Larsen, 2011).

SKILLED NURSING FACILITIES

Skilled nursing facilities, sometimes called nursing homes, may also provide rehabilitation and can be housed in acute care hospitals, in independent specialty units, or within long-term care facilities. Not all skilled nursing facilities provide the same level of rehabilitation services, with services ranging from Commission on Accreditation of Rehabilitation Facilities (CARF)–accredited programs to restorative care. Thus consumers should carefully evaluate their options when choosing a facility (Forster, Lambley, & Young, 2010; Larsen, 2011).

Several benefits are seen with skilled nursing facilities. First, the pace is generally slower. Second, patients often have more continuity of care with nursing staff than in an acute care hospital. Third, length of stay is generally longer, perhaps weeks or months instead of days. The focus of treatment is on individual outcomes with less regard to speed of progress.

HOSPITALS AND FREESTANDING FACILITIES

Acute rehabilitation is often provided in acute care hospitals or freestanding rehabilitation facilities. A person requiring inpatient rehabilitation is not just in need of therapy—if that was the only service required, it could be done on an outpatient basis, as often occurs with such conditions as joint replacement surgery. Rather, the person needing intensive inpatient rehabilitation also requires 24-hour nursing care to address such problems as medication management, complex comorbidities, nutrition, swallowing disorders, behavior issues, skin care, and bowel and bladder retraining. Clients in acute rehabilitation may be admitted for a specific diagnosis, such as stroke, but also have preexisting or coexisting conditions that complicate recovery, such as hypertension, cancer, diabetes, and renal disease. In addition, the majority of clients treated in acute rehabilitation are older adults. Older adults as a population have unique needs with or without undergoing acute rehabilitation. Generally, to qualify for the acute intensive rehabilitation services offered in these facilities, clients must be able to tolerate at least 3 hours of therapy per day, have a goal of discharge to home, and be able to demonstrate progress toward mutually established goals (Amann & LeBlanc, 2014). They should also have private insurance or Medicare coverage to cover the high cost of the interdisciplinary services provided by multiple therapies and nursing.

LONG-TERM CARE FACILITIES OR RETIREMENT COMMUNITIES

Although long-term care facilities often carry a negative stigma with the general public, the rehabilitative services offered in these facilities may be quite appropriate for assisting adults to regain independence and function. Long-term care facilities, especially those offering multiple levels of care, may have accredited rehabilitation units housed within them. Persons making a retirement community their home may also avail themselves of therapeutic services offered within the facility. An increasing number of continuous care retirement communities (CCRCs) have physical or other therapists available to assist with rehabilitation after an accident, surgery, or illness so as to help older adults "age in place" by offering a tiered approach to aging (AARP, 2014). In addition, many CCRCs offer health promotion activities that include state-of-the-art fitness centers with personal trainers to foster primary prevention as well as rehabilitation.

COMMUNITY-BASED REHABILITATION

Community-based rehabilitation may involve a rehabilitation team or involve only nursing. Community-based nurses may work in outpatient rehabilitation clinics, senior centers, assisted-living facilities, home health care, public schools, or churches; they may also function as case managers. Community-based rehabilitation is used in a variety of settings, including home health care, subacute care, long-term care, and independent living.

Home health care provides services to clients of all ages and emphasizes primary care and case management. It allows individuals and families to remain in the home and still receive services that focus on health restoration and maximizing function. Home care is considered a cost-effective service for those recuperating from an injury or illness who are not able to completely care for themselves (Larsen, 2011). Unique models may even allow CCRCs to provide homecare services covered by Medicare (L. Mullet, personal communication, October 22, 2013).

Subacute care in the community-based model generally provides services to adults through a team-nursing delivery system, with most of the daily care being provided by nursing assistants, but with supervision by licensed practical nurses and case management by RNs. In the long-term care setting, services are offered mainly to geriatric residents using a team approach, with the RN as the case manager. In independent living settings, older adults may receive care from personal care attendants. Once again, the RN serves as a care manager and client advocate (Parker & Neal-Boylan, 2007).

Rehabilitation Specialties

Within the discipline of rehabilitation, many subspecialties have emerged. Although most traditional rehabilitation programs provide care to a mixed group of clients, both population- and diagnosis-specific units may exist that cater to the needs of smaller, more narrowly defined groups of patients. These types of specialty programs, which may be conducted on an inpatient or outpatient basis, may include geriatric patients, pediatric patients, and patients with cardiac, pulmonary, cancer, HIV, and Alzheimer's diseases.

GERIATRIC REHABILITATION

By 2030, it is estimated that there will be more than 72 million Americans older than age 65, accounting for 19.3% of the U.S. population

(Administration on Aging, 2010). The top chronic illnesses among older people that are considered the greatest health burden to society include arthritis, heart disease and stroke, diabetes, and cancer, and more recently obesity and tobacco-related disease (National Center for Chronic Disease Prevention and Health Promotion, 2007). Heart disease, cancer, and stroke account for more than 50% of all deaths in the United States (CDC, 2013b). Of the six leading causes of death in older Americans, five involve chronic illnesses, indicating that rehabilitation in geriatric clients should be a priority.

Geriatric rehabilitation focuses on restoring and maintaining optimal function while considering holistically the unique effects of aging on the person (Mauk & Patel, 2011). Programs specifically designed for older adults may have adjusted expectations such as requiring less intensive rehabilitation and preventing potential complications that occur more frequently in older adults, such as falls, dehydration, pressure sores, immobility, delirium, and polypharmacy (Mauk, Hanson, & Hain, 2014; Mauk & Patel, 2011). Geriatric rehabilitation also focuses on enhancing quality of life through the strengthening of social support systems, family involvement, client education, and connection with community resources.

There are two ways in which disability affects older adults: (1) acquiring disability at an advanced age and (2) aging with an earlier-onset disability (Mauk & Lehman, 2007). Factors that may affect an older adult's rehabilitation potential include age, frailty, the normal aging process, effects of chronic disease, functional and cognitive status, the use of multiple medications, and the presence of social support (Charles & Lehman, 2006; Guse, 2014; Mauk & Patel, 2011). The more commonly acquired disabilities in older adults include stroke, head injury, and fractures from falls. In addition, the various syndromes that are seen more often in older adults (such as delirium, dizziness, incontinence, dehydration, and functional loss) can negatively impact the rehabilitation process (Mauk & Patel, 2011).

Persons aging with a disability tend to experience a greater degree of complications over time. For example, a man with a lower-extremity amputation that occurred in his 20s is much more likely to have arthritis and range-of-motion problems in his shoulders from overuse of a non–weight-bearing joint than the person who has lost this limb later in life. However, the person with lower-extremity amputation later in life as a result of peripheral vascular disease secondary to diabetes is at an increased risk for complications because of advanced age and the diabetes disease process. As these examples demonstrate, both the disability and the aging process contribute to a person's overall rehabilitation potential. Rehabilitation can positively impact older adults by providing services to strengthen both physical and psychosocial functioning.

Pediatric Rehabilitation

Children with functional limitations have different needs and development concerns than adults do. Pediatric rehabilitation involves the collaboration of an interprofessional team to provide a continuum of care for children from the onset of injury or illness until adulthood. The focus of treatment is on adaptation and maximum function to promote independence within the family and society. The ARN (2007) defines pediatric rehabilitation nursing as "the specialty practice committed to improving the quality of life for children and adolescents with disabilities and their families" (p. 1). Professionals working with children practice family-centered care, must be knowledgeable about normal growth and development, and must be able to work with an interdisciplinary team to address interventions that include physical, emotional, cultural, educational, socioeconomic, and spiritual dimensions (Hertzberg & Sapp, 2011).

Some of the common disorders associated with the need for pediatric rehabilitation are traumatic brain injury, spinal cord injury, burns, cancer, congenital diseases and birth defects, and chronic illness. Nevertheless, whether a child sustains a brain injury from an accident or is born with cerebral palsy, the interventions from the interdisciplinary rehabilitation team are designed to maximize function and help the child attain adulthood as a well-adjusted member of society.

Cardiac Rehabilitation

According to the American Heart Association (AHA, 2011), one in six deaths in the United States is caused by coronary heart disease. Cardiac rehabilitation programs "usually provide education and counseling services to help heart patients increase physical fitness, reduce cardiac symptoms, improve health and reduce the risk of future heart problems, including heart attack" (AHA, 2013). Cardiac rehabilitation is appropriate for persons with congenital or acquired heart disease, such as those with myocardial infarction, chronic angina, or cardiomyopathy, or postsurgical patients. The aims are to improve functional capacity and to reduce related morbidity and mortality (Madison, 2011). Cardiac rehabilitation following a myocardial infarction has four phases:

- Phase I: acute phase—during the inpatient stay
- Phase II: restoration phase—early post-discharge
- Phase III: training phase—outpatient structured and supervised exercise program
- Phase IV: maintenance phase—post training and lifestyle changes (American Association of Cardiovascular and Pulmonary Rehabilitation, 2010)

Measures employed in cardiac rehabilitation include risk-factor modification along with medication management and medical interventions. Risk-factor management focuses on smoking cessation, controlling hypertension, decreasing cholesterol, management of diabetes, increasing physical activity, and decreasing stress (AHA, 2013). Client participation in cardiac rehabilitation is an ongoing problem, with recent research suggesting that the strength of the physician recommendation, gender (men participate more than women), and disease severity may be the best predictors of whether clients participate in cardiac rehabilitation (Shanks, Moore, & Zeller, 2007).

PULMONARY REHABILITATION

COPD, which includes chronic bronchitis and emphysema, is the third leading cause of death in the United States (American Lung Association [ALA], 2014). When asthma and other pulmonary problems are factored in, chronic respiratory problems are a leading cause of functional disability in this country. The primary risk factor for COPD is smoking, and 80% to 90% of deaths from COPD are attributed to this cause (ALA, 2014). Because of the large number of Americans experiencing pulmonary problems, specific programs have been developed to address their needs. The essential components of a pulmonary rehabilitation program include assessment, patient education, exercise, psychosocial interventions, and follow-up (Madison, 2011). Smoking cessation programs are a major focus in both prevention and rehabilitative treatment of respiratory problems.

In a recent meta-analysis of 18 randomized controlled trials, Liu and colleagues (2014) found that home-based pulmonary rehabilitation programs were effective in relieving respiratory symptoms associated with COPD. Such programs benefited patients through increased exercise capacity, improved respiratory function, and increased reports of well-being. Home-based pulmonary rehabilitation programs expand the role of the rehabilitation nurse, and are an important part of long-term management for patients with COPD.

CANCER REHABILITATION

According to the CDC (2013c), the types of cancer associated with the largest number of deaths among both males and females across all races are prostate, female breast, lung and bronchus, colon and rectum, uterus, and bladder. Given these statistics, many cancers detected early appear to be highly treatable and need not be viewed as a terminal diagnosis. These data suggest that persons with cancer will not only survive, but also may require rehabilitation to enhance quality

of life and return to optimal functioning after their diagnosis and as part of their treatment. Cancer rehabilitation can improve quality of life, promote strength, help persons adjust to losses, reduce sleep problems, and decrease rehospitalizations (Cancer.net Editorial Board, 2009; McMahon, 2011). The goals of cancer rehabilitation include maximizing independence in mobility and ADLs, preserving dignity, and promoting quality of life (Gillis, Cheville, & Worsowicz, 2001; McMahon, 2011).

Rehabilitation programs are individualized to each person, given the stage of his or her disease. The cancer rehabilitation team includes all of the usual team members of rehabilitation as well as the oncologist. Quality of life is enhanced through cancer rehabilitation by assistance with ADLs, pain management, improving nutrition, smoking cessation, stress reduction, and improved coping strategies. In one study of women with breast cancer, exercise therapy significantly enhanced quality of life (Dale, Crank, Saxton, Mutrie, Coleman, & Roalfe, 2007).

DEMENTIA AND/OR ALZHEIMER'S DISEASE PROGRAMS

Alzheimer's disease is a progressive and fatal brain disease that currently affects more than 5 million Americans and is the sixth leading cause of death in the United States (Alzheimer's Association, 2014). The National Institutes of Health estimate that one in seven Americans older than the age of 71 has some type of dementia (Plassman et al., 2007). Although Alzheimer's disease typically occurs in older adults, there are believed to be between 220,000 and 500,000 cases of early-onset Alzheimer's disease, which affects persons in their 30s, 40s, and 50s (Alzheimer's Association, 2014). Alzheimer's disease is the most common type of dementia and has no cure. Although Alzheimer's disease is not generally considered a rehabilitation diagnosis, it certainly fits the profile of a chronic illness. Persons with early-onset Alzheimer's disease are likely to avail themselves of all treatments possible—including interventions from the rehabilitation team—to postpone the inevitable effects of this progressive illness.

Rehabilitation nurses are often found working in long-term care facilities that serve residents with dementia, and the need for their services is likely to grow. Although the focus of care for older persons with Alzheimer's disease includes rehabilitation goals, realistic outcome planning as the disease progresses will not likely include discharge to home. Persons with Alzheimer's disease may receive services in assisted-living facilities, nursing homes, and/or special care units (Alzheimer's Association, 2014). The Alzheimer's unit within the nursing home often becomes the last home that a person with dementia will know. The number of Alzheimer's units within long-term care facilities is increasing due to the demand for services that occurs as the disease progresses and family caregivers are no longer able to manage persons at home.

A recent study found that "elevated stroke risk at midlife is associated with accelerated cognitive decline over 10 years" (Kaffashian et al., 2013), suggesting that those persons with dementia are at higher risk for stroke and may have additional challenges as disease burden increases. As a person's condition deteriorates with advancing dementia, the fundamental principles of rehabilitation still apply to these residents: to assist individuals to remain as independent as possible for as long as possible, to maintain function, and to prevent complications.

HIV/AIDS

An estimated 1,178,350 persons aged 13 and older were living with HIV or acquired immunodeficiency syndrome (AIDS) in the United States in 2009 (aids.gov, 2012a). It is estimated that 25 million people worldwide have died from HIV or AIDS (aids.gov, 2012b), including 636,000 Americans. Although current treatments have dramatically increased the life expectancy for many persons with HIV, those developing AIDS may experience many associated neurologic, pulmonary, cardiac, and

rheumatologic problems. Rehabilitation programs designed to address all levels of prevention along with the associated health problems inherent with HIV/AIDS are becoming more common. Rehabilitation nurses may work with infected patients before diagnosis through end of life (Fan, Conner, & Villarreal, 2011). Rehabilitation goals depend on the stage of illness, whether symptomatic, asymptomatic, or terminal. Interventions include careful assessment, addressing psychological needs and responses, balancing energy with rest, medication management, education regarding prevention of transmission, emotional support, and counseling for the person and family.

Ensuring Quality in Rehabilitation Facilities

There are two primary accrediting bodies for rehabilitation providers: The Joint Commission and CARF. Although The Joint Commission accreditation is expected for inpatient rehabilitation providers, CARF accreditation is viewed as a mark of distinction that signifies meeting higher standards for rehabilitation.

THE JOINT COMMISSION

The oldest and best-known accrediting body is The Joint Commission, previously known as the Joint Commission on the Accreditation of Healthcare Organizations. The mission of The Joint Commission is "to continuously improve health care for the public, in collaboration with other stakeholders, by evaluating health care organizations and inspiring them to excel in providing safe and effective care of the highest quality and value" (Joint Commission, 2014, p. 1). This organization has developed current, professionally based standards for hospitals, long-term care, home health care, and other organizations, and it uses a survey process to evaluate the compliance of healthcare organizations with these standards. The Joint Commission has a cooperative agreement with CARF regarding the evaluation of rehabilitation facilities. In 1997, the ORYX initiative allowed the integration of outcomes and standard performance measures into the accreditation process and helped organizations identify care issues that required attention (Black, 2007). The Joint Commission accredits organizations responsible for providing safe care that meets the standards of the industry and protects public safety. Benefits of Joint Commission accreditation and certification include strengthening the trust of the public in the organization, improving risk management, promoting patient safety and comfort, and enhancing staff recruitment into the organization (Joint Commission, 2014).

COMMISSION ON ACCREDITATION OF REHABILITATION FACILITIES

CARF is an independent, not-for-profit organization that accredits rehabilitation programs and services. It provides accreditation services for organizations throughout the world. The standards for CARF accreditation are high so that persons seeking treatment who choose a CARF-accredited facility can have confidence in its ability to provide quality care and positive outcomes (CARF, 2014). There are six divisions in CARF's organizational structure: medical rehabilitation; behavioral health; employment and community services; aging services; child and youth services; and durable medical equipment, prostheses, orthotics, and supplies suppliers (Black & Cournan, 2011). Recent publications from this organization include the *Child and Youth Standards Manual* and *Aging Services Standards Manual* (CARF, 2011a, 2011b).

Outcome Measurement and Performance Improvement

According to Black and Cournan (2011), outcomes of care are being emphasized as never before. They list the following benefits of monitoring outcomes (p. 529):

- Track efficiency and effectiveness
- Identify trends
- Facilitate communication between the patient, family, treatment team, payers, referral source, and other stakeholders

- Assess follow-up measures to determine whether progress is continuing after discharge
- Identify areas for improvement
- Measure access to programs

In rehabilitation, outcomes are key to ensuring that goals are being met. Goal setting in rehabilitation should be mutual, between the client and the interprofessional team. Individual goals for clients are reviewed systematically at team conferences. Outcomes measurement can be used to look at trends within an organization, benchmarked against industry standards, and compared with best practices.

There are many ways that outcomes can be measured. Accreditation provides one way to ensure that facilities are meeting the industry standards. A variety of tools can also be used to monitor individual and collective rehabilitation outcomes. One of the most commonly used is the FIM instrument (Figure 24-2), which provides a quantitative measure of function on admission, discharge, and follow-up so that data may be compared across time and with other cohorts (Uniform Data System for Medical Rehabilitation, 1997). This information often proves useful in justifying insurance coverage by demonstrating continued improvement by the client.

Many other tools and models address performance improvement in health care. Most of these focus on devices to assist team members in improving the quality of care for clients. Diagrams, flow sheets, checklists, charts, and other visual aids can all be used to enhance performance. Standards setting by national organizations provides another means of quality improvement, as organizations strive to meet these standards and, therefore, industry aims.

Outcomes measurement and documentation of performance improvement are critical because reimbursement under present payment systems requires rehabilitation providers to provide evidence of the effectiveness of their programs and services.

Evidence-Based Practice Box

A critical appraisal of the literature has demonstrated that education increases knowledge in a specialty area. This evidence was tested in an inpatient rehabilitation setting through an evidence-based educational intervention. Sixteen nurses on a new inpatient rehabilitation unit completed author-developed self-study modules on 15 rehabilitation competencies. Outcomes were evaluated using pre- and post-tests via ARN's online Competency Assessment Tool (CAT). The results showed a statistically significant increase between pre- and post-test scores on 14 of the 15

competencies measured. Even experienced nurses who did not have specific rehabilitation nursing education were found to lack this specialized knowledge. The findings suggested that rehabilitation knowledge is not part of basic nursing preparation and that education of nursing staff in basic rehabilitation nursing competencies results in increased knowledge that could promote quality of care.

Source: Mauk, K. L. (2013). The effect of advanced practice nurse-modulated education on rehabilitation nursing staff knowledge. *Rehabilitation Nursing, 38*(2), 99–111. doi: 10.1002/rnj.70.

CASE STUDY 24-1 ADJUSTMENT TO A LIFE-ALTERING CONDITION

Major Nealy, a 32-year-old soldier, was injured by an improvised explosive device (IED) and experienced polytrauma that included traumatic brain injury, blast lung, eye trauma, amputation of his right arm, and third-degree burns to his trunk and arms (total area of 11%). Major Nealy is married, with a wife and two small children. He is being treated at a polytrauma center in Texas. The APRN consults with his wife and parents about Major Nealy's treatment and prognosis. His wife is concerned about permanent brain damage, and his parents are most concerned about his appearance after the burns and what that long-term treatment will entail.

Discussion Questions

1. Which team members would have been involved in Major Nealy's rehabilitation in the inpatient rehabilitation unit after his polytrauma injury?
2. Which goals are appropriate for Major Nealy in the long term? In the short term?
3. Name two tools or classification systems that would be appropriate in evaluating Major Nealy's functional ability.
4. How would you address the wife's concern about his brain injury? The parents' questions about burn rehabilitation? Which outcomes are realistic for this patient and his family?
5. If you developed a long-term plan of care for this patient, which outcomes would be appropriate over a 10-year period?

CASE STUDY 24-2 TECHNOLOGICAL ADVANCES

Ms. Lurie was a 19-year-old Olympic snowboarder who suffered a serious accident during a major competition. She sustained a mild brain injury, from which she had a complete recovery, and an eventual amputation of her left lower leg as a result of a crushing injury that became infected after her first major reconstructive surgery, which involved numerous internal fixations. After extensive time in rehabilitation, she was fitted with a specially engineered prosthetic limb with the hopes of returning to snowboarding. Ms. Lurie is considering entering the Paralympics, but one of her major goals is to compete in the Olympic Winter Games with the able-bodied individuals with whom she competed before her accident. Ms. Lurie has the support of her parents, coaches, and sponsors to accomplish this goal.

Discussion Questions

1. How would the interprofessional team assist Ms. Lurie in developing a long-term plan to achieve her goals using her new technologically advanced prosthetic limb?
2. Which rehabilitation issues and concerns would be involved in Ms. Lurie's situation? Which psychosocial and emotional factors should be addressed?
3. How should the family and her coach be involved in the plan of care for her?
4. Is Ms. Lurie's goal of competing in the Paralympics realistic? What about competing in the Olympic Winter Games as she did before with her prior competitors? Which factors should be considered for this outcome to be realized?

STUDY QUESTIONS

1. Rehabilitation is both a philosophy and an approach to treatment. Describe the philosophy of rehabilitation, and explain how it relates to treatment from an interdisciplinary team of professionals.
2. Define the following rehabilitation terms in relationship to chronic illness: *impairment, functional limitation, disability,* and *community reintegration*.
3. Identify three problems in the provision of rehabilitation services to patients with chronic illness.
4. Describe the different settings where rehabilitation services can be provided, and explain why certain clients might be at one facility versus another.
5. Which specific issues in rehabilitation complicate the research process?
6. Discuss the advantages and disadvantages of the major functional assessment tools mentioned in this chapter.

Internet Resources

Alzheimer's Association: http://www.alz.org

American Heart Association: http://www.aha.org

American Stroke Association: http://www.strokeassociation.org

Association of Rehabilitation Nurses: http://www.rehabnurse.org

Centers for Medicare and Medicaid Services: http://www.cms.hhs.gov/medicare/

National Institute of Neurological Disorders and Stroke: http://www.ninds.nih.gov

National Rehabilitation Association: http://www.nationalrehab.org

National Rehabilitation Information Center: http://www.naric.com

National Stroke Association: http://www.stroke.org

The State of Aging and Health in America: http://www.cdc.gov/aging/data/stateofaging.htm

References

AARP. (2014). Continuing care retirement communities. http://www.aarp.org/relationships/caregiving-resource-center/info-09-2010/ho_continuing_care_retirement_communities.html

Adams, P. F., Dey, A. N., & Vickerie, J. L. (2007). Summary health statistics for the US population National Health Interview Survey, 2005. National Center for Health Statistics. *Vital Health Statistics*, *19*(233). Hyattsville, MD: U.S. Department of Health and Human Services.

Adams, P. F., Kirzinger, W. K., & Martinez, M. E. (2011). Summary health statistics for the U.S. population: National Health Interview Survey, 2011. National Center for Health Statistics. *Vital Health Statistics*, *10*(255). Hyattsville, MD: U.S. Department of Health and Human Services.

Administration on Aging. (2010). A profile of older Americans, 2010. http://www.aoa.gov/aoaroot/aging_statistics/profile/2010/docs/2010profile.pdf

AIDS.gov. (2012a). HIV/in the U.S.: At a glance. http://aids.gov/hiv-aids-basics/hiv-aids-101/statistics/

AIDS.gov. (2012b). Global statistics. http://aids.gov/hiv-aids-basics/hiv-aids-101/global-statistics/

Al-Krenawi, A., Graham, J. R., & Al Gharaibeh, F. (2011). The impact of intellectual disability, caregiver burden, family functioning, marital quality, and sense of coherence. *Disability & Society*, *26*(2), 139–150.

Alzheimer's Association. (2014). Alzheimer's disease. http://www.alz.org/alzheimers_disease_facts_and_figures.asp#quickFacts

Amann, C. A., & LeBlanc, R. G. (2014). Caring across the continuum. In K. L. Mauk (Ed.), *Gerontological nursing: Competencies for care* (3rd ed. pp. 857–878). Burlington, MA: Jones & Bartlett Learning.

American Academy of Physical Medicine and Rehabilitation. (2014). Home page. http://www.aapmr.org/Pages/default.aspx

American Association of Cardiovascular and Pulmonary Rehabilitation. (2010). Cardiac and pulmonary rehabilitation fundamentals. www.aacvpr.org/Resources/CardiacPulmonaryRehabFundamentals/tabid/256/Default.aspx

American Heart Association (AHA). (2011). Heart disease and stroke statistics: 2011 update. http://cire.ahajournals.org/content/123/4/el8.full.pdf

American Heart Association (AHA). (2013). What is cardiac rehabilitation? http://www.heart.org/HEARTORG/Conditions/More/CardiacRehab/What-is-Cardiac-Rehabilitation_UCM_307049_Article.jsp

American Lung Association (ALA). (2014). COPD. http://www.lungusa.org/lung-disease/copd/

Arbour, K. P., Latimer, A. E., Ginis, K. A., & Jung, M. E. (2007). Moving beyond the stigma: The impression formation benefits of exercise for individuals with a physical disability. *Adapted Physical Activity Quarterly*, *24*(2), 144–159.

Association of Academic Physiatrists. (2014). About AAP. http://www.physiatry.org/

Association of Rehabilitation Nurses (ARN). (2007). ARN positional statement on the role of the nurse in the rehabilitation team. http://www.rehabnurse.org/pdf/PS-Role.pdf

Association of Rehabilitation Nurses (ARN). (2008). *Standards and scope of rehabilitation nursing practice*. Glenview, IL: Author.

Association of Rehabilitation Nurses (ARN). (2010). Role description brochures. http://www.rehabnurse.org/pubs/role/index.html

Association of Rehabilitation Nurses (ARN). (2012). History: What do rehabilitation nurses do? http://www.rehabnurse.org/about/content/History/html

Association of Rehabilitation Nurses (ARN). (2013). Strategic plan. http://www.rehabnurse.org/about/content/ARN-Strategic-Plan.html

Bayen, E., Pradat-Diehl, P., Jourdan, C., Ghout, I., Bosserelle, V., Azerad, S., … Azouvi, P. (2013). Predictors of informal care burden 1 year after a severe traumatic brain injury: Results from the PariS-TBI study. *Journal of Head Trauma Rehabilitation*, *28*(6), 408–418.

Beauchamp, T. L., & Childress, J. F. (2008). *Principles of biomedical ethics*. New York, NY: Oxford University Press.

Behm, J., & Gray, N. (2012). Interdisciplinary rehabilitation team. In K. L. Mauk (Ed.), *Rehabilitation nursing: A contemporary approach to practice* (5th ed., pp. 51–63). Sudbury, MA: Jones and Bartlett.

Black, T. (2007). Outcomes measurement and performance improvement. In K. L. Mauk (Ed.), *The specialty practice of rehabilitation nursing: A core curriculum* (5th ed., pp. 395–411). Glenview, IL: Association of Rehabilitation Nurses.

Black, T., & Cournan, M. (2011). Outcomes measurement and performance improvement. In C. Jacelon (Ed.), *The specialty practice of rehabilitation nursing: A core curriculum* (6th ed., pp. 529–546). Glenview, IL: Association of Rehabilitation Nurses.

Brandt, E., & Pope, A. (1997). *Enabling America: Assessing the role of rehabilitation science and engineering*. Committee on Assessing Rehabilitation Science and Engineering, Division of Health Policy, Institute of Medicine. Washington, DC: National Academies Press.

Bratcher, R., Farrell, J. J., Stevens, K. A., & Vanderground, K. W. (2012). Ethical and legal issues. In K. L. Mauk (Ed.), *Rehabilitation nursing: A contemporary approach to practice.* (pp. 386–401). Sudbury, MA: Jones and Bartlett.

Buchanan, L. (1996). Community-based rehabilitation nursing. In S. Hoeman (Ed.), *Rehabilitation nursing: Process and application* (2nd ed., pp. 114–129). St. Louis, MO: Mosby.

Buse, N. A., Burker, E. J., & Bernacchio, C. (2013). Cultural variation in resilience as a response to traumatic experience. *Journal of Rehabilitation*, *79*(2), 15–23.

Bushnik, T., Wright, J., & Burdsall, D. (2007). Personal attendant turnover: Association with level of injury, burden of care, and psychosocial outcome. *Topics in Spinal Cord Injury Rehabilitation*, *12*(3), 66–76.

Campinha-Bacote, J. (2001). A model of practice to address cultural competence. *Rehabilitation Nursing*, *26*(1), 8–11.

Cancer.Net Editorial Board. (2009). Rehabilitation. http://www.cancer.net/patient/Survivorship/Rehabilitation

Cecil, R., Thompson, K., Parahoo, K., & McCaughan, E. (2013). Towards an understanding of the lives of families affected by stroke: A qualitative study of home carers. *Journal of Advanced Nursing*, *69*(8), 1761–1770.

Centers for Disease Control and Prevention (CDC). (2009). Chronic disease and health promotion. http://www.cdc.gov/chronicdisease/overview/index/htm

Centers for Disease Control and Prevention. (2013a). American Indians and Alaska Native populations. http://www.cdc.gov/minorityhealth/populations/REMP/aian.html

Centers for Disease Control and Prevention (CDC). (2013b). Chronic disease prevention and health promotion. http://www.cdc.gov/chronicdisease/overview/index.htm

Centers for Disease Control and Prevention (CDC). (2013c). United States cancer statistics. http://www.cdc.gov/Features/CancerStatistics/

Centers for Disease Control and Prevention (CDC). (2014). Definitions. http://www.cdc.gov/minorityhealth/populations/atrisk.html

Centers for Disease Control and Prevention (CDC), Office of Minority Health and Health Equity (2013). CDC Health disparities and inequalities report (CHDR). http://www.cdc.gov/minorityhealth/CHDIReport.html

Centers for Medicare and Medicaid Services (CMS). (2011). Overview of inpatient rehabilitation facility PPS. http://www.cms.gov/InPatientRehabFacPPS/

Centers for Medicare and Medicaid Services (CMS). (2013). Spotlight. https://www.cms.gov/Medicare/Medicare-Fee-for-Service-Payment/InpatientRehabFacPPS/Spotlight.html

Centers for Medicare and Medicaid Services (CMS). (2014). Medicare and you, 2014. http://www.medicare.gov/Pubs/pdf/10050.pdf

Charles, C. V., & Lehman, C. (2006). Medications and laboratory values. In K. L. Mauk (Ed.), *Gerontological nursing: Competencies for care* (pp. 293–320). Sudbury, MA: Jones and Bartlett.

Commission on Accreditation of Rehabilitation Facilities International (CARF). (2011a). 2011 aging services program descriptions. http://www.carf.org/ASprogramDescriptions/

Commission on Accreditation of Rehabilitation Facilities International (CARF). (2011b). 2011 child and youth services program descriptions. http://www.carf.org/WorkArea/DownloadAsset.aspx?

Commission on Accreditation of Rehabilitation Facilities (CARF). (2014). CARF accreditation focuses on quality, results. http://www.carf.org/home/

Cook, C., Stickley, L., Ramey, K., & Knotts, V. J. (2005). Variables associated with occupational and physical therapy stroke rehabilitation utilization and outcomes. *Journal of Allied Health, 34*(1), 3–10.

Cot, D. (2013). Intercultural communication in health care: Challenges and solutions in work rehabilitation practices and training: A comprehensive review. *Disability & Rehabilitation, 35*(2), 153–163.

Dale, A. J., Crank, H., Saxton, J. M., Mutrie, N., Coleman, R., & Roalfe, A. (2007). Randomized trial of exercise therapy in women treated for breast cancer. *Journal of Clinical Oncology, 25*(13), 1713–1721.

De Souza Olivereira, A. R., Cordeiro Rodrigues, R., Carvalho De Sousa, V. E., De Sousa Costa, A. G., De Olivereira Lopes, M V., & De Araujo, T. L. (2013). Clinical indicators of "caregiver role strain" in caregivers of stroke patients. *Contemporary Nurse: A Journal for the Australian Nursing Profession, 44*(2), 215–224.

Deutsch, A., & Dean-Baar, S. (2007). Economics and health policy in rehabilitation. In K. L. Mauk (Ed.), *The specialty practice of rehabilitation nursing: A core curriculum* (5th ed., pp. 35–53). Glenview, IL: Association of Rehabilitation Nurses.

Dijkers, M. P. (2014). Rehabilitation treatment taxonomy: Establishing common ground. *Archives of Physical Medicine and Rehabilitation, 95*(1 suppl), S1–S5.

Dijkers, M. P., Hart, T., Tsaousides, T., Whyte, J., & Zanca, J. M. (2014). Treatment taxonomy for rehabilitation: Past, present, and prospects. *Archives of Physical Medicine and Rehabilitation, 95*(1 suppl 1), S6–S16.

Dijkers, M. P., Hart, T., Whyte, J., Zanca, J. M., Packel, A., & Tsaousides, T. (2014). Rehabilitation treatment taxonomy: Implications and continuations. *Archives of Physical Medicine and Rehabilitation, 95*(1 suppl 1), S45–S54.

Disability Statistics Compendium. (2013). Annual disability statistics compendium. http://www.disability-compendium.org/compendium-statistics

Draper, B., Bowring, G., Thompson, C., Van Heyst, J., Conroy, P., & Thompson, J. (2007). Stress in caregivers of aphasic stroke patients: A randomized controlled trial. *Clinical Rehabilitation, 21*(2), 122–130.

Edwards, P. (2007). Rehabilitation nursing: Past, present and future. In K. Mauk (Ed.), *The specialty practice of rehabilitation nursing: A core curriculum* (5th ed., pp. 455–466). Glenview, IL: Association of Rehabilitation Nurses.

Family Caregiver Alliance. (2012). Selected caregiver statistics. http://www.caregiver.org/jsp/content_node.jsp?nodeid=439

Fan, H. Y., Conner, R. F., & Villarreal, L. P. (2011). *AIDS science and society* (6th ed.). Sudbury, MA: Jones and Bartlett.

Fasoli, S. E., & Chen, C. C. (2014). What do clinicians need from a rehabilitation treatment taxonomy? An alternate approach for describing treatment content versus process. *Archives of Physical Medicine and Rehabilitation, 95*(1 suppl), 74–76. doi: 10.1016/j.aprmr.2013.06.037

Forster, A., Lambley, R., & Young, J. B. (2010). Is physical rehabilitation for older people in long-term care effective? Findings from a systematic review. *Age and Aging, 39*, 169–175.

Gillis, T. A., Cheville, A. L., & Worsowicz, G. M. (2001). Cardiopulmonary rehabilitation and cancer rehabilitation: Oncologic rehabilitation. *Archives of Physical Medicine and Rehabilitation, 83*(suppl 1), S47–S51.

Greene, J. V. (2013). *Exploring the role of culture and race in stroke rehabilitation disparities.* Doctoral dissertation, University of South Carolina, Columbia, SC.

Grunfeld, E., Coyle, D., Whelan, T., Clinch, J., Reyno, L., Earle, C.C., ... Glossop, R. (2004). Family caregiver burden: Results of a longitudinal study of breast cancer patients and their principal caregivers. *Canadian Medical Association Journal, 170*(12), 1795–1801.

Guse, L. W. (2014). Comprehensive assessment of the older adult. In K. L. Mauk (Ed.), *Gerontological nursing: Competencies for care* (pp. 149–186). Burlington, MA: Jones & Bartlett Learning.

Hackman, D. (2011). What's the point? Exploring rehabilitation for people with primary CNS tumours using ethnography: Patients' perspectives. *Physiotherapy Research International, 16*(4), 201–217.

Hall, W. (2013). Gov't spends more on disability than food stamps, welfare combined. http://www.breitbart.com/Big-Government/2013/03/25/Govt-Spends-More-On-Disability-Than-Food-Stamps-And-Welfare-Combined

Halm, M. A., Treat-Jacobson, D., Lindquist, R., & Savik, K. (2007). Caregiver burden and outcomes of caregiving of spouses of patient who undergo coronary artery bypass graft surgery. *Heart & Lung, 36*(3), 170–187.

Hart, T., Tsaousides, T., Zanca, J. M., Whyte, J., Packel, A., Ferraro, M., & Dijkers, M. P. (2014). Toward a theory-driven classification of rehabilitation treatment. *Archives of Physical Medicine and Rehabilitation, 95*(1 suppl 1), S33–S44.

Herrera, A. P., George, R., Angel, J. L., Markides, K., & Torres-Gil, F. (2013). Variation in Older Americans

Act caregiver service use, unmet hours of care, and independence among Hispanics, African Americans, and whites. *Home Health Care Services Quarterly, 32*(1), 35–56.

Hertzberg, D., & Sapp, L. (2011). Pediatric rehabilitation. In C. Jacelon (Ed.), *The specialty practice of rehabilitation nursing: A core curriculum* (pp. 449–473). Glenview, IL: Association of Rehabilitation Nurses.

Hooten, W. M., Knight-Brown, M., Townsend, C. O., & Laures, H. J. (2012). Clinical outcomes of multidisciplinary pain rehabilitation among African American compared with Caucasian patients with chronic pain. *Pain Management, 13*(11),1499–1508.

Indian Health Services. (2014). Fact sheet. http://www .ihs.gov/newsroom/factsheets/quicklook/

Inman, J., McGurk, E., & Chadwick, J. (2007). Is vocational rehabilitation a transition to recovery? *British Journal of Occupational Therapy, 70*(2), 60–66.

Jacelon, C. (2011a). Health care, rehabilitation, and rehabilitation nursing. In C. Jacelon (Ed.), *The specialty practice of rehabilitation nursing* (pp. 1–14). Glenview, IL: Association of Rehabilitation Nurses.

Jacelon, C. (2011b). Psychosocial healthcare patterns and nursing interventions. In C. Jacelon (Ed.), *The specialty practice of rehabilitation nursing* (pp. 145–168). Glenview, IL: Association of Rehabilitation Nurses.

The Joint Commission. (2014). About The Joint Commission. http://www.jointcommission.org /AboutUs/

Kaffashian, S., Dugravot, A., Brunner, E. J., Sabia, S., Ankri, J., Kivimäki, M., & Singh-Manoux, A. (2013). Midlife stroke risk and cognitive decline: A 10-year follow-up of the Whitehall II cohort study. *Alzheimer's & Dementia, 9*(5), 572–579.

Kaiser Commission. (2007). Medicaid and the uninsured. http://www.kff.org/medicaid/upload/7682.pdf

Kent, B., & Smith, S. (2006). They only see it when the sun shines in my ears: Exploring perceptions of adolescent hearing aid users. *Journal of Deaf Studies & Deaf Education, 11*(4), 461–476.

King, R. B., Hartke, R. J., & Denby, F. (2007). Problem-solving early intervention: A pilot study of stroke caregivers. *Rehabilitation Nursing, 32*(2), 68–76.

Koenig, S., Teixeira, J., & Yetzer, E. (2014). Promoting mobility and function. In K. L. Mauk (Ed.), *Rehabilitation nursing: A contemporary approach to practice* (pp. 136–146). Burlington, MA: Jones & Bartlett Learning.

Kosciulek, J. F. (2007). A test of the theory of informed consumer choice in vocational rehabilitation. *Journal of Rehabilitation, 73*(2), 41–49.

Kothe, M. (2014). Legal aspects of gerontological nursing. In K. L. Mauk (Ed.), *Gerontological nursing: Competencies for care.* Burlington, MA: Jones & Bartlett Learning.

Kottke, F., Stillwell, G., & Lehmann, J. (Eds.). (1982). *Krusen's handbook of physical medicine and rehabilitation* (3rd ed.). Philadelphia, PA: Saunders.

LaPlante, M., Kaye, H. S., Kang, T., & Harrington, C. (2004). Unmet need for personal assistance services: Estimating the shortfall in hours of help and adverse consequences. *Journal of Gerontology, Series B, Psychological Science and Social Science, 59*(2), S98–S108.

Larsen, P. (2011). The environment for rehabilitation nursing. In C. Jacelon (Ed.), *The specialty practice of rehabilitation nursing: A core curriculum* (pp. 507–511). Glenview, IL: Association of Rehabilitation Nurses.

Lehman, C. A., & Wirt, A. (2014). The aging population. In K. L. Mauk (Ed.), *Gerontological nursing: Competencies for care* (pp. 28–60). Burlington, MA: Jones & Bartlett Learning.

Liu, X., Tan, J., Wang, T., Zhang, Q., Zhang, M., Yao, L., & Chen, J. (2014). Effectiveness of home-based pulmonary rehabilitation for patients with chronic obstructive pulmonary disease: A meta-analysis of randomized controlled trials. *Rehabilitation Nursing, 39*(1), 36–59. doi: 10.1002/rjn.112

Lloyd, C., & Waghorn, G. (2007). The importance of vocation in recovery for young people with psychiatric disabilities. *British Journal of Occupational Therapy, 70*(2), 50–59.

Lutz, B. J., & Bowers, B. J. (2003). Understanding how disability is defined and conceptualized in the literature. *Rehabilitation Nursing, 28*(3), 74–78.

Madison, H. E. (2011). Cardiac and pulmonary rehabilitation: Acute and long-term management. In C. Jacelon (Ed.), *The specialty practice of rehabilitation nursing: A core curriculum* (pp. 365–382). Glenview, IL: Association of Rehabilitation Nurses.

Masters-Ferrell, P. A. (2007). Ethical, moral, and legal considerations. In K. L. Mauk (Ed.), *The specialty practice of rehabilitation nursing: A core curriculum* (pp. 27–34). Glenview, IL: Association of Rehabilitation Nurses.

Mauk, K. L. (2012). *Rehabilitation nursing: A contemporary approach to practice.* Burlington, MA: Jones & Bartlett Learning.

Mauk, K. L. (2013). The effect of advanced practice nurse–modulated education on rehabilitation nursing staff knowledge. *Rehabilitation Nursing, 38*(2), 99–111. doi: 10.1002/rnj.70

Mauk, K. L., Hanson, P., & Hain, D. (2014). Management of common illnesses, diseases, and health conditions. In K. L. Mauk (Ed.), *Gerontological nursing: Competencies for care* (pp. 270–376). Burlington, MA: Jones & Bartlett Learning.

Mauk, K. L., & Lehman, C. (2007). Geriatric rehabilitation. In K. L. Mauk (Ed.), *The specialty practice of rehabilitation nursing: A core curriculum* (5th ed., pp. 359–383). Glenview, IL: Association of Rehabilitation Nurses.

Mauk, K. L., & Patel, U. (2011). Geriatric rehabilitation. In C. Jacelon (Ed.), *The specialty practice of rehabilitation nursing: A core curriculum,* (pp. 475–504). Glenview, IL: Association of Rehabilitation Nurses.

McMahon, J. C. (2011). Specific disease processes requiring rehabilitation interventions. In C. Jacelon (Ed.), *The specialty practice of rehabilitation nursing: A core curriculum* (pp. 397–429). Glenview, IL: Association of Rehabilitation Nurses.

Monisvais, D. (2011). Promoting culturally competent chronic pain managements using the clinically relevant continuum model. *Nursing Clinics of North America,* 46(2), 163–169.

Monisvais, D., & Engebretson, J. (2011). Cultural cues: Review of qualitative evidence of patient-centered care in patients with non-malignant chronic pain. *Rehabilitation Nursing,* 36(4), 166–171.

Morgan, J. E. (2007). *Successful outcomes in vocational rehabilitation: The effects of stage of change and relational development.* Doctoral dissertation, Brandeis University, Waltham, MA.

Mpofu, E., & Harley, D. A. (2006). Racial and disability identity: Implications for the career counseling of African Americans with disabilities. *Rehabilitation Counseling Bulletin,* 50(1), 14–23.

National Alliance for Caregiving & AARP. (2009). Caregiving in the United States. http://www.caregiving.org/pdf/research/CaregivingUSAllAgesExecSum.pdf

National Center for Chronic Disease Prevention and Health Promotion, Centers for Disease Control and Prevention. (2007). Quick facts: Economic and health burden of chronic disease. www.cdc.gov/nccdphp/press/#4

National Center for Chronic Disease Prevention and Health Promotion, Centers for Disease Control and Prevention. (2009). Healthy aging. http://www.cdc.gov/nccdphp/publications/aag/pdf/healthy_aging.pdf

Parker, B. J., & Neal-Boylan, L. (2007). Community and family-centered rehabilitation nursing. In K. L. Mauk (Ed.), *The specialty practice of rehabilitation nursing: A core curriculum* (5th ed., pp. 13–26). Glenview, IL: Association of Rehabilitation Nurses.

Pescosolido, B. A., Martin, J. K., Lang, A., & Olafsdottir, S. (2008). Rethinking theoretical approaches to stigma: A Framework Integrating Normative Influences on Stigma (FINIS). *Social Science & Medicine,* 67(3), 431–440.

Plassman, B. L., Langa, K. M., Fisher, G. G., Heeringa, S. G., Weir, D. R., Ofstedal, M. B., ... Wallace, R.B. (2007). Prevalence of dementia in the United States: The aging, demographics, and memory study. *Neuroepidemiology,* 29, 125–132.

Podsiadlo, D., & Richardson, S. (1991). The timed "up & go": A test of basic functional mobility for frail elderly persons. *Journal of the American Geriatric Society,* 39, 142–148.

Pope, A. M., & Tarlov, A. R. (1991). *Disability in America: Toward a national agenda for prevention.* Washington, DC: National Academies Press.

President's Committee for People with Intellectual Disabilities. (2009). About the committee. http://www.acf.hhs.gov/programs/pcpid/pcpid_about.html

Rattanasuk, D., Nantachaipan, P., Sucamvang, K., & Moongtui, W. (2013). A causal model of well-being among caregivers of people with spinal cord injury. *Pacific Rim International Journal of Nursing Research,* 17(3), 342–355.

Rehabilitation Services Administration. (2014). About RSA. https://rsa.ed.gov/

Remsburg, R., & Carson, B. (2006). Rehabilitation. In I. Lubkin & P. Larsen (Eds.), *Chronic illness: Impact and Intervention* (pp. 579–616). Sudbury, MA: Jones and Bartlett.

Resnick, B., Galik, E., Bolz, M., & Pretzer-Aboff, I. (Eds.) (2012). *Restorative care for nursing for older adults: A guide for all care settings.* New York, NY: Springer.

Robert Wood Johnson Foundation. (2012). United States in search of nurses with geriatrics training. http://www.rwjf.org/en/about-rwjf/newsroom/newsroom-content/2012/02/united-states-in-search-of-nurses-with-geriatrics-training.html

Rusk, H. (1965). Preventive medicine, curative medicine: The rehabilitation. *New Physician,* 59(4), 156–160.

Scott, J. R. (2010). Two new pilot programs stem from healthcare bill. http://www.rehabnurse.org/enews/11junjuly/11junjulyadvocacy.html

Shanks, L. C., Moore, S. M., & Zeller, R. A. (2007). Predictors of cardiac rehabilitation initiation. *Rehabilitation Nursing,* 32(4), 152–157.

Shannon, M. P., & Hassler, L. J. (2014). Culture and spirituality. In K. L. Mauk (Ed.), *Gerontological nursing: Competencies for care* (pp. 734–791). Burlington, MA: Jones & Bartlett Learning.

Ski, C., & O'Connell, B. (2007). Stroke: The increasing complexity of carer needs. *Journal of Neuroscience Nursing*, *39*(3), 172–179.

Social Security Administration. (2014). Social Security. http://www.ssa.gov/dibplan/index.htm#a0=0

Stuart, H. (2006). Mental illness and employment discrimination. *Current Opinion in Psychiatry*, *5*, 522–526.

Tapper, E. B., Vercler, C. J., Cruze, D., & Sexson, W. (2010). Ethics consultation at a large urban public teaching hospital. *Mayo Clinic Proceedings*, *85*(5), 433–438.

Thompson, T. L., Emrich, K., & Moore, G. (2003). The effect of curriculum on the attitudes of nursing students toward disability. *Rehabilitation Nursing*, *28*(1), 27–30.

Uniform Data System for Medical Rehabilitation. (1997). FIM Instrument. University at Buffalo, Buffalo, NY, 14214.

U.S. Department of Education. (2014). Office of Special Education and Rehabilitation Services, Rehabilitation Services Administration. http://www2.ed.gov/about /offices/list/osers/rsa/index.html

U.S. Department of Health and Human Services (HHS). (2013). *Vital and health statistics. Summary health statistics for the U.S. population: National Health Interview Survey, 2012*. Hyattsville, MD: Author.

U.S. Department of Labor. (2014). Worker's compensation. http://www.dol.gov/dol/topic/workcomp/

U.S. Department of Veterans Affairs. (2010). Federal benefits for veterans, survivors, and dependents. http://www1.va.gov/opa/publications/benefits_book /federal_benefits.pdf

U.S. Department of Veterans Affairs. (2011). Vocational rehabilitation and employment services. http://www .vba.va.gov/bln/vre/

U.S. Department of Veterans Affairs. (2014). Vocational rehabilitation and employment. http://www.benefits .va.gov/vocrehab/index.asp

U.S. Equal Employment Opportunity Commission. (2008). Americans with Disabilities Act. http://www .eeoc.gov/facts/fs-ada.html

Velcoff, J., Hernandez, B., & Keys, C. (2010). Employment and vocational rehabilitation experiences of Latinos with disabilities with differing patterns of acculturation. *Journal of Vocational Rehabilitation*, *33*(1), 51–64.

Ward, R. L., Nichols, A., & Freedman, R. I. (2010). Uncovering health care inequalities among adults with intellectual and developmental disabilities. *Health & Social Work*, *35*(4), 280–290.

Whyte, J. (1998). Enabling America: A report from the Institute of Medicine on rehabilitation science and engineering. *Archives of Physical Medicine and Rehabilitation*, *79*(11), 1477–1480.

Whyte, J. (2014). Contributions of treatment theory and enablement theory to rehabilitation research and practice. *Archives of Physical Medicine and Rehabilitation*, *95*(1 suppl 1), S17–S23.

Williams, D. (2011). Health care, rehabilitation, and rehabilitation nursing. In C. Jacelon (Ed.), *The specialty practice of rehabilitation nursing* (6th ed., pp.15–30). Glenview, IL: Association of Rehabilitation Nurses.

Williams, D., & Doeschot, K. (2011). Rehabilitation nursing and case management. In C. Jacelon (Ed.), *The specialty practice of rehabilitation nursing: A core curriculum* (6th ed., pp. 65–74). Glenview, IL: Association of Rehabilitation Nurses.

World Health Organization (WHO). (1980). *International classification of impairments, disabilities and handicaps*. Geneva, Switzerland: Author.

World Health Organization (WHO). (2002). Towards a common language for functioning, disability and health ICF. http://www.who.int/classifications/icf /training/icfbeginnersguide.pdf

World Health Organization (WHO). (2007). International classification of functioning, disability, and health. http://www.who.int/classifications/icf/en

Index